Endocrine Hypertension

Endocrine Hypertension
From Basic Science to Clinical Practice

Edited by

Joseph M. Pappachan
Department of Endocrinology & Metabolism, Royal Preston Hospital, The Lancashire Teaching Hospitals NHS Foundation Trust, Preston, United Kingdom; The University of Manchester, Manchester, United Kingdom; Faculty of Science, Manchester Metropolitan University, Manchester, United Kingdom

Cornelius J. Fernandez
Department of Endocrinology & Metabolism, Pilgrim Hospital, United Lincolnshire Hospitals NHS Trust, Boston, United Kingdom

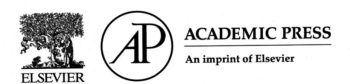

ACADEMIC PRESS
An imprint of Elsevier

Academic Press is an imprint of Elsevier
125 London Wall, London EC2Y 5AS, United Kingdom
525 B Street, Suite 1650, San Diego, CA 92101, United States
50 Hampshire Street, 5th Floor, Cambridge, MA 02139, United States
The Boulevard, Langford Lane, Kidlington, Oxford OX5 1GB, United Kingdom

ISBN: 978-0-323-96120-2

For information on all Academic Press publications visit our website at
https://www.elsevier.com/books-and-journals

Publisher: Stacy Masucci
Acquisitions Editor: Patricia M. Osborn
Editorial Project Manager: Timothy J. Bennett
Production Project Manager: Omer Mukthar
Cover Designer: Vicky Pearson Esser

Typeset by TNQ Technologies

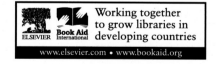

Foreword

Endocrine causes of hypertension are among the most frequent causes of secondary hypertension, and with the recognition of the increased prevalence of primary aldosteronism, could represent a sizable percentage, perhaps up to 20% of the aetiologies of hypertension. Accurate diagnosis of these conditions is critical because of the complications associated with the persistence of disease in cases in which diagnosis is not made, and because many of these conditions may be cured, in contrast to primary hypertension, which can be controlled but not cured in present times. There are guidelines for diagnosis and treatment of endocrine hypertension from many organizations, such as those of the Endocrine Society of the USA, the 2017 AHA/ACC Guideline, and the latest European Guidelines, both for the management of hypertension in general but including recommendations for endocrine hypertension, and many other sources of recommendations that include how to diagnose and manage endocrine hypertension. However, there is a need for a treatise on endocrine hypertension that addresses in-depth the etiology, pathophysiology and the molecular underpinnings, the differential diagnosis, and the management of endocrine hypertension, including the more practical aspects of treatment and follow-up.

Endocrine Hypertension, from Basic Science to Clinical Practice, edited by Joseph M. Pappachan and Cornelius James Fernandez does precisely that. With X chapters written by authorities in the field, Endocrine Hypertension provides an in-depth description of all aspects of hypertension with endocrine connotations. From adrenal hyperplasia to acromegaly, and from paragangliomas and pheochromocytoma to Cushing's, through hyperaldosteronism in its different types to the role of the renin-angiotensin system and the many forms of monogenic hypertension, no aspect of endocrine hypertension is left unexamined. The genetics, molecular and cellular aspects, etiopathogenesis, pathophysiology, clinical description, screening, and diagnosis, and finally management and follow-up including practical tips, all are addressed in clear and readable prose that makes it not only attractive and entertaining but also hugely easy to incorporate into everyday practice.

Chapters on catecholamines and the renin-angiotensin system are followed by ones on pheochromocytoma, paragangliomas and different forms of adrenal hypertension, including recent findings on aldosterone-producing cell clusters and somatic mutations in genes encoding for ion channels and ATPases found in aldosteronomas and aldosterone-producing cell clusters, and all the genetic, cellular, and molecular heterogeneity in adrenals with an aldosterone-producing adenoma, including the familial forms of primary aldosteronism.

Rarer forms of endocrine hypertension such as acromegaly and Cushing's syndrome, as well as the monogenic forms of hypertension, require high clinical suspicion but it is important that they be diagnosed. The same applies to the notion of the high frequency of primary aldosteronism, which requires testing in most cases of hypertension because it often has more subtle manifestations than the classical Conn's syndrome, and its diagnosis and treatment can be extremely gratifying and beneficial to patients, with prevention of target organ damage and complications.

Anyone interested in hypertension, from genetics to pathophysiology and molecular and cellular manifestations to diagnosis and treatment should be interested in endocrine hypertension and should read this volume if they want to have adequate knowledge of these conditions and be able to practice evidence-based diagnosis and management of hypertensive patients, many of whom will have some form of endocrine hypertension, very often primary aldosteronism, but occasionally some of the more rare forms of endocrine hypertension.

Ernesto L. Schiffrin, C.M., MD, Ph.D., FRSC, FRCPC, FACP
Physician-in-Chief, Sir Mortimer B. Davis-Jewish General Hospital, Director, Hypertension and Vascular Research Unit, Lady Davis Institute for Medical Research, Distinguished James McGill Professor and Associate Chair, Department of Medicine, McGill University Editor-in-Chief, The American Journal of Hypertension

Contents

Contributors   xv
Editors' brief resumes   xvii
Invited senior authors' profiles   xix
Preface   xxvii

1. Endocrine hypertension—an overview

Joseph M. Pappachan and
Cornelius J. Fernandez

Introduction   2
Primary hypertension versus secondary hypertension   2
Individual chapters   3
Catecholamines and blood pressure regulation   3
Adrenocortical hormones and BP regulation   3
Hypothalamic—pituitary—adrenal axis and blood pressure regulation   3
Renin-angiotensin—aldosterone system and blood pressure regulation   4
Monogenic hypertension: an overview   4
Primary aldosteronism (Conn's syndrome)   4
Familial hyperaldosteronism   5
Congenital adrenal hyperplasia and hypertension   5
Endocrine hypertension: discovering the inherited causes   5
Pheochromocytomas and hypertension   6
Paragangliomas and hypertension   6
ACTH-dependent Cushing syndrome   6
Adrenal Cushing's syndrome   7
Hypertension in growth hormone excess (acromegaly) and deficiency   7
Hypertension in thyroid disease and hyperparathyroidism   7
Obesity, insulin resistance, and obstructive sleep apnea   7
Endocrine hypertension in children   8
Endocrine hypertension in pregnant woman   8

Imaging for patients with endocrine hypertension   8
Systematic approach for the diagnosis and management of endocrine hypertension   9
Recent trends/emerging concepts   9
Genetic testing for familial PPGL   10
Genetic testing for familial hyperparathyroidism   10
Genetic testing for familial hyper-aldosteronism especially GRA   11
Conclusions   13
References   14

2. Catecholamines and blood pressure regulation

Cornelius J. Fernandez, Fahmy W.F. Hanna,
Karel Pacak and Matthew A. Nazari

Introduction   20
Catecholamines and autonomic physiology   20
The synthesis, storage, and regulation of catecholamines   20
Metabolism of catecholamines   22
Adrenoceptors, subtypes, and associated second messenger systems   23
Neuroendocrine effects of catecholamines on blood pressure   25
Metabolic regulation by catecholamines   26
Biologic effects   26
Summarizing the net effect of catecholamines on vascular hemodynamics   26
PPGLs and excess catecholamine states   28
Deleterious cardiac effects of excess catecholamines: CICMP   28
Stress cardiomyopathy: impaired adrenoceptor and second messenger signaling   28
Hypertrophic cardiomyopathy: load-dependent and nonload-dependent remodeling   29
Dilated cardiomyopathy: cardiotoxic effects of catecholamines   29
Deleterious vascular effects of catecholamines   31

Catecholamines and alterations in renal
physiology   31
Catecholamines and other organs   31
Catecholamines and autonomic failure   31
Summary and conclusions   32
Learning points   32
References   32

3. Adrenal cortical hormones and blood pressure regulation

Anna Sanders, Cornelius J. Fernandez and Rousseau Gama

Introduction   36
Physiological aspects   36
An overview of adrenal steroid synthetic
pathways   36
Regulation of steroidogenesis: cholesterol,
StAR, and p450scc   36
Aldosterone synthesis in the zona
glomerulosa   37
Cortisol synthesis in the zona fasciculata   38
Adrenal androgen synthesis and regulation
in the zona reticularis   39
The glucocorticoid receptor (GR)   40
*Glucocorticoid receptor and blood
pressure regulation*   41
The mineralocorticoid receptor   42
*MR and blood pressure regulation:
genomic effects*   42
*MR and blood pressure: non-genomic
actions*   42
Androgens, receptors, and cardiovascular
system effects   43
**Pathophysiological alterations in
adrenocortical hormones and effects on
cardiovascular homeostasis**   45
Glucocorticoid excess states (including
non-neoplastic Cushing's)   45
Mineralocorticoid excess states: primary
aldosteronism (PA) and familial
hyperaldosteronism   45
Apparent mineralocorticoid excess   46
Androgen deficiency/excess states
(including congenital disorders such as
CAH)   46
Emerging research questions   46
Summary and conclusions   47
Learning points   47
References   47

**4. Hypothalamic–pituitary–adrenal
axis and blood pressure
regulation**

*Joseph M. Pappachan, Cornelius J. Fernandez
and Constantine A. Stratakis*

Introduction   54
**Physiology of blood pressure regulation
and HPA axis**   54
POMC (pro-opiomelanocortin): its role in
metabolism and energy balance   54
CRH (corticotropin-releasing hormone) and
AVP (arginine vasopressin) control the
expression of POMC (pro-
opiomelanocortin)   55
**Pathophysiology of hypertension and HPA
axis**   55
HPA axis and autonomic nervous system
(in relation to BP)   56
HPA axis, adrenal hormones, and blood
pressure   57
HPA axis and metabolic syndrome   57
HPA axis, various hormonal disorders, and
hypertension   57
Summary and conclusions   60
Learning points   60
References   60

**5. Renin–angiotensin–aldosterone
system and blood pressure
regulation**

Gino Seravalle and Guido Grassi

Introduction   64
Physiological aspects of RAAS   65
RAAS, inflammation, and remodeling   66
**RAAS blocking agents and
cardiovascular protection in
hypertension**   67
ACE inhibitors   67
ARBs   68
Direct renin inhibitors   69
Dual RAAS inhibition   69
ACEI versus ARBs   69
**Mineralocorticoid receptor
antagonists**   70
Conclusions   71
Learning points   71
References   71

6. Monogenic hypertension: an overview

Cornelius J. Fernandez, Joseph M. Pappachan and Ute I. Scholl

Introduction	78
Genetics of monogenic hypertension	79
Summary	85
Learning points	85
References	85

7. Primary aldosteronism (Conn's syndrome)

Filippo Ceccato, Irene Tizianel, Giacomo Voltan and Franco Mantero

Introduction	90
The renin–angiotensin–aldosterone system	91
Who should be screened? (The epidemiology of primary aldosteronism)	92
Aldosterone–renin ratio as screening test	92
Confirmatory test after positive ARR	93
Subtyping in primary aldosteronism: adrenal vein sampling or imaging?	95
Laparoscopic surgery and peri-operative management	96
Medical therapy of primary aldosteronism	96
Familial forms of primary aldosteronism	98
Conclusions	99
Learning points	99
References	100

8. Familial hyperaldosteronism   105

Joseph M. Pappachan, Cornelius J. Fernandez and David S. Geller

Introduction	106
Pathophysiology of familial hyperaldosteronism	106
Subtypes of familial hyperaldosteronism	106
Familial hyperaldosteronism type 1	106
Familial hyperaldosteronism type 2	108
Familial hyperaldosteronism type 3	109
Familial hyperaldosteronism type 4	109
PASNA syndrome	110
Emerging research questions/future research	110
Summary and conclusions	110
Learning points	110
References	111

9. Congenital adrenal hyperplasia and hypertension

Busra Gurpinar Tosun and Tulay Guran

Introduction	114
Genetics of CAH (in general—all forms)	114
Pathophysiology of hypertension in CAH	116
11β-hydroxylase deficiency	118
Clinical presentations	118
Diagnostic approach for 11β-hydroxylase deficiency	118
Management algorithm	119
Therapeutic targets	119
17α-hydroxylase deficiency	119
Clinical presentation	119
Diagnostic approach	120
Management algorithm	120
Therapeutic targets	120
Overtreatment of CAH	120
When to suspect of CAH in patients with hypertension	121
Future research	121
Summary and conclusions	122
Learning points	122
References	122

10. Endocrine hypertension: discovering the inherited causes

Farahnak Assadi, Nakysa Hooman, Mojgan Mazaheri and Fatemeh Ghane Sharbaf

Introduction	128
Inherited disorders of endocrine hypertension	129
Monogenic hypertension associated with suppressed PAC and PRA	131
Liddle syndrome	131
Congenital adrenal hyperplasia (CAH)	134
Apparent mineralocorticoid excess (AME)	135
Geller syndrome	137
Monogenic hypertension associated with normal PAC and low PRA	137
Pseudohypoaldosteronism type II (Gordon syndrome)	137
Monogenic hypertension associated with high PAC and low PRA	138
Familial hyperaldosteronism type 1 (FH-1) or glucocorticoid suppressible aldosteronism	138
Familial hyperaldosteronism type 2 (FH-2)	139
Familial hyperaldosteronism type 3 (FH-3)	139

Familial hyperaldosteronism type 4 (FH-4)   140

Monogenic hypertension associated with elevated PAC and PRA   140

Renin-secreting juxtaglomerular cell tumors (JGCT)   140

Monogenic hypertension associated with normal PAC and PRA   141

Familial pheochromocytoma and paragangliomas   141

Primary generalized glucocorticoid resistance (Chrousos syndrome)   142

Carney complex   142

Summary and conclusions   143

Learning points   144

References   144

11.   **Pheochromocytomas and hypertension**

Iuri Martin Goemann and Ana Luiza Maia

Introduction   150

Molecular and genetic aspects of PCCs   150

Tumor clusters   150

Clinical and biochemical characteristics of PCC: genotype-phenotype correlations   151

Pathophysiology   151

Metastatic risk   152

Clinical presentation   153

Diagnostic workup   153

Biochemical testing   153

Diagnostic imaging   154

MEN2 and VHL PCCs   155

Molecular diagnosis   157

Management   157

Presurgical and surgical management of PCC   157

Locoregional approaches   158

External beam radiotherapy   158

Other approaches   158

Systemic therapy   158

Chemotherapy   158

Radionuclide therapy   158

Tyrosine kinase inhibitors (TKIs)   158

Other agents   159

Follow-up   159

Areas of uncertainty/emerging concepts   159

Summary and conclusions   160

Learning points   160

References   160

12.   **Paragangliomas and hypertension**

Tomáš Zelinka and Ondřej Petrák

Introduction   166

Epidemiology of paragangliomas and hypertension   166

Pathophysiology of paraganglioma and hypertension   167

Genetics of paragangliomas   168

Clinical presentation   168

Biochemical investigations   171

Anatomical and functional imaging studies   171

Perioperative medical management of paragangliomas   174

Surgery for management of paragangliomas   175

Curative surgery   175

Metastatic paragangliomas   175

Palliative surgery   176

Systemic therapy   176

Radionuclide therapy   176

Local ablative therapy   177

Follow-up care of patients with paragangliomas   177

Management in special populations   177

Children   177

Pregnancy   177

Elderly   178

Areas of uncertainty/emerging research   178

Summary and conclusions   178

Learning points   178

References   179

13.   **ACTH-dependent Cushing's syndrome**

Stuti Fernandes, Elena V. Varlamov and Maria Fleseriu

Introduction   184

Clinical presentation, screening, and diagnosis of Cushing's syndrome   184

Localization testing: distinguishing between ACTH-dependent and ACTH-independent Cushing's syndrome   185

Epidemiology of hypertension in Cushing's syndrome   187

Pathophysiology of hypertension in Cushing's syndrome   187

Other complications of Cushing's syndrome   189

Treatment of Cushing's syndrome and associated hypertension   190

Antihypertensive therapy in Cushing's
syndrome 190
Role of medical therapy for CS in the
treatment of hypertension 195
Adrenal steroidogenesis inhibitors 195
Pituitary targeted agents 195
Glucocorticoid receptor blockers 196
Follow up of Cushing syndrome and
hypertension 196
Summary 197
Learning points 197
References 197

14. Adrenal Cushing's syndrome

Oskar Ragnarsson

Introduction 202
Causes and epidemiology of adrenal
Cushing syndrome 202
Genetic syndromes associated with adrenal
Cushing syndrome 203
Genetics of ACTH -independent Cushing
syndrome 203
Clinical features 204
Pathophysiology of hypertension in adrenal
Cushing syndrome 205
Investigations for adrenal CS 206
Treatment of adrenal CS 207
Preoperative treatment of adrenal CS 208
Postoperative treatment of adrenal CS 208
Long-term outcome of adrenal CS 208
Autonomous cortisol secretion in adrenal
incidentaloma 210
Areas of uncertainty/emerging
concepts 211
Summary and conclusions 211
Learning points 211
References 212

15. Hypertension in growth hormone excess and deficiency

Gabriela Mihai and Márta Korbonits

GH and IGF-1 physiological effects 218
GH and IGF-1 in the blood vessels 218
The role of GH and IGF-1 in the
myocardium 218
The role of GH and IGF-1 in the kidney 219
Acromegaly and hypertension 219
Epidemiology 219
Pathophysiology of hypertension in
acromegaly 220

Hypertension phenotype and car-
diovascular comorbidities 223
Characteristics of acromegaly related
hypertension 223
Acromegaly and comorbidities 224
Screening for acromegaly in hypertensive
patients 226
When to suspect acromegaly in hyper-
tensive patients 226
Treatment 227
Therapeutical options in acromegaly 227
The effect of disease activity on blood
pressure 227
Hypertension management 229
Growth hormone deficiency and
hypertension 229
Epidemiology 229
Pathophysiology of hypertension in AGHD 231
Phenotype of AGHD and characteristics of
blood pressure profile 232
AGHD and comorbidities 234
Screening for AGHD 236
When to suspect AGHD in hypertension? 236
AGHD diagnosis 237
Treatment 237
Impact of AGHD management on blood
pressure 237
Summary and closing remarks 239
Learning points 239
References 239

16. Hypertension in thyroid disease and primary hyperparathyroidism

Naomi Szwarcbard and Duncan J. Topliss

Introduction 250
Thyroid disease 250
Physiology of hypothalamo—pituitary
—thyroid axis and cardiovascular system 250
Pathophysiology of hypertension in thyroid
dysfunction 251
Subclinical or overt hypothyroidism and
associated hypertension 253
Subclinical or overt hyperthyroidism and
associated hypertension 253
When to suspect hypothyroidism and
hyperthyroidism in hypertensive
subjects? 255
Parathyroid disease 255
Physiology of parathyroid hormone action 255
Pathophysiology of hypertension in
primary hyperparathyroidism 255

Bidirectional relation between renin
—angiotensin—aldosterone system
and PTH 256
When to suspect PHPT in hypertensive
subjects? 258
Summary and conclusions 259
Learning points 259
References 259

17. Obesity, insulin resistance, and obstructive sleep apnea

*Dominic Oduro-Donkor and
Thomas M. Barber*

Introduction 264
Epidemiology of OSA 264
OSA and obesity 265
Diagnosis of OSA 266
**Pathophysiology of OSA-related
secondary hypertension** 266
Nocturnal sympathetic overdrive 266
Chronic inflammation and oxidative
stress driven by hypoxia 267
Nocturnal fluid shifts 267
Cardiac effects of nocturnal negative
intrathoracic pressure 268
Activation of the RAAS 268
OSA and insulin resistance 268
Management of OSA 269
Conservative management 270
CPAP 270
Oral appliances 271
Surgical management 271
Weight loss therapies 271
Conclusions 271
Learning points 272
Acknowledgments 272
References 272

18. Endocrine hypertension in children

Badhma Valaiyapathi and Ambika P. Ashraf

Introduction 278
**Primary versus secondary hypertension
in children** 278
Endocrine hypertension in children 279
**Clinical presentation of endocrine
hypertension in children** 280
Catecholamine producing tumors 280
Cushing's syndrome in children 281
Biochemical phenotype of mineralocorti-
coid excess in children 283

Congenital adrenal hyperplasia and
hypertension in children 286
Excessive growth hormone production 286
Thyroid and parathyroid disorders and
hypertension in children 287
**Diagnostic approach to endocrine
hypertension in children** 288
**Management of endocrine hypertension
in children** 290
Summary and conclusions 290
Learning points 290
References 290

19. Endocrine hypertension in pregnancy

Felix Jebasingh and Nihal Thomas

Introduction 294
Primary hyperaldosteronism in pregnancy 294
Cushing syndrome in pregnancy 295
Pheochromocytoma and paraganglioma
(PPGL) in pregnancy 298
Primary hyperparathyroidism 299
Hyperthyroidism and hypothyroidism in
pregnancy 300
Acromegaly in pregnancy 301
Rare causes of endocrine hypertension in
pregnancy 302
Adrenal cortical carcinoma/deoxy-
corticosterone-secreting adrenal tumor 303
Liddle's syndrome 303
Hypopituitarism 303
Familial hyperaldosteronism 304
Geller syndrome 304
Summary and conclusions 304
Learning points 304
References 304
Further reading 307

20. Imaging for patients with endocrine hypertension 309

Katherine Ordidge and Anju Sahdev

Introduction 310
Adrenal computed tomography (CT) 310
Adrenal magnetic resonance imaging
(MRI) 311
Adrenal venous sampling (AVS) 312
Positron-emission tomography (PET)/CT to
localize an ectopic source of ACTH
secretion 315
Neck ultrasound 318
4D computed tomography (CT) 319

SPECT/CT imaging with 99mTc-sestamibi 319
PET/CT with 18-fluorine labeled choline
    analogues 320
Thyroid ultrasound 322
Planar scintigraphy 322
MRI of the pituitary 326
Summary and conclusions 327
Learning points 327
References 328

**21. Systematic approach to the
       diagnosis and management of
       endocrine hypertension**

*Michael Stowasser, Pieter Jansen
and Martin Wolley*

Introduction 332
Primary aldosteronism (PA) 332
Clinical diagnosis 332
Management 338
**Other mineralocorticoid forms of
hypertension** 341
11β-hydroxylase deficiency 341
17α-hydroxylase deficiency 342
Primary glucocorticoid resistance (PGR)
    or Chrousos syndrome 342
Syndrome of apparent mineralocorticoid
    excess (SAME) 343
DOC-secreting tumors 343
Ectopic ACTH syndrome 343
Activating mutations of the MR
    or Geller syndrome 344
Liddle syndrome 344
Familial hyperkalemic hypertension
    (Gordon syndrome) 344

Pheochromocytoma and paraganglioma 345
Management 346
Cushing's syndrome 347
Prevalence, pathophysiology and clinical
    presentation 347
Diagnosis 348
Management 349
Acromegaly 350
Prevalence, pathophysiology, and clinical
    presentation 350
Diagnosis 351
Management 351
Thyroid disorders 352
Hypothyroidism 352
Hyperthyroidism 353
Primary hyperparathyroidism 354
Prevalence, pathophysiology, and clinical
    presentation 354
Diagnosis 355
Management 355
**Renal artery stenosis and other rare
forms of renin driven hypertension** 355
Clinical presentation 356
Diagnostic approach 356
Management 357
Page kidney 357
Reninoma 357
Conclusion 359
Learning points 359
References 359

Index 369

Contributors

Ambika P. Ashraf, Director, Division of Pediatric Endocrinology and Diabetes, University of Alabama at Birmingham, Birmingham, AL, United States

Farahnak Assadi, Rush University of Medical Center, Department of Pediatrics, Division of Nephrology, Chicago, IL, United States

Thomas M. Barber, Warwickshire Institute for the Study of Diabetes, Endocrinology and Metabolism, University Hospitals Coventry and Warwickshire, Coventry, United Kingdom; Division of Biomedical Sciences, Warwick Medical School, University of Warwick, Coventry, United Kingdom

Filippo Ceccato, Endocrinology Unit, Department of Medicine DIMED, University Hospital of Padova, Padova, Italy

Stuti Fernandes, Department of Medicine, Division of Endocrinology, Diabetes & Clinical Nutrition, Oregon Health and Science University and VA Hospital, Portland, OR, United States

Cornelius J. Fernandesz, Department of Endocrinology and Metabolism, Pilgrim Hospital, United Lincolnshire Hospitals NHS Trust, Boston, United Kingdom

Maria Fleseriu, Departments of Medicine (Division of Endocrinology, Diabetes and Clinical Nutrition) and Neurological Surgery, and Pituitary Center, Oregon Health & Science University, Portland, OR, United States

Rousseau Gama, Department of Clinical Biochemistry, Black Country Pathology Services, The Royal Wolverhampton NHS Trust, Wolverhampton, United Kingdom; Department of Laboratory and Metabolic Medicine, The University of Wolverhampton, Wolverhampton, United Kingdom

David S. Geller, Department of Nephrology, West Haven VA Hospital, West Haven and Yale University School of Medicine, New Haven, CT, United States

Iuri Martin Goemann, Universidade Federal do Rio Grande do Sul, Endocrinology, Porto Alegre, Brazil; Universidade do Vale do Rio dos Sinos, Porto Alegre, Brazil

Guido Grassi, Clinica Medica, University Milano-Bicocca, Milano, Italy

Tulay Guran, Department of Pediatric Endocrinology and Diabetes, Marmara University, School of Medicine, Istanbul, Turkey

Fahmy W.F. Hanna, Department of Diabetes and Endocrinology, University Hospitals of North Midlands NHS Trust and Centre for Health and Development, Staffordshire University, Stoke-on-Trent, United Kingdom

Nakysa Hooman, Aliasghar Clinical Research Development Center, Iran University of Medical Sciences, Pediatric Nephrology, Tehran, Iran

Pieter Jansen, Department of Diabetes and Endocrinology, Princess Alexandra Hospital, Woolloongabba, QLD, Australia

Felix Jebasingh, Christian Medical College Vellore, India

Márta Korbonits, Centre for Endocrinology, William Harvey Research Institute, Barts and The London School of Medicine and Dentistry, Queen Mary University of London, London, United Kingdom

Ana Luiza Maia, Universidade Federal do Rio Grande do Sul, Endocrinology, Porto Alegre, Brazil

Franco Mantero, Endocrinology Unit, Department of Medicine DIMED, University Hospital of Padova, Padova, Italy

Mojgan Mazaheri, Semnan University of Medical Sciences, Pediatric Nephrology, Semnan, Iran

Gabriela Mihai, Centre for Endocrinology, William Harvey Research Institute, Barts and The London School of Medicine and Dentistry, Queen Mary University of London, London, United Kingdom

Matthew A. Nazari, Section on Medical Neuroendocrinology, Eunice Kennedy Shriver National Institute of Child Health and Human Development, National Institutes of Health, Bethesda, MD, United States

Dominic Oduro-Donkor, Warwickshire Institute for the Study of Diabetes, Endocrinology and Metabolism, University Hospitals Coventry and Warwickshire,

Coventry, United Kingdom; Division of Biomedical Sciences, Warwick Medical School, University of Warwick, Coventry, United Kingdom

Katherine Ordidge, Consultant Radiologist, Department of Imaging, St Bartholomew's Hospital, Barts Health NHS Trust, London, United Kingdom

Karel Pacak, Section on Medical Neuroendocrinology, Eunice Kennedy Shriver National Institute of Child Health and Human Development, National Institutes of Health, Bethesda, MD, United States

Joseph M. Pappachan, Department of Endocrinology and Metabolism, Royal Preston Hospital, The Lancashire Teaching Hospitals NHS Foundation Trust, Preston, United Kingdom; The University of Manchester, Manchester, United Kingdom; Faculty of Science, Manchester Metropolitan University, Manchester, United Kingdom

Ondřej Petrák, Department of Medicine — Department of Endocrinology and Metabolism, General Faculty Hospital and First Faculty of Medicine, Charles University in Prague, Prague, Czech Republic

Oskar Ragnarsson, Department of Internal Medicine and Clinical Nutrition, Institute of Medicine at Sahlgrenska Academy, University of Gothenburg, Gothenburg, Sweden; Department of Endocrinology, Sahlgrenska University Hospital, Gothenburg, Sweden

Anju Sahdev, Consultant Radiologist, Department of Imaging, St Bartholomew's Hospital, Barts Health NHS Trust and Clinical Professor of Diagnostic Imaging, Barts Cancer Institute, Queen Mary University Hospital, London, United Kingdom

Anna Sanders, Department of Clinical Biochemistry, Russells Hall Hospital, Black Country Pathology Services, The Royal Wolverhampton NHS Trust, Wolverhampton, United Kingdom

Ute I. Scholl, Center of Functional Genomics, Berlin Institute of Health at Charité—Universitätsmedizin Berlin, Berlin, Germany

Gino Seravalle, Cardiology Department, IRCCS Istituto Auxologico Italiano, and University Milano-Bicocca, Milano, Italy

Fatemeh Ghane Sharbaf, Pediatric Nephrology, Mashhad University of Medical Sciences, Mashhad, Iran

Michael Stowasser, Endocrine Hypertension Research Centre, University of Queensland, Brisbane, QLD, Australia

Constantine A. Stratakis, Human Genetics and Precision Medicine, IMMB, FORTH & ELPEN Research Institute, Pikermi, Greece

Naomi Szwarcbard, Department of Endocrinology & Diabetes, Alfred Health, Melbourne, VIC, Australia

Nihal Thomas, Christian Medical College Vellore, India

Irene Tizianel, Endocrinology Unit, Department of Medicine DIMED, University Hospital of Padova, Padova, Italy

Duncan J. Topliss, Department of Endocrinology & Diabetes, Alfred Health, Melbourne, VIC, Australia; Monash University, Melbourne, VIC, Australia

Busra Gurpinar Tosun, Department of Pediatric Endocrinology and Diabetes, Marmara University, School of Medicine, Istanbul, Turkey

Badhma Valaiyapathi, University of Alabama at Birmingham, Birmingham, AL, United States

Elena V. Varlamov, Departments of Medicine (Division of Endocrinology, Diabetes and Clinical Nutrition) and Neurological Surgery, and Pituitary Center, Oregon Health & Science University, Portland, OR, United States

Giacomo Voltan, Endocrinology Unit, Department of Medicine DIMED, University Hospital of Padova, Padova, Italy

Martin Wolley, Endocrine Hypertension Research Centre, University of Queensland, Brisbane, QLD, Australia

Tomáš Zelinka, Department of Medicine — Department of Endocrinology and Metabolism, General Faculty Hospital and First Faculty of Medicine, Charles University in Prague, Prague, Czech Republic

Editors' brief resumes

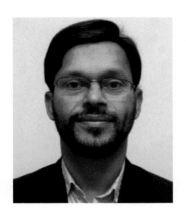

Professor Joseph M. Pappachan MD, FRCP is a consultant endocrinologist at Lancashire Teaching Hospitals NHS Trust and an honorary professor at the Manchester Metropolitan University, UK. He is also a section editor (endocrinology and metabolism) to "Current Drug Safety" and associate editor to the "World Journal of Diabetes" and "Frontiers in Clinical Diabetes and Healthcare." He has vast editing experience including editing journal special issues since 2010 and has authored more than 100 peer-reviewed articles in various medical journals and textbooks. He also has extensive academic collaboration across the globe and is a principal investigator in several ongoing clinical trials in endocrinology and metabolism. His research special interests include endocrine hypertension, neuroendocrinology, parathyroid disease, bone mineral metabolism, diabetic foot disease, and diabesity.

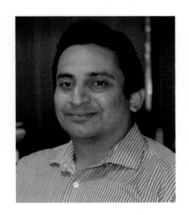

Dr. Cornelius J. Fernandez MD, MRCP is a consultant endocrinologist at Pilgrim Hospital, United Lincolnshire Hospitals NHS Trust, Boston, UK. He graduated from Kottayam Medical College, and underwent internal medicine postgraduate training from Coimbatore Medical College (India) with further specialist training in Endocrinology in the UK. He is a review editor to "Frontiers in Clinical Diabetes and Healthcare" and scientific peer reviewer to several other medical journals. He has authored 35 peer-reviewed scientific papers to date in different medical journals and actively involves in clinical research programs in his hospital. His research special interests include endocrine hypertension, diabetic foot disease, and diabesity.

Invited senior authors' profiles

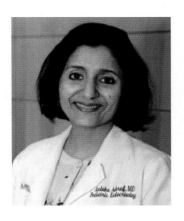

Professor Ambika P. Ashraf MD FACE is the Division Director of Pediatric Endocrinology and Diabetes at the University of Alabama at Birmingham (UAB), Ralph Frohsin Endowed Chair in Pediatric Endocrinology and the Director of the Pediatric Lipid Clinic at the Children's of Alabama, Co-Director of the multidisciplinary Pediatric Metabolic Bone clinic, and an Associate Director of the UAB Comprehensive Diabetes Center. She is board certified in Pediatrics, Pediatric Endocrinology, and Clinical Lipidology. Prof. Ashraf is a member of multiple professional societies, including the American Academy of Pediatrics, Pediatric Endocrine Society, ASBMR, Society for Pediatric Research, and National Lipid Association. She has served as the Chairperson for the AAP National Conference and Exhibition of the Section on Endocrinology and program co-chair of Pediatric Endocrine Society. She is active in clinical research investigating lipid, bone and mineral homeostasis, and diabetes. Prof. Ashraf also serves on the subboard of Endocrinology for the American Board of Pediatrics.

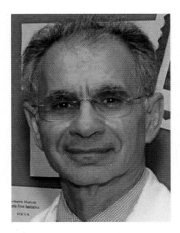

Professor Faranak Assadi MD is distinguished Emeritus Professor of pediatrics at Rush University Medical College. He served as professor of pediatrics and medical director of Children's Program at Children's Hospital of Philadelphia, University of Pennsylvania, and chief of pediatric nephrology at duPont Hospital's for Children, Thomas Jefferson University Medical College from 1990 to 2000 prior to joining the faculty of Rush University Medical Center. Prof. Assadi has an impressive record of scholarly activity. His research interests are in aspects of newborn developmental renal physiology, fluid-electrolytes and acid-base disorders, hypertension, and chronic renal disease prevention. As a testament to his excellence, he received over 25 teaching, mentoring, and patients' care awards. He has also served as a senior member of the Society for Pediatric Research, American Society of Pediatric Nephrology, National Kidney Foundation, North America Renal Transplant Society, and the International Society of Pediatric Nephrology.

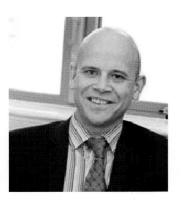

Dr. Thomas M. Barbar DPhil, FRCP is an Associate Professor and Honorary Consultant Endocrinologist at University of Warwick and University Hospitals Coventry and Warwickshire (UHCW). He has a research background in the genetic and metabolic features of Polycystic Ovary Syndrome and ethnic-specific cut-points for obesity. He was awarded of the prestigious "Society for Endocrinology Clinical Prize Lecture" and "University of Oxford Medical Sciences Divisional Research Prize" in 2009. He has published >110 papers in leading peer-reviewed journals Dr. Barber presents regularly as an invited speaker at scientific meetings both nationally and internationally and engages regularly with national media on topics relating to human metabolism and Obesity. As scientific lead for the Human Metabolism Research Unit, his current research interests include the impact of human metabolism on the development of Obesity, and novel strategies to prevent and manage Obesity and Diabetes Mellitus within the populace. As Clinical Lead for the Obesity service at UHCW, Dr. Barber combines clinical duties with clinical and translational research.

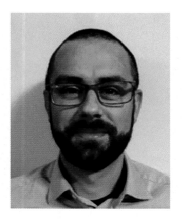

Dr. Filippo Ceccato MD, PhD is an Associate Professor in Endocrinology at the Department of Medicine DIMED, University of Padova, and a consultant in Clinical Endocrinology at the Endocrine Unit (expertise in pituitary and adrenal diseases), University-Hospital of Padova. His research activity is focused on the diagnosis of pituitary and adrenal neoplasms, on clinical application of mass spectrometry for cortisol-related diseases, on the management of disease-related complications and identification of genetic alterations in inherited diseases and endocrine tumors. He is invited speaker in more than 40 lectures in International and National Congresses/ Symposia. He is author of more than 100 publications in peer-reviewed journal (H-Index 25, 1600 citation index.) In 2019, he received Best Researcher in Endocrinology under 35 Award from the Italian Society of Endocrinology.

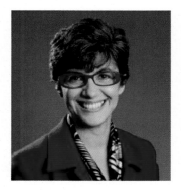

Professor Maria Fleseriu, MD, FACE is a Professor of Medicine and Neurological Surgery and Director of the Pituitary Center at Oregon Health and Science University in Portland, Oregon, USA and Past President of the Pituitary Society. Dr. Fleseriu has a long-standing clinical and research interest in pituitary and adrenal disorders and has been global principal investigator in many international Cushing's and acromegaly clinical trials for development of novel therapies. She has published extensively in prestigious journals, including guidelines, consensus papers, and book chapters and she is a frequent plenary guest speaker at national and international meetings. Major research focus currently is individualized treatment of Cushing's and acromegaly with the goal of improving patients' outcomes and quality of life.

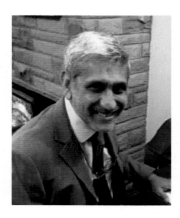

Professor Rousseau Gama MD, FRCPath is a consultant chemical pathologist at Black country pathology services, the Royal Wolverhampton NHS Trust, and professor of laboratory and metabolic medicine at the University of Wolverhampton. He is an Associate Editor for Journal of Laboratory and Precision Medicine and on the Editorial Board for the Journal of Clinical Pathology having previously been Best Practice Editor (Chemical Pathology). He serves and has served in several academic and professional roles for the Association of Clinical Pathologists, Royal College of Pathologists, Association of Clinical Biochemistry and Health Education England, West Midlands. He provides clinical care for patients with dyslipidemia, endocrine disease, and metabolic disorders. His research interest relates to laboratory healthcare delivery leading to improvements in patient safety, care, and outcomes. He has authored/coauthored over 150 highly cited publications.

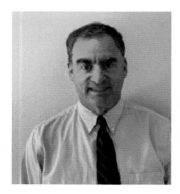

Dr. David Geller MD, PhD is a Nephrologist and Associate Professor of Clinical Medicine at Yale University School of Medicine and at the West Haven Veterans Administration Hospital. He graduated *summa cum laude* from Dartmouth College in Hanover, New Hampshire and received his MD and PhD in Biochemistry from the New York University School of Medicine. He is recognized for his work on the genetics of hypertension, having described the molecular basis of Autosomal Dominant Pseudohypoaldosteronism type 1 as well as Hypertension Exacerbated by Pregnancy (now known as Geller's Syndrome).

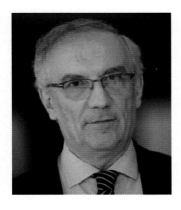

Professor Guido Grassi MD, PhD is the director of the Clinica Medica Institute at Saint Gerardo Hospital-Monza/Milano and the director of the Post-graduate School of Internal Medicine and of the PHD course in Public Health, University of Milan-Bicocca, Italy. He had been the Chairman (2004—06) of the Working Group "Hypertension and the Heart" of the European Society of Cardiology. He served as expert member to many hypertension societies and guideline makers across the world. In 2009, he has received the Bjorn Folkow Award and Lecture from the European Society of Hypertension. His research areas include the pathophysiology, clinical pharmacology and treatment of hypertension, obesity and metabolic syndrome, cardiac arrhythmias, and heart failure. He has published more than 600 original papers and reviews in major scientific international journals (H index 98). He is also an Editor of several journals on hypertension and other medical journals. In 2014, he has been included in the Top Ten Hypertension Expert Ranking made by Expertscape Ranks World's Top Scientists. In 2017, he received the Talaj Zein Award from the European Society of Hypertension and in 2018 the Paul Korner Award from the International Society of Hypertension. In 2018, he has been appointed by ESC/ESH expert Reviewer of the 2018 ESC/ESH Guidelines document on Hypertension. He is the president of Italian Society of Hypertension 2019—22.

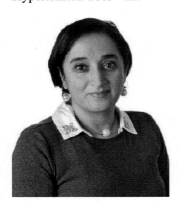

Professor Tulay Guran MD is a Pediatric Endocrinologist at Marmara University, Turkey. She received fellowship from European Society of Pediatric Endocrinology (ESPE) for training at University of Cambridge, and EU Marie Curie postdoc fellowship at the Birmingham University, School of Medicine (both in the UK). In 2015, she received the Young Investigator Award by ESPE. She has more than 130 peer-reviewed articles in the field of pediatric endocrinology. The focus of her research has been to investigate the pathogenesis of adrenal insufficiency, disorders of steroidogenesis and DSD. She is currently coordinating the ESPE DSD working group. She is a member of steering committee of the I-DSD Registry Network, ESPE research fellowship reviewer board associate editorial board of Hormone Research in Pediatrics journal. She holds a member position in the Scientific Advisory Board of Turkish Ministry of Health Neonatal CAH screening program. She is also the general secretary of Turkish Society of Pediatric Endocrinology and Diabetes since June 2021.

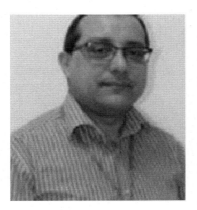

Professor Fahmy F.W. Hanna MD, FRCP is a senior consultant endocrinologist at University Hospitals of North Midlands and professor of Endocrinology and Metabolism at University of North Staffordshire. With his extensive research and academic publishing experience, he was appointed the honorary clinical chair in Endocrinology at the Staffordshire University in 2016. He is applicant/coapplicant on several research grants. His research interests are in adrenal diseases in addition to gestational diabetes mellitus, as a model for evolving type 2 diabetes. Professor Hanna and his collaborators have developed a track record in the process of managing adrenal incidentalomas and have been exploring options to streamline and expedite the management process, reducing the burden on healthcare systems.

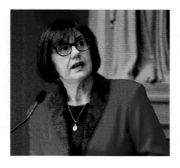

Professor Márta Korbonits PhD FRCP is Professor of Endocrinology and Metabolism at Barts and the London School of Medicine and Dentistry, Queen Mary University of London. She was a Medical Research Council Clinician Scientist Fellow working on ghrelin and the hormonal regulation of the metabolic enzyme AMP-activated protein kinase and her latest study in the field showed the beneficial effects of AMPK stimulator metformin on glucocorticoid-treated patients. She also works on endocrine tumorigenesis, especially the genetic origin of pituitary adenomas and other endocrine tumor syndromes. She studies both the clinical characterization as well as molecular aspects of pituitary diseases and leads a large international consortium to study the genetic background of endocrine tumors. She published over 200 original papers (H-index 80 at Google Scholar). She was a recipient of several national and international awards and is an elected Member of the Hungarian Academy of Sciences. She is Deputy Editor of *Endocrine-Related Cancer,* Director of the *HARP* Clinical Doctoral Training Programme, and President-Elect for the Society for Endocrinology.

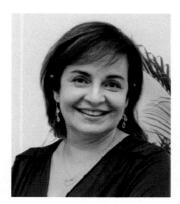

Professor Ana Luiza Maia MD, PhD is the chief of Thyroid Unit at the Hospital de Clínicas de Porto Alegre (HCPA), Universidade Federal do Rio Grande do Sul. She obtained her PhD in thyroid hormone metabolism at the Harvard Medical School. She joined the Endocrinology Division (HCPA) in 1997 and implemented the molecular diagnosis of Multiple Endocrine Neoplasia Type 2 (MEN2), thenceforth considered as a reference to the management of medullary thyroid carcinoma (MTC). She coordinates studies on the molecular and clinical aspects of MEN2 and differentiated thyroid carcinomas. She published over 170 papers to date and received numerous awards such as The Knoll Young Investigator, Latin American Thyroid Society (LATS) Prize, and Fogarty award. She served as Coordinator of the Advisory Committee on Medicine on the Brazilian National Research Council (CNPq). Prof. Maia has an active role at the Brazilian Endocrine Society, being the past President of the Thyroid Department (2002–05). She served as a member of the Executive and Scientific Committees and past President (2019–21) of LATS. She is a member of the American Thyroid Association and Endocrine Society, where she has served as a member of task forces and committees.

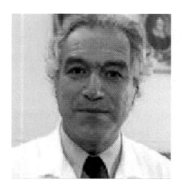

Professor Franco Matero MD received his MD at the University of Padua, Italy and underwent his postdoctoral training in the University of Geneva, Switzerland and University of California, USA. He also had research training in the UK and France. Since 2000, he is the Chair and Chief of the Endocrinology Unit of the Department of Medicine, the University of Padua, Italy. He has received several national and international honors, including a Doctor Honoris Causa at the Semmelweis University, Budapest, Hungary. He has been Editorial Board Member of several scientific Journals such as *Clinical Endocrinology, Endocrinology, Journal of Hypertension, Journal of Endocrinological Investigations and Steroids.* He has served as Member of the Council of several international scientific Societies (including *International Society of Endocrinology, International Aldosterone Conference, Journee Klotz d'Endocrinologie Clinique,ENS@T*) and one of the founders of the European Network for the Study of Adrenal Tumors. His research interests include clinical and basic endocrinology of the adrenal gland and endocrinology of hypertension, in particular pathophysiology of mineralocorticoids and primary aldosteronism. He has authored about 500 peer-reviewed articles and edited several books and proceedings.

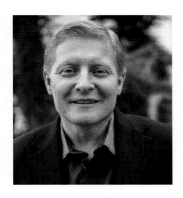

Professor Karel Pacak PhD, DSc is an endocrinologist and tenured Chief of the Section on Medical Neuroendocrinology at *Eunice Kennedy Shriver* National Institute of Child Health and Human Development (NICHD), NIH, Bethesda, MD, USA. He is recognized for patient-oriented pheochromocytoma and paraganglioma (PPGL) research programs. He and his colleagues described the role of a new *HIF2A* gain-of-function somatic mutation in the pathogenesis of paraganglioma, somatostatinoma, and polycythemia (known as the Pacak-Zhuang syndrome). He and his colleagues also discovered other genes including *SUCLG2*, *PHD1*, and *IRP1* in the pathogenesis of PPGL. He and his team introduced into clinical practice genotype-specific functional imaging approaches for PPGL. He has received distinguished awards from the International Association of Endocrine Surgeons, Australian Endocrine Society, Irish Endocrine Society, the Outstanding Clinical Endocrinologist Award and Frontiers in Science and Distinction in Endocrinology from AACE, the Gold Jessenius Medal from the Slovak Academy of Sciences, Purkyne Medal from the Czech Medical Society, the Outstanding Clinical Investigator Award from the US Endocrine Society, and the Directors' award from the NIH and NICHD.

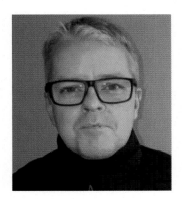

Associate professor Oskar Ragnarsson MD, PhD is a consultant in endocrinology and the chief physician of the in-patient department of Endocrinology at Sahlgrenska University Hospital, Gothenburg, Sweden. His research relates to pituitary and adrenal diseases, especially long-term consequences in patients with Cushing's syndrome and patients with adrenal insufficiency. He is an author to more than 100 highly cited research/review papers and has involved in various international clinical trials related to adrenal and pituitary disorders.

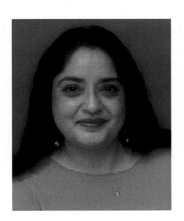

Professor Anju Sahdev MRCP, FRCR Professor Anju Sahdev is a Professor of Clinical Diagnostic Imaging, a Uro-Gynae Specialist Radiology Consultant, and a Director for Research at St Bartholomew's Hospital, Barts Health, London. Professor Sahdev's specialties are imaging in oncology, particularly gynaecological and uro-oncology, endocrine diseases and benign gynecological diseases using all imaging modalities. She has authored and coauthored 89 peer-reviewed publications and has authored more than 20 chapters in clinical and imaging textbooks. She has delivered over 65 lecturers at national and international meetings. She is the senior editor for the reference textbook *Husband and Reznek Imaging in Oncology 2021*. She is an associate editor for British Journal Radiology and Cancer Imaging, and a member of educational subcommittee of International Cancer Imaging Society. She is the gynecological imaging module lead for UK National RITI e-learning program. She is also the Director for Imaging research, clinical radiation expert, and imaging guardian for North Thames Clinical Research Network and principal investigator and coinvestigator for several clinical imaging trials.

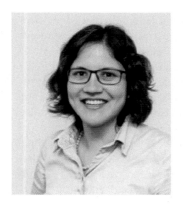

Professor Ute I. Scholl MD, PhD is BIH Johanna Quandt Professor for Hypertension and Molecular Biology of Endocrine Tumors at the Berlin Institute of Health at Charité Universitätsmedizin Berlin, Germany. She graduated with an M.D. *summa cum laude* from RWTH Aachen University, Germany and trained as a postdoc at Yale University, followed by an Assistant Professorhip in Düsseldorf, Germany. She is recognized for her work on the genetics and pathophysiology of primary aldosteronism. She and her colleagues discovered and investigated several primary aldosteronism disease genes including *KCNJ5, CACNA1D, CACNA1H,* and *CLCN2.* Among others, she has received awards from the German Research Foundation (DFG) and the German Society of Nephrology.

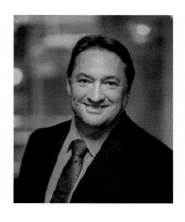

Professor Michael Stowasser MD FRACP has >30 years clinical research experience in pathogenesis and management of hypertension (HT), including endocrine varieties such as primary aldosteronism (PA). With his mentor Richard Gordon, Prof Stowasser demonstrate that PA accounts for up to 10% of HT, making it the commonest specifically treatable, potentially curable variety, and in the description of a new familial form (FH-II) which recently led to the elucidation of its genetic basis. His HT Unit has possibly the largest series (>2200) worldwide of patients with PA who have been thoroughly documented and meticulously studied, helping him to become internationally recognized as an authority on pathogenesis/genetics, diagnostic workup, and management of PA. In 2006, MS served as a member of an international Task Force sponsored by the US Endocrine Society to develop the first guidelines for diagnosis and management of PA he conceived, developed, and validated the seated saline suppression test which has since become the favored method for definitively confirming the diagnosis of PA. He has published one textbook, 16 chapters for textbooks of medicine, and >220 highly cited papers in scientific journals. Since 2013, MS has received ∼$16 million in research grant support. MS has collaborated with researchers in >30 international Units. He is currently one of six chief investigators on a highly prestigious Leducq Foundation Transatlantic Networks of Excellence Program Grant examining the mechanisms by which potassium lowers blood pressure. Prof Stowasser is immediate Past President of the Asian-Pacific Society of Hypertension and of the High Blood Pressure Research Council of Australia.

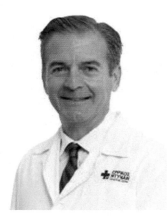

Professor Constantine Stratakis MD, PhD is an internationally recognized researcher with more than 800 publications, editorial roles many journals and winner of several awards such as Excellence Published Clinical Research award in 1999 and Ernst Oppenheimer Award in 2009 from Endocrine Society, and the 2019 Dale Medal from the Society for Endocrinology. His laboratory identified genes for adrenal and pituitary tumors, the genetic defects responsible for Carney complex, Carney Triad, the dyad of paragangliomas and gastric stromal sarcomas (Carney-Stratakis syndrome), and described new entities such as X-LAG (X-linked acrogigantism) and 3-PAs (the 3 Ps association of paragangliomas pheochromocytomas and PA), GPR101 defects in gigantism, and succinate dehydrogenase (SDH) mutations in gastric stromal sarcomas (GIST). He served as the 2018−19 President of the Society for Pediatric Research, and as NICHD, NIH Scientific Director from 2009 to 2020, where he oversaw one of the largest NIH intramural research programs in the USA. Prof. Stratakis was recently selected to serve as CSO of ELPEN and the Director of a new Research Institute in Athens, Greece, a position he assumed on March 1, 2021, along with his appointment as Research Director at FORTH, also in Greece.

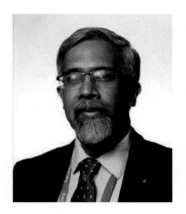

Professor Nihal Thomas PhD, FRCP was former Vice Principal (Research) and Associate Director at Christian Medical College Vellore and is currently Prof and Head of Unit-1, Endocrinology. He has more than 300 indexed publications, several chapters, and two books in his credit and a Google Citation index of 22,000+. He has given around 20 orations. His areas of interest involve the Pathogenesis of Diabetes in India, and General Endocrinology. He has initiated projects to train medical and paramedical staff from 200 rural hospitals for diabetes. He has completed around 70 multinational/in-house clinical trials. He has supported the initiation of laboratory and basic science expertise for next-generation sequencing, and spearheaded basic science research in Diabetes, with indirect calorimetry, hyperinsulinemic euglycemic clamp studies, body composition, and NMR spectroscopy. He has generated around 10 million US dollars in Research grants. Has had extensive overseas networks with several Foreign Universities. He has received the Lourd-Yedanapalli Award for Outstanding researcher in 2009. The department was recognized by the BMJ for Diabetology team of the year 2015 and The Royal College of Physicians award for Excellence in teaching and training of the 2017.

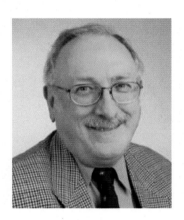

Professor Duncan Topliss MD FRACP is a Senior Endocrinologist in the Department of Endocrinology and Diabetes, at the Alfred Hospital, Melbourne, and Professor of Medicine in the Department of Medicine, Monash University, Melbourne, Australia. He was the Director of the Department from 1996 to 2020. He trained in clinical endocrinology in Melbourne before undertaking research fellowships at the University of Toronto on the immunology of thyroid disease, then at the University of Minnesota on cellular mechanisms of thyroid hormone action. He has a particular interest in advanced thyroid cancer as a site principal investigator for SELECT, COSMIC-311, and LIBRETTO-511. He has a long interest in drug regulation and safety as an advisor to the Therapeutic Goods Administration (Australia), both as a member of the Advisory Committee on Medicine for the since 1999 and as chairman of the Adverse Drug Reaction Advisory Committee (2002–10).

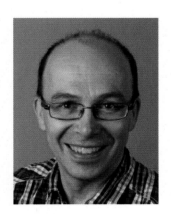

Professor Tomáš Zelinka MD, PhD graduated at the first Medical Faculty, Charles University in Prague, Czech Republic. Since the end of his studies, he has been working at the third Medical Department of the first Medical Faculty of the Charles University and General University Hospital in Prague. Currently, he acts as a chief of the clinical ward which is a part of the Hypertension Excellence Center. He received here his medical (cardiology, endocrinology, and internal medicine) and scientific degrees. His research is mainly focused on endocrine hypertension—pheochromocytoma and primary aldosteronism and has published more than 120 outstanding articles in various high-profile journals.

He has received scientific awards from the Czech Society of Hypertension, and the Czech Endocrinological Society.

Preface

According to the latest estimate of the world health organization, 1.28 billion adults worldwide suffer from hypertension, which substantially increases the morbidity and mortality from cardiovascular and renal diseases. 10%—15% of these patients have secondary hypertension, the majority of whom have dysfunction of one or more of the endocrine systems which causes high blood pressure. Accurate diagnosis of endocrine hypertension is of paramount importance because of the risk of potential complications in undiagnosed cases, the likelihood of optimal control with pharmacotherapy, and the probability of a surgical cure with a timely diagnosis. Even though about 10% of hypertensive individuals suffer from endocrine hypertension, the diagnosis is often delayed or even never made because of inadequate awareness among physicians. This textbook, written by the global experts in the field, is a treatise on endocrine hypertension that addresses, in-depth, the etiology, pathophysiology, and molecular underpinnings, the differential diagnosis, and the management of endocrine hypertension, including all the practical aspects of treatment and follow-up.

Understanding hormone science is difficult without adequate knowledge about the complexities involved in the physiological, biochemical, molecular, and genetic aspects of endocrine disease therefore, we have planned chapters in this book with four basic science chapters immediately after the editorial (Chapter 1) to improve reader experience. Every attempt is made by each of our renowned authors to provide a clear understanding of their chapters by compiling the best and up-to-date evidence with optimal numbers of tables, figures, flow charts, illustrations and graphical abstracts and we are indebted to all our authors.

We are thankful to the Elsevier acquisition editor Ms. Ana Claudia Abad Garcia for her initial approach to us to edit this textbook and her continued support during the initial processes of making the plan and formatting of this book. We also extend our sincere gratitude to Ms. Patricia Osbourne, the senior content acquisition editor, Mr. Timothy Bennett, the editorial project manager and Mr. Omer Mukhtar, the production manager, without whose timely actions, this long-cherished dream of ours would not have come to fruition so well. We are also thankful to Dr. Marina George Kudiyirickal BDS, MJDF (RCS), Ph.D., for providing us with the audio summary for the video abstract of this textbook.

We dedicate this textbook to our beloved teachers during our graduate and postgraduate medical career whose excellent commitment and passion to instil knowledge in their trainees motivated us to make this humble contribution to the scientific world.

Joseph M. Pappachan MD, FRCP,
Cornelius J. Fernandez MD, MSc, MRCP,
Editors

Chapter 1

Endocrine hypertension—an overview

Joseph M. Pappachan[1,2,3] and Cornelius J. Fernandez[4]

[1]Department of Endocrinology & Metabolism, Royal Preston Hospital, The Lancashire Teaching Hospitals NHS Foundation Trust, Preston, United Kingdom; [2]The University of Manchester, Manchester, United Kingdom; [3]Faculty of Science, Manchester Metropolitan University, Manchester, United Kingdom; [4]Department of Endocrinology & Metabolism, Pilgrim Hospital, United Lincolnshire Hospitals NHS Trust, Boston, United Kingdom

Visit the *Endocrine Hypertension: From Basic Science to Clinical Practice, First Edition* companion web site at: https://www.elsevier.com/books-and-journals/book-companion/9780323961202.

Graphical Abstract

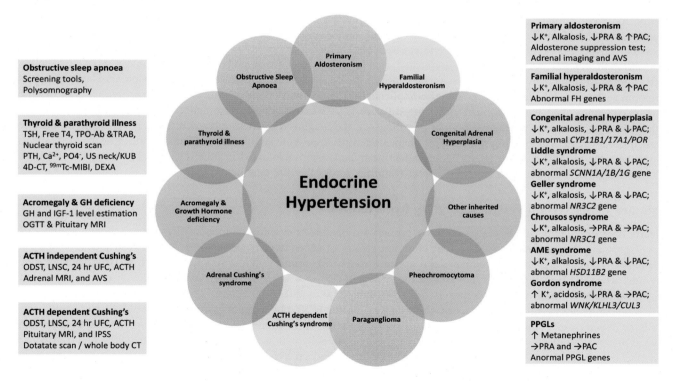

Endocrine Hypertension. https://doi.org/10.1016/B978-0-323-96120-2.00022-4

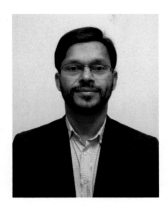

Joseph M. Pappachan

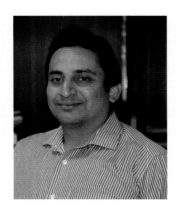

Cornelius J. Fernandez

Introduction

Hypertension is a major risk factor for cardiovascular disease (CVD) and chronic kidney disease among the global population. The disease affects about 45% of the US population and significantly increases the risk of chronic morbidity and mortality among the sufferers [1]. Similar prevalence figures are likely to exist in the other regions of the world also owing to the rising prevalence of sedentary lifestyles and adverse nutritional habits. 85% to 90% of patients with hypertension have primary or essential hypertension (without an identifiable cause), while the remainder have secondary hypertension, of whom the majority have dysfunction of one or more endocrine systems [2]. The most common causes of secondary hypertension are renal disease and endocrine disorders.

Although adrenal disease is often implicated as the cause of endocrine hypertension, pituitary as well as other extraadrenal disorders are also identified as the cause of the disease. Correct diagnosis of these disorders is of paramount importance because of the risk of potential complications in undiagnosed cases, the likelihood of optimal control with pharmacotherapy, and the probability of a surgical cure [3]. Even though the prevalence of endocrine hypertension is relatively high compared to many other chronic illnesses, the diagnosis is often delayed or even never made because of inadequate awareness among physicians. This chapter attempts to provide an overview of some of the basic science aspects along with the clinical practice pearls about endocrine hypertension elaborated in other chapters of this textbook by the global experts in the field from twelve different countries across the five continents.

Primary hypertension versus secondary hypertension

Nearly 85% of patients with hypertension have primary (idiopathic or essential) hypertension, whereas the remaining 15% have secondary hypertension [4]. The four common causes of secondary hypertension with their prevalence in the hypertensive subjects include obstructive sleep apnea (>5−15%), primary aldosteronism (PA) (1.4−10%), renal parenchymal disease (1.6−8.0%), and renovascular hypertension (1.0−8.0%) [5]. Among patients with resistant hypertension, the prevalence of these four etiologies is >30.0%, 6.0−23.0%, 2.0−10.0%, and 2.5−20.0%, respectively. The less common causes include thyroid disorders, Cushing's syndrome (CS), pheochromocytoma, coarctation of aorta, and drug-induced hypertension. A recently published retrospective analysis from China observed a change in the trend in secondary hypertension etiology [6]. They observed that though renal parenchymal disease contributed to nearly 50% and obstructive sleep apnea to nearly 25% of hospitalized patients with secondary hypertension, there is a downward trend for renal parenchymal disease and an upward trend for obstructive sleep apnea, endocrine hypertension, renovascular hypertension, and aortic disease, from 2013 to 2016 ($P < .001$).

The prevalence of secondary hypertension varies depending on age. The common causes in children are renal parenchymal disease and coarctation of aorta; in young adults are renovascular hypertension caused by fibromuscular dysplasia (especially in women), and renal parenchymal disease; in middle-age are PA, obstructive sleep apnea, CS, and pheochromocytoma; and in older adults are atherosclerotic renovascular hypertension, renal failure, and hypothyroidism [7]. Marked discrepancies in the reported prevalence of secondary hypertension are due to the wide variations in the approach to diagnostic workup, inadequate awareness among physicians, and the resource strain for appropriate investigations in many population groups. For the same reasons, correct estimation of the actual prevalence of endocrine hypertension in the global population is difficult.

Once the clinical suspicion of endocrine hypertension arises, semiurgent diagnostic workup and the plan for appropriate management should be enforced to avoid catastrophic complications related to some of these disorders, with the probability of complete cure, or marked improvement of the disease, their complications, and hypertension. However, we must bear in mind that the clinical presentation of some of these disorders can be quite vague and can mimic many other systemic diseases, and therefore, the diagnosis is often delayed by several months to years. A thorough understanding of the basic science aspects, pathophysiology, clinical profile, diagnostic workup, and the management algorithm of endocrine hypertension are crucial for an appropriate scientific approach to patients with hypertension that we encounter in our day-to-day clinical practice. With the help of the most up-to-date evidence, the best global experts in the field of fundamental and clinical research elaborate on these aspects of endocrine hypertension in the subsequent chapters.

Individual chapters

Catecholamines and blood pressure regulation

Catecholamines (epinephrine, norepinephrine, and dopamine) are monoamine neurotransmitters and circulating hormones which play various vital roles in the maintenance of body homeostasis and BP regulation through different effector organs especially the cardiovascular system [8]. These neurochemicals exert their wide variety of physiological and pathophysiological effects through three types of G-protein-coupled receptors viz. α-adrenoreceptors, β-adrenoreceptors, and dopamine receptors distributed throughout the body organs, tissues, and cells. While a steady physiological output of catecholamines is crucial for the maintenance of normal health, their excess production as seen in some patients with pheochromocytomas and paragangliomas (PPGLs), and deficiency states as in autonomic failure may be associated with catastrophic consequences. In their review of the role of catecholamines in BP regulation, Fernandez et al. provide a detailed analysis of these basic science aspects in Chapter 2.

Adrenocortical hormones and BP regulation

Blood pressure in human beings is maintained in the normal physiological range through highly complex and interconnected mechanisms involving the symapthoadrenergic (central and peripheral) pathways that also include the chemoreceptors and baroreceptors, renin—angiotensin—aldosterone system (RAAS) that involves kidney and the adrenal cortical hormones (principally aldosterone), antidiuretic hormone from the hypothalamus, atrial natriuretic peptide (ANP) from the heart, and local factors from the blood vessel such as nitric oxide (NO) [9—11]. Although the role of RAAS in BP regulation was known to man from the first half of the 20th century [12], more light on this area was shed in our understanding during the latter half [13]. Much more subsequent research input has been invested by the global scientific fraternity on to this important hormonal circuitry with many more newer discoveries that markedly changed our current approach to the management of hypertension.

Though aldosterone is the principal mineralocorticoid involved in the regulation of BP, other hormones of the adrenal cortex also play important roles in the human BP homeostasis. There is evidence to show the interrelationship between glucocorticoids [14] and sex steroids [15], and BP regulation in physiological and disease states. In their extensive review of the topic "Adrenocortical hormones and blood pressure regulation," Sanders et al. provide us the current evidence on the mechanisms involved in this complex neuro-endocrine circuitry in health and disease (Chapter 3). This chapter also highlights the importance of ongoing and future research in this area.

Hypothalamic—pituitary—adrenal axis and blood pressure regulation

Historically, the human hypothalamic—pituitary—adrenal (HPA) axis was an area of immense scientific research input in the past two centuries though we are still in an infantile stage of our understanding of its protean functions including those involved in human neurohumoral responses, endocrine homeostasis, and metabolic regulation. Ongoing research is expected to provide us with more rewarding output to unmask these mysteries in near future. The central regulation of BP is mainly through two unique neuro-endocrine circuitries, viz. the central sympathetic nervous system and the neuro-endocrine signals through the HPA axis while these two pathways are closely interlinked [14,16,17]. In addition, the biological clock mechanisms in the brain and peripheral organs are also connected to these complex pathways and play significant roles in the neuro-endocrine signaling cascade which controls homeostatic equilibrium in healthy individuals.

Various physiological, metabolic, hormonal, and psychological stressors can alter this equilibrium state that may affect BP regulation and thereby result in hypertension.

In their concise review "Hypothalamic-pituitary-adrenal axis and blood pressure regulation," Pappachan, Fernandez, and Stratakis portray the complex mechanisms involved in the control of human BP in health and disease (Chapter 4). Various factors that alter the physiological, psychological, and metabolic adaptive stress responses in health and disease states have been revealed in recent years [18,19]. However, considering the complexity and the current inadequate knowledge about these biological mechanisms, more research input is necessary for this area in the future as suggested by the authors of the chapter.

Renin-angiotensin—aldosterone system and blood pressure regulation

The history of RAAS began with the initial experiments of Tigerstedt and Bergman of the Karolinska Institute in 1898 showing the effects of rabbit's renal tissue on arterial BP which led to the discovery of renin—angiotensin system in the early 20th century [12,20]. The puzzling effects of RAAS as an endocrine and neurohumoral effector circuit in the control of human health, well-being, and illness are still being evolved through the 21st century, improving some of our understanding of its complexities. Several physical, pharmaceutical, and surgical interventions can alter the functions of RAAS that may modulate homeostatic equilibrium and pathological states in man including hypertension, CVD, and infectious diseases like COVID-19 [21—24].

The mechanisms of BP regulation by the RAAS are mostly elucidated in the recent years through decades of immense research. In their chapter "Renin—angiotensin—aldosterone system and blood pressure regulation," Seravalle and Grassi outline the normal and pathophysiological mechanisms involved in RAAS and BP variations in health and disease (Chapter 5). The role of RAAS in regulating systemic vascular resistance, and blood volume through the effects on salt-fluid balance, and vascular inflammation and remodeling is narrated in this chapter with up-to-date evidence. In addition, they highlight the importance of pharmacological modulation of RAAS as a key strategy in the treatment of hypertension, CVD, and chronic renal disease. The emerging role of mineralocorticoid antagonist therapy in the modern approach to management of resistant hypertension is also emphasized in this chapter.

Monogenic hypertension: an overview

The concept "monogenic hypertension" encompasses a group of genetic disorders associated with hypertension that follow a Mendelian inheritance pattern with a strong family history of the disease in affected individuals. Essential hypertension, on the other hand, is polygenic without a clear inheritance pattern. Although with some heterogeneity in its phenotypic expression depending on the degree of penetrance, monogenic hypertension usually presents with unique clinical and pathophysiological characteristics [25]. With the help of modern DNA sequencing technology, several of the genes associated with monogenic hypertension are recently identified which improved our understanding of the pathobiology of these disorders making the clinical profiling, diagnostic evaluation, and management options easier. Most forms of monogenic hypertension syndromes are associated with dysfunction of sympathoadrenal or renal mechanisms of BP control owing to gain-of-function or loss-of-function mutations in the mineralocorticoid, glucocorticoid, or autonomic pathways [26].

In their comprehensive and concise chapter "Monogenic Hypertension: An Overview," Fernandez, Pappachan, and Scholl outline the classification, genetic associations, and diagnostic approach to monogenic hypertension (Chapter 6). The algorithms demonstrated by the authors in this chapter along with a more detailed discussion on the genetic aspects of the inherited syndromes associated with hypertension in several other chapters of this textbook are expected to equip the readers with reasonable knowledge in working up and managing patients with endocrine hypertension. Ongoing research is expected to further improve our understanding of monogenic hypertension.

Primary aldosteronism (Conn's syndrome)

PA results from overproduction of the mineralocorticoid hormone aldosterone from the adrenal cortex, usually from the zona glomerulosa layer. PA is the most common form of endocrine hypertension accounting for $\approx 10\%$ of patients with elevated BP attending hypertension clinics and $\approx 20\%$ of those with resistant hypertension [27,28]. Although the prevalence of PA is relatively high for a chronic disease state affecting a significant proportion of individuals in the society, the diagnosis of this condition in the community and even in the secondary care settings is alarmingly low because of the poor awareness of PA among the healthcare workers, difficulty with its diagnostic work-up in resource-poor settings in most underdeveloped economies, and the physician inertia to appropriately evaluate patients with hypertension to exclude PA. Correct identification and appropriate management of PA can potentially cure or improve the adverse outcomes associated with the disease, and therefore, a proactive approach from the endocrinologists to heighten the awareness of this enigmatic disease among healthcare providers is an urgent need of our time.

The chapter "Primary aldosteronism (Conn's syndrome)" by Ceccato et al. brings forth the current evidence base on the clinical profile, diagnostic approach, and management algorithms with a brief discussion on the familial forms of PA to enable readers to have a better knowledge about the disease (Chapter 7). Of the patients with PA, nearly one third only have unilateral disease with the remainder having bilateral adrenal involvement (with a small proportion having inherited monogenic forms of PA described below). A timely and accurate diagnosis of PA is of paramount importance as resection of an aldosterone-producing adenoma (APA) is associated with a cure of hypertension in 50 to 60% of individuals, and with significant improvement in the remainder [29,30]. However, the correct identification of cases through appropriate biochemical workup and subtyping the disease through investigations such as adrenal venous sampling (AVS) in those with PA often pose significant challenges to clinicians. Through the detailed and precise narrative of the diagnostic and therapeutic approaches to PA in their chapter, Ceccato et al. enable the readers to overcome these challenges.

Familial hyperaldosteronism

The genetic landscape of PA has been largely disclosed in recent years making use of next-generation sequencing (NGS) methods which identify several somatic and germline mutations improving our understanding of the pathobiology of the disease [31]. Familial hyperaldosteronism (FH) forms a group of monogenic hypertensive disorders associated with PA that shows a clear inheritance pattern with phenotypic variability depending on the degree of penetrance of the culprit gene. There are 4 main forms of FH (FH-I, II, III, and IV) currently known, with an additional disorder known as PASNA (PA with seizures and neurological abnormalities) syndrome described recently. Because of the dominant inheritance nature, patients with FH present early in life (usually before the age of 20 years) with hypertension and sometimes a hypertensive complication such as hemorrhagic stroke. In their chapter "Familial Hyperaldosteronism," Pappachan, Fernandez, and Geller discuss the pathobiological aspects, diagnosis, and management of FH with the aid of latest research evidence (Chapter 8).

Congenital adrenal hyperplasia and hypertension

Congenital adrenal hyperplasia (CAH) is a group of genetic disorders characterized by abnormalities in the enzymes catalyzing adrenal steroidogenesis. CAH is inherited as an autosomal recessive disorder, and there are 7 different types depending on the enzyme deficiency involved, viz. 21-hydroxylase (21OH), 11β-hydroxylase (11βOH), 17α-hydroxylase/17,20-lyase (17OH), 3β-hydroxysteroid dehydrogenase type 2 (3βHSD2), steroidogenic acute regulatory protein (StAR), P450 cholesterol side-chain cleavage enzyme (P450scc), and P450 oxidoreductase (POR) [32]. CAH secondary to 21-OH deficiency (from *CYP21A2* mutation) is the most common form of the disease accounting for $\sim$95% of cases with an incidence of $\sim$1 in 15,000, and is not usually associated with hypertension as a part of the primary disease [33]. Of the CAH subtypes, those due to 11β-hydroxylase and 17α-hydroxylase deficiencies are associated with hypertension in the affected individuals [34]. Very rarely POR deficiency may also result in hypertension in the affected individuals [35]. However, among patients with monogenic hypertension, CAH accounts for only a small proportion of cases.

In their chapter "Congenital Adrenal Hyperplasia and Hypertension," Gurpinar and Guran provide a detailed account of these uncommon disorders of monogenic hypertension that often presents during childhood (Chapter 9). However, we must bear in mind that hypertensive forms of CAH can also be associated with variable phenotypic expression, and therefore, some of these patients may present to the clinician for the first time with hypertension during early adult life. In their detailed monograph, the authors provide us with the clinical features, diagnostic approach, management algorithms, and follow-up plan for patients with these subtypes of CAH associated with hypertension.

Endocrine hypertension: discovering the inherited causes

As mentioned in the section on monogenic hypertension, there are several inherited monogenic disorders which result in endocrine hypertension. More than 30 genes and $\sim$1500 single nucleotide polymorphisms have been identified to date in association with monogenic forms of hypertension or hypotension syndromes which mainly involve abnormalities in the RAAS and adrenal steroidogenic pathways and some uncommon neuroendocrine tumors [36]. Each of these endocrine hypertensive disorders may invoke enthusiasm in the readers to understand their pathophysiology, clinical profile, diagnostic evaluation, and management algorithm. Assadi and colleagues in their chapter "Endocrine hypertension: discovering the inherited causes" do that job in a very concise and precise way (Chapter 10) summarizing the complex topic with the aid of multiple tables and figures.

Pheochromocytomas and hypertension

Although the prevalence of PPGLs among patients with adrenal incidentalomas is 5—7% [37], they are rare endocrine tumors with an estimated prevalence of 2 to 8 per million in the general population [38] and account for only 0.1—0.6% of cases of hypertension attending general medical outpatient clinics [6,39]. PPGLs are unique in their secretory behavior with vasoactive catecholamine production and often present with sustained and/or episodic hypertension. The molecular and genetic landscapes of PPGLs are clearer in recent years with the discovery of several mutations and tumor syndromes which give us a better understanding of their clinical, epidemiological, and pathobiological characteristics to enable the development of more scientific diagnostic, prognostic, and management algorithms [40]. With the aid of up-to-date evidence, Goemann and Maia elaborate on these algorithms in their comprehensive chapter "Pheochromocytomas and hypertension" (Chapter 11).

Paragangliomas and hypertension

Paragangliomas (PGLs) are rare neuroendocrine tumors originating from the embryonic neural crest cells which form the extra-adrenal autonomic paraganglia dispersed from the skull base to the pelvic floor [41]. Though many of the clinical, pathophysiological, and genetic nature simulate those of adrenal pheochromocytomas, PGLs show certain unique clinical, familial, and pathophysiological characteristics [40]. These include sustained arterial hypertension or rarely normotension (dopamine-secreting tumors), malignant/metastatic potential, genetic characteristics (predominantly Cluster 1-related gene mutations), and relatively silent clinical behavior (often detected as incidentalomas in imaging studies or during open surgery). Majority of the functional PGLs (70—80%) arise from the infradiaphragmatic sympathetic ganglia, whereas the head and neck PGLs are rarely hormone producing. With the help of a couple of case vignettes, Petrák and Zelinka give us a detailed account of PGLs in their chapter "Paragangliomas and hypertension" enabling the readers to have a very thorough understanding of these rare neoplasms causing endocrine hypertension (Chapter 12).

ACTH-dependent Cushing syndrome

CS resulting from glucocorticoid administration for pharmacotherapy of various disease states is common. However, endogenous CS is a rare endocrine disorder associated with protean manifestations that may vary from subclinical hypercortisolemia without significant major clinical abnormalities to florid multiorgan dysfunction and cushingoid appearance. Approximately 70—80% of endogenous CS cases result from excess production of adrenocorticotrophin (ACTH) from the pituitary ($\approx$60—70%; Cushing's disease/CD) or from an extrapituitary source (5—10%), while the remainder are caused by primary adrenal disorders [42]. Endogenous hypercortisolemia resulting from ACTH overproduction is termed ACTH-dependent CS. Hypertension is the most common sequel of CS regardless of the etiology and can occur in 75—85% of adults and 47—51% of children and adolescents [43,44]. The severity of hypertension in patients with CS may be related to multiple factors including the age of the patient and the duration and degree of cortisol exposure [43]. However, the prevalence of CS in hypertensive population is relatively low at 0.5%, and only <1% of cases with resistant hypertension result from CS [5].

The pathophysiological factors involved in the causation of hypertension in patients with CS are not fully elusive though various mechanisms are proposed to explain this important comorbidity, mostly based on small-scale studies [45]. The diagnosis and management of CS can often be challenging and require close multidisciplinary association with different specialties such as biochemistry, radiology, surgery, and endocrinology. A recently updated international consensus on evaluation and management of CD gives us insight into the complexities of this approach [46]. Currently, there are no guidelines exclusively for the management of hypertension in patients with CS, and therefore, we must rely upon the general guidelines for managing essential hypertension in any patient to treat such cases. In their concise and comprehensive chapter "ACTH-dependent Cushing's syndrome," Fernandes, Varlamov, and Fleseriu successfully fill these evidence gaps (Chapter 13).

Adrenal Cushing's syndrome

Approximately, 20—30% of endogenous CS is ACTH-independent resulting from adrenal disease (adrenal CS) as mentioned above. The annual incidence of adrenal CS is 1.3 per million as reported by a large recent series from Korea [47]. Adrenal CS results from cortisol producing adrenal adenoma (most common; >50%), adrenocortical carcinoma, and bilateral micro and macronodular adrenal hyperplasia [48]. Several genetic disorders and syndromes have been implicated in the causation of these types of CS [42]. In his chapter "Adrenal Cushing's syndrome", Ragnarsson provides us with the latest evidence on epidemiology, genetic aspects, clinical profile, diagnostic evaluation, pathophysiology of hypertension, and management of patients with adrenal CS (Chapter 14).

Hypertension in growth hormone excess (acromegaly) and deficiency

Growth hormone excess that results in acromegaly had been a puzzling hormonal disorder for modern medical practice historically, and continues to pose significant diagnostic and management challenges even in the 21st century. Acromegaly is a rare endocrinopathy with a disease prevalence of 28—137 cases per million and an annual incidence ranging between 2 and 11 cases per million people [49]. Although hypertension is the most common comorbidity among patients with acromegaly, this endocrine disorder contributes only a negligible proportion to the global hypertensive population. Recent estimates show a hypertension prevalence of 11—55% in patients with acromegaly [50]. Hypertension in acromegaly is multifactorial and the mechanisms involved are increased plasma volume from fluid retention, increased vascular resistance, and endothelial dysfunction [50], along with other factors such as sleep apnea, insulin resistance, and increased cardiac output [51]. Hypertension is one of the most important comorbidities in acromegaly associated with excess mortality from associated CVD.

Adult growth hormone deficiency (AGHD) on the other hand is also associated with a high risk of CVD mainly because of the development of metabolic syndrome, an integral component of which is hypertension [52]. AGHD is a rare disease with an estimated annual incidence of 16.5 per million population [53]. Therefore, AGHD also accounts for a negligible proportion of patients with hypertension in the general population. As in acromegaly, the pathophysiology of hypertension in AGHD also is not fully understood and various mechanisms have been proposed by different authors.

In their detailed review of the currently available literature for diagnosis and management of acromegaly and growth hormone deficiency (GHD), Mihai and Korbonits provide extensive scientific evidence-base to enable clinicians to approach these uncommon endocrine problems. Therefore, the chapter "Hypertension in patients with growth hormone excess and deficiency" (Chapter 15) is an invaluable resource to this textbook.

Hypertension in thyroid disease and hyperparathyroidism

Thyroid disease forms the second most common type of endocrine disorder after diabetes mellitus, while primary hyperparathyroidism forms the third. Large studies show the prevalence of hypothyroidism at 4—7% [54], hyperthyroidism at 0.5—2.1% (overt hyperthyroidism 0.1—0.5%) [55], and primary hyperparathyroidism at ≈1% of adults [56] among the general population. Both types of thyroid diseases and primary hyperparathyroidism are directly associated with an increased prevalence of hypertension. Considering the relatively high prevalence of these endocrinopathies in the population, they constitute important causes of hypertension, and therefore, a thorough understanding of the pathophysiology, clinical presentation, and management of thyroid disease and primary hyperparathyroidism is crucial while approaching patients with endocrine hypertension. Szwarcbard and Topliss in their chapter "Hypertension in thyroid disease and hyperparathyroidism" provide readers with this wonderful opportunity (Chapter 16).

Obesity, insulin resistance, and obstructive sleep apnea

The prevalence of obesity in the global population has been steadily increasing over the past 5—6 decades because of the adverse lifestyles and modernization of food industry that resulted in a fast-food culture across the world. Numerous complex mechanisms have been proposed to explain how overweight and obesity result in hypertension [57]. One of the key components of metabolic syndrome, commonly observed in obese individuals, is hypertension. There is also clear evidence to show that weight gain usually increases BP, while weight loss is associated with reduction of BP [58]. Obesity-related primary hypertension was found to affect 78% and 65% of men and women, respectively, in the Framingham Heart Study [59]. Obesity also results in insulin resistance and obstructive sleep apnea (OSA), the other important risk factors for the development of hypertension.

OSA, the commonest form of sleep-disordered breathing, increases the risk of hypertension by several mechanisms. The estimated prevalence of OSA is 15−24% among the adult population [60]. Considering the inadequate awareness among healthcare professionals about the high prevalence of the disease, and the inertia for appropriate diagnostic evaluation from physicians, there is a high likelihood of under-reporting of OSA. In addition to the higher risk of essential hypertension related to obesity, patients can also develop OSA-related secondary hypertension (ORSH), often resistant to usual pharmacotherapy [61]. Clear understanding of the pathophysiology, clinical presentation, diagnostic evaluation, and management of OSA and ORSH is important in managing patients with endocrine and secondary hypertension. This task is very efficiently performed by Oduro-Donkor and Barber in their chapter "Obesity, Insulin Resistance and Obstructive Sleep Apnea" to enable the readers of this textbook to look for and to treat OSA, if present, in individuals with resistant hypertension (Chapter 17).

Endocrine hypertension in children

Hypertension is becoming a major health problem among children and adolescents with a recently estimated prevalence of 4% in those younger than 19 years [62]. Approximately 60% of cases of hypertension in children are from secondary causes such as CVD and renal disorders [63]. Endocrinopathies as a cause account for only 0.05−6% of cases of hypertension in the pediatric population [64]. Therefore, a more vigilant clinical and diagnostic approach should be practiced by the clinicians while dealing with these patients as the signs and symptoms can be subtle, and may not be often familiar to many professionals. Prompt suspicion and urgent clinical workup of all children with hypertension are mandatory to avoid hypertension-related complications including premature mortality.

The pathophysiological features, clinical characteristics, and laboratory parameters of endocrine hypertension in childhood and the approach for diagnostic workup are also often different from those in the adult population with the disease. Reading the chapter "Endocrine Hypertension in Children" by Valaiyapathi and Ashraf (Chapter 18) would enable us to obtain a clear evidence-based understanding of how to approach and manage children and adolescents with these uncommon disorders associated with high morbidity and mortality.

Endocrine hypertension in pregnant woman

Pregnancy is a physiological state with marked variations in the maternal body metabolism, circulation, and chemical composition to accommodate the physiological needs of the growing fetus. Therefore, there shall be significant variations in the neurohumoral and hormonal balance in a pregnant woman compared to a nonpregnant female. Output of normal female hormones like estrogens and progesterone shall be very different during pregnancy compared to nonpregnant states, and several placental hormones such as human placental lactogen and human chorionic gonadotropin also come into play in the maternal circulation [65]. Marked alterations in the HPA, and hypothalamic−pituitary−gonadal (HPG) axes, also occur during pregnancy compounding the situation further [66]. Moreover, there shall be mechanical factors such as compression of other abdominal organs including the kidneys and the adrenals by the gravid uterus that may result in exacerbation of the preexisting diseases of these organs present prior to pregnancy.

Approximately, 30% increase in the blood and plasma volume occur during pregnancy, and therefore, the hormone assays are expected to have different cut-offs especially with the interference from alterations in the HPA/HPG axes and placental hormones as mentioned above. Several of the imaging modalities utilizing ionizing radiations (e.g., CT scan) and compounds (e.g., nuclear imaging techniques) are contraindicated during pregnancy, and some of the pharmacotherapeutic agents used for the management of hypertension are unsafe. All these issues make diagnosis and management of endocrine hypertension during pregnancy complicated in ordinary clinical settings. To address these issues, and to empower readers with the best evidence, Jebasingh and Thomas compiled their chapter "Endocrine Hypertension in Pregnancy" which has turned out to be an invaluable resource (Chapter 19) to this textbook.

Imaging for patients with endocrine hypertension

Imaging studies for confirmation of the disease are integral and final components of the diagnostic algorithms in hormone science. Full laboratory workup to reach the biochemical diagnosis is almost always followed by imaging studies to identify the structural and/or functional abnormalities in the endocrine glands which help us to plan definitive treatment that may lead to a surgical cure of the disease. Endocrine hypertension is often caused by tumoral involvement of one or more of the hormone-producing glands which can be detected by an anatomical imaging modality such as CT, MRI, or ultrasonography scans for disease localization. For example, primary hyperaldosteronism is caused by an APA in about one third of individuals which may be localized by a CT scan of the adrenal gland with subsequent lateralization (for aldosterone overproduction) study by an image-assisted AVS to pinpoint the site for surgical target [67−69]. Adrenalectomy in such cases is associated with a cure rate of hypertension in 50−60% and improvement in most of the remainder [30].

Another important group of imaging studies which assist final diagnosis in patients with endocrine hypertension is functional imaging to localize the abnormal gland(s) causing hormone overproduction. Several nuclear imaging techniques utilizing radioisotopes have been made use of in the past few decades for imaging the adrenal, thyroid, parathyroid, and pituitary glands for disease localization/detecting functional hyperactivity. For example, ^{68}Ga-DOTATATE PET/CT scan has emerged as the best imaging modality in recent years for the detection and staging of neuroendocrine tumors with a reported sensitivity of 93% and specificity of 95% [70]. Anatomical and functional imaging studies are also important for prognostication and follow-up management of patients after initial treatment. For example, ^{123}I-MIBG (^{123}Iodine-labeled metaiodobenzylguanidine)-avid malignant pheochromocytomas are more likely to respond to radionuclide therapy with ^{131}I-MIBG [71]. Basic understanding of the relevant imaging studies and adequate knowledge about diagnostic performance of each imaging modality are essential among physicians who workup patients with endocrine hypertension for appropriate patient care and optimal resource utilization. With the back-up of up-to-date evidence through extensive literature review and several good quality images, Ordidge and Sahdev did a wonderful job through their chapter "Imaging for Patients with Endocrine Hypertension" (Chapter 20) in enabling the readers of the textbook to gain thorough ideas on "whom," "what," and "when" to image when endocrine hypertension is suspected.

Systematic approach for the diagnosis and management of endocrine hypertension

"Last but not the least chapter" of this textbook is "Systematic Approach for the Diagnosis and Management of Endocrine Hypertension" by Stowasser, Jansen, and Wolley (Chapter 21). A structured and systematic approach to any clinical problem is expected to give the best answer to every puzzling disorder in our day-to-day medical practice in the diagnostic workup and management options. This approach is very crucial in practicing hormone science with a special emphasis on working up and treating patients with endocrine hypertension considering the diagnostic and therapeutic complexities involved in such cases. For example, diagnosis and disease localization in PA can be often difficult and a vast majority of cases in the community, and even in the secondary care settings, are underdiagnosed considering the relatively high prevalence rates of ≈10% in patients attending hypertension clinics and ≈20% with resistant hypertension [27]. Moreover, there is ongoing debate even among endocrinologists about the screening criteria for patients, the appropriateness of individual cut offs regarding plasma renin activity (PRA), direct renin concentration (DRC), plasma aldosterone concentration (PAC), and aldosterone renin ratio (ARR), the need for AVS in each case for definitive therapeutic planning and individualizing medical therapy [72].

To add more complexity to the above conundrum regarding the approach to patients with PA, several authors also reported marked ethnic variations in the RAAS activity with differences in the plasma levels of renin and aldosterone especially in African and African American ethnic groups [73−75]. This fact would demand ethic-specific approach to patients and the necessity of changing the current international guidelines accordingly. With their extensive experience in developing real-world practical algorithms for the diagnosis and management of PA in Australia, backed up by the latest and extensive literature review, Stowasser et al. fill in the evidence gap in this controversial area at large through Chapter 21.

An individualized approach to patients with hormonal disorders is highly important for planning diagnostic workup and management while dealing with cases of endocrine hypertension. In the subsequent sections of the chapter, this task has been very effectively performed by Stowasser et al. For example, by the discussion regarding the change in age-standardized incidence rate for the incidence of PPGLs, the authors provide guidance to enable an individualized approach while reviewing patients [76,77]. Overall, Chapter 21 would serve as a quick reference guide within this textbook to empower the readers with the best evidence to manage their patients with endocrine hypertension.

Recent trends/emerging concepts

Many of the conditions associated with endocrine hypertension have a genetic/familial background of inheritance that makes it essential for appropriate testing to prognosticate/follow-up the patients and families with the disease gene. These tests can be labor-intensive and expensive, and therefore, endocrinologists should use them very judiciously. Recent guidelines and emerging testing algorithms help us to approach such cases more pragmatically as discussed briefly in the following sections.

Genetic testing for familial PPGL

Large number of susceptibility genes are implicated in the diagnosis of familial PPGLs. NGS technology is ideally suited for genetic testing of patients with PPGL [78]. NGS involves DNA sequencing using a disease-specific gene panel including *SDHA, SDHB, SDHC, SDHD, SDHAF2, RET, TMEM127, MAX, FH, VHL,* and *MEN1* [79]. The gene panel used might vary between laboratories: basic panel—looking for germline mutations with highest evidence, extended panel—looking for germline mutations at basic panel genes and at candidate susceptibility genes with low evidence, and comprehensive panel—looking for somatic mutations in addition to the extended panel [80]. Any sequence variants observed would be classified as pathogenic, benign, or variants of uncertain significance (VUS) by the reporting laboratory. NGS has high risk of false positivity as they detect many VUS [79].

NGS is not capable of detecting large deletions or insertions, thereby causing false negative results [79]. Multiplex ligation-dependent probe analysis (MLPA) together with NGS can improve the sensitivity [81,82]. If no pathogenic variants are detected on NGS, then MLPA should be done for *SDHB, SDHC, SDHD, VHL,* and *MEN1* as 10%—12% variants in these genes will have large deletions [79]. Germline mutations in *SDHA, SDHB, SDHC,* and *SDHD* account for 30% of all hereditary PPGL cases [83]. They are associated with high risk of malignancy, with increased lifetime risk of multifocal and synchronous tumors. These mutations predispose to PPGL, gastrointestinal stromal tumor (GIST), renal cell carcinoma (RCC), and pituitary tumors.

Indications for genetic testing in PPGL as per NHS England national genomic test registry are as follows (if patient meets one of the criteria): [84]

1. All patients <60 years with a diagnosis of pheochromocytoma
2. Patients at any age with bilateral pheochromocytoma
3. Patients at any age with pheochromocytoma and RCC
4. Patients at any age with any paraganglioma
5. Patients with pheochromocytoma/paraganglioma with loss of staining for SDH proteins on immunohistochemistry
6. Patients at any age with pheochromocytoma/paraganglioma and a family history of pheochromocytoma/paraganglioma/RCC/GIST

Fig. 1.1 shows an algorithm for genetic testing for familial PPGL.

Genetic testing for familial hyperparathyroidism

Familial hyperparathyroidism represents only <5% of total cases [85]. A history of pituitary adenomas, pancreatic neuroendocrine tumors, bronchial carcinoid, or duodenal endocrine tumors in the patient or first-degree relative favors the

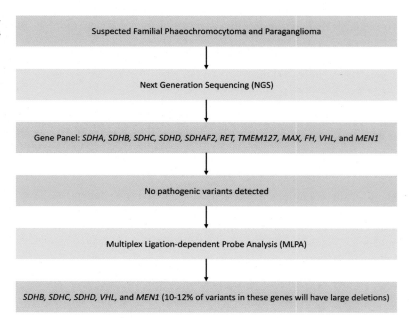

FIGURE 1.1 An algorithm for genetic testing for suspected familial pheochromocytoma paragangliomas (PPGLs).

Suspected Familial Phaeochromocytoma and Paraganglioma

Next Generation Sequencing (NGS)

Gene Panel: *SDHA, SDHB, SDHC, SDHD, SDHAF2, RET, TMEM127, MAX, FH, VHL,* and *MEN1*

No pathogenic variants detected

Multiplex Ligation-dependent Probe Analysis (MLPA)

SDHB, SDHC, SDHD, VHL, and *MEN1* (10-12% of variants in these genes will have large deletions)

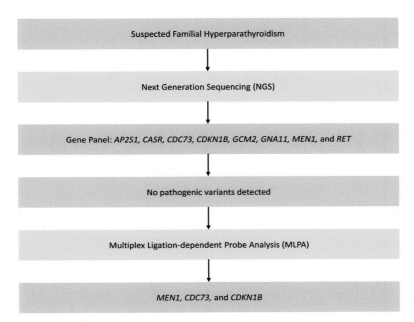

FIGURE 1.2 An algorithm for genetic evaluation of suspected familial hyperparathyroidism.

diagnosis of multiple endocrine neoplasia type 1 (MEN1). A history of medullary thyroid carcinoma or pheochromocytoma in the patient or a family member favors the diagnosis of MEN2A. History of parathyroid cancer, maxillary or mandibular tumors, Wilms' tumor, or uterine abnormalities requiring early hysterectomy in the patient, or another family member raise the possibility of hyperparathyroidism-jaw tumor syndrome (HPT-JTS). Persistent hypercalcemia following parathyroidectomy, hypocalciuria, hypermagnesemia, and hypercalcemia in family members <10 years of age would favor diagnosis of familial hypocalciuric hypercalcemia (FHH). NGS panel in these patients includes genes currently implicated in primary hyperparathyroidism including *MEN1, CDC73, RET, CDKN1B, GCM2,* and *CASR* and/or the genes implicated in FHH including *CASR, GNA11,* and *AP2S1*. If no pathogenic variants are detected on NGS, then MLPA should be done for *MEN1, CDC73,* and *CDKN1B* [86,87].

Indications for genetic testing for familial hyperparathyroidism as per NHS England national genomic test registry (if patient meets one of the following criteria): [84]

1. All patients <35 years
2. Patients <45 years with multiglandular involvement, or hyperplasia on histology, or ossifying fibroma(s) of maxilla and/or mandible, or at least one first degree relative with unexplained hyperparathyroidism
3. Patients with clinical features of endocrine neoplasia syndromes which include hyperparathyroidism (e.g., MEN1, MEN2A, MEN4, HPT-JTS)
4. Patients at any age with hypocalciuric hypercalcemia (calcium clearance/creatinine clearance ratio <0.02).

An algorithm for evaluation of suspected familial hyperparathyroidism is shown in Fig. 1.2.

Genetic testing for familial hyperaldosteronism especially GRA

Indications for genetic testing for GRA as per NHS England national genomic test registry (if patient meets one of the criteria): [84]

1. Age of presentation <30 years or
2. Family history of primary hyperaldosteronism or stroke <40 years.

Genetic testing for familial pituitary tumors (MEN1, FIPA, X-LAG, and Carney complex)

Indications for genetic testing for MEN1 as per NHS England national genomic test registry (patients who meets one of the criteria): [84]

FIGURE 1.3 An algorithm for diagnostic evaluation suspected familial pituitary tumors.

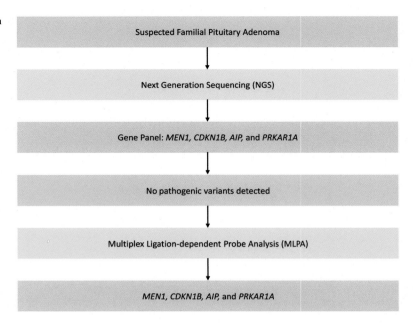

1. Patients with pituitary adenoma or insulinoma <20 years
2. Patients with pituitary macroadenoma <30 years
3. Patients with parathyroid multiglandular disease (hyperplasia/adenoma) < 35 years
4. Patients at any age with ≥2 MEN1-related endocrine abnormalities
5. Patients at any age with ≥1 MEN1-related endocrine abnormality and ≥1 MEN1-related nonendocrine tumors
6. Patients at any age with ≥1 MEN1-related endocrine abnormality and a first degree relative having ≥1 MEN1-related endocrine abnormality

MEN1-related endocrine abnormalities include parathyroid hyperplasia/multiglandular adenoma, pituitary tumors, gastro-entero-pancreatic neuroendocrine neoplasms, carcinoid tumors, and adrenocortical tumors, whereas MEN1-related nonendocrine tumors include facial angiofibroma, collagenoma, and meningioma [84].

Indication for genetic testing for familial isolated pituitary adenoma (FIPA) as per NHS England national genomic test registry [84] includes isolated pituitary adenoma <35 years with at least one first-degree relative with an isolated pituitary adenoma. Indication for genetic testing for X-linked acrogigantism (X-LAG) as per NHS England national genomic test

FIGURE 1.4 Algorithm for genetic diagnosis of X-linked acrogigantism.

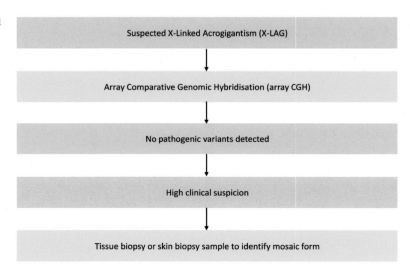

registry [84] includes growth hormone excess diagnosed by the age of 20 years in male patients with increased growth velocity or tall stature.

For all patients with suspected familial pituitary tumors except X-LAG, do NGS for *MEN1, CDKN1B, AIP,* and *PRKAR1A* [88]. If no pathogenic variants are identified, do MLPA for *MEN1, CDKN1B, AIP,* and *PRKAR1A*. For diagnosis of X-LAG, do array CGH (array comparative genomic hybridization), a competitive fluorescence in situ hybridization technique for abnormalities of chromosome number. If no pathogenic variants are identified, and clinical suspicion is high, send tissue sample or skin biopsy sample to identify a mosaic form [89].

An algorithm for suspected familial pituitary tumors is shown in Fig. 1.3 and that for X-LAG is shown in Fig. 1.4.

Conclusions

Endocrine hypertension is caused by various unique hormonal disorders which are often difficult to diagnose and manage in the primary care and even specialist care settings. Approximately 10% of patients with hypertension may have an endocrine cause which necessitates prompt diagnostic evaluation, and appropriate and timely management to prevent complications including those from hypertension and other comorbidities associated with these disorders. Several of these diseases are potentially curable by surgical interventions or are optimally controllable by medical therapy which makes the need for urgent evaluation highly important. An individualized patient evaluation algorithm for endocrine hypertension is provided by most of the authors of this textbook in their chapters. A pragmatic individualized algorithm for diagnostic evaluation of patients suspected to have endocrine hypertension is provided in Fig. 1.5.

Writing this editorial chapter was a herculean task for us considering the academic caliber of the contributing authors who provided individual chapters (Chapters 2 to 21) to this textbook. We must say that the fervor with which the authors worked toward the fruition of this project is highly remarkable. Several of our authors are attributed with the discovery of various diseases and/or the associated genes implicated in the etiology of endocrine hypertension. We hope that each of the chapters would enable the readers to approach individual hormonal disorders more pragmatically to offer a better chance of cure to their patients. It will be the best reward for the hard work and collective effort behind the creation of this textbook.

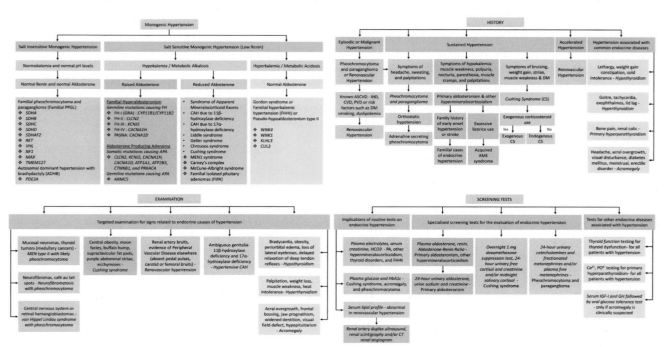

FIGURE 1.5 A pragmatic algorithm for individualized diagnostic evaluation of patients with suspected endocrine hypertension. *AME,* apparent mineralocorticoid excess; *ASCVD,* atherosclerotic cardiovascular disease; *CT,* computed tomography; *CAH,* congenital adrenal hyperplasia; *CVD,* cardiovascular disease; *DM,* diabetes mellitus; *FH,* familial hyperaldosteronism; *FHHt,* familial hyperkalemic hypertension; *GRA,* glucocorticoid remediable aldosteronism; *HCO₃⁻,* bicarbonate; *HbA1c,* glycated hemoglobin; *IHD,* ischemic heart disease; *MEN,* multiple endocrine neoplasia; *PA,* primary aldosteronism; *PVD,* peripheral vascular disease; *PASNA,* primary aldosteronism seizures and neurologic abnormalities.

References

[1] US Preventive Services Task Force, Krist AH, Davidson KW, Mangione CM, Cabana M, Caughey AB, Davis EM, et al. Screening for hypertension in adults: US Preventive Services task force reaffirmation recommendation statement. JAMA April 27, 2021;325(16):1650−6. https://doi.org/10.1001/jama.2021.4987. PMID: 33904861.

[2] Manosroi W, Williams GH. Genetics of human primary hypertension: focus on hormonal mechanisms. Endocr Rev June 1, 2019;40(3):825−56. https://doi.org/10.1210/er.2018-00071. PMID: 30590482.

[3] O'Shea PM, Griffin TP, Fitzgibbon M. Hypertension: the role of biochemistry in the diagnosis and management. Clin Chim Acta 2017;465:131−43. https://doi.org/10.1016/j.cca.2016.12.014. PMID: 28007614.

[4] Young Jr WF, Calhoun DA, Lenders JWM, Stowasser M, Textor SC. Screening for endocrine hypertension: an endocrine society scientific statement. Endocr Rev 2017;38:103−22. https://doi.org/10.1210/er.2017-00054.

[5] Rimoldi SF, Scherrer U, Messerli FH. Secondary arterial hypertension: when, who, and how to screen? Eur Heart J May 14, 2014;35(19):1245−54. https://doi.org/10.1093/eurheartj/eht534. PMID: 24366917.

[6] Zhang L, Li J, Li N, Sun N, Xie L, Han Q, et al. Trends in cause-related comorbidities in hospitalized patients with secondary hypertension in China from 2013 to 2016: a retrospective analysis of hospital quality monitoring system data. J Hypertens October 1, 2021;39(10):2015−21. https://doi.org/10.1097/HJH.0000000000002891. PMID: 33973956.

[7] Viera AJ, Neutze DM. Diagnosis of secondary hypertension: an age-based approach. Am Fam Physician December 15, 2010;82(12):1471−8. PMID: 21166367.

[8] Motiejunaite J, Amar L, Vidal-Petiot E. Adrenergic receptors, and cardiovascular effects of catecholamines. Ann Endocrinol (Paris) 2021;82(3−4):193−7. https://doi.org/10.1016/j.ando.2020.03.012. PMID: 32473788.

[9] Chopra S, Baby C, Jacob JJ. Neuro-endocrine regulation of blood pressure. Indian J Endocrinol Metab October 2011;15(Suppl. 4):S281−8. https://doi.org/10.4103/2230-8210.86860. PMID: 22145130.

[10] Antunes-Rodrigues J, de Castro M, Elias LL, Valença MM, McCann SM. Neuroendocrine control of body fluid metabolism. Physiol Rev January 2004;84(1):169−208. https://doi.org/10.1152/physrev.00017.2003. PMID: 14715914.

[11] Savić B, Murphy D, Japundžić-Žigon N. The paraventricular nucleus of the hypothalamus in control of blood pressure and blood pressure variability. Front Physiol March 16, 2022;13:858941. https://doi.org/10.3389/fphys.2022.858941. PMID: 35370790.

[12] Basso N, Terragno NA. History about the discovery of the renin-angiotensin system. Hypertension December 1, 2001;38(6):1246−9. https://doi.org/10.1161/hy1201.101214. PMID: 11751697.

[13] MacGregor GA, Markandu ND, Roulston JE, Jones JC, Morton JJ. Maintenance of blood pressure by the renin-angiotensin system in normal man. Nature May 28, 1981;291(5813):329−31. https://doi.org/10.1038/291329a0. PMID: 7015149.

[14] al'Absi M, Arnett DK. Adrenocortical responses to psychological stress and risk for hypertension. Biomed Pharmacother 2000;54(5):234−44. https://doi.org/10.1016/S0753-3322(00)80065-7. PMID: 10917460.

[15] Rossi GP, Caroccia B, Seccia TM. Role of estrogen receptors in modulating aldosterone biosynthesis and blood pressure. Steroids 2019;152:108486. https://doi.org/10.1016/j.steroids.2019.108486. PMID: 31499072.

[16] Tsigos C, Kyrou I, Kassi E, Chrousos GP. Stress: endocrine physiology and pathophysiology. 2020 Oct 17. In: Feingold KR, Anawalt B, Boyce A, Chrousos G, de Herder WW, Dhatariya K, et al., editors. Endotext [Internet]. South Dartmouth (MA: MDText.com, Inc.; 2000. PMID: 25905226.

[17] Jayasinghe SU, Lambert GW, Torres SJ, Fraser SF, Eikelis N, Turner AI. Hypothalamo-pituitary adrenal axis and sympatho-adrenal medullary system responses to psychological stress were not attenuated in women with elevated physical fitness levels. Endocrine February 2016;51(2):369−79. https://doi.org/10.1007/s12020-015-0687-6. PMID: 26206752.

[18] Deussing JM, Chen A. The corticotropin-releasing factor family: physiology of the stress response. Physiol Rev 2018;98(4):2225−86. https://doi.org/10.1152/physrev.00042.2017. PMID: 30109816.

[19] Peeters B, Langouche L, Van den Berghe G. Adrenocortical stress response during the course of critical illness. Compr Physiol December 12, 2017;8(1):283−98. https://doi.org/10.1002/cphy.c170022. PMID: 293571C29.

[20] Tigerstedt R, Bergman PG. Niere und Kreislauf. Skand Arch Physiol 1898;8:223−71.

[21] Jeong JH, Sprick JD, DaCosta D, Quyyumi AA, Park J. Renin-angiotensin system blockade is associated with exercise capacity, sympathetic activity, and endothelial function in patients with chronic kidney disease. Kidney Blood Press Res 2022;47(2):103−12. https://doi.org/10.1159/000520760. PMID: 34758473.

[22] Hansen E, Grimm D, Wehland M. Current knowledge about the new drug firibastat in arterial hypertension. Int J Mol Sci January 27, 2022;23(3):1459. https://doi.org/10.3390/ijms23031459. PMID: 35163378.

[23] Wu H, Sun Q, Yuan S, Wang J, Li F, Gao H, Chen X, Yang R, Xu J. AT1 receptors: their actions from hypertension to cognitive impairment. Cardiovasc Toxicol April 2022;22(4):311−25. https://doi.org/10.1007/s12012-022-09730-0. PMID: 35211833.

[24] Vaduganathan M, Vardeny O, Michel T, McMurray JJV, Pfeffer MA, Solomon SD. Renin-angiotensin-aldosterone system inhibitors in patients with covid-19. N Engl J Med April 23, 2020;382(17):1653−9. https://doi.org/10.1056/NEJMsr2005760. PMID: 32227760.

[25] Lu YT, Fan P, Zhang D, Zhang Y, Meng X, Zhang QY, Zhao L, Yang KQ, Zhou XL. Overview of monogenic forms of hypertension combined with hypokalemia. Front Pediatr January 25, 2021;8:543309. https://doi.org/10.3389/fped.2020.543309. PMID: 33569358.

[26] Burrello J, Monticone S, Buffolo F, Tetti M, Veglio F, Williams TA, et al. Is there a role for genomics in the management of hypertension? Int J Mol Sci 2017;18(6):1131. https://doi.org/10.3390/ijms18061131. PMID: 28587112.

[27] Sabbadin C, Fallo F. Hyperaldosteronism: screening and diagnostic tests. High Blood Press Cardiovasc Prev 2016;23(2):69−72. https://doi.org/10.1007/s40292-016-0136-5.

[28] Williams TA, Reincke M. Management of endocrine disease: diagnosis and management of primary aldosteronism: the Endocrine Society guideline 2016 revisited. Eur J Endocrinol 2018;179(1):R19−29. https://doi.org/10.1530/EJE-17-0990.

[29] Rutherford JC, Taylor WL, Stowasser M, Gordon RD. Success of surgery for primary aldosteronism judged by residual autonomous aldosterone production. World J Surg 1998;22:1243−5.

[30] Stowasser M, Gordon RD. Primary aldosteronism-careful investigation is essential and rewarding. Mol Cell Endocrinol 2004;217:33−9.

[31] Scholl UI. Genetics of primary aldosteronism. HYPERTENSIONAHA12116498 Hypertension February 2022;10. https://doi.org/10.1161/HYPERTENSIONAHA.121.16498. PMID: 35139664.

[32] El-Maouche D, Arlt W, Merke DP. Congenital adrenal hyperplasia. Lancet November 11, 2017;390(10108):2194−210. https://doi.org/10.1016/S0140-6736(17)31431-9. Erratum in: Lancet. 2017 Nov 11;390(10108):2142. PMID: 28576284.

[33] Claahsen-van der Grinten HL, Stikkelbroeck N, Falhammar H, Reisch N. Management of endocrine disease: gonadal dysfunction in congenital adrenal hyperplasia. Eur J Endocrinol March 2021;184(3):R85−97. https://doi.org/10.1530/EJE-20-1093. PMID: 33320831.

[34] Raina R, Krishnappa V, Das A, Amin H, Radhakrishnan Y, Nair NR, Kusumi K. Overview of monogenic or Mendelian forms of hypertension. Front Pediatr July 1, 2019;7:263. https://doi.org/10.3389/fped.2019.00263. PMID: 31312622.

[35] Tomalik-Scharte D, Maiter D, Kirchheiner J, Ivison HE, Fuhr U, Arlt W. Impaired hepatic drug and steroid metabolism in congenital adrenal hyperplasia due to P450 oxidoreductase deficiency. Eur J Endocrinol December 2010;163(6):919−24. https://doi.org/10.1530/EJE-10-0764. PMID: 20844025.

[36] Padmanabhan S, Dominiczak AF. Genomics of hypertension: the road to precision medicine. Nat Rev Cardiol April 2021;18(4):235−50. https://doi.org/10.1038/s41569-020-00466-4. PMID: 33219353.

[37] Young Jr WF. Management approaches to adrenal incidentalomas. A view from Rochester, Minnesota. x Endocrinol Metab Clin North Am March 2000;29(1):159−85. https://doi.org/10.1016/s0889-8529(05)70122-5. PMID: 10732270.

[38] Crona J, Taïeb D, Pacak K. New perspectives on pheochromocytoma and paraganglioma: toward a molecular classification. Endocr Rev December 1, 2017;38(6):489−515. https://doi.org/10.1210/er.2017-00062. PMID: 28938417.

[39] Pappachan JM, Tun NN, Arunagirinathan G, Sodi R, Hanna FWF. Pheochromocytomas and hypertension. Curr Hypertens Rep January 22, 2018;20(1):3. https://doi.org/10.1007/s11906-018-0804-z. PMID: 29356966.

[40] Nölting S, Bechmann N, Taieb D, Beuschlein F, Fassnacht M, Kroiss M, Eisenhofer G, Grossman A, Pacak K. Personalized management of pheochromocytoma and paraganglioma. Endocr Rev March 9, 2022;43(2):199−239. https://doi.org/10.1210/endrev/bnab019. Erratum in: Endocr Rev. 2021 Dec 14;: Erratum in: Endocr Rev. 2021 Dec 14;: PMID: 34147030.

[41] Lenders JWM, Kerstens MN, Amar L, Prejbisz A, Robledo M, Taieb D, et al. Genetics, diagnosis, management and future directions of research of phaeochromocytoma and paraganglioma: a position statement and consensus of the Working Group on Endocrine Hypertension of the European Society of Hypertension. J Hypertens August 2020;38(8):1443−56. https://doi.org/10.1097/HJH.0000000000002438. PMID: 32412940.

[42] Lacroix A, Feelders RA, Stratakis CA, Nieman LK. Cushing's syndrome. Lancet August 29, 2015;386(9996):913−27. https://doi.org/10.1016/S0140-6736(14)61375-1. PMID: 26004339.

[43] Schernthaner-Reiter MH, Siess C, Gessl A, Scheuba C, Wolfsberger S, Riss P, et al. Factors predicting long-term comorbidities in patients with Cushing's syndrome in remission. Endocrine April 2019;64(1):157−68. https://doi.org/10.1007/s12020-018-1819-6. Erratum in: Endocrine. 2019 Jan 24;: PMID: 30467627.

[44] Magiakou MA, Mastorakos G, Zachman K, Chrousos GP. Blood pressure in children and adolescents with Cushing's syndrome before and after surgical care. J Clin Endocrinol Metab June 1997;82(6):1734−8. https://doi.org/10.1210/jcem.82.6.3985. PMID: 9177372.

[45] Isidori AM, Graziadio C, Paragliola RM, Cozzolino A, Ambrogio AG, Colao A, Corsello SM, Pivonello R, Study Group ABC. The hypertension of Cushing's syndrome: controversies in the pathophysiology and focus on cardiovascular complications. J Hypertens January 2015;33(1):44−60. https://doi.org/10.1097/HJH.0000000000000415. PMID: 25415766.

[46] Fleseriu M, Auchus R, Bancos I, Ben-Shlomo A, Bertherat J, Biermasz NR, et al. Consensus on diagnosis and management of Cushing's disease: a guideline update. Lancet Diabetes Endocrinol December 2021;9(12):847−75. https://doi.org/10.1016/S2213-8587(21)00235-7. PMID: 34687601.

[47] Ahn CH, Kim JH, Park MY, Kim SW. Epidemiology and comorbidity of adrenal Cushing syndrome: a nationwide cohort study. J Clin Endocrinol Metab March 8, 2021;106(3):e1362−72. https://doi.org/10.1210/clinem/dgaa752. PMID: 33075802.

[48] Wengander S, Trimpou P, Papakokkinou E, Ragnarsson O. The incidence of endogenous Cushing's syndrome in the modern era. Clin Endocrinol (Oxf) August 2019;91(2):263−70. https://doi.org/10.1111/cen.14014. PMID: 31094003.

[49] Lavrentaki A, Paluzzi A, Wass JA, Karavitaki N. Epidemiology of acromegaly: review of population studies. Pituitary February 2017;20(1):4−9. https://doi.org/10.1007/s11102-016-0754-x. PMID: 27743174.

[50] Puglisi S, Terzolo M. Hypertension and acromegaly. Endocrinol Metab Clin North Am December 2019;48(4):779−93. https://doi.org/10.1016/j.ecl.2019.08.008. PMID: 31655776.

[51] Kasuki L, Rocha PDS, Lamback EB, Gadelha MR. Determinants of morbidities and mortality in acromegaly. Arch Endocrinol Metab 2019;63(6):630−7. https://doi.org/10.20945/2359-3997000000193. PMID: 31939488.

[52] Gazzaruso C, Gola M, Karamouzis I, Giubbini R, Giustina A. Cardiovascular risk in adult patients with growth hormone (GH) deficiency and following substitution with GH–an update. J Clin Endocrinol Metab January 2014;99(1):18−29. https://doi.org/10.1210/jc.2013-2394. PMID: 24217903.

[53] Stochholm K, Gravholt CH, Laursen T, Jørgensen JO, Laurberg P, Andersen M, et al. Incidence of GH deficiency - a nationwide study. Eur J Endocrinol July 2006;155(1):61−71. https://doi.org/10.1530/eje.1.02191. PMID: 16793951.

[54] Gottwald-Hostalek U, Schulte B. Low awareness and under-diagnosis of hypothyroidism. Curr Med Res Opin January 2022;38(1):59−64. https://doi.org/10.1080/03007995.2021.1997258. PMID: 34698615.

[55] Aoki Y, Belin RM, Clickner R, Jeffries R, Phillips L, Mahaffey KR. Serum TSH and total T4 in the United States population and their association with participant characteristics: National Health and Nutrition Examination Survey (NHANES 1999-2002). Thyroid December 2007;17(12):1211−23. https://doi.org/10.1089/thy.2006.0235. PMID: 18177256.

[56] Best CAE, Krishnan R, Malvankar-Mehta MS, MacNeil SD. Echocardiogram changes following parathyroidectomy for primary hyperparathyroidism: a systematic review and meta-analysis. Medicine (Baltimore) October 2017;96(43):e7255. https://doi.org/10.1097/MD.0000000000007255. PMID: 29068975.

[57] Hall JE, do Carmo JM, da Silva AA, Wang Z, Hall ME. Obesity-induced hypertension: interaction of neurohumoral and renal mechanisms. Circ Res March 13, 2015;116(6):991−1006. https://doi.org/10.1161/CIRCRESAHA.116.305697. PMID: 25767285.

[58] Appel LJ, Brands MW, Daniels SR, Karanja N, Elmer PJ, Sacks FM, American Heart Association. Dietary approaches to prevent and treat hypertension: a scientific statement from the American Heart Association. Hypertension February 2006;47(2):296−308. https://doi.org/10.1161/01.HYP.0000202568.01167.B6. PMID: 16434724.

[59] Garrison RJ, Kannel WB, Stokes 3rd J, Castelli WP. Incidence and precursors of hypertension in young adults: the Framingham Offspring Study. Prev Med March 1987;16(2):235−51. https://doi.org/10.1016/0091-7435(87)90087-9. PMID: 3588564.

[60] Patel AR, Patel AR, Singh S, Singh S, Khawaja I. The association of obstructive sleep apnea and hypertension. Cureus June 7, 2019;11(6):e4858. https://doi.org/10.7759/cureus.4858. PMID: 31410341.

[61] Pedrosa RP, Drager LF, Gonzaga CC, Sousa MG, de Paula LK, Amaro AC, et al. Obstructive sleep apnea: the most common secondary cause of hypertension associated with resistant hypertension. Hypertension November 2011;58(5):811−7. https://doi.org/10.1161/HYPERTENSIONAHA.111.179788. PMID: 21968750.

[62] Song P, Zhang Y, Yu J, Zha M, Zhu Y, Rahimi K, Rudan I. Global prevalence of hypertension in children: a systematic review and meta-analysis. JAMA Pediatr December 1, 2019;173(12):1154−63. https://doi.org/10.1001/jamapediatrics.2019.3310. PMID: 31589252.

[63] Gartlehner G, Vander Schaaf EB, Orr C, Kennedy SM, Clark R, Viswanathan M. Screening for hypertension in children and adolescents: updated evidence report and systematic review for the US Preventive Services task force. JAMA November 10, 2020;324(18):1884−95. https://doi.org/10.1001/jama.2020.11119. PMID: 33170247.

[64] Bouhanick B, Sosner P, Brochard K, Mounier-Véhier C, Plu-Bureau G, Hascoet S, et al. Hypertension in children and adolescents: a position statement from a panel of multidisciplinary experts coordinated by the French Society of Hypertension. Front Pediatr July 7, 2021;9:680803. https://doi.org/10.3389/fped.2021.680803. PMID: 34307254.

[65] Napso T, Yong HEJ, Lopez-Tello J, Sferruzzi-Perri AN. The role of placental hormones in mediating maternal adaptations to support pregnancy and lactation. Front Physiol August 17, 2018;9:1091. https://doi.org/10.3389/fphys.2018.01091. PMID: 30174608.

[66] Behura SK, Dhakal P, Kelleher AM, Balboula A, Patterson A, Spencer TE. The brain-placental axis: therapeutic and pharmacological relevancy to pregnancy. Pharmacol Res November 2019;149:104468. https://doi.org/10.1016/j.phrs.2019.104468. PMID: 31600597.

[67] Funder JW, Carey RM, Mantero F, Murad MH, Reincke M, Shibata H, Stowasser M, Young Jr WF. The management of primary aldosteronism: case detection, diagnosis, and treatment: an endocrine society clinical practice guideline. J Clin Endocrinol Metab May 2016;101(5):1889−916. https://doi.org/10.1210/jc.2015-4061. PMID: 26934393.

[68] Jakobsson H, Farmaki K, Sakinis A, Ehn O, Johannsson G, Ragnarsson O. Adrenal venous sampling: the learning curve of a single interventionalist with 282 consecutive procedures. Diagn Interv Radiol 2018 ;24(2):89−93. https://doi.org/10.5152/dir.2018.17397. PMID: 29467114.

[69] Naruse M, Katabami T, Shibata H, Sone M, Takahashi K, Tanabe A, et al. Japan Endocrine Society clinical practice guideline for the diagnosis and management of primary aldosteronism 2021. Endocr J April 2022;69(4):327−59. https://doi.org/10.1507/endocrj.EJ21-0508. PMID: 35418526.

[70] Geijer H, Breimer LH. Somatostatin receptor PET/CT in neuroendocrine tumours: update on systematic review and meta-analysis. Eur J Nucl Med Mol Imaging October 2013;40(11):1770−80. https://doi.org/10.1007/s00259-013-2482-z. PMID: 23873003.

[71] Carrasquillo JA, Chen CC, Jha A, Ling A, Lin FI, Pryma DA, Pacak K. Imaging of pheochromocytoma and paraganglioma. J Nucl Med August 1, 2021;62(8):1033−42. https://doi.org/10.2967/jnumed.120.259689. PMID: 34330739.

[72] Kim JH, Ahn CH, Kim SJ, Lee KE, Kim JW, Yoon HK, et al. Outcome-based decision-making algorithm for treating patients with primary aldosteronism. Endocrinol Metab (Seoul) April 2022;14. https://doi.org/10.3803/EnM.2022.1391. PMID: 35417953.

[73] Joseph JJ, Pohlman NK, Zhao S, Kline D, Brock G, Echouffo-Tcheugui JB, et al. Association of serum aldosterone and plasma renin activity with ambulatory blood pressure in African Americans: the Jackson Heart Study. Circulation June 15, 2021;143(24):2355−66. https://doi.org/10.1161/CIRCULATIONAHA.120.050896. PMID: 33605160.

[74] Rifkin DE, Khaki AR, Jenny NS, McClelland RL, Budoff M, Watson K, Ix JH, Allison MA. Association of renin and aldosterone with ethnicity and blood pressure: the Multi-Ethnic Study of Atherosclerosis. Am J Hypertens June 2014;27(6):801−10. https://doi.org/10.1093/ajh/hpt276. PMID: 24436325.

[75] Brown MJ. Hypertension and ethnic group. BMJ April 8, 2006;332(7545):833−6. https://doi.org/10.1136/bmj.332.7545.833. Erratum in: BMJ. 2006 May 13;332(7550):1138. PMID: 16601044.

[76] Leung AA, Pasieka JL, Hyrcza MD, et al. Epidemiology of pheochromocytoma and paraganglioma: population-based cohort study. Eur J Endocrinol 2021;184:19−28.

[77] Ebbehoj A, Stochholm K, Jacobsen SF, et al. Incidence and clinical presentation of pheochromocytoma and sympathetic paraganglioma: a population-based study. J Clin Endocrinol Metab 2021;106:e2251−61.

[78] Jhawar S, Arakawa Y, Kumar S, Varghese D, Kim YS, Roper N, et al. New insights on the genetics of pheochromocytoma and paraganglioma and its clinical implications. Cancers (Basel) January 25, 2022;14(3):594. https://doi.org/10.3390/cancers14030594. PMID: 35158861.

[79] Andrews KA, Ascher DB, Pires DEV, Barnes DR, Vialard L, Casey RT, et al. Tumour risks and genotype-phenotype correlations associated with germline variants in succinate dehydrogenase subunit genes SDHB, SDHC and SDHD. J Med Genet June 2018;55(6):384—94. https://doi.org/10.1136/jmedgenet-2017-105127. Erratum in: J Med Genet. 2019 Jan;56(1):50-52. PMID: 29386252.

[80] NGS in PPGL (NGSnPPGL) Study Group, Toledo RA, Burnichon N, Cascon A, Benn DE, Bayley JP, Welander J, et al. Consensus statement on next-generation-sequencing-based diagnostic testing of hereditary phaeochromocytomas and paragangliomas. Nat Rev Endocrinol April 2017;13(4):233—47. https://doi.org/10.1038/nrendo.2016.185. PMID: 27857127.

[81] Ma X, Li M, Tong A, Wang F, Cui Y, Zhang X, Zhang Y, Chen S, Li Y. Genetic and clinical profiles of pheochromocytoma and paraganglioma: a single center study. Front Endocrinol (Lausanne) December 11, 2020;11:574662. https://doi.org/10.3389/fendo.2020.574662. PMID: 33362715.

[82] Muth A, Crona J, Gimm O, Elmgren A, Filipsson K, Stenmark Askmalm M, et al. Genetic testing, and surveillance guidelines in hereditary pheochromocytoma and paraganglioma. J Intern Med February 2019;285(2):187—204. https://doi.org/10.1111/joim.12869. PMID: 30536464.

[83] MacFarlane J, Seong KC, Bisambar C, Madhu B, Allinson K, Marker A, et al. A review of the tumour spectrum of germline succinate dehydrogenase gene mutations: beyond phaeochromocytoma and paraganglioma. Clin Endocrinol (Oxf). November 2020;93(5):528—38. https://doi.org/10.1111/cen.14289. PMID: 32686200.

[84] National genomic test directory: testing criteria for rare and inherited disease. https://www.england.nhs.uk/wp-content/uploads/2018/08/rare-and-inherited-disease-eligibility-criteria-v2.pdf Assessed: 16/05/2022.

[85] Blau JE, Simonds WF. Familial hyperparathyroidism. Front Endocrinol (Lausanne) February 25, 2021;12:623667. https://doi.org/10.3389/fendo.2021.623667. PMID: 33716975.

[86] Pardi E, Borsari S, Saponaro F, Bogazzi F, Urbani C, Mariotti S, et al. Mutational and large deletion study of genes implicated in hereditary forms of primary hyperparathyroidism and correlation with clinical features. PLoS One October 16, 2017;12(10):e0186485. https://doi.org/10.1371/journal.pone.0186485. PMID: 29036195.

[87] De Sousa SMC, Carroll RW, Henderson A, Burgess J, Clifton-Bligh RJ. A contemporary clinical approach to genetic testing for heritable hyperparathyroidism syndromes. Endocrine 2022;75(1):23—32. https://doi.org/10.1007/s12020-021-02927-3. PMID: 34773560.

[88] Chang M, Yang C, Bao X, Wang R. Genetic and epigenetic causes of pituitary adenomas. Front Endocrinol (Lausanne) January 26, 2021;11:596554. https://doi.org/10.3389/fendo.2020.596554. PMID: 33574795.

[89] Daly AF, Yuan B, Fina F, Caberg JH, Trivellin G, Rostomyan L, et al. Somatic mosaicism underlies X-linked acrogigantism syndrome in sporadic male subjects. Endocr Relat Cancer April 2016;23(4):221—33. https://doi.org/10.1530/ERC-16-0082. PMID: 26935837.

Chapter 2

Catecholamines and blood pressure regulation

Cornelius J. Fernandez[1], Fahmy W.F. Hanna[2], Karel Pacak[3] and Matthew A. Nazari[3]

[1]Department of Endocrinology and Metabolism, Pilgrim Hospital, United Lincolnshire Hospitals NHS Trust, Boston, United Kingdom; [2]Department of Diabetes and Endocrinology, University Hospitals of North Midlands NHS Trust and Centre for Health and Development, Staffordshire University, Stoke-on-Trent, United Kingdom; [3]Section on Medical Neuroendocrinology, Eunice Kennedy Shriver National Institute of Child Health and Human Development, National Institutes of Health, Bethesda, MD, United States

Visit the *Endocrine Hypertension: From Basic Science to Clinical Practice, First Edition* companion web site at: https://www.elsevier.com/books-and-journals/book-companion/9780323961202.

Graphical Abstract

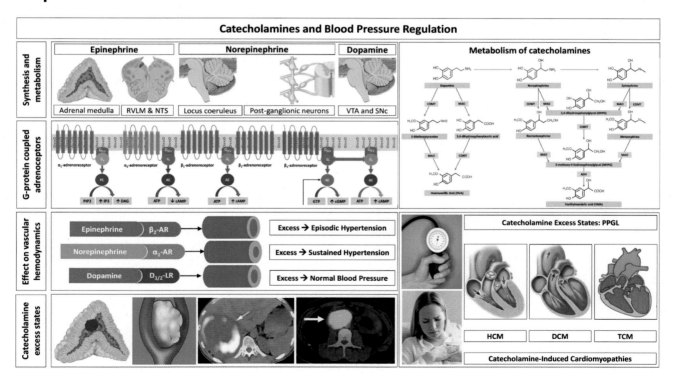

Endocrine Hypertension. **https://doi.org/10.1016/B978-0-323-96120-2.00010-8**

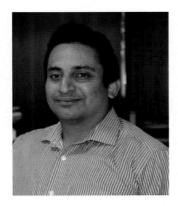

Cornelius J. Fernandez

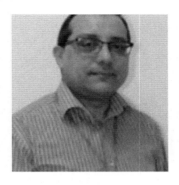

Fahmy F.W. Hanna

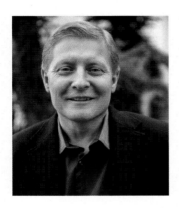

Karel Pacak

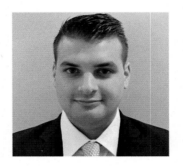

Matthew A. Nazari

Introduction

Catecholamines are monoamine neurotransmitters and circulating hormones derived from the amino acid tyrosine, produced by the sympathetic nervous system, brain, and adrenal medulla [1]. The three physiologically active catecholamines synthesized in the human body are epinephrine (adrenaline), norepinephrine (noradrenaline), and dopamine. As neurotransmitters and hormones, catecholamines play vital roles for the maintenance of body homeostasis through the autonomic nervous system [2]. The wide range of effects of catecholamines on blood pressure regulation have been well known for more than half a century. These very powerful neurochemicals exert their protean effects through three main types of G-protein-coupled receptors widely distributed on effector organs, tissues, and cells. These are α-adrenoreceptors, β-adrenoreceptors, and dopamine receptors [3,4]. This chapter describes the physiological aspects, biological effects (as hormones as well as neurotransmitters), and pathophysiologic alterations of catecholamines in relation to blood pressure regulation.

Catecholamines and autonomic physiology

The synthesis, storage, and regulation of catecholamines

Catecholamines contain a catechol (1,2-dihydroxy benzene) moiety, an ethylamine side chain, and an amine group with additional substitutions [5]. The chemical structure of the catecholamines, the steps involved in the catecholamine biosynthetic pathway, and the enzymes involved are depicted in Fig. 2.1. The first step incatecholamine biosynthesis is the conversion of phenylalanine to tyrosine. Tyrosine is further converted to L-DOPA (L-3,4-dihydroxyphenylalanine) by

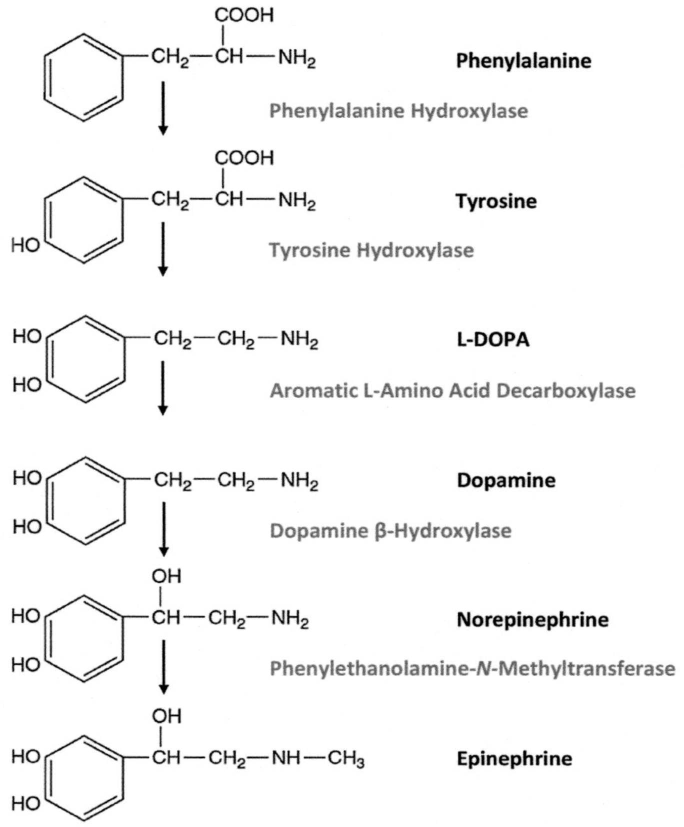

FIGURE 2.1 The chemical structure of the catecholamines, the steps involved in the catecholamine biosynthetic pathway, and the enzymes involved. L-DOPA: L-3,4-dihydroxyphenylalanine.

tyrosine hydroxylase, the rate-limiting step of catecholamine biosynthesis. This is followed by decarboxylation of L-DOPA into dopamine by the enzyme L-aromatic amino acid decarboxylase. The pathway stops here in the dopaminergic neurons located in the midbrain nuclei, namely the ventral tegmental area and the substantia nigra pars compacta [6].

In the postganglionic neurons of the sympathetic nervous system and in the clusters of noradrenergic neurons (the largest cluster being the locus coeruleus) located in the pons and the medulla, further hydroxylation of dopamine by the enzyme dopamine β-hydroxylase (DBH) leads to formation of norepinephrine [6]. Subsequent N-methylation of norepinephrine yields epinephrine [7]. This process is catalyzed by the enzyme phenylethanolamine-N-methyltransferase (PNMT) which uses S-adenosyl-L-methionine as the methyl donor. This conversion of norepinephrine to epinephrine occurs within chromaffin cells of the adrenal medulla, neurons of the rostral ventrolateral medulla (RVLM), and neurons of the nucleus tractus solitarius (NTS).

Sympathetic neurons, unlike chromaffin cells within the adrenal medulla, do not possess PNMT and therefore cannot synthesize epinephrine [8]. Therefore, the adrenal medulla is the major source of epinephrine released into systemic circulation. The adrenal medulla releases predominantly epinephriine (80%), followed by norepinephrine (19%) and dopamine (1%). The function of PNMT is potentiated by the presence of glucocorticoids, which are produced and released by the adrenal cortex, creating a physiologic link between the adrenal cortex, medulla, and the release of epinephrine [8]. The organ of Zuckerkandl (chromaffin cells located around the aorta from the level of the superior mesenteric artery to the level of the aortic bifurcation), neurons of the amygdala, and neurons of the retina also express PNMT and can produce epinephrine [9−11].

The RVLM is one of the most important regions involved in the maintenance of sympathetic tone [12−14]. The RVLM sends direct monosynaptic projections to the intermediolateral columns of the thoracolumbar spinal cord (from T1 to L2) where the sympathetic preganglionic neurons are located.

In the postganglionic neurons of the sympathetic nervous system, norepinephrine is stored in vesicles and released into the synaptic cleft by exocytosis. This exocytosis is prompted by acetylcholine released by preganglionic neurons—which are themselves stimulated to do so [5,15]. The norepinephrine that is released from these vesicles binds to postsynaptic adrenoceptors present on either target cells or on presynaptic adrenoceptors to modulate the presynaptic neuronal activity [5]. Norepinephrine also undergoes reuptake either into the noradrenergic neurons or into the target cells through the norepinephrine transporter (NET). Nearly 80%—95% of norepinephrine that is released from vesicles will undergo active reuptake into noradrenergic neurons [16]. This reuptake subsequently returns norepinephrine to storage vesicles. Ultimately, only a minority of norepinephrine binds to corresponding adrenoceptors [16].

In chromaffin cells of the adrenal medulla, catecholamines are stored in vesicles and released into the bloodstream by exocytosis [5]. Exocytosis of these catecholamines occurs when acetylcholine released by preganglionic sympathetic nerve fibers binds to nicotinic cholinergic receptors present on chromaffin cells, leading to pursuant depolarization of chromaffin cells which activates voltage-gated calcium channels. The consequent rise in intracellular calcium leads to vesicular exocytosis. Upon release, these circulating catecholamines bind to their cognate adrenoceptors on target organs (discussed below). Notably, epinephrine and norepinephrine have short half-lives due to their rapid metabolism into inactive products thus leading to often short-lived physiologic responses.

Metabolism of catecholamines

Under physiologic conditions catecholamines are metabolized mainly by catechol-O-methyltransferase (COMT, COMT-MB and COMT-S for membrane bound and soluble COMT enzymes, respectively) and monoamine oxidase (MAO-A and MAO-B) [17]. Catecholamine metabolism is depicted in Fig. 2.2. COMT catalyzes the O-methylation of dopamine into methoxytyramine, norepinephrine into normetanephrine, and epinephrine into metanephrine. MAO catalyzes the oxidative deamination of dopamine into 3,4 dihydroxyphenylacetic acid (DOPAC), and norepinephrine and epinephrine into 3,4 dihydroxyphenylglycol (DHPG). The metabolites catalyzed by MAO can be metabolized further by COMT, and those metabolites catalyzed by COMT can be metabolized further by MAO. The final product of dopamine metabolism is homovanillic acid, and that of norepinephrine and epinephrine metabolism is vanillic acid.

COMT is absent in sympathetic nerves; therefore, norepinephrine in sympathetic nerves is metabolized by deamination rather than O-methylation [18]. On the other hand, due to the presence of COMT within the cytoplasm of the adrenal medullary and extraadrenal chromaffin cells, O-methylation metabolites are relatively specific to chromaffin cells. In normal individuals, at least 90% of metanephrine and nearly 25% of normetanephrine are produced within adrenal chromaffin cells. Of the remaining 75% of normetanephrine, nearly 15% is derived from extraadrenal

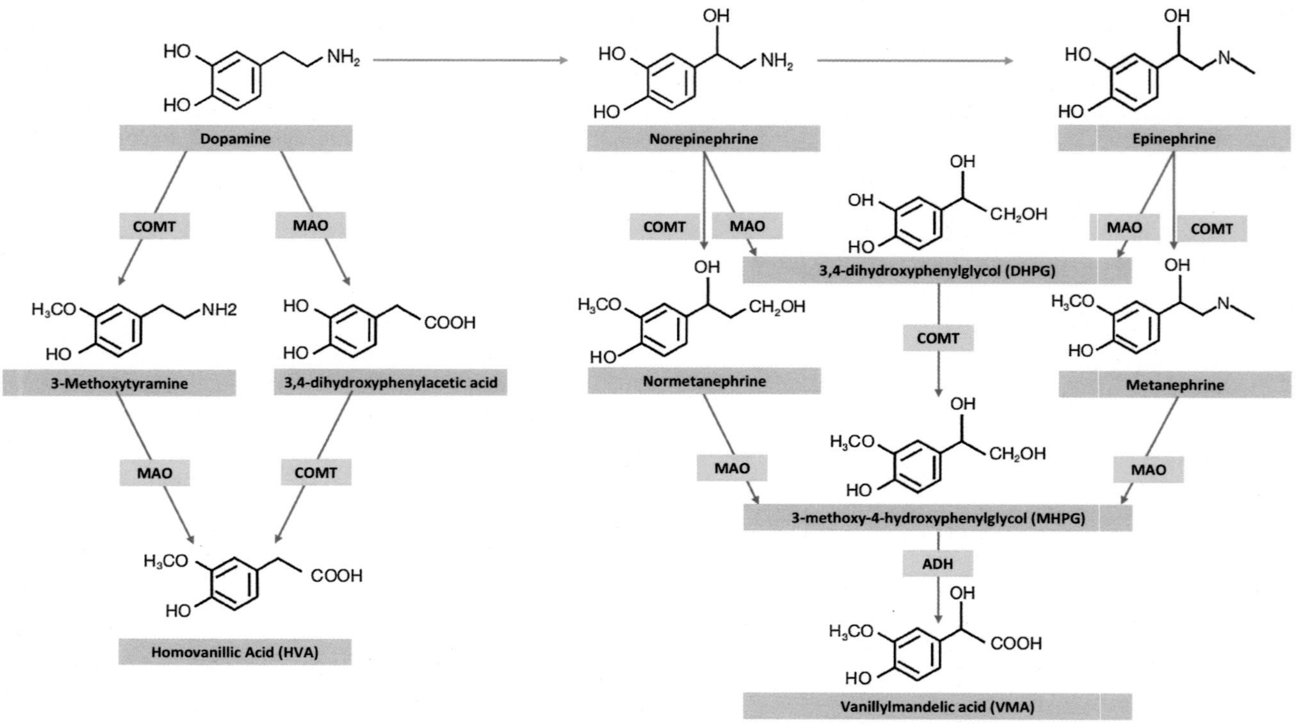

FIGURE 2.2 The metabolic fate of catecholamines. *ADH*, alcohol dehydrogenase; *COMT*, catechol-O-methyltransferase; *MAO*, monoamine oxidase.

chromaffin cells, while 60% is derived from the metabolism (by extraneuronal cells) of norepinephrine released by sympathetic nerves.

Adrenoceptors, subtypes, and associated second messenger systems

Adrenoceptors are G-protein-coupled receptors (GPCRs) which are composed of (1) an extracellular element that binds catecholamines, (2) seven transmembrane domains (which anchor the protein to the cell membrane), and (3) an intracellular element that allows the bound receptor to interact with the G-protein present within the cell [19]. This structure lends to the functional ability to transduce an extracellular signal into an intracellular signal. Functionally, a catecholamine (the ligand) binds to the GPCR resulting in a conformational change, causing an interaction with a G-protein. This G-protein in turn then modulates the activity of the enzyme attached to the G-protein and it is these enzymes and their downstream effectors that define canonical second messenger pathways (elaborated upon below). These G-proteins are composed of three distinct subunits: α, β, and γ. It is the α subunit that confers the name of the G-protein. Accordingly, the G_s protein has a stimulatory α subunit that activates the enzyme adenylyl-cyclase; the G_i protein has an inhibitory α subunit that inhibits the enzyme adenylyl-cyclase; and the G_q protein has a stimulatory α subunit that activates the enzyme phospholipase C [20]. The physiology of the GPCR signaling pathway is depicted in Fig. 2.3.

Adrenoceptors are divided into α_1, α_2, β_1, β_2, and β_3 receptor subtypes. The α_1-adrenoceptors are subdivided into three subtypes namely α_{1A}, α_{1B}, and α_{1D} [21]. Similarly, the α_2-adrenoceptors have at least three subtypes namely α_{2A}, α_{2B}, and α_{2C} [22]. However, this text will focus on the major functions of α_1- and α_2-adrenoceptors. α_1-adrenoceptor stimulation of vascular smooth muscle cells, present within blood vessels, results in their contraction. This contraction of smooth muscle cells, oriented radially within the tunica media of arteries and veins, leads to inward narrowing of the vascular lumen or vasoconstriction. Moreover, α_1-adrenoceptor stimulation of the heart mediates positive inotropic effects and coronary artery vasoconstriction. On the other hand, α_2-adrenoceptor stimulation within the central nervous system (presynaptic neurons) reduces sympathetic outflow and consequent sympathetic tone (by inhibiting the release of norepinephrine). This results in a decrease in blood pressure [23]. α_2-adrenoceptor stimulation also causes coronary vasoconstriction.

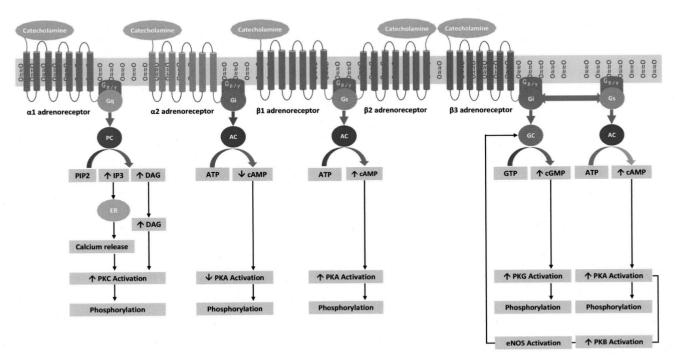

FIGURE 2.3 The molecular mechanisms of catecholamine action in the body. *AC*, adenylyl-cyclase; *ATP*, adenosine triphosphate; *cAMP*, cyclic adenosine monophosphate; *cGMP*, cyclic guanosine monophosphate; *DAG*, diacylglycerol; *ER*, endoplasmic reticulum; *eNOS*, endothelial nitric oxide synthase; G_q, G_q alpha subunit; G_s, G_s alpha subunit; G_i, G_i alpha subunit; $G_{\beta/\gamma}$, β and γ subunits of the G-protein; *GC*, guanylyl-cyclase; *GTP*, guanosine triphosphate; *IP3*, inositol 1,4,5-trisphosphate; *PC*, phospholipase C; *PIP2*, phosphatidylinositol 4,5-bisphosphate; *PKC*, protein kinase C; *PKA*, protein kinase A; *PKG*, protein kinase G; *PKB*, protein kinase B.

The stimulation of β_1-adrenoceptors in the heart (which account for nearly 80% of the β-adrenoceptors of the heart) results in a positive inotropic (increased force of contraction), chronotropic (increased heart rate), dromotropic (increased electrical conduction velocity), and lusitropic (increased ventricular relaxation) effects [24]. In addition, stimulation of β_1-adrenoceptors mediates coronary artery vasodilatation and increases automaticity while decreasing refractory period within cardiomyocytes. In the juxtaglomerular cells of the kidneys, β_1-adrenoceptor stimulation mediates renin release.

The stimulation of β_2-adrenoceptors within vascular smooth muscle cells results in radial relaxation of blood vessels and resultant peripheral arterial and venous vasodilatation [25]. β_2-adrenoceptor stimulation also affects bronchodilatation and relaxation of muscles of the uterus (tocolytic effect), urinary bladder, and gastrointestinal tract. The stimulation of β_2-adrenoceptors in the heart (which accounts for nearly 20% of the β-adrenoceptors of the heart) results in positive inotropic and chronotropic effects with enhanced lusitropy. In addition, it increases the automaticity and decreases the refractory period within cardiomyocytes and mediates coronary artery vasodilatation.

The effect of adrenoceptor stimulation on a particular vascular bed or blood vessel is determined by the distribution of adrenoceptors and the affinities of those adrenoceptors for epinephrine and norepinephrine. β_2-adrenoceptors are present on blood vessels feeding skeletal muscles, whereas α_1-adrenoceptors are present on metarterioles [26,27]. At high concentrations, epinephrine acts on both β_2- and α_1-adrenoceptors. Through this mechanism, it can cause a decrease in diastolic blood pressure (mediated through β_2-adrenoceptor stimulation), but an increase in systolic blood pressure (mediated through α_1-adrenoceptor stimulation).

Though both epinephrine and norepinephrine can bind to and stimulate β_1-adrenoceptors, the tendency to cause a tachyarrhythmia in catecholamine excess states differs between these two catecholamines [28]. Epinephrine has a greater tendency to cause tachyarrhythmias given its relatively high affinity for β_1- compared to α_1-adrenoceptors. On the contrary, norepinephrine has less of a tendency to cause tachyarrhythmias and a greater tendency to cause hypertension due to its high affinity for α_1- compared to β_1-adrenoceptors. Further, in some instances, epinephrine may lead to hypotension due to excessive β_2-adrenoceptor-mediated vasodilation. This phenomenon can be seen in epinephrine secreting pheochromocytomas and paragangliomas (PPGLs) and during preoperative treatment of pheochromocytomas with sole α_1-adrenoceptor blockade due to a relative excess of catecholamines available to bind β_2-adrenoceptors.

The β_3-adrenoceptors are most abundant in white and brown adipose tissue, where they mediate lipolysis, fatty acid oxidation, and thermogenesis [29]. In the cardiovascular system, the β_3-adrenoceptors are present in the cardiomyocytes where they modulate cardiac function (positive lusitropy—with improved diastolic function and negative inotropy—with decreased myocardial oxygen consumption), and in the vasculature where they modulate vasodilatation and angiogenesis—with enhanced oxygen supply. β_3-adrenoceptor stimulation requires a higher catecholamine concentration (at the receptor level) than is required for β_1- and β_2-adrenoceptors activation, indicating that it could act as a brake to prevent β_1- and β_2-adrenoceptor overactivation. β_3-adrenoceptors are an "up and coming" area of research in cardiac function and heart failure but they are still being researched. The β_3-adrenoceptor response to catecholamine stimulation seems to be preserved even after prolonged catecholamine stimulation. On the other hand, the β_1- and β_2-adrenoceptor responses are diminished by excessive stimulation leading to desensitization.

In cardiomyocytes, the desensitization to sustained β_1- and β_2-adrenoceptor stimulation is mediated by adrenoceptor phosphorylation via G-protein-coupled receptor kinases (GRKs), followed by binding to β-arrestin2 [30,31]. The GRK2/β-arrestin2 complex facilitates uncoupling of G-proteins from their respective β_1- and β_2-adrenoceptors leading to internalization of β_1-and β_2-adrenoceptors. In addition, a switch from G_s to G_i protein occurs in β_2- and not β_1-adrenoreceptors [31]. The coupling of β_2-adrenoceptors to the G_i protein results in decreased cardiac contractility. Moreover, the switch happens only with epinephrine excess, not with norepinephrine excess (given differing affinities for the β_2-adrenoceptor). Epinephrine activates both the G_s and G_i pathways (G_s at lower and G_i at higher concentrations), whereas norepinephrine activates only the G_s pathway through the β_2-adrenoceptor. Furthermore, norepinephrine exhibits a 20-fold lower affinity toward β_2-adrenoceptors compared to β_1-adrenoceptors. This difference in affinity likely explains why epinephrine-secreting PPGLs are commonly associated with catecholamine-induced stress cardiomyopathy in comparison to norepinephrine-secreting and dopamine-secreting PPGLs.

There are at least five dopamine receptors (D1—D5), which are GPCRs that are divided into two subfamilies: the D1-like receptor subfamily that corresponds to the original D1 dopamine receptor is comprised of D1 and D5 receptors and the D2-like receptor subfamily corresponds to the original D2 receptor and is comprised of D2, D3, and D4 receptors [32]. The D1-like subfamily of dopamine receptors is coupled to the G_s protein that activates adenylyl-cyclase, which increases the generation of the second messenger cyclic adenosine monophosphate (cAMP), activating protein kinase A (PKA) leading to phosphorylation of downstream proteins. On the other hand, the D2-like subfamily of dopamine receptors is coupled to the G_i protein that inhibits adenylyl-cyclase, decreasing the generation of cAMP and PKA-mediated phosphorylation of downstream proteins.

Neuroendocrine effects of catecholamines on blood pressure

Ultimately, a simple signal, a rise in a given catecholamine, can lead to a complex coordinated response from the cardiovascular system. Adrenoceptors modulate cell function by influencing intracellular second messenger systems. This occurs because of adrenoceptor subtypes, each with differing affinities for catecholamines. These adrenoceptor subtypes are themselves present with varying levels of expression and differing spatial densities on end-organs (namely throughout the vasculature and the heart). This system ramifies a binary signal into multiple different subsignals all acting together with one unifying prerogative, to stimulate cardiovascular performance. In this way, a rise in epinephrine may enact vasoconstriction of certain vessels via α_1-adrenoceptor stimulation, while paradoxically leading to vasodilation of other vessels due to stimulation of β_2-adrenoceptors, and finally augmenting cardiac output via its effect on β_1- and β_2-adrenoceptors. Though seemingly haphazard, these functions unify to direct an increase in cardiac output (mediated by β_1- and β_2-adrenoceptor stimulation) toward vital tissues (for example, via β_2-adrenoceptor-mediated vasodilation) and away from nonessential tissues (for example, via α_1-adrenoceptor-mediated vasoconstriction). Thus, to fully understand the effects of catecholamines upon blood pressure and cardiac performance, one must be familiar with the predominant adrenoceptor present within a given vascular bed or blood vessel, its paired second messenger system, and its final effect on downstream effectors, namely ion channels and the actin—myosin cross-bridge. These relationships are elaborated upon in Fig. 2.3 and are discussed below [33].

Different vascular beds or blood vessels have varying expression of adrenoceptors—allowing each to act in a specific manner in response to a given catecholamine. However, three major patterns exist regarding adrenoceptor expression throughout the vasculature and consequent effects on blood pressure. Stimulation of α_1-adrenoceptors on metarterioles leads to vasoconstriction and is a major determinant of increasing blood pressure. β_2-adrenoceptor stimulation on blood vessels feeding skeletal muscle can allow for improved blood flow in times of stress; however, excessive stimulation may lead to a decrease in blood pressure. Finally, α_2-adrenoceptor expression on presynaptic terminals establishes a negative feedback pathway. Stimulation of α_2-adrenoceptors may then blunt the release of norepinephrine (for example at metarterioles) which can lead to a decrease in blood pressure.

The α_1-adrenoceptors present upon vascular smooth muscle cells are coupled to the G_q protein that activates the enzyme phospholipase C, which cleaves phosphatidylinositol 4,5-bisphosphate yielding inositol triphosphate (IP3) and diacylglycerol [34]. Among other pathways, IP3 binds to its cognate receptor on the endoplasmic reticulum leading to a release of calcium into the cytoplasm. Calcium then augments actin—myosin cross-bridge cycling by leading to downstream phosphorylation of myosin. Increased actin—myosin cross-bridge cycling leads to sarcomere contraction at metarterioles on precapillary sphincters, increasing total peripheral resistance. By maintaining more blood within the arterial compartment, this leads to a rise in blood pressure. The net result of α_1-adrenoceptor activation by norepinephrine or epinephrine is vasoconstriction and hypertension.

Stimulation of α_2-adrenoceptors on presynaptic terminals, via catecholamines, defines a negative feedback pathway [35]. The α_2-adrenoceptor stimulation inhibits adenylyl-cyclase via the G_i protein; this leads to a decrease in cAMP, in turn, reducing the stimulation of PKA leading to less vesicular exocytosis of catecholamines. In this way, α_1-adrenoceptor stimulation via canonical second messengers increases the blood pressure, while α_2-adrenoceptor stimulation via a negative feedback pathway decreases the blood pressure.

The β_2-adrenoceptors present on vascular smooth muscle and the heart are coupled to the G_s protein. When stimulated by epinephrine, the coupled G_s protein increases cAMP levels in both cardiomyocytes and vascular smooth muscle cells. In vascular smooth muscle cells, the rise in cAMP leads to downstream inhibition of myosin light chain kinase (MLCK) [36]. This action on MLCK reduces phosphorylation of myosin and reduces actin—myosin cross-bridge cycling leading to vasodilation and increasing blood flow to skeletal muscle. When epinephrine levels are elevated, as previously mentioned, excessive vasodilation can lead to a drop in diastolic blood pressure. On the contrary, in cardiomyocytes, the G_s-mediated rise in cAMP activates MLCK with resultant phosphorylation of myosin; this increases the force of myocardial contraction [37].

Within the heart, β_1- and β_2-adrenoceptors are present on cardiac conductive cells within the sinoatrial node (SA Node) and the atrioventricular node (AV Node) as well as the atrial- and ventricular cardiomyocytes. β_1-adrenoceptors are heavily expressed upon conductive cells of the SA and AV node and their stimulation has a dromotropic and chronotropic effect. Within the SA node, stimulation of β_1-adrenoceptors by catecholamines leads to a rise in cAMP which stimulates the hyperpolarization-activated cyclic nucleotide-gated (HCN) channel leading to an influx of positive ions augmenting the rate of spontaneous depolarization and therefore the heart rate (increased chronotropy) [28]. Within the AV node, stimulation of β_1-adrenoceptors by catecholamines leads to a rise in cAMP, stimulating PKA and leading to phosphorylation of L-type voltage-gated calcium channels (L-type VGCCs). This leads to a rise in intracytoplasmic calcium leading to more brisk depolarization and a quickening of conduction velocity through the atrioventricular node (increased dromotropy). Regarding force of contraction, catecholamines increase inotropy by binding to and stimulating β_2-adrenoceptors present upon cardiomyocytes, while enhancing lusitropy via β_1 and β_2-adrenoceptors. This leads to a rise in cAMP and PKA-mediated phosphorylation of L-type VGCCs, the pursuant influx of calcium augments inotropy [38,39]. Finally, both β_1- and β_2-adrenoceptor stimulation on ventricular cardiomyocytes increases ventricular relaxation (lusitropy) allowing for enhanced diastolic filling, which upon contraction leads to increased ejection fraction and forward delivery of blood into the arterial system [40].

The β_3-adrenoceptor is coupled to both the G_s and G_i protein [41]. β_3-adrenoceptor-mediated stimulation via G_s activates both adenylyl-cyclase and guanylyl-cyclase. This enhances the generation of cAMP and cyclic guanosine monophosphate (cGMP) which, in turn, activates PKA and protein kinase G (PKG), respectively. On the other hand, the β_3-adrenoceptor-mediated G_i pathway stimulation activates guanylyl-cyclase, generating cGMP, and activating PKG in isolation. Both PKA and PKG stimulate the phosphorylation of the myofilament components like cTnI and calcium handling proteins like phospholamban. In addition, PKA phosphorylates and activates L-type VGCCs, whereas PKG inactivates them. The β_3-adrenoceptor-mediated G_s pathway stimulation with resultant PKA activation leads to the activation of protein kinase B (PKB) and endothelial nitric oxide synthase (eNOS) leading to nitric oxide generation. Nitric oxide generation can occur via enhanced eNOS mediated by both the G_s and G_i pathway, and from enhanced neuronal nitric oxide synthase via the G_i pathway. The rise in nitric oxide levels, mediated by β_3-adrenoceptor stimulation, enhances myocardial lusitropy and reduces myocardial inotropy. Thus, targeting β_3-adrenoceptors could provide a novel approach to improving cardiac function, metabolism, and deleterious cardiac remodeling [41].

Metabolic regulation by catecholamines

Catecholamines, predominantly epinephrine, less so norepinephrine, cause a hypermetabolic state with significant insulin resistance [42]. Catecholamines stimulate aerobic glycolysis, glycogenolysis, and gluconeogenesis, and inhibit glycogen synthesis. They stimulate lipolysis, ketogenesis, and proteolysis to provide sufficient glucose precursor molecules, such as fatty acids and alanine. These together will result in hyperglycemia and hyperlactatemia. In the mitochondria, they promote mitochondrial uncoupling, and aggravate oxidative stress either through an accelerated glycolytic pathway, or through catecholamine autooxidation, thereby contributing to mitochondrial dysfunction. Catecholamines lower the potassium level due to β_2-adrenoceptor activation which stimulates potassium uptake into cells.

Biologic effects

Summarizing the net effect of catecholamines on vascular hemodynamics

As previously mentioned, the physiologic effects of catecholamines depend on the concentration of a catecholamine, the tissue distribution of adrenoceptors, and differences in affinity toward adrenoceptors [43]. These cardiovascular effects of catecholamines are summarized in Table 2.1. In blood vessels, at low epinephrine levels, preferential activation of β-adrenoceptors—especially the β_2-adrenoceptors—mediates a hypotensive response. On the other hand, at high epinephrine levels, the preferential activation of α-adrenoceptors (especially α_1-adrenoceptors) mediates a hypertensive response. In the heart, the epinephrine-mediated β_1-adrenoceptor stimulation results in a positive inotropic and chronotropic effect, whereas the epinephrine-mediated β_2-adrenoceptor stimulation results in improved coronary circulation. This improved coronary circulation persists even at higher epinephrine levels despite greater α_1-adrenoceptor mediated coronary artery vasoconstriction. This is because coronary blood flow is enhanced due to an increased relative duration of diastole and through local release of vasodilators from adrenoceptor-stimulated myocardium. These effects largely counterbalance the direct α_1-adrenoceptor-mediated increase in coronary arterial tone.

Norepinephrine, released from postganglionic sympathetic nerves, has a high affinity for α_1-adrenoceptors, and a low affinity for β-adrenoceptors [43]. Norepinephrine primarily increases the systolic and diastolic blood pressure as well as the pulse pressure through an α_1-adrenoceptor-mediated increase in peripheral vascular resistance as well as venoconstriction, the latter increases venous return to the heart and resultant cardiac output. The norepinephrine-mediated increase in blood pressure is not associated with an increase in heart rate (no chronotropic effect). Instead, norepinephrine stimulation may be associated with a decrease in heart rate due to baroreceptor activation (e.g., the baroreceptor reflex). Hence, intravenous norepinephrine can be provided to support cardiovascular performance in situations where tachycardia is undesirable. Notably, norepinephrine also induces coronary artery vasodilatation, increasing delivery of blood to the heart.

TABLE 2.1 Cardiovascular and other effects of catecholamines.

	α₁-AR	α₂-AR	β₁-AR	β₂-AR
G-protein	G_q	G_i	G_s	G_s
Chronotropic effect	–	–	↑	↑
Inotropic effect	↑	–	↑	↑
Lusitropic effect	–	–	↑	↓*(via G_i)
Dromotropic effect	–	–	↑	–
Automaticity	–	–	↑	↑
Refractoriness	–	–	↓	↑
Ventricular hypertrophy	↑	↓	↑↑	↑
Coronary artery tone	↑	↑	↓	↓↓
Blood vessel tone	Constriction	Relaxation		Relaxation
Blood pressure	↑↑	↓	↑	↓
Other effects	Mydriasis, ↑ urinary bladder sphincter tone	↓ Release of NE, Ach and insulin	↑ Renin ↑ Lipolysis	Bronchodilatation Tocolytic effect ↑ Glycogenolysis ↑ Glucagon release
Adrenoceptor affinities				
Epinephrine (low)	–	–	++	+++
Epinephrine (high)	+++	+++	++	+++
Norepinephrine	+++	+++	++	+/–

Ach, acetylcholine; α₁-AR, α₁-adrenoceptor; α₂-AR, α₂-adrenoceptor; β₁-AR, β₁-adrenoceptor; β₂-AR, β₂-adrenoceptor; E, epinephrine; NE, norepinephrine.

Dopamine is the immediate precursor of norepinephrine in the catecholamine synthetic pathway. It has a dose-dependent effect on the cardiovascular system [43]. At low levels, it acts on the dopaminergic receptors located in the renal, mesenteric, coronary, and cerebral vascular beds to promote vasodilatation and increase blood flow to these vascular beds. Dopamine, at lower levels, is therefore associated with a decrease in blood pressure. At intermediate levels, it stimulates β_1-adrenoceptors, augmenting inotropy and chronotropy leading to an increase in cardiac output. At high levels, α_1-adrenoceptor-mediated vasoconstriction prevails leading to hypertension.

PPGLs and excess catecholamine states

PPGLs are rare tumors that secrete various catecholamines including epinephrine, norepinephrine, and dopamine. Pheochromocytomas arising from the adrenal medulla account for nearly 80%—85% of PPGLs, whereas paragangliomas arising from autonomic neural ganglia account for 15%—20% of PPGLs [44]. While normal adrenal glands predominantly secrete epinephrine, the majority of PPGLs predominantly secrete norepinephrine with only about 15% secreting predominantly epinephrine [45]. Pheochromocytomas and paragangliomas that predominantly secrete dopamine are rare. These tumors are often malignant and lack the dopamine decarboxylase enzyme [46]. Up to 70% of PPGLs can have a genetic basis [47]. The PPGLs related to *VHL* and *SDHx* mutations predominantly secrete norepinephrine, those metastatic PPGLs related to *SDHB* and *SDHD* mutations predominantly secrete dopamine, and those related to *RET* and *NF1* mutations predominantly secrete epinephrine [48].

The clinical presentation of PPGL includes a classical triad (headache, hyperhidrosis, and palpitations), in addition to tachycardia, tremor, anxiety, pallor, chest pain, dyspnea, and sometimes local tumoral symptoms like abdominal pain, although many patients can be asymptomatic [49]. Hypertension is present in nearly 95% of patients with PPGL, with sustained hypertension in 55% and episodic hypertension in 45% [50]. The PPGLs predominantly secreting norepinephrine present with sustained hypertension (owing to continuous release of norepinephrine), those predominantly secreting epinephrine present with episodic hypertension (owing to episodic release of epinephrine), and those predominantly secreting dopamine usually present without any hypertension and occasionally with hypotension. Patients with PPGLs may be hypotensive (e.g., from a dopamine-releasing tumor) or normotensive as well. PPGL patients may be normotensive (1) as their tumors, despite producing an excess of catecholamines, have very high levels of intratumoral metabolism, leading to the metabolic inactivation of catecholamines before release, (2) as their tumors may secrete other molecules together with catecholamines that oppose hypertension—for example, vascular endothelial growth factor that suppresses catecholamine action, (3) as there may be desensitization to catecholamines due to chronically elevated levels (as previously mentioned), and/or (4) if there is a significant reduction in cardiac function due to a catecholamine-induced cardiomyopathy (CICMP) [51].

The activities of tyrosine hydroxylase, L-aromatic amino acid decarboxylase, and dopamine β-hydroxylase are elevated in pheochromocytoma in comparison to the normal adrenal medulla [17]. Moreover, patients with pheochromocytoma do not exhibit the normal negative feedback mechanism through tyrosine hydroxylase and these patients exhibit unstable catecholamine degradation mechanisms in comparison to patients with normal adrenal medullas. Furthermore, in patients with pheochromocytoma, nearly 94% of catecholamine metabolism occurs through the COMT enzyme resulting in raised plasma free metanephrines, with the conversion to plasma free metanephrines primarily occurring within the tumor cells rather than in the blood.

Deleterious cardiac effects of excess catecholamines: CICMP

The impact of catecholamines upon the myocardium can be reversible such as in early stages of remodeling or such as in stress cardiomyopathy (also known as Takotsubo cardiomyopathy) or irreversible such as when hypertrophy has sufficiently progressed, or myocardial fibrosis has occurred. Understanding these distinctions allows for early recognition and prompt intervention to mitigate the progression toward permanent hypertrophic or dilated cardiomyopathy and associated heart failure with preserved or reduced ejection fraction.

Stress cardiomyopathy: impaired adrenoceptor and second messenger signaling

Catecholamine excess states, as in PPGL, are associated with impaired β_1- and β_2-adrenoceptor signaling. This process can occur by desensitization which is mediated by uncoupling of G proteins from their β_1- and β_2-adrenoreceptors, internalization of β_1- and β_2-adrenoreceptors, and/or a switch from G_s to G_i protein in states of excessive β_2-adrenoreceptor stimulation [31]. These mechanisms are depicted in Fig. 2.4. This G_s to G_i switch predominantly occurs in the apical

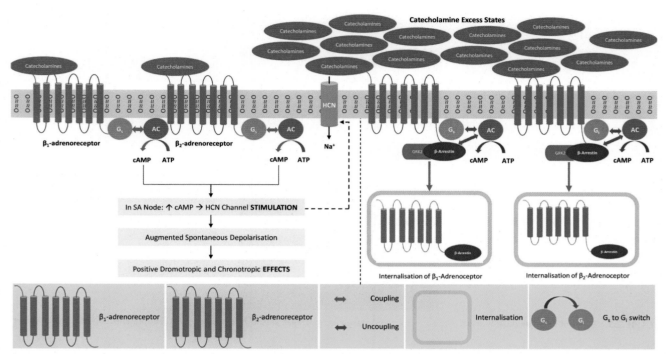

FIGURE 2.4 Mechanism of catecholamine excess states causing tissue injury. *AC*, adenylyl-cyclase; *ATP*, adenosine triphosphate; *cAMP*, cyclic adenosine monophosphate; *GRK2*, G-protein-coupled receptor kinase 2; G_s, G_s alpha subunit; G_i, G_i alpha subunit.

segments of the ventricular myocardium, leading to apical ballooning associated with compensatory stimulation of the basal segments of the ventricle, characteristic of stress cardiomyopathy [49,52]. Although the G_s to G_i switch in β_2-adrenoreceptors is mechanically detrimental as it impairs cardiac contractility, it protects the heart against β_1- and β_2-adrenoreceptor-mediated proapoptotic and proarrhythmogenic effects during states of catecholamine excess. This stress cardiomyopathy is often transient and self-resolving, though in some cases, it may lead to irreversible damage, often leading to a dilated cardiomyopathy.

Hypertrophic cardiomyopathy: load-dependent and nonload-dependent remodeling

A sustained rise in cardiac workload due to hypertension can lead to the development of a load-dependent remodeling within the myocardium with eventual development of cardiac hypertrophy. Separately, a nonload-dependent remodeling can also occur due to direct adrenoceptor stimulation. This remodeling can affect the heart and the blood vessels [53]. In the heart, a sustained α_1- and β-adrenoceptor stimulation enhances the synthesis of cardiomyocyte proteins leading to catecholamine-induced cardiac hypertrophy, which in the initial compensated stage is associated with preserved or even enhanced ventricular systolic function due to increased sarcoplasmic reticulum calcium content and calcium release. However, hypertrophy may progress to the extent where it is irreversible (hypertrophic cardiomyopathy) or may eventually lead to abnormalities in calcium handling, myocardial necrosis, and fibrosis (or dilated cardiomyopathy) [36].

Dilated cardiomyopathy: cardiotoxic effects of catecholamines

As previously mentioned, catecholamine excess states may lead to irreversible hypertrophic or dilated cardiomyopathy (see Fig. 2.5 for elaboration). The latter is often the result of catecholamine excess states leading to eventual cardiomyocyte apoptosis/necrosis (usually mediated by excessive β_1- and β_2-adrenoceptor stimulation) and eventual myocardial fibrosis [54].

In catecholamine excess states, catecholamines undergo oxidation to form reactive oxygen species, aminochromes (active metabolite) and aminolutins (inactive metabolite). Please see Fig. 2.6 for more details. These mediators ultimately lead to mitochondrial dysfunctin and to increased sarcolemmal permeability which increases intracellular calcium.

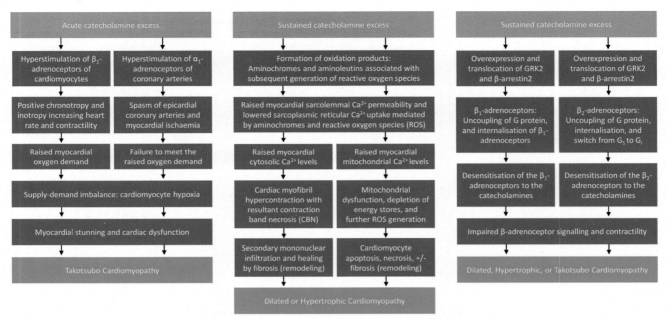

FIGURE 2.5 Types of catecholamine-induced cardiac injury and corresponding mechanisms. Ca^{2+}, calcium; $GRK2$, G-protein-coupled receptor kinase 2.

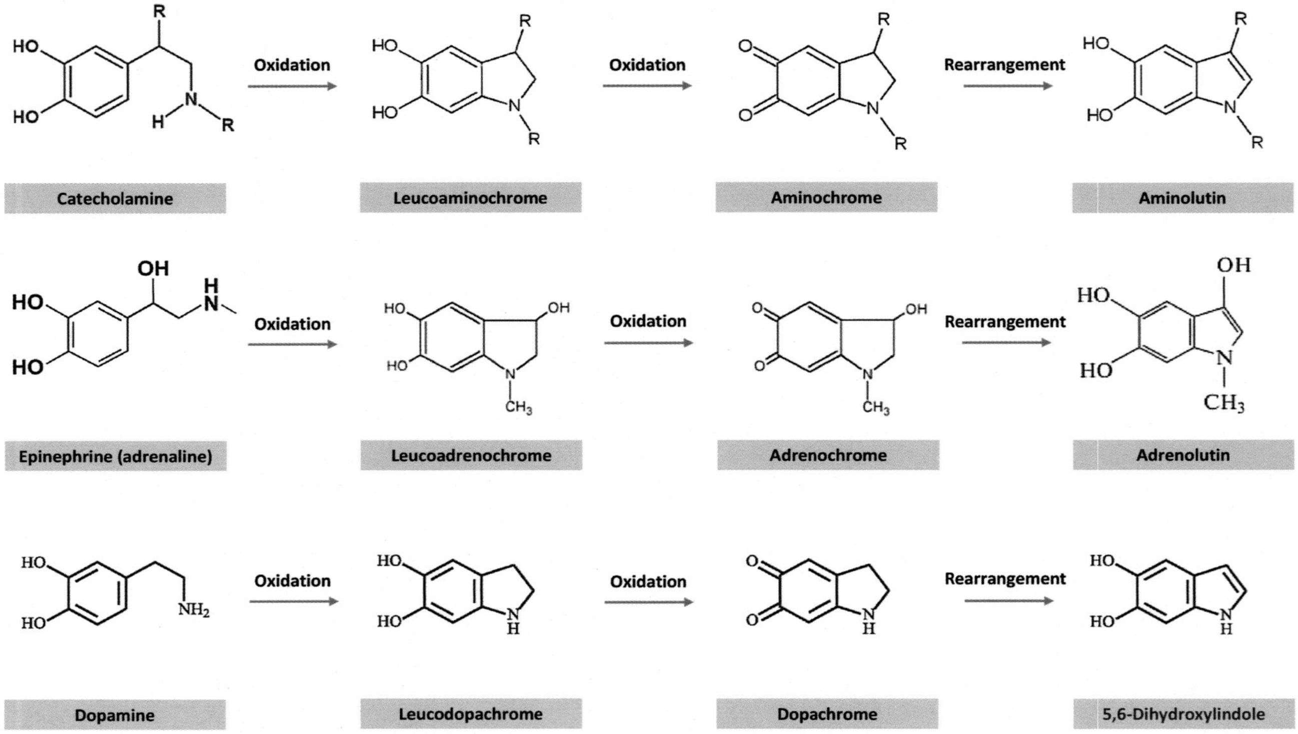

FIGURE 2.6 The metabolic fate of catecholamines in the body.

Together, these effects lead to depletion of energy stores, myocardial edema, inflammation, apoptosis, and necrosis (see Fig. 2.5 for elaboration) [55].

Early intervention is critical when treating CICMPs. Thus, with early diagnosis, the provision of treatment, and surgical removal of PPGLs the prognosis can be quite favorable in most cases—especially in cases of stress cardiomyopathy [49].

Deleterious vascular effects of catecholamines

Similarly, excessive α_1-adrenoceptor stimulation leads to a rise in intracellular calcium levels within vascular smooth muscle cells. Acutely, this can result in coronary artery vasospasm, myocardial ischemia, and contractile dysfunction [56]. See Fig. 2.5 for further details. Chronically, sustained α_1-adrenoceptor stimulation can increase arterial stiffness via deleterious remodeling [57,58], while sustained β_2-adrenoceptor stimulation can predispose to vascular calcification [59,60]. These vascular modifications decrease the tensile strength of the vessels contributing to hypertension and predisposing to potential rupture of blood vessels (e.g., a hemorrhagic stroke).

Catecholamines and alterations in renal physiology

Hypertension is characterized by a rise in renal sympathetic nerve activity (RSNA), which in turn perpetuates hypertension and contributes to the development of hypertensive kidney disease [61]. Moreover, sustained RSNA is associated with the development of end organ damage such as cardiac hypertrophy and deterioration of kidney function [35]. RSNA increases the amount of norepinephrine release from the prejunctional renal sympathetic nerves. Another factor that determines norepinephrine release is the presence of prejunctional α_{2A}-adrenoceptors which, when activated by norepinephrine that is released from the renal sympathetic nerve endings, inhibits the subsequent release of norepinephrine. Acting through the β_1-adrenoceptors, norepinephrine stimulates renin release from the juxtaglomerular apparatus, thereby activating the renin—angiotensin—aldosterone cascade. Acting through the vascular α_1- and α_2-adrenoceptors, norepinephrine mediates vasoconstriction, and an increase in renal vascular resistance which leads to compensatory vascular hypertrophy, renal vascular stiffness, and a decrease in renal blood flow with consequent reduction in glomerular filtration rate. Acting through the α_1-, α_2-, and β_1-adrenoceptors on renal tubules, norepinephrine modulates the activity of various sodium transporters like the sodium hydrogen exchanger 3, sodium chloride cotransporter, and epithelial sodium channel leading to reduced sodium and water excretion. In addition, norepinephrine enhances immune cell infiltration and release of proinflammatory cytokines including tumor necrosis factor alpha, interleukin-17, and interferon gamma causing renal fibrosis and perpetuation of hypertension.

Catecholamines and other organs

Catecholamines are associated with both proinflammatory and antiinflammatory effects [42]. Catecholamines have an immunosuppressive effect, increasing susceptibility to secondary infections. Catecholamines tip the coagulation—fibrinolysis balance toward hypercoagulability leading to an increased risk of thrombosis. Catecholamines are also associated with impaired gastrointestinal motility and a decrease in splanchnic perfusion due to their vasoconstrictive properties. Catecholamines do not cross the blood—brain barrier; so their central nervous system effects including anxiety and agitation are indirect.

Catecholamines and autonomic failure

The baroreflex is a feedback loop that provides a continuous and instantaneous regulation of blood pressure [62]. Any increase in blood pressure leads to activation of arterial baroreceptors. This leads to activation of the NTS. The NTS then simultaneously reduces sympathetic tone by inhibiting the RVLM and enhances parasympathetic tone by stimulating the dorsal nucleus of the vagus nerve. This results in a reduction in blood pressure due to vasodilatation and a decrease in cardiac output due to a reduction in heart rate. The same mechanism can also augment blood pressure. For example, when standing, venous blood pools in the lower limbs and the lower abdomen. This is associated with a transient decrease in blood pressure. This results in baroreflex-mediated activation of sympathetic tone and inhibition of parasympathetic tone, effectively leading to increased blood pressure from vasoconstriction and a rise in cardiac output.

Primary neurodegenerative autonomic disorders often lead to a failure to regulate blood pressure. These disorders can lead to orthostatic hypotension (neurogenic orthostatic hypotension) and supine hypertension (an often-overlooked presentation). In patients with neurodegenerative autonomic disorders, autonomic failure results from either the neurodegeneration of central autonomic pathways (as in multiple system atrophy) or peripheral postganglionic noradrenergic fibers (as in pure autonomic failure and Parkinson's disease). In either case, these patients with neurodegenerative disorders lose their baroreflex mechanisms which leads to profound neurogenic orthostatic hypotension.

Neurogenic orthostatic hypotension develops due to the absence of the noradrenergic stimulation that normally occurs in the upright posture. Therefore, mechanistically, noradrenergic agents including midodrine (α_1-agonist) and droxidopa (synthetic prodrug of norepinephrine that is converted in the body to norepinephrine) are often used in the management of these patients. An alternative method is to induce the release of endogenous norepinephrine by increasing the residual sympathetic tone that may still be present using drugs like pyridostigmine (a cholinesterase inhibitor) or yohimbine (a selective α_2-adrenoceptor antagonist). The second approach seems to be more physiologic as these agents preferentially improve blood pressure in the upright posture, whereas the first approach improves both supine and upright blood pressure.

Summary and conclusions

Catecholamines are powerful neurochemicals that exert their biologic effects via dopamine and adrenergic GPCRs. These GPCRs are widely distributed throughout the body with a substantial influence upon the cardiovascular system. It is the understanding of catecholamine synthesis and action via these GPCRs that informs the appropriate recognition and management of many diseases involving the cardiovascular system.

Learning points

- Catecholamines are powerful vasoactive neurochemicals produced by the autonomic nervous system and ganglia (including the adrenal medulla) with protean physiologic effects. These effects are mediated through various G-protein-coupled receptors that are distributed throughout the body and are heavily expressed on the heart and vasculature.
- Catecholamine excess states, like PPGL, can lead to hemodynamic derangements, and when prolonged, deleterious structural abnormalities of the heart and vasculature. With early recognition and intervention, these conditions can be treated, often with a favorable prognosis.
- Autonomic neurodegenerative disorders may result in underproduction/abnormal processing of catecholamines within the body, commonly leading to neurogenic orthostatic hypotension and supine hypertension.

References

[1] Joh TH, Hwang O. Dopamine beta-hydroxylase: biochemistry and molecular biology. Ann N Y Acad Sci 1987;493:342−50. https://doi.org/10.1111/j.1749-6632.1987.tb27217.x. PMID: 3473965.

[2] Young WF. Endocrine hypertension. In: Melmed S, Koenig R, Rosen C, Auchus R, Goldfine A, editors. In Williams textbook of endocrinology. 14th ed. Elsevier; 2019. p. 542−72. e7.

[3] Mannelli M, Pupilli C, Lanzillotti R, Ianni L, Serio M. Catecholamines and blood pressure regulation. Horm Res 1990;34(3−4):156−60. https://doi.org/10.1159/000181816. PMID: 2104398.

[4] Venugopalan VV, Ghali Z, Senecal J, Reader TA, Descarries L. Catecholaminergic activation of G-protein coupling in rat spinal cord: further evidence for the existence of dopamine and noradrenaline receptors in spinal grey and white matter. Brain Res 2006;1070(1):90−100. https://doi.org/10.1016/j.brainres.2005.10.101. PMID: 16423330.

[5] Motiejunaite J, Amar L, Vidal-Petiot E. Adrenergic receptors, and cardiovascular effects of catecholamines. Ann Endocrinol 2021;82(3−4):193−7. https://doi.org/10.1016/j.ando.2020.03.012. PMID: 32473788.

[6] Ranjbar-Slamloo Y, Fazlali Z. Dopamine, and noradrenaline in the brain; overlapping or dissociate functions? Front Mol Neurosci 2020;12:334. https://doi.org/10.3389/fnmol.2019.00334. PMID: 32038164.

[7] Minson J, Llewellyn-Smith I, Neville A, Somogyi P, Chalmers J. Quantitative analysis of spinally projecting adrenaline-synthesising neurons of C1, C2 and C3 groups in rat medulla oblongata. J Auton Nerv Syst 1990;30(3):209−20. https://doi.org/10.1016/0165-1838(90)90252-e. PMID: 2172354.

[8] Kutikov A, Crispen PL, Uzzo RG. Pathophysiology, evaluation, and medical management of adrenal disorders. Campbell's Urology. In: Wein AJ, Kavoussi LR, Novick AC, Partin AW, editors. Peters CA: Elsevier Saunders; 2012. p. 1685−736.

[9] Ziegler MG, Bao X, Kennedy BP, Joyner A, Enns R. Location, development, control, and function of extraadrenal phenylethanolamine N-methyltransferase. Ann N Y Acad Sci October 2002;971:76−82. https://doi.org/10.1111/j.1749-6632.2002.tb04437.x. PMID: 12438093.

[10] Palkovits M, Mezey E, Skirboll LR, Hokfelt T. Adrenergic projections from the lower brainstem to the hypothalamic paraventricular nucleus, the lateral hypothalamic area and the central nucleus of the amygdala in rats. J Chem Neuroanat 1992;5(5):407−15. https://doi.org/10.1016/0891-0618(92)90057-w. PMID: 1418754.

[11] Osborne NN, Nesselhut T. Adrenaline: occurrence in the bovine retina. Neurosci Lett August 19, 1983;39(1):33−6. https://doi.org/10.1016/0304-3940(83)90161-1. PMID: 6633936.

[12] Abbott SB, Kanbar R, Bochorishvili G, Coates MB, Stornetta RL, Guyenet PG. C1 neurons excite locus coeruleus and A5 noradrenergic neurons along with sympathetic outflow in rats. J Physiol 2012;590(12):2897−915. https://doi.org/10.1113/jphysiol.2012.232157. PMCID: PMC3448155.

[13] Card JP, Sved JC, Craig B, Raizada M, Vazquez J, Sved AF. Efferent projections of rat rostroventrolateral medulla C1 catecholamine neurons: implications for the central control of cardiovascular regulation. J Comp Neurol December 10, 2006;499(5):840−59. https://doi.org/10.1002/cne.21140. PMID: 17048222.

[14] Ross CA, Ruggiero DA, Park DH, Joh TH, Sved AF, Fernandez-Pardal J, Saavedra JM, Reis DJ. Tonic vasomotor control by the rostral ventrolateral medulla: effect of electrical or chemical stimulation of the area containing C1 adrenaline neurons on arterial pressure, heart rate, and plasma catecholamines and vasopressin. J Neurosci February 1984;4(2):474−94. https://doi.org/10.1523/JNEUROSCI.04-02-00474.1984. PMID: 6699683; PMCID: PMC6564896.

[15] Carandini T, Mancini M, Bogdan I, Rae CL, Barritt AW, Sethi A, Harrison N, Rashid W, Scarpini E, Galimberti D, Bozzali M, Cercignani M. Disruption of brainstem monoaminergic fibre tracts in multiple sclerosis as a putative mechanism for cognitive fatigue: a fixel-based analysis. Neuroimage Clin 2021;30:102587. https://doi.org/10.1016/j.nicl.2021.102587. PMID: 33610097; PMCID: PMC7903010.

[16] Nakamura T, Sobue G. Noradrenaline and 123I-meta-iodobenzylguanidine kinetics in the sympathetic nervous system. In: Iwase S, Hayano J, Orimo S, editors. Clinical assessment of the autonomic nervous system. Tokyo: Springer; 2017. https://doi.org/10.1007/978-4-431-56012-8_13.

[17] Pacak K. Phaeochromocytoma: a catecholamine and oxidative stress disorder. Endocr Regul 2011;45(2):65−90. https://doi.org/10.4149/endo_2011_02_65.

[18] Eisenhofer G, Klink B, Richter S, Lenders JW, Robledo M. Metabologenomics of phaeochromocytoma and paraganglioma: an integrated approach for personalised biochemical and genetic testing. Clin Biochem Rev April 2017;38(2):69−100. PMID: 29332973; PMCID: PMC5759086.

[19] Ritter SL, Hall RA. Fine-tuning of GPCR activity by receptor-interacting proteins. Nat Rev Mol Cell Biol December 2009;10(12):819−30. https://doi.org/10.1038/nrm2803. PMID: 19935667; PMCID: PMC2825052.

[20] Mizuno N, Itoh H. Functions, and regulatory mechanisms of Gq-signaling pathways. Neurosignals 2009;17(1):42−54. https://doi.org/10.1159/000186689. PMID: 19212139.

[21] Perez DM, Doze VA. Cardiac and neuroprotection regulated by α(1)-adrenergic receptor subtypes. J Recept Signal Transduct Res 2011;31(2):98−110. https://doi.org/10.3109/10799893.2010.550008. PMID: 21338248; PMCID: PMC3623295.

[22] Evdokimovskii EV, Jeon R, Park S, Pimenov OY, Alekseev AE. Role of α2-adrenoceptor subtypes in suppression of L-type Ca^{2+} current in mouse cardiac myocytes. Int J Mol Sci 2021;22(8):4135. PMID: 33923625; PMCID: PMC8072751.

[23] Kanagy NL. Alpha(2)-adrenergic receptor signalling in hypertension. Clin Sci (Lond) November 2005;109(5):431−7. https://doi.org/10.1042/CS20050101. PMID: 16232127.

[24] Sandilands AJ, O'Shaughnessy KM. β1-Adrenoreceptor polymorphisms and blood pressure: 49S variant increases plasma renin but not blood pressure in hypertensive patients. Am J Hypertens 2019;32(5):447−51. https://doi.org/10.1093/ajh/hpz019. PMID: 30753253; PMCID: PMC6475877.

[25] Lymperopoulos A. Physiology and pharmacology of the cardiovascular adrenergic system. Front Physiol September 4, 2013;4:240. https://doi.org/10.3389/fphys.2013.00240. Retraction in: Front Physiol. 2015;6:379. PMID: 24027534; PMCID: PMC3761154.

[26] Joyner MJ, Casey DP. Regulation of increased blood flow (hyperemia) to muscles during exercise: a hierarchy of competing physiological needs. Physiol Rev April 2015;95(2):549−601. https://doi.org/10.1152/physrev.00035.2013. PMID: 25834232; PMCID: PMC4551211.

[27] Sakai T, Hosoyamada Y. Are the precapillary sphincters and metarterioles universal components of the microcirculation? An historical review. J Physiol Sci September 2013;63(5):319−31. https://doi.org/10.1007/s12576-013-0274-7. PMID: 23824465; PMCID: PMC3751330.

[28] Nazari MA, Rosenblum JS, Haigney MC, Rosing DR, Pacak K. Pathophysiology and acute management of tachyarrhythmias in pheochromocytoma: JACC review topic of the week. J Am Coll Cardiol July 28, 2020;76(4):451−64. https://doi.org/10.1016/j.jacc.2020.04.080. PMID: 32703516; PMCID: PMC7454044.

[29] Gauthier C, Rozec B, Manoury B, Balligand JL. Beta-3 adrenoceptors as new therapeutic targets for cardiovascular pathologies. Curr Heart Fail Rep September 2011;8(3):184−92. https://doi.org/10.1007/s11897-011-0064-6. PMID: 21633786.

[30] Murga C, Arcones AC, Cruces-Sande M, Briones AM, Salaices M, Mayor Jr F. G protein-coupled receptor kinase 2 (GRK2) as a potential therapeutic target in cardiovascular and metabolic diseases. Front Pharmacol February 19, 2019;10:112. https://doi.org/10.3389/fphar.2019.00112. PMID: 30837878; PMCID: PMC6390810.

[31] Nakano T, Onoue K, Nakada Y, Nakagawa H, Kumazawa T, Ueda T, et al. Alteration of β-adrenoceptor signalling in left ventricle of acute phase Takotsubo syndrome: a human study. Sci Rep 2018;8(1):12731. https://doi.org/10.1038/s41598-018-31034-z. PMID: 30143703.

[32] Beaulieu JM, Gainetdinov RR. The physiology, signaling, and pharmacology of dopamine receptors. Pharmacol Rev March 2011;63(1):182−217. https://doi.org/10.1124/pr.110.002642. PMID: 21303898.

[33] Antal CE, Newton AC. Spatiotemporal dynamics of phosphorylation in lipid second messenger signaling. Mol Cell Proteomics 2013;12(12):3498−508. https://doi.org/10.1074/mcp.R113.029819. PMID: 23788531; PMCID: PMC3861703.

[34] Wier WG, Morgan KG. Alpha1-adrenergic signaling mechanisms in contraction of resistance arteries. Rev Physiol Biochem Pharmacol 2003;150:91−139. https://doi.org/10.1007/s10254-003-0019-8. Epub 2003 Jul 17. PMID: 12884052.

[35] Hering L, Rahman M, Potthoff SA, Rump LC, Stegbauer J. Role of α2-adrenoceptors in hypertension: focus on renal sympathetic neurotransmitter release, inflammation, and sodium homeostasis. Front Physiol November 9, 2020;11:566871. https://doi.org/10.3389/fphys.2020.566871. PMID: 33240096; PMCID: PMC7680782.

[36] Castle-Kirszbaum M, Lai L, Maingard J, Asadi H, Danks RA, Goldschlager T, et al. Intravenous milrinone for treatment of delayed cerebral ischaemia following subarachnoid haemorrhage: a pooled systematic review. Neurosurg Rev December 2021;44(6):3107−24. https://doi.org/10.1007/s10143-021-01509-1. PMID: 33682040.

[37] Zaugg M, Schaub MC. Cellular mechanisms in sympatho-modulation of the heart. Br J Anaesth July 2004;93(1):34−52. https://doi.org/10.1093/bja/aeh159. PMID: 15145820.

[38] Locatelli J, de Assis LV, Isoldi MC. Calcium handling proteins: structure, function, and modulation by exercise. Heart Fail Rev March 2014;19(2):207−25. https://doi.org/10.1007/s10741-013-9373-z. PMID: 23436107.

[39] Barefield D, Sadayappan S. Phosphorylation, and function of cardiac myosin binding protein-C in health and disease. J Mol Cell Cardiol May 2010;48(5):866−75. https://doi.org/10.1016/j.yjmcc.2009.11.014. PMID: 19962384; PMCID: PMC6800196.

[40] Katz AM, Lorell BH. Regulation of cardiac contraction and relaxation. Circulation November 14, 2000;102(20):IV69−74. https://doi.org/10.1161/01.cir.102.suppl_4.iv-69. PMID: 11080134.

[41] Cannavo A, Koch WJ. Targeting β3-adrenergic receptors in the heart: selective agonism and β-blockade. J Cardiovasc Pharmacol 2017;69(2):71−8. https://doi.org/10.1097/FJC.0000000000000444. PMID: 28170359; PMCID: PMC5295490.

[42] Hartmann C, Radermacher P, Wepler M, Nußbaum B. Non-hemodynamic effects of catecholamines. Shock 2017;48(4):390−400. https://doi.org/10.1097/SHK.0000000000000879. PMID: 28915214.

[43] Overgaard CB, Dzavík V. Inotropes, and vasopressors: review of physiology and clinical use in cardiovascular disease. Circulation 2008;118(10):1047−56. https://doi.org/10.1161/CIRCULATIONAHA.107.728840. PMID: 18765387.

[44] Pappachan JM, Tun NN, Arunagirinathan G, Sodi R, Hanna FWF. Pheochromocytomas and hypertension. Curr Hypertens Rep 2018;20:3.

[45] Soltani A, Pourian M, Davani BM. Does this patient have pheochromocytoma? A systematic review of clinical signs and symptoms. J Diabetes Metab Disord 2016;15:6.

[46] Hamidi O, Young WF, Iniguez-Ariza NM, Kittah NE, Gruber L, Bancos C, et al. Malignant pheochromocytoma and paraganglioma: 272 patients over 55 years. J Clin Endocrinol Metabol 2017;102:3296−305.

[47] Nölting S, Bechmann N, Taieb D, Beuschlein F, Fassnacht M, Kroiss M, et al. Personalized management of pheochromocytoma and paraganglioma. bnab019 Endocr Rev 2022;43(2):199−239. https://doi.org/10.1210/endrev/bnab019. Erratum in: Endocr Rev. 2021 Dec 14; Erratum in: Endocr Rev. 2021 Dec 14; PMID: 34147030; PMCID PMC8905338.

[48] Costa MH, Ortiga-Carvalho TM, Violante AD, Vaisman M. Pheochromocytomas and paragangliomas: clinical and genetic approaches. Front Endocrinol 2015;6:126. https://doi.org/10.3389/fendo.2015.00126. PMID: 26347711; PMCID: PMC4538298.

[49] Kumar A, Pappachan JM, Fernandez CJ. Catecholamine-induced cardiomyopathy: an endocrinologist's perspective. Rev Cardiovasc Med 2021;22(4):1215−28. https://doi.org/10.31083/j.rcm2204130. PMID: 34957765.

[50] Malindretos PM, Sarafidis PA, Geropoulou EZ, Kapoulas S, Paramythiotis DD, Lasaridis AN. Sustained hypotension complicating an extra-adrenal pheochromocytoma. Am J Hypertens 2008;21:840−2.

[51] Kaneto H, Kamei S, Tatsumi F, Shimoda M, Kimura T, Nakanishi S, et al. Case report: malignant pheochromocytoma without hypertension accompanied by increment of serum VEGF level and catecholamine cardiomyopathy. Front Endocrinol 2021;12:688536.

[52] Moady G, Atar S. Stress-induced cardiomyopathy-considerations for diagnosis and management during the COVID-19 pandemic. Medicina (Kaunas) January 27, 2022;58(2):192. https://doi.org/10.3390/medicina58020192. PMID: 35208516; PMCID: PMC8875249.

[53] Barki-Harrington L, Perrino C, Rockman HA. Network integration of the adrenergic system in cardiac hypertrophy. Cardiovasc Res August 15, 2004;63(3):391−402. https://doi.org/10.1016/j.cardiores.2004.03.011. PMID: 15276464.

[54] Amin P, Singh M, Singh K. β-Adrenergic receptor-stimulated cardiac myocyte apoptosis: role of β1 integrins. J Signal Transduct 2011;2011:179057. https://doi.org/10.1155/2011/179057. PMID: 21776383; PMCID: PMC3135092.

[55] Hašková P, Kovaříková P, Koubková L, Vávrová A, Macková E, Šimůnek T. Iron chelation with salicylaldehyde isonicotinoyl hydrazone protects against catecholamine autoxidation and cardiotoxicity. Free Radic Biol Med February 15, 2011;50(4):537−49. https://doi.org/10.1016/j.freeradbiomed.2010.12.004. PMID: 21147217.

[56] Dhalla NS, Adameova A, Kaur M. Role of catecholamine oxidation in sudden cardiac death. Fundam Clin Pharmacol October 2010;24(5):539−46. https://doi.org/10.1111/j.1472-8206.2010.00836.x. PMID: 20584205.

[57] Erami C, Zhang H, Tanoue A, Tsujimoto G, Thomas SA, Faber JE. Adrenergic catecholamine trophic activity contributes to flow-mediated arterial remodeling. Am J Physiol Heart Circ Physiol 2005;289(2):H744−53. https://doi.org/10.1152/ajpheart.00129.2005. PMID: 15849236.

[58] Chalothorn D, Zhang H, Clayton JA, Thomas SA, Faber JE. Catecholamines augment collateral vessel growth and angiogenesis in hindlimb ischemia. Am J Physiol Heart Circ Physiol 2005;289(2):H947−59. https://doi.org/10.1152/ajpheart.00952.2004. PMID: 15833801.

[59] Moser B, Poetsch F, Estepa M, Luong TTD, Pieske B, Lang F, et al. Increased β-adrenergic stimulation augments vascular smooth muscle cell calcification via PKA/CREB signalling. Pflügers Archiv 2021;473(12):1899−910. https://doi.org/10.1007/s00424-021-02621-3. PMID: 34564739; PMCID: PMC8599266.

[60] Osadchii OE. Cardiac hypertrophy induced by sustained beta-adrenoreceptor activation: pathophysiological aspects. Heart Fail Rev 2007;12(1):66−86. https://doi.org/10.1007/s10741-007-9007-4. PMID: 17387610.

[61] Sata Y, Head GA, Denton K, May CN, Schlaich MP. Role of the sympathetic nervous system and its modulation in renal hypertension. Front Med 2018;5:82. https://doi.org/10.3389/fmed.2018.00082. PMID: 29651418; PMCID: PMC5884873.

[62] Biaggioni I. The pharmacology of autonomic failure: from hypotension to hypertension. Pharmacol Rev January 2017;69(1):53−62. https://doi.org/10.1124/pr.115.012161. PMID: 28011746; PMCID: PMC6047298.

Chapter 3

Adrenal cortical hormones and blood pressure regulation

Anna Sanders[1], Cornelius J. Fernandez[2] and Rousseau Gama[3,4]

[1]Department of Clinical Biochemistry, Russells Hall Hospital, Black Country Pathology Services, The Royal Wolverhampton NHS Trust, Wolverhampton, United Kingdom; [2]Department of Endocrinology and Metabolism, Pilgrim Hospital, United Lincolnshire Hospitals NHS Trust, Boston, United Kingdom; [3]Department of Clinical Biochemistry, Black Country Pathology Services, The Royal Wolverhampton NHS Trust, Wolverhampton, United Kingdom; [4]Department of Laboratory and Metabolic Medicine, The University of Wolverhampton, Wolverhampton, United Kingdom

Visit the *Endocrine Hypertension: From Basic Science to Clinical Practice, First Edition* companion web site at: https://www.elsevier.com/books-and-journals/book-companion/9780323961202.

Graphical Abstract

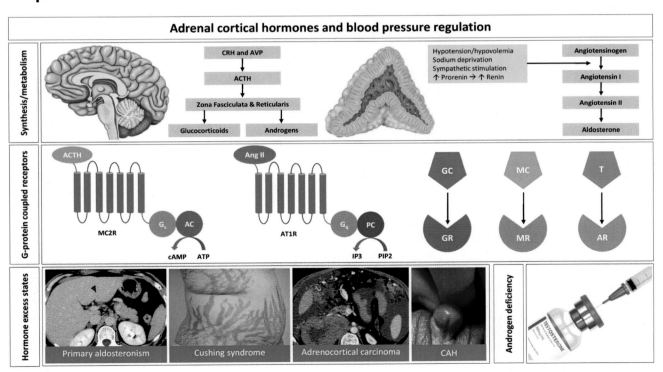

Endocrine Hypertension. https://doi.org/10.1016/B978-0-323-96120-2.00019-4

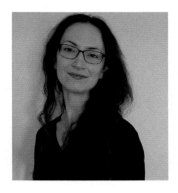

Anna Sanders

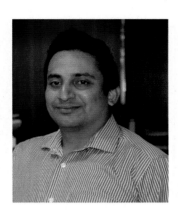

Cornelius J. Fernandez

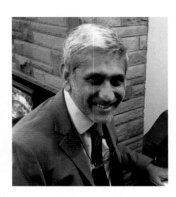

Rousseau Gama

Introduction

The human adrenal cortex has three distinct layers; the outer zona glomerulosa producing mineralocorticoids, the central zona fasciculata producing glucocorticoids, and inner zona reticularis producing androgens and some glucocorticoids [1]. These steroid hormones alter the vascular hemodynamics and play key roles in the regulation of blood pressure and cardiovascular homeostasis. Excessive production of these hormones may lead to hypertension [2], whereas deficiency may cause life-threatening illness including profound hemodynamic failure [3,4]. This chapter describes the physiological aspects, the biological effects, and pathophysiological alterations of adrenal cortical hormones in relation to human blood pressure regulation.

Physiological aspects

An overview of adrenal steroid synthetic pathways

A depiction of the adrenal steroid synthesis pathways and their sites of synthesis is shown in Fig. 3.1.

Regulation of steroidogenesis: cholesterol, StAR, and p450scc

Common to steroidogenic pathways is the initial conversion of cholesterol to pregnenolone by P450scc (cholesterol side chain cleavage enzyme, steroid 20−22 lyase, cholesterol 20−22 desmolase, or CYP11A1) that is present on the inner mitochondrial membrane. While adrenocortical cells are capable of de novo cholesterol synthesis, the majority comes from the uptake of LDL particles. Cholesterol esters are transferred to lysosomes where they are either converted into free cholesterol, or stored as cytosolic lipid particles to be released when required by hormone-sensitive lipase (HSL). Steroidogenic acute regulatory (StAR) protein facilitates the transfer of cholesterol across the mitochondrial membrane where P450scc resides. While not essential for steroidogenesis, the absence or dysfunction of StAR protein due to gene mutations results in severe and sometimes fatal hyposteroidaemia [5,6].

Adrenal steroidogenesis is regulated by rapid "nongenomic" cell signaling processes, as well as slower "genomic" processes that are dependent on gene expression. The predominant regulator of adrenal steroidogenesis is adrenocorticotropic hormone (adrenocorticotropin; ACTH) secreted from the anterior pituitary. ACTH binds to the transmembrane bound melanocortin type-2 receptor (MC2R), a G-protein-coupled receptor that exerts its effect through downstream cyclic adenosine monophosphate (cAMP). While the MC2R is predominantly found in the zona fasciculata, it is also located in the zona glomerulosa and to a lesser extent, the zona reticularis [7]. ACTH regulates the activity and expression of various steroidogenic enzymes especially that of HSL and StAR protein which control levels of intracellular cholesterol and its transport within the mitochondrial matrix, respectively [8]. This regulation occurs predominantly through cyclic adenosine monophosphate/protein kinase A (cAMP/PKA) pathway, resulting in rapid phosphorylation of proteins involved in steroidogenesis, including HSL and StAR proteins (nongenomic response). In addition to the classical cAMP/PKA pathway, the cAMP can cross-talk with other signaling pathways such as mitogen-activated protein kinase/extracellular signal-regulated protein kinase (MEK/ERK) pathway to mediate phosphorylation of proteins involved in steroidogenesis [9].

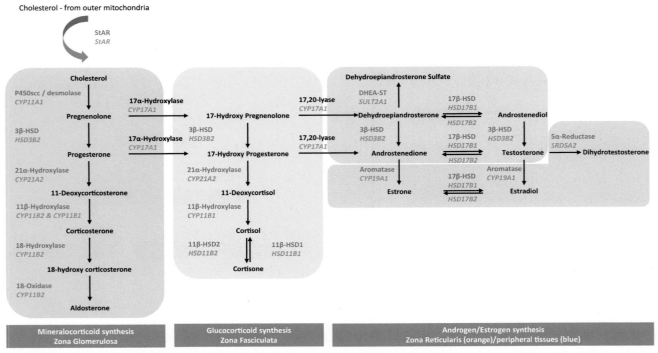

FIGURE 3.1 Schematic of the principal pathways of steroid biosynthesis in the adrenal. The pathways to sex steroids in peripheral tissues are also depicted. Common enzyme names are in orange font, and the corresponding gene names are in *blue* font.

Simultaneously, ACTH also triggers a slower genomic response by stimulating the expression of various steroidogenic genes including *StAR, CYP11A, MC2R,* and melanocortin-2 receptor accessory protein which serve to upregulate the steroid synthesis. The half-life of StAR protein is very short, approximately 5 to 15 minutes. Hence, in addition to the rapid phosphorylation of steroidogenic enzymes, stimulation of expression of steroidogenic genes is important to replenish and maintain StAR protein expression. ACTH can directly activate the cAMP-responsive element binding protein (CREB), which is a key transcription factor involved in the regulation of Star transcription, through pulsatile phosphorylation. Additionally, ACTH can indirectly activate CREB through posttranscriptional modification of cotranscription factors [8]. Fig. 3.2 shows the genomic and nongenomic pathways involved in the adrenal steroidogenesis under the influence of ACTH [10−12].

Aldosterone synthesis in the zona glomerulosa

Aldosterone synthesis is usually confined to the zona glomerulosa. Its regulation and synthesis is dependent on the high levels of expression of angiotensin II type 1 receptors (AT1Rs) and aldosterone synthase (CYP11B2) found in this zone. CYP11B2 has both 11-hydroxylase and 18-hydroxylase activity and is responsible for the final stages of aldosterone synthesis (Fig. 3.1). The other three steroidogenic enzymes required for aldosterone biosynthesis are P450scc, 3β-hydroxysteroid dehydrogenase (3β-HSD), and 21α-hydroxylase. These three enzymes are found in all adrenocortical zones; however, absent expression of CYP11B1 and CYP17A1 genes in the zona glomerulosa which encode 11β-hydroxylase and 17α-hydroxylase, respectively, prevents diversion of steroid synthesis toward cortisol or androgens [13].

Aldosterone synthesis is stimulated predominantly by angiotensin II and plasma K^+ but is also acutely regulated by ACTH and locally produced endothelin-1 [14]. Angiotensin-II acting via the AT1R and ACTH acting via the MC2R both lead to an increase in the availability of precursors, such as cholesterol and NADPH, the latter of which is an essential cofactor for CYP450 activity [15]. Long-term upregulation of aldosterone synthesis involves the increased expression of StAR protein and aldosterone synthase [15,16].

In vitro studies indicate that angiotensin II binding to the AT1R induces activation of several signaling pathways in zona glomerulosa cells. Angiotensin II binding to the AT1R induces G-protein-mediated Ca^{2+} signal generation and protein kinase C (PKC) activation, which activates diverse signaling pathways, including stimulation of MAPK, tyrosine

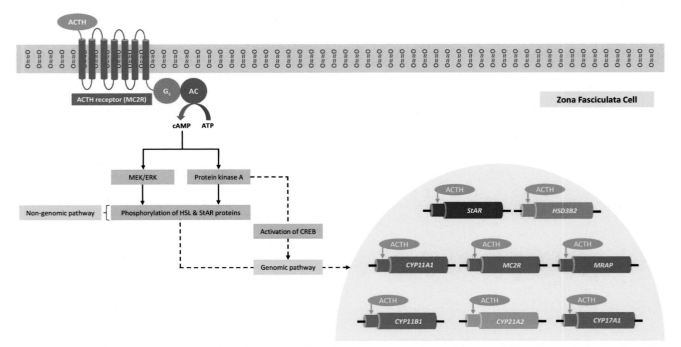

FIGURE 3.2 Schematic depicting the downstream effects of ACTH binding to the melanocortin type 2 receptor (MC2R) binding in the zona fasciculata cell. *AC*, adenylate cyclase; *CREB*, cAMP-responsive element binding protein; *Gs*, stimulatory G-protein; *HSL*, hormone sensitive lipase; *MRAP*, melanocortin receptor accessory protein.

kinases, lipoxygenase production, phospholipase D, and phospholipase A2 [17]. Angiotensin II, however, also induces G protein-independent signaling pathways, such as β-arrestin-mediated activation of MAPK [18]. Specifically, upregulation of aldosterone synthase involves Ca^{2+} signal-mediated activation of calmodulin kinases (CAMKs), which regulates the transcription and/or activity of early transcription factors [16,17].

Like angiotensin II, K^+ shares calcium signaling as a key regulator of aldosterone production, with K^+ increasing intracellular calcium activating voltage-sensitive L- and T-type calcium channels resulting in the influx of calcium from extracellular sources [19]. Adrenal zona glomerulosa cells are typically hyperpolarized by a predominant K^+ conductance facilitated by the "leak" K^+ channels of the 2-pore domain/transmembrane family, TASK1 (KCNK3) [20]. Membrane polarity is also under the control of different Kir (K^+ inward rectifying) channels, many of which are G-protein coupled. An increase in K^+ functionally results in increased mobilization of intracellular calcium and the activation of the calcium-CAMK system signal cascade [21,22].

Although angiotensin II and K^+ regulate aldosterone production independently, they also act synergistically. When both angiotensin II and K^+ levels are low, they attenuate the effect of the other agonist on aldosterone production, whereas when the concentration of angiotensin II or K^+ is modest to high, small changes in the concentration of the other agonist elicit large increases in aldosterone production [23]. Fig. 3.3 outlines the pathways involved in aldosterone synthesis regulated by angiotensin II [24].

Cortisol synthesis in the zona fasciculata

The zona fasciculata does not express AT1R nor aldosterone synthase but expresses the MC2R and 11β-hydroxylase (CYP11B1), which, unlike CYP11B2, does not have 18-hydroxylase activity and thus cannot convert 18-hydroxycorticosterone to aldosterone and has minimal capacity to convert corticosterone to 18-hydroxycorticosterone [25]. Both the zona glomerulosa and zona fasciculata express 21α-hydroxylase, but the expression of 17α-hydroxylase in the zona fasciculata selectively permits cortisol synthesis. Very little, if any, cytochrome *b*5 is expressed in the zona fasciculata. Cytochrome *b*5 is an important regulator of CYP17 side-chain cleavage activity and its presence is required for the efficient side chain cleavage activity of CYP17, but not for 17α-hydroxylase function. In consequence, the 17α-hydroxylation but not 17,20-lyase activity of CYP17 predominates in zona fasciculata resulting in the production of glucocorticoids (cortisol and corticosterone) but very little dehydroepiandrosterone (DHEA) [26].

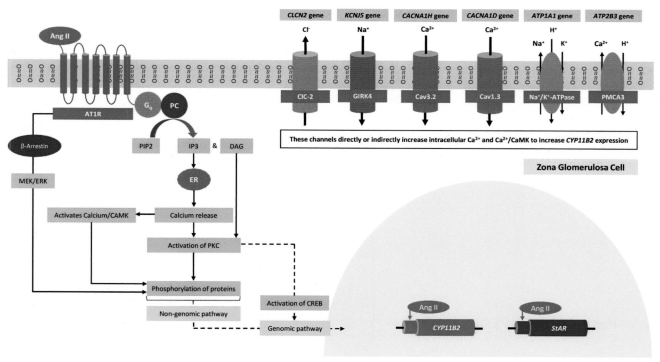

FIGURE 3.3   Schematic showing the pathways involved in the regulation of aldosterone synthesis. *Ang II*, Angiotensin II; *AT1R*, angiotensin II type 1 receptor; Ca^{2+}, calcium; *CAMK*, calmodulin kinase; *CREB*, cAMP-responsive element binding protein; *DAG*, diacylglycerol; *ER*, endoplasmic reticulum; G_q, G-protein; *IP3*, inositol triphosphate; *PC*, phospholipase C; *PIP2*, phosphatidylinositol biphosphate; *PKC*, protein kinase C;.

De novo biosynthesis of adrenal steroid hormones (adrenal steroidogenesis) is a dynamic process that is tightly regulated by multiple mechanisms including transcriptional and posttranslational modification of steroidogenic enzymes and proteins involved in the substrate transportation [27]. In addition, various proteins involved in the cholesterol biosynthesis and uptake also function as regulatory factors of adrenal steroidogenesis. These regulatory mechanisms are extremely vital, as glucocorticoid hormones (cortisol in humans and corticosterone in rodents) are the key regulators of variety of physiological functions including blood pressure, inflammation, glucose metabolism, and stress. The endoplasmic reticulum-associated degradation (ERAD) is a mechanism to remove misfolded or unfolded proteins to maintain protein quality. Small vasolin-containing protein-interacting protein (SVIP) is an endogenous ERAD (endoplasmic reticulum associated protein degradation pathway) inhibitor. SVIP overexpression increases the cortisol and DHEA biosynthesis, whereas exaggerated overexpression led to apoptosis and diminished adrenal steroidogenesis. This indicates that SVIP is a novel regulator of adrenal cortisol and DHEA biosynthesis [27].

Corticotrophin-releasing hormone (CRH) secreted by the paraventricular nucleus of the hypothalamus predominantly coordinates the central regulation of glucocorticoid secretion, potentiated by other hypothalamic products most importantly vasopressin [28]. CRH activates CRH receptors on the corticotrophs of anterior pituitary to enhance ACTH secretion, which in turn stimulates glucocorticoid-secreting cells within the adrenal cortex signaling. The glucocorticoids send inhibitory feedback signs to the hypothalamic–pituitary–adrenal (HPA) axis, especially at the level of the anterior pituitary, but also at the level of the hippocampus and hypothalamus. The HPA axis has a characteristic dynamic ultradian rhythm manifested by oscillating levels of ACTH and glucocorticoid hormones, so that adrenal glands release glucocorticoids in near-hourly pulses. This ultradian rhythm becomes disrupted during aging and in stress-related disease such as major depression. The ultradian rhythm results from a sub-HPA system that functions as a peripheral hormone oscillator [28].

Adrenal androgen synthesis and regulation in the zona reticularis

Unlike the zona glomerulosa and zona fasciculata, which replace the fetal adrenal zones early in the neonatal period, the zona reticularis develops slowly, becoming active in producing androgens at adrenarche at around 6–8 years [29], and peaking in androgen production at around 30 years [30]. During adrenarche, the gene expression profile of the zona reticularis changes leading to an increase in the synthesis of 17α-hydroxylase, cytochrome *b*5, and P450 cytochrome oxidoreductase (POR) enzymes, and a decrease in synthesis of 3β-hydroxysteroid dehydrogenase type II (HSD3B2) [29].

Cytochrome *b*5 and POR form a quaternary complex with 17α-hydroxylase, which maximizes its 17—20 lyase activity. This pattern of expression of steroidogenic enzymes and cofactors in combination with the relatively low levels of 21α-hydroxylase and 11β-hydroxylase and the greater affinity of 17α-hydroxylase for pregnenolone and 17-hydroxypregnenolone over HSD3B2 enable DHEA synthetic pathways to predominate over those of cortisol synthesis in zona reticularis [13].

DHEA is largely converted to its sulfated form, DHEAS, by the high levels of sulfotransferase 2A1 (SULT2A1) found in the zona reticularis [31]. A small proportion of the DHEA produced is converted to androstenedione, some of which is converted into testosterone, presumably due to the presence of 17β-hydroxysteroid dehydrogenase-5 (HSD5) [32]. The clinical significance, however, of these small quantities of adrenal testosterone is not established.

The regulation of adrenal androgen synthesis is predominantly dependent on the ACTH/cAMP/PKA and the MEK/ERK signaling pathways [30]. Inhibition of MEK/ERK signaling affects CYP17 and HSD3B2 expression and thus androgen synthesis [30].

In summary, the differential expression of enzymes in each zone of the adrenal cortex is responsible for zonal selectivity of the type of steroid synthesis and secretion.

Glucocorticoids, receptors, and cardiovascular system effects

Glucocorticoids and their actions via the glucocorticoid receptor (GR) have a role in the genesis and development of cardiovascular disease (CVD). Glucocorticoids are essential for life, coordinating a multitude of fundamental processes including metabolic homeostasis, immune and inflammatory responses, reproduction, development, cell proliferation, and cognitive function [33]. Glucocorticoid actions are largely mediated through their binding to the GR, but newer studies indicating non-GR activity demonstrate a more complex interplay of corticosteroid action [34]. The GR is evolutionarily related to the mineralocorticoid receptor (MR), another member of the nuclear receptor (NR) superfamily and steroid receptor subfamily that includes the progesterone receptor (PR), estrogen receptors (E2), and androgen receptors (ARs), and as such, there are emerging data showing cross-talk between steroid receptors and physiological and pathophysiological function [35—37].

The glucocorticoid receptor (GR)

The GR, like the other steroid hormone receptors, is a member of the NR superfamily, which share common features and mechanisms of action, and mainly act as ligand-inducible transcription factors that directly bind DNA and influence the expression of target genes. The GR is encoded by the *NR3C1* gene located on chromosome 5q31-32 [34]. Like other NRs, the GR consists of an N-terminal transactivation domain (NTD), a central DNA-binding domain (DBD), a C-terminal ligand-binding domain (LBD), and a linker domain connecting the DBD and LBD [38]. The LBD contains the site for glucocorticoid binding as well as an activation function site (AF2) which undergoes a conformational change upon ligand binding enabling additional interaction with an array of coactivators or corepressors. The NTD binds a diverse range of coregulators and components of the transcriptional machinery through activation function domain 1 (AF1). It is the most varied region of gene and subject to greater polymorphism as a result of posttranslational modifications. The NTD cooperates synergistically with the LBD to reinforce the receptor structure [39,40]. Conversely, the DBD is a highly conserved two zinc finger motif that mediates dimerization and subsequent binding to specific genomic sequences called glucocorticoid response elements (GREs).

The GR exists in several isoforms generated by alternative splicing. To date, this includes GR-α (8 subisoforms), GR-β (8 subisoforms), GR-γ, GR-A, and GR-P. The GR-α isoforms have similar affinities for glucocorticoids and similar interaction abilities with GREs. In vitro studies, however, have demonstrated isoform specific differences in function [41]. Unlike other GR isoforms, the GR-β isoform is located to the nucleus; it does not bind glucocorticoids and yet binds to GREs acting as a negative inhibitor of GR-α [42]. Increased expression of GR-β has been associated with glucocorticoid resistance, which may be due to competition for GRE binding, competition for transcriptional co-regulators, or the formation of inactive isoform heterodimers. The ability of GR-β and other GRs to inhibit the activity of GR-α is suggestive of a key role in glucocorticoid resistance and insensitivity [43]. The GR-γ, GR-A, and GR-P have low transactivation activities. It has been postulated that the tissue-specific and the individual differences in relative abundances of GR isoforms could be of significance in glucocorticoid action [38].

Glucocorticoid receptor and blood pressure regulation

Blood pressure is dependent on the combined efforts of cardiac output and systemic vascular resistance and is regulated by baroreceptors. Hypertension is an established major risk factor for CVD. Glucocorticoids regulate the blood pressure and may cause hypertension [44]. While it is traditionally believed that glucocorticoids influence blood pressure through activation of the MR, the presence of GRs in the vascular smooth muscle cells (VSMCs) and vascular endothelial cells (VECs) has shifted focus to the role of these tissue-specific receptors in modulating BP [45,46]. VSMC GR knock out (GRKO) mouse model studies demonstrate that while both control and GRKO mice had similar BP at baseline, the GRKO mice had attenuated acute and chronic hypertensive responses to dexamethasone in comparison to control mice suggesting a role for the GRs in VSMC in mediating the hypertensive response [45]. Similarly, in a vascular endothelial GRKO mouse model, the GRKO mice had slightly elevated baseline BP but were moderately resistant to dexamethasone-induced hypertension compared to control mice, indicating the important role of GRs in VECs in BP regulation [46].

In cell culture experiments, glucocorticoids increase the expression of angiotensin II receptor type I (AT-1) in VSMCs, which have been postulated as a mechanism for increasing BP [47,48]. Studies have also demonstrated a role for both the GR and the MR in BP regulation by mediating the influx of Ca^{2+} and/or Na^+ into VSMCs [49]. Cell culture studies have also indicated that glucocorticoids may regulate BP through alternative pathways in VECs. One such study demonstrated that through nongenomic GR cell signaling, glucocorticoids influence generation of nitric oxide (NO) in VECs via nitric oxide synthase (NOS) activity, which induces vasodilation in VSMCs as well as acts locally to prevent platelet and leukocyte aggregation and inhibit VSMC proliferation [50]. Fig. 3.4 shows graphical representation of the role of glucocorticoids and GR in the regulation of human blood pressure [51,52].

Mineralocorticoids, receptors, and effects on the cardiovascular system

The primary function of aldosterone, the main mineralocorticoid, is to increase sodium reabsorption, and subsequent water reuptake in the kidney, thus maintaining normal blood pressure. The classic understanding of how aldosterone mediates its effect is through binding to the MR, which acts as a transcription factor for responsive genes, including that of the

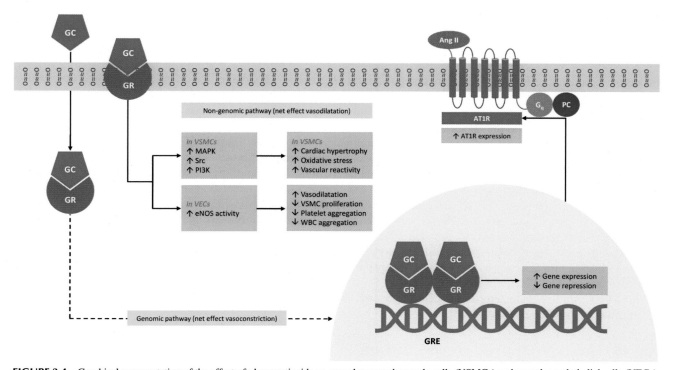

FIGURE 3.4 Graphical representation of the effect of glucocorticoids on vascular smooth muscle cells (VSMCs) and vascular endothelial cells (VECs). *Ang II*, angiotensin II; *AT1R*, angiotensin II type 1 receptor; *eNOS*, endothelial nitric oxide synthase; *Gq*, G-protein; *GC*, glucocorticoid; GR, glucocorticoid receptor; *GRE*, glucocorticoid response element; *MAPK*, mitogen-activated protein kinase; *PC*, phospholipase C, *PI3K*, Phosphoinositide 3-kinase; *WBC*, white blood cell.

epithelial sodium channel, ENaC. Increased number of ENaC channels in the apical membrane results in enhanced reabsorption of sodium, which in turn promotes water reuptake [53].

Unlike other steroids with cross-(steroid) receptor affinity, aldosterone binds only to the MR. Interestingly, the emergence of the MR preexisted aldosterone synthase, which coincided with the emergence of land vertebrates, and therefore, it is presumed that other steroid ligands are likely to have physiological effects [54]. In fact, it is long established that 11-deoxycortisol and cortisol also act as MR agonists and have similar affinities to the MR as that of aldosterone. However, aldosterone is still the primary ligand for the MR in epithelial tissues at least, despite the significantly more abundant cortisol. This is due to the presence of colocalized 11β-hydroxysteroid dehydrogenase type 2 (11βHSD2) that converts cortisol to the inactive cortisone [55–57].

The MR is widely distributed in a range of epithelial and nonepithelial tissues [58], including the kidney, the cardiovascular system, the central nervous system, the gonads, and the colon [59]. The function of the MR in many of these tissues is not fully elucidated, but in tissues where there is an absence of colocalized 11βHSD2, it is suggested that the MR acts as an additional or alternative GR [60].

The mineralocorticoid receptor

The human MR (encoded by *NR3C2* gene) is the longest of the NRs, containing 984 amino acids, and like the other members of the NR superfamily, it is comprised of three main functional domains: an N-terminal domain (NTD), a highly conserved DBD, and an LBD [61,62]. The NTD is intrinsically disordered allowing structural flexibility and diverse protein interactions [63]. Like the GR, the MR contains an activation function (AF-1) region that is refuted to be able to bind a wide array of corepressors [64].

When unbound to a ligand, the MR is localized to the cytoplasm where it is complexed with several chaperone proteins [65,66] which play a dynamic role in determining ligand-affinity [66]. The LBD interacts with chaperone proteins which retain the inactive MR in the cytoplasm, in a high affinity state [67]. Ligand binding induces a conformational change in the LBD, which (1) releases the chaperones enabling translocation to the nucleus and (2) creates the activation function-2 region (AF-2) which is a site for binding of transcriptional coregulators. In the nucleus, the dimerized MR−ligand complex recruits coregulators and transcription machinery and binds to hormone response element (HRE) in the promoter of MR-regulated genes [68].

MR and blood pressure regulation: genomic effects

In kidney epithelial cells, MR activation upregulates the expression of proteins important in electrolyte homeostasis including ENaC, Na$^+$/K$^+$ ATPase, renal outer medullary potassium channel, and serum- and glucocorticoid-inducible protein kinase 1 (SGK-1) [69]. SGK-1 is a signaling molecule, upregulated as early as 30 min after the MR activation whose synthesis is related to the increased cell surface density of ENaC [70]. SGK-1 inhibits the ENaC degradation [71]. Coexpression of SGK-1 and ENaC increases the sodium channel activity by fourfold [70].

SGK-1 is upregulated in several fibrotic diseases including myocardial fibrosis, lung fibrosis, liver cirrhosis, diabetic nephropathy, and glomerulonephritis [72]. In the myocardium, SGK-1 promotes myocardial fibrosis by increasing fibrotic mediators such as connective tissue growth factor and transforming growth factor-β (TGF-β); proinflammatory cytokines such as tumor necrosis factor-α (TNF-α), and interleukin-1β (IL-1β); and NADPH oxidase [73].

Apart from mineralocorticoids, SGK-1 is upregulated by a variety of hormones including glucocorticoids (GR activation), 1,25-dihydroxyvitamin D3, gonadotropins, and TGFβ [74]. Cardiomyocytes have both glucocorticoid and mineralocorticoid receptors. Glucocorticoid receptor agonist dexamethasone activates both GRs and MRs to upregulate SGK-1, which in turn activates a wide variety of transporters including Na$^+$/H$^+$ exchanger 1 (Nhe1), which is a key factor in cardiac remodeling [74].

In VSMC studies, aldosterone has been demonstrated to stimulate the expression of genes involved in fibrosis, calcification, and inflammation [75,76].

MR and blood pressure: non-genomic actions

Beyond these classic genomic effects, aldosterone also stimulates other, more rapid molecular pathways, which can be MR-independent or involve cross-talk between MR and other receptors [77]. In renal epithelia, aldosterone has been shown to cause tyrosine kinase c-Src-mediated transactivation of the epidermal growth factor receptor and the subsequent

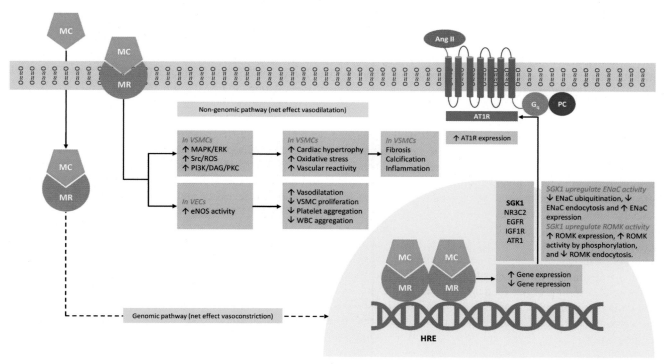

FIGURE 3.5   Schematic of the effects of mineralocorticoid on vascular smooth muscle cells (VSMCs) and vascular endothelial cells (VECs) via genomic and nongenomic pathways. *Ang II*, Angiotensin II; *ATR1*, angiotensin II type 1 receptor; *DAG*, diacylglycerol; *EGFR*, epidermal growth factor; *ENaC*, Epithelial sodium channel; *eNOS*, endothelial nitric oxide synthase; G_q, G-protein; *HRE*, hormone response element; *IGF1R*, Insulin-like growth factor 1 receptor; *MAPK*, mitogen-activated protein kinase; *MC*, mineralocorticoid; *MR*, mineralocorticoid receptor; NR3C2, MC2R gene; *PC*, phospholipase C; *PI3K*, Phosphoinositide 3-kinase; *PKC*, protein kinase C; *SGK1*, serum- and glucocorticoid-inducible protein kinase 1; *ROMK*, renal outer medullary potassium channel.

activation of the extracellular signal-regulated kinase 1/2 (ERK 1/2) and a rapid and transient increase in intracellular Ca^{2+} [78,79].

In VSMCs, stimulation with aldosterone has been shown to cause an increase in phosphorylation of tyrosine kinase c-Src via both G-protein-dependent and independent pathways, leading to subsequent activation of ERK 1/2, MAPK, and NADPH oxidase pathways resulting in profibrotic and proinflammatory pathways [80]. Interestingly, ERK activation can be blocked by an AT1R blocker [77], and several reports [81,82], in disparate cell lines, have demonstrated cross-talk between these two receptors: MR and AT1R. In cardiomyocytes, aldosterone also stimulates apoptosis via the activation of ERK 1/2 and mitochondrial superoxide formation [77]. Activation of PI3K pathways leads to increased endothelial nitric oxide synthase activity in VECs, and increased contractility of VSMCs [83]. Fig. 3.5 depicts the role of mineralocorticoids and MR in the blood pressure regulation [84,85].

Androgens, receptors, and cardiovascular system effects

Androgens exert their effect through binding to the AR. The most potent activator of the AR is dihydrotestosterone, followed by testosterone, and then much weaker stimulation from androstenedione [86]. DHEA, the predominant adrenal androgen, does not bind to the AR. Instead, it largely serves as a precursor to androgen and estrogen synthesis in other tissues. In adult males, the gonad is by far the predominant source of androgens, whereas in adult females, approximately 50% of androgens originates from the adrenal androgen synthetic pathway [87]. Normal androgen synthesis is needed for pubertal development, sexual life, and fertility in both males and females. Thus, androgen biosynthesis must be tightly regulated during fetal and postnatal life. Among vertebrates, androgen production is regulated in a species-, sex-, organ-, and mostly cell-specific manner. However, its regulation is still not fully understood.

The physiological role and clinical significance of adrenal androgen production remains unknown, and interestingly, the process of adrenarche is only observed in humans and higher primates, which means animal models studies are difficult. The development of enhanced adrenal androgen production such as in premature adrenarche as well as specific steroidogenic enzyme defects or in androgen secreting tumors are regarded as pathological states, and interestingly, premature adrenarche has been linked to PCOS in later life [30].

Androgens exert their biological actions via genomic or nongenomic mechanisms [86]. The genomic mechanism involves androgen entering the cells binding to the AR; the ligand-bound AR subsequently dimerizes, translocates into the nucleus, and binds to specific androgen response element sites located within the promoter regions of target genes to modulate transcription. The nongenomic mechanisms include upregulation of cAMP, and cytosolic Ca^{2+} levels, and activation of PKA, PKC, and MAPK. The expression of ARs is found in cardiac myocytes, endothelial cells, VSMCs, and fibroblasts.

The impact of sex differences on CVD is well established, with clear sex differences in all types of CVD. Males have higher prevalence of CVD in comparison to premenopausal women. After menopause, male and female incidence of CVD becomes comparable. The protective effect of estrogen has been long discussed and studied. Although androgens have been considered to have adverse CVD risk in previous animal and human studies, recent studies have revealed favorable effects on cardiovascular remodeling, indicating that at least physiological levels of androgens are required for cardiovascular homeostasis in males [86].

Studies using androgen receptor-knockout (ARKO) mice observed that angiotensin II-treated ARKO mice showed the reduced activation of ERKs 1,2 and 5, cardiac hypertrophy-related signaling pathways, acceleration of TGF-β1-Smad pathway, and increased expression of profibrotic genes in the heart, indicating that androgens regulate the physiological cardiac growth and modulates the cardiac adaptive hypertrophy and fibrosis [88]. The ARKO mice experiments on vascular remodeling observed that the male ARKO mice showed exaggerated angiotensin II-induced medial thickening and perivascular fibrosis, as well as angiotensin II-induced oxidative stress, and decreased the nitric oxide bioavailability in the coronary artery and aorta, thus, indicating that androgens influence angiotensin II-induced vascular remodeling by suppressing oxidative stress and preserving nitric oxide production [89]. Fig. 3.6 shows the role of androgens and their receptors in human blood pressure regulation [90,91].

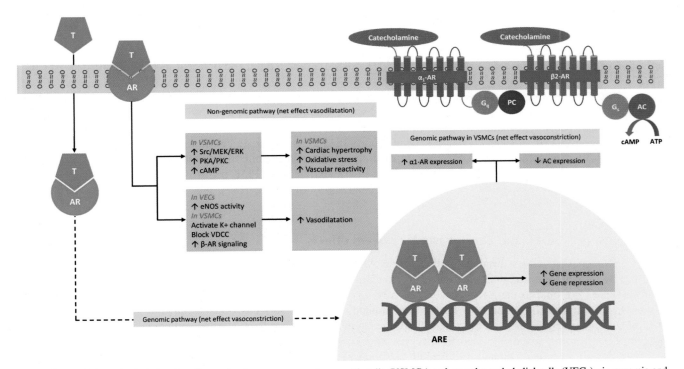

FIGURE 3.6 Schematic depicting the effects of androgens on vascular smooth cells (VSMCs) and vascular endothelial cells (VECs) via genomic and nongenomic pathways. *AC*, adenylate cyclase; *AR*, androgen receptor; *ARE*, androgen response element; *ATP*, adenosine triphosphate; *cAMP*, cyclic adenosine monophosphate; *α1-AR*, α1-adrenergic receptor; *β2-AR*, β2-adrenergic receptor; *eNOS*, endothelial nitric oxide synthase; G_q, G-protein; G_s, stimulatory G-protein; *MAPK*, mitogen-activated protein kinase; *PC*, phospholipase C; *PKA*, protein kinase A; *PKC*, protein kinase C; *T*, testosterone (androgen); *VDCC*, voltage gated calcium channel.

Pathophysiological alterations in adrenocortical hormones and effects on cardiovascular homeostasis

Glucocorticoid excess states (including non-neoplastic Cushing's)

Cushing's syndrome refers to signs and symptoms of hypercortisolism due to either the endogenous overproduction of cortisol predominantly, but also of other glucocorticoids and metabolites, or the overreplacement/use of exogenous corticosteroids (iatrogenic Cushing's). While endogenous Cushing's is relatively uncommon, with a reported worldwide prevalence of ~3/1,000,000 [92], iatrogenic Cushing's is relatively common with ~1% of the population on steroids, and approximately two thirds of those using systemic glucocorticoids showing symptoms related to excess exposure [93]. Cushing's syndrome is broadly categorized as either ACTH-dependent due to pituitary or ectopic overproduction of ACTH or rarely CRH producing tumors; or as ACTH-independent, which includes adrenal adenoma, adrenal carcinoma, adrenal hyperplasia, or exogenous glucocorticoids.

Cardiovascular events are the main cause of mortality in Cushing's syndrome, with patients displaying signs of advanced CVD including increased carotid artery intima-media thickness [94] as well as atherosclerotic plaques, hypertension, left ventricular hypertrophy, dyslipidaemia, glucose intolerance (or overt diabetes mellitus), and visceral fat deposition. Hypertension is the second most common symptom after weight gain, affecting $\approx 80\%$ of patients at diagnosis [95]. Presumably because of irreversible changes to the heart and vasculature, cardiovascular risk remains even after cure [96]. Glucocorticoids are thought to cause hypertension through several different mechanisms: (1) their intrinsic mineralocorticoid activity; (2) through activation of the renin—angiotensin system; (3) by enhancement of vasoactive substances; and (4) by causing suppression of the vasodilatory systems. In addition, glucocorticoids may exert some hypertensive effects on cardiovascular regulation through the CNS via both glucocorticoid and mineralocorticoid receptors. Glucocorticoid excess also increases risk of thrombotic events through alterations in clotting factors along with other risk factors such as obesity and increased likelihood for invasive procedures. For further reading on Cushing's syndrome, refer Chapters 13 and 14.

Mineralocorticoid excess states: primary aldosteronism (PA) and familial hyperaldosteronism

PA is increasingly recognized as a relatively common, and yet underdiagnosed cause of hypertension, with a prevalence of 5%—10% in hypertensive patients and 12%—20% of patients with resistant hypertension [97—99].

PA is the autonomous aldosterone overproduction from the adrenal gland, which in most cases is due to a unilateral aldosterone-producing adenoma (APA) or due to bilateral adrenal hyperplasia [100]. Most cases of PA are sporadic, while a small proportion of patients carry a familial form of the disease. To date, the familial forms have been classified into four different types that are associated with different genetic defects [101]. Familial hyperaldosteronism 1 (FH1), also known as glucocorticoid—remedial hyperaldosteronism (GRA), is caused by a chimeric gene: a crossing-over event that fuses the regulatory regions of CYP11B1 (11β-hydroxylase), to the coding sequence of CYP11B2 (aldosterone synthase). As a result, aldosterone synthesis occurs across multiple layers of the adrenals under the regulation of ACTH [101]. FH types 2, 3, and 4 are a result of mutations in the genes encoding ion channels and pumps, which lead to increased cytosolic concentrations of calcium in zona glomerulosa cells, and subsequently autonomous CYP11B2 expression [101]. For more reading on PA, please read Chapters 7, 8 and 21.

Large numbers of in vitro cell studies and animal model studies have demonstrated the proinflammatory and profibrotic effects of aldosterone. Constitutive activation of the MR in various tissues including cardiac myocytes, VSMCs, VECs, and macrophages has been found to promote oxidative stress, endothelial inflammation, fibrosis, and remodeling [102,103].

Disproportionately high rates of CVD are observed in patients with PA when compared to those with essential hypertension. Evidence indicates that the activation of the MR in tissues such as the heart and vasculature may help to explain this difference [102—104]. Patients with PA have higher rates of myocardial fibrosis [104,105] and increased left ventricular mass and hypertrophy when compared to blood pressure-matched patients with essential hypertension [105—107]. It is therefore unsurprising that multiple observational studies comparing PA and essential hypertension have consistently demonstrated substantially higher rates of congestive heart failure, atrial fibrillation, stroke, MI, diabetes, and cardiovascular mortality, when compared to blood pressure-matched patients with essential hypertension [98,108—115].

Surgical adrenalectomy is the recommended treatment for suitable patients [100] and is curative for most patients with unilateral PA [116—118]. Regarding longer-term outcomes, studies show that surgical adrenalectomy lowers the risk for cardiovascular events and atrial fibrillation compared with essential hypertension [110] and seemingly reduces the risk of diabetes mellitus and mortality [113]. Optimal outcomes are however mixed regarding MR antagonist therapy [110,113], with recent studies highlighting that the excess risk reported for CVD when compared to those with essential hypertension was limited to those whose renin remained suppressed on treatment [110].

Apparent mineralocorticoid excess

The syndrome of apparent mineralocorticoid excess (AME) is a genetic disorder that manifests clinically as PA (hypertension, hypokalaemia, metabolic alkalosis, and low plasma renin); however, plasma aldosterone and renin levels are both low in this condition. In AME, mutations in the CYP11B2 gene result in absent or impaired activity of the enzyme 11β-hydroxysteroid dehydrogenase Type 2, leading to cortisol-mediated activation of the MR. In severe forms, apart from findings of primary PA, signs and symptoms include low birth weight, failure to thrive, early childhood severe hypertension with target organ damage, hypercalciuria and nephrocalcinosis (unknown mechanism), and renal failure [119]. Milder forms may present with a phenotype indistinguishable from essential hypertension [120].

Androgen deficiency/excess states (including congenital disorders such as CAH)

Androgen deficiency and blood pressure

Androgens have an important role to play in metabolism, adipose tissue, and endothelial cell function. Androgen deficiency is associated with increased visceral fat deposition, promotion of a chronic inflammatory state through various mechanisms including nuclear factor kappa B (NF-kB) activation, adipocyte dysfunction with reduced adiponectin/leptin ratio, altered endothelial function, and hypertension [121]. Thus, in men and postmenopausal women, androgen deficiency is associated with an increased prevalence of hypertension and CVD. In men with androgen deficiency, androgen replacement reduces both systolic as well as diastolic blood pressure [122]. On the other hand, in men without androgen deficiency, androgen replacement exacerbates the hypertension and the cardiovascular risk.

Androgen excess and blood pressure

In children and adolescents with congenital adrenal hyperplasia due to 21-hydroxylase deficiency, an increased prevalence of systolic blood pressure (12.2% vs. 3.5% in normal children and adolescents) noted was not related to the androgen levels (androgen excess states) but related to the glucocorticoid treatment [123]. On the other hand, contrary to the previous belief that hyperandrogenism has little effect per se in inducing hypertension in young women of reproductive age, a recent study on women with androgen excess polycystic ovary syndrome (AE-PCOS) observed that the androgen excess state is associated with decreased NO production, increased endothelin-1 production, and endothelial dysfunction [124]. Although women with AE-PCOS commonly manifest with a spectrum of risk factors like obesity, insulin resistance, and hypertension, the androgen excess itself is a driver of endothelial dysfunction [125].

Causes of androgen excess in men can be endogenous (CAH, or tumors) or exogenous (androgenic steroid abuse including testosterone, DHEA, or androstenedione). Causes of androgen excess in women can be endogenous (PCOS or CAH) or exogenous (rare) [30].

Various pathophysiological mechanisms with which androgen excess causes hypertension (especially in premenopausal women) include modulation of vascular endothelial growth factor (VEGF), extracellular matrix proteins like matrix metalloproteinase-9 (MMP-9), and vasoconstricting metabolite of arachidonic acid known as 20-hydroxyeicosatetraenoic acid [126]. These can increase the renal microvascular reactivity, activate NF-kB, increase reactive oxygen species (ROS) production, and deplete NO bioavailability, resulting in hypertension [127]. Similarly, androgen excess states with upregulation of ARs can cause activation of renin−angiotensin system (RAAS) in kidneys and adipose tissue. Androgens can induce VSMC migration via NADPH oxidase-derived ROS production and c-Src−dependent pathways. Finally, in the VSMCs, androgens can increase α1-adrenergic receptor and decrease adenylate cyclase expression, favoring hypertension [91].

Emerging research questions

The complex interplay of genomic and nongenomic stimulatory and inhibitory cellular signaling pathways makes it unsurprising that clinical data are often confounded by overlapping genetic and environmental factors. Animal studies, especially gene knock out studies, have provided invaluable information but sometimes report conflicting results, and may limit applicability to humans. Studies into the tissue-specific effects of mineralocorticoid receptors and their subsequent inhibition raise tantalizing prospects of novel therapeutic agents for reducing blood pressure and atherosclerotic plaque formation and progression. Closing the gap on sex differences in CVD may also lead to interesting insights and novel agents. Determining the benefits in terms of long-term health outcomes in seeking to identify or screen patients for early and mild PA should be a priority, especially since the long-term sequelae of PA are well understood.

Summary and conclusions

Mineralocorticoids, predominantly aldosterone, through the RAAS, regulate BP through several different mechanisms: predominantly through the MR receptor, but also via other nongenomic pathways, including oxidative stress, inflammation, fibrosis, vascular tonicity, and endothelial dysfunction.

Glucocorticoids, predominantly cortisol, affect blood pressure through several different mechanisms: (1) intrinsic mineralocorticoid activity; (2) activation of the RAAS; (3) enhancement of vasoactive substances; and (4) suppression of the vasodilatory systems. In addition, glucocorticoids may exert some hypertensive effects on cardiovascular regulation through the CNS via both glucocorticoid and mineralocorticoid receptors.

Both androgen deficiency and excess may be associated with hypertension. The physiological role of adrenal androgens is likely to be of greater significance in women since the major source of androgens in men are the testes. Various pathophysiological mechanisms with which androgen excess causes hypertension (especially premenopausal women) include modulation of VEGF, extracellular matrix proteins like matrix metalloproteinase-9 (MMP-9), and vasoconstricting metabolite of arachidonic acid known as 20-hydroxyeicosatetraenoic acid.

Learning points

1. Aldosterone, the predominant mineralocorticoid, via the mineralocorticoid receptor (MR), is the main steroid hormone involved in BP regulation.
2. Aldosterone secretion is largely regulated by the renin–angiotensin system, and to a lesser extent, extracellular K^+ ion concentration.
3. The MR has a similar affinity for aldosterone and glucocorticoids. In epithelial tissues, endothelial cells, and smooth muscle cells, the enzyme 11β-hydroxysteroid dehydrogenase type 2 (11HSD2) rapidly converts endogenous glucocorticoids to inactive metabolites, thus providing MR selectivity for aldosterone.
4. Several nongenomic pathways induced by mineralocorticoids and glucocorticoids may have a role in BP regulation.
5. The physiological role, if any, of adrenal androgens on BP regulation is unclear. Low levels of androgens in men and increased levels of androgens in women, however, are associated with increased risk of hypertension and CVD.

References

[1] Baranowski ES, Arlt W, Idkowiak J. Monogenic disorders of adrenal steroidogenesis. Horm Res Paediatr 2018;89(5):292−310. https://doi.org/10.1159/000488034. PMID: 29874650.

[2] Genest J, Biron P, Koiw E, Nowaczynski W, Chretien M, Boucher R. Adrenocortical hormones in human hypertension and their relation to angiotensin. Circ Res 1961;9:775−91. https://doi.org/10.1161/01.res.9.3.775. PMID: 13704360.

[3] Husebye ES, Pearce SH, Krone NP, Kämpe O. Adrenal insufficiency. Lancet 2021;397(10274):613−29. https://doi.org/10.1016/S0140-6736(21)00136-7. PMID: 33484633.

[4] Puar TH, Stikkelbroeck NM, Smans LC, Zelissen PM, Hermus AR. Adrenal crisis: still a deadly event in the 21st century. Am J Med 2016;129(3):339.e1−9. https://doi.org/10.1016/j.amjmed.2015.08.021. PMID: 26363354.

[5] Kraemer FB, Shen WJ. Hormone-sensitive lipase: control of intracellular tri-(di) acylglycerol and cholesteryl ester hydrolysis. J Lipid Res 2002;43:1585−94.

[6] Lin D, et al. Role of steroidogenic acute regulatory protein in adrenal and gonadal steroidogenesis. Science 1995;267:1828−31.

[7] Abdel-Malek ZA. Melanocortin receptors: their functions and regulation by physiological agonists and antagonists. Cell Mol Life Sci 2001;58:434−41.

[8] Smith LIF, Zhao Z, Walker J, Lightman S, Spiga F. Activation and expression of endogenous CREB-regulated transcription coactivators (CRTC) 1, 2 and 3 in the rat adrenal gland. J Neuroendocrinol January 2021;33(1):e12920. https://doi.org/10.1111/jne.12920. PMID: 33314405; PMCID: PMC7900988.

[9] Vargas VE, Kaushal KM, Monau TR, Myers DA, Ducsay CA. Extracellular signal-regulated kinases (ERK1/2) signaling pathway plays a role in cortisol secretion in the long-term hypoxic ovine fetal adrenal near term. Am J Physiol Regul Integr Comp Physiol April 15, 2013;304(8):R636−43. https://doi.org/10.1152/ajpregu.00318.2012. PMID: 23427082.

[10] Chung S, Son GH, Kim K. Circadian rhythm of adrenal glucocorticoid: its regulation and clinical implications. Biochim Biophys Acta May 2011;1812(5):581−91. https://doi.org/10.1016/j.bbadis.2011.02.003. PMID: 21320597.

[11] Xing Y, Parker CR, Edwards M, Rainey WE. ACTH is a potent regulator of gene expression in human adrenal cells. J Mol Endocrinol July 2010;45(1):59−68. https://doi.org/10.1677/JME-10-0006. PMID: 20460446.

[12] Ruggiero C, Lalli E. Impact of ACTH signaling on transcriptional regulation of steroidogenic genes. Front Endocrinol March 29, 2016;7:24. https://doi.org/10.3389/fendo.2016.00024. PMID: 27065945.

[13] Miller WL, Auchus RJ. The molecular biology, biochemistry, and physiology of human steroidogenesis and its disorders. Endocr Rev 2011;32(1):81−151.

[14] El Ghorayeb N, Bourdeau I, Lacroix A. Role of ACTH and other hormones in the regulation of aldosterone production in primary aldosteronism. Front Endocrinol June 27, 2016;7:72. https://doi.org/10.3389/fendo.2016.00072. PMID: 27445975.

[15] Hattangady NG, Olala LO, Bollag WB, Rainey WE. Acute and chronic regulation of aldosterone production. Mol Cell Endocrinol 2012;350(2):151−62.

[16] Bassett MH, White PC, Rainey WE. The regulation of aldosterone synthase expression. Mol Cell Endocrinol 2004;217(1−2):67−74.

[17] Spät A, Hunyady L. Control of aldosterone secretion: a model for convergence in cellular signaling pathways. Physiol Rev April 2004;84(2):489−539. https://doi.org/10.1152/physrev.00030.2003. PMID: 15044681.

[18] Lymperopoulos A, Rengo G, Zincarelli C, Kim J, Soltys S, Koch WJ. An adrenal beta-arrestin 1-mediated signaling pathway underlies angiotensin II-induced aldosterone production in vitro and in vivo. Proc Natl Acad Sci U S A April 7, 2009;106(14):5825−30. https://doi.org/10.1073/pnas.0811706106. PMID: 19289825.

[19] Spat A. Glomerulosa cell—a unique sensor of extracellular K^+ concentration. Mol Cell Endocrinol 2004;217(1−2):23−6.

[20] Nogueira EF, Gerry D, Mantero F, Mariniello B, Rainey WE. The role of TASK1 in aldosterone production and its expression in normal adrenal and aldosterone-producing adenomas. Clin Endocrinol 2010;73:22−9.

[21] Nanba K, Chen A, Nishimoto K, Rainey WE. Role of Ca^{2+}/calmodulin-dependent protein kinase in adrenal aldosterone production. Endocrinology 2015;156(5):1750−6. https://doi.org/10.1210/en.2014-1782.

[22] Condon JC, Pezzi V, Drummond BM, Yin S, Rainey WE. Calmodulin-dependent kinase I regulates adrenal cell expression of aldosterone synthase. Endocrinology 2002;143(9):3651−7.

[23] Young DB, Smith MJ, Jackson TE, Scott RE. Multiplicative interaction between angiotensin II and K concentration in stimulation of aldosterone. Am J Physiol 1984;247:E328−35.

[24] Pereira SS, Lobato CB, Monteiro MP. Cell signaling within endocrine glands: thyroid, parathyroids and adrenal glands. In: Silva J, Freitas M, Fardilha M, editors. Tissue-specific cell signaling. Cham: Springer; 2020. https://doi.org/10.1007/978-3-030-44436-5_3.

[25] Mulatero P, Curnow KM, Aupetit-Faisant B, Foekling M, Gomez-Sanchez C, Veglio F, et al. Recombinant CYP11B genes encode enzymes that can catalyze conversion of 11-deoxycortisol to cortisol, 18-hydroxycortisol, and 18-oxocortisol. J Clin Endocrinol Metab 1998;83:3996−4001.

[26] Vinson GP. Functional zonation of the adult mammalian adrenal cortex. Front Neurol 2016;10:238.

[27] Ilhan R, Üner G, Yilmaz S, Atalay Sahar E, Cayli S, Erzurumlu Y, Gozen O, Ballar Kirmizibayrak P. Novel regulation mechanism of adrenal cortisol and DHEA biosynthesis via the endogen ERAD inhibitor small VCP-interacting protein. Sci Rep January 18, 2022;12(1):869. https://doi.org/10.1038/s41598-022-04821-y. PMID: 35042898.

[28] Walker JJ, Spiga F, Waite E, Zhao Z, Kershaw Y, Terry JR, Lightman SL. The origin of glucocorticoid hormone oscillations. PLoS Biol 2012;10(6):e1001341. https://doi.org/10.1371/journal.pbio.1001341. PMID: 22679394.

[29] Havelock JC, Auchus RJ, Rainey WE. The rise in adrenal androgen biosynthesis: adrenarche. Semin Reprod Med 2004;22:337−47.

[30] Udhane SS, Flück CE. Regulation of human (adrenal) androgen biosynthesis—new insights from novel throughput technology studies. Biochem Pharmacol February 15, 2016;102:2−33. https://doi.org/10.1016/j.bcp.2015.10.010. PMID: 26498719.

[31] Auchus RJ, Rainey WE. Adrenarche—physiology, biochemistry, and human disease. Clin Endocrinol 2004;60:288−96.

[32] Nakamura Y, Hornsby PJ, Casson P, Morimoto R, Satoh F, Xing Y, Kennedy MR, Sasano H, Rainey WE. Type 5 17β-hydroxysteroid dehydrogenase (AKR 1C3) contributes to testosterone production in the adrenal reticularis. J Clin Endocrinol Metab 2009;94:2192−8.

[33] Whirledge S, DeFranco DB. Glucocorticoid signaling in health and disease: insights from tissue-specific GR knockout mice. Endocrinology 2018;159(1):46−64. https://doi.org/10.1210/en.2017-00728. PMID: 29029225.

[34] Zhou J, Cidlowski JA. The human glucocorticoid receptor: one gene, multiple proteins and diverse responses. Steroids 2005;70(5−7):407−17.

[35] Heery DM, Kalkhoven E, Hoare S, Parker MG. A signature motif in transcriptional co-activators mediates binding to nuclear receptors. Nature 1997;387(6634):733−6.

[36] Kino T, De Martino MU, Charmandari E, Mirani M, Chrousos GP. Tissue glucocorticoid resistance/hypersensitivity syndromes. J Steroid Biochem Mol Biol 2003;85(2−5):457−67.

[37] Hunter RW, Ivy JR, Bailey MA. Glucocorticoids and renal Na^+ transport: implications for hypertension and salt sensitivity. J Physiol April 15, 2014;592(8):1731−44. https://doi.org/10.1113/jphysiol.2013.267609. PMID: 24535442.

[38] Vandevyver S, Dejager L, Libert C. Comprehensive overview of the structure and regulation of the glucocorticoid receptor. Endocr Rev August 2014;35(4):671−93. https://doi.org/10.1210/er.2014-1010. PMID: 24937701.

[39] de Lange P, Segeren CM, Koper JW, Wiemer E, Sonneveld P, Brinkmann AO, et al. Expression in hematological malignancies of a glucocorticoid receptor splice variant that augments glucocorticoid receptor-mediated effects in transfected cells. Cancer Res May 15, 2001;61(10):3937−41. PMID: 11358809.

[40] Gaitan D, DeBold CR, Turney MK, Zhou P, Orth DN, Kovacs WJ. Glucocorticoid receptor structure and function in an adrenocorticotropin-secreting small cell lung cancer. Mol Endocrinol 1995;9:1193−201.

[41] Lu NZ, Collins JB, Grissom SF, Cidlowski JA. Selective regulation of bone cell apoptosis by translational isoforms of the glucocorticoid receptor. Mol Cell Biol October 2007;27(20):7143−60. https://doi.org/10.1128/MCB.00253-07. PMID: 17682054.

[42] Kino T, Su YA, Chrousos GP. Human glucocorticoid receptor isoform beta: recent understanding of its potential implications in physiology and pathophysiology. Cell Mol Life Sci November 2009;66(21):3435−48. https://doi.org/10.1007/s00018-009-0098-z. PMID: 19633971.

[43] Lewis-Tuffin LJ, Cidlowski JA. The physiology of human glucocorticoid receptor beta (hGRbeta) and glucocorticoid resistance. Ann N Y Acad Sci June 2006;1069:1−9. https://doi.org/10.1196/annals.1351.001. PMID: 16855130.

[44] Goodwin JE, Geller DS. Glucocorticoid-induced hypertension. Pediatr Nephrol 2012;27:1059−66.

[45] Goodwin JE, Zhang J, Geller DS. A critical role for vascular smooth muscle in acute glucocorticoid-induced hypertension. J Am Soc Nephrol 2008;19:1291−9.

[46] Goodwin JE, Zhang J, Gonzalez D, Albinsson S, Geller DS. Knockout of the vascular endothelial glucocorticoid receptor abrogates dexamethasone-induced hypertension. J Hypertens 2011;29:1347−56.

[47] Yang S, Zhang L. Glucocorticoids, and vascular reactivity. Curr Vasc Pharmacol 2004;2:1−12.

[48] Sato A, Suzuki H, Nakazato Y, Shibata H, Inagami T, Saruta T. Increased expression of vascular angiotensin ii type 1a receptor gene in glucocorticoid-induced hypertension. J Hypertens 1994;12:511−6.

[49] Kornel L, Prancan AV, Kanamarlapudi N, Hynes J, Kuzianik E. Study on the mechanisms of glucocorticoid-induced hypertension: glucocorticoids increase transmembrane Ca^{2+} influx in vascular smooth muscle in vivo. Endocr Res 1995;21:203−10.

[50] Hafezi-Moghadam A, Simoncini T, Yang Z, Limbourg FP, Plumier JC, Rebsamen MC, Hsieh CM, Chui DS, Thomas KL, Prorock AJ, Laubach VE, Moskowitz MA, French BA, Ley K, Liao JK. Acute cardiovascular protective effects of corticosteroids are mediated by non-transcriptional activation of endothelial nitric oxide synthase. Nat Med May 2002;8(5):473−9. https://doi.org/10.1038/nm0502-473. PMID: 11984591.

[51] Nicolaides NC, Charmandari E. Primary generalized glucocorticoid resistance and hypersensitivity syndromes: a 2021 update. Int J Mol Sci October 7, 2021;22(19):10839. https://doi.org/10.3390/ijms221910839. PMID: 34639183.

[52] Meduri GU, Chrousos GP. General adaptation in critical illness: glucocorticoid receptor-alpha master regulator of homeostatic corrections. Front Endocrinol April 22, 2020;11:161. https://doi.org/10.3389/fendo.2020.00161. PMID: 32390938.

[53] Verrey F. Transcriptional control of sodium transport in tight epithelial by adrenal steroids. J Membr Biol March 1995;144(2):93−110. https://doi.org/10.1007/BF00232796. PMID: 7595948.

[54] Baker ME, Katsu Y. 30 years OF the mineralocorticoid receptor: evolution of the mineralocorticoid receptor: sequence, structure, and function. J Endocrinol July 2017;234(1):T1−16. https://doi.org/10.1530/JOE-16-0661. PMID: 28468932.

[55] Edwards CR, Stewart PM, Burt D, Brett L, McIntyre MA, Sutanto WS, de Kloet ER, Monder C. Localisation of 11 beta-hydroxysteroid dehydrogenase—tissue specific protector of the mineralocorticoid receptor. Lancet October 29, 1988;2(8618):986−9. https://doi.org/10.1016/s0140-6736(88)90742-8. PMID: 2902493.

[56] Funder JW, Pearce PT, Smith R, Smith AI. Mineralocorticoid action: target tissue specificity is enzyme, not receptor, mediated. Science October 28, 1988;242(4878):583−5. https://doi.org/10.1126/science.2845584. PMID: 2845584.

[57] Odermatt A, Kratschmar DV. Tissue-specific modulation of mineralocorticoid receptor function by 11β-hydroxysteroid dehydrogenases: an overview. Mol Cell Endocrinol March 24, 2012;350(2):168−86. https://doi.org/10.1016/j.mce.2011.07.020. PMID: 21820034.

[58] Viengchareun S, Le Menuet D, Martinerie L, Munier M, Pascual-Le Tallec L, Lombès M. The mineralocorticoid receptor: insights into its molecular and (patho)physiological biology. Nucl Recept Signal November 30, 2007;5:e012. https://doi.org/10.1621/nrs.05012. PMID: 18174920.

[59] Fuller PJ, Verity K. Mineralocorticoid receptor gene expression in the gastrointestinal tract: distribution and ontogeny. J Steroid Biochem July 4, 1990;36(4):263−7. https://doi.org/10.1016/0022-4731(90)90215-e. PMID: 2168006.

[60] Rickard AJ, Morgan J, Tesch G, Funder JW, Fuller PJ, Young MJ. Deletion of mineralocorticoid receptors from macrophages protects against deoxycorticosterone/salt-induced cardiac fibrosis and increased blood pressure. Hypertension September 2009;54(3):537−43. https://doi.org/10.1161/HYPERTENSIONAHA.109.131110. PMID: 19635989.

[61] Arriza JL, Simerly RB, Swanson LW, Evans RM. The neuronal mineralocorticoid receptor as a mediator of glucocorticoid response. Neuron November 1988;1(9):887−900. https://doi.org/10.1016/0896-6273(88)90136-5. PMID: 2856104.

[62] Savory JG, Préfontaine GG, Lamprecht C, Liao M, Walther RF, Lefebvre YA, Haché RJ. Glucocorticoid receptor homodimers and glucocorticoid-mineralocorticoid receptor heterodimers form in the cytoplasm through alternative dimerization interfaces. Mol Cell Biol February 2001;21(3):781−93. https://doi.org/10.1128/MCB.21.3.781-793.2001. PMID: 11154266.

[63] McEwan IJ, Lavery D, Fischer K, Watt K. Natural disordered sequences in the amino terminal domain of nuclear receptors: lessons from the androgen and glucocorticoid receptors. Nucl Recept Signal March 9, 2007;5:e001. https://doi.org/10.1621/nrs.05001. PMID: 17464357.

[64] Fischer K, Kelly SM, Watt K, Price NC, McEwan IJ. Conformation of the mineralocorticoid receptor N-terminal domain: evidence for induced and stable structure. Mol Endocrinol October 2010;24(10):1935−48. https://doi.org/10.1210/me.2010-0005. PMID: 20685853.

[65] Binart N, Lombès M, Baulieu EE. Distinct functions of the 90 kDa heat-shock protein (hsp90) in oestrogen and mineralocorticosteroid receptor activity: effects of hsp90 deletion mutants. Biochem J November 1, 1995;311(Pt 3):797−804. https://doi.org/10.1042/bj3110797. PMID: 7487934.

[66] Huyet J, Pinon GM, Fay MR, Rafestin-Oblin ME, Fagart J. Structural determinants of ligand binding to the mineralocorticoid receptor. Mol Cell Endocrinol March 24, 2012;350(2):187−95. https://doi.org/10.1016/j.mce.2011.07.035. PMID: 21820032.

[67] Faresse N, Ruffieux-Daidie D, Salamin M, Gomez-Sanchez CE, Staub O. Mineralocorticoid receptor degradation is promoted by Hsp90 inhibition and the ubiquitin-protein ligase CHIP. Am J Physiol Ren Physiol December 2010;299(6):F1462−72. https://doi.org/10.1152/ajprenal.00285.2010. PMID: 20861078.

[68] Lombès M, Binart N, Oblin ME, Joulin V, Baulieu EE. Characterization of the interaction of the human mineralocorticosteroid receptor with hormone response elements. Biochem J June 1, 1993;292(Pt 2):577—83. https://doi.org/10.1042/bj2920577. PMID: 8389140.

[69] Bhargava A, Wang J, Pearce D. Regulation of epithelial ion transport by aldosterone through changes in gene expression. Mol Cell Endocrinol March 31, 2004;217(1—2):189—96. https://doi.org/10.1016/j.mce.2003.10.020. PMID: 15134817.

[70] Shigaev A, Asher C, Latter H, Garty H, Reuveny E. Regulation of sgk by aldosterone and its effects on the epithelial Na$^+$ channel. Am J Physiol Ren Physiol April 2000;278(4):F613—9. https://doi.org/10.1152/ajprenal.2000.278.4.F613. PMID: 10751222.

[71] Snyder PM, Olson DR, Thomas BC. Serum and glucocorticoid-regulated kinase modulates Nedd4-2-mediated inhibition of the epithelial Na$^+$ channel. J Biol Chem January 4, 2002;277(1):5—8. https://doi.org/10.1074/jbc.C100623200. PMID: 11696533.

[72] Terada Y, Kuwana H, Kobayashi T, Okado T, Suzuki N, Yoshimoto T, Hirata Y, Sasaki S. Aldosterone-stimulated SGK1 activity mediates profibrotic signaling in the mesangium. J Am Soc Nephrol February 2008;19(2):298—309. https://doi.org/10.1681/ASN.2007050531. PMID: 18184857.

[73] Gan W, Ren J, Li T, Lv S, Li C, Liu Z, et al. The SGK1 inhibitor EMD638683, prevents Angiotensin II-induced cardiac inflammation and fibrosis by blocking NLRP3 inflammasome activation. Biochim Biophys Acta (BBA)—Mol Basis Dis January 2018;1864(1):1—10. https://doi.org/10.1016/j.bbadis.2017.10.001. PMID: 28986310.

[74] Voelkl J, Pasham V, Ahmed MS, Walker B, Szteyn K, Kuhl D, Metzler B, Alesutan I, Lang F. Sgk1-dependent stimulation of cardiac Na$^+$/H$^+$ exchanger Nhe1 by dexamethasone. Cell Physiol Biochem 2013;32(1):25—38. https://doi.org/10.1159/000350120. PMID: 23860121.

[75] Jaffe IZ, Tintut Y, Newfell BG, Demer LL, Mendelsohn ME. Mineralocorticoid receptor activation promotes vascular cell calcification. Arterioscler Thromb Vasc Biol April 2007;27(4):799—805. https://doi.org/10.1161/01.ATV.0000258414.59393.89. PMID: 17234727.

[76] Wu SY, Yu YR, Cai Y, Jia LX, Wang X, Xiao CS, Tang CS, Qi YF. Endogenous aldosterone is involved in vascular calcification in rat. Exp Biol Med January 2012;237(1):31—7. https://doi.org/10.1258/ebm.2011.011175. PMID: 22185918.

[77] Cannavo A, Liccardo D, Eguchi A, Elliott KJ, Traynham CJ, Ibetti J, et al. Myocardial pathology induced by aldosterone is dependent on non-canonical activities of G protein-coupled receptor kinases. Nat Commun March 2, 2016;7:10877. https://doi.org/10.1038/ncomms10877. PMID: 26932512.

[78] Markos F, Healy V, Harvey BJ. Aldosterone rapidly activates Na$^+$/H$^+$ exchange in M-1 cortical collecting duct cells via a PKC-MAPK pathway. Nephron Physiol 2005;99(1):p1—9. https://doi.org/10.1159/000081796. PMID: 15637466.

[79] Grossmann C, Benesic A, Krug AW, Freudinger R, Mildenberger S, Gassner B, Gekle M. Human mineralocorticoid receptor expression renders cells responsive for nongenotropic aldosterone actions. Mol Endocrinol July 2005;19(7):1697—710. https://doi.org/10.1210/me.2004-0469. PMID: 15761031.

[80] Callera GE, Touyz RM, Tostes RC, Yogi A, He Y, Malkinson S, Schiffrin EL. Aldosterone activates vascular p38MAP kinase and NADPH oxidase via c-Src. Hypertension 2005;45:773—9.

[81] Rautureau Y, Paradis P, Schiffrin EL. Crosstalk between aldosterone and angiotensin signaling in vascular smooth muscle cells. Steroids August 2011;76(9):834—9. https://doi.org/10.1016/j.steroids.2011.02.015. PMID: 21371487.

[82] Tsai CF, Yang SF, Chu HJ, Ueng KC. Crosstalk between mineralocorticoid receptor/angiotensin II type 1 receptor and mitogen-activated protein kinase pathways underlies aldosterone-induced atrial fibrotic responses in HL-1 cardiomyocytes. Int J Cardiol October 25, 2013;169(1):17—28. https://doi.org/10.1016/j.ijcard.2013.06.046. PMID: 24120080.

[83] Mutoh A, Isshiki M, Fujita T. Aldosterone enhances ligand-stimulated nitric oxide production in endothelial cells. Hypertens Res September 2008;31(9):1811—20. https://doi.org/10.1291/hypres.31.1811. PMID: 18971560.

[84] Ong GS, Young MJ. Mineralocorticoid regulation of cell function: the role of rapid signalling and gene transcription pathways. J Mol Endocrinol January 2017;58(1):R33—57. https://doi.org/10.1530/JME-15-0318. PMID: 27821439.

[85] Valinsky WC, Touyz RM, Shrier A. Aldosterone, SGK1, and ion channels in the kidney. Clin Sci (Lond) January 19, 2018;132(2):173—83. https://doi.org/10.1042/CS20171525. PMID: 29352074.

[86] Ikeda Y, Aihara K, Yoshida S, Akaike M, Matsumoto T. Effects of androgens on cardiovascular remodeling. J Endocrinol July 2012;214(1):1—10. https://doi.org/10.1530/JOE-12-0126. PMID: 22493003.

[87] Puurunen J, Piltonen T, Jaakkola P, Ruokonen A, Morin-Papunen L, Tapanainen JS. Adrenal androgen production capacity remains high up to menopause in women with polycystic ovary syndrome. J Clin Endocrinol Metab June 2009;94(6):1973—8. https://doi.org/10.1210/jc.2008-2583. PMID: 19318449.

[88] Ikeda Y, Aihara K, Sato T, Akaike M, Yoshizumi M, Suzaki Y, et al. Androgen receptor gene knockout male mice exhibit impaired cardiac growth and exacerbation of angiotensin II-induced cardiac fibrosis. J Biol Chem August 19, 2005;280(33):29661—6. https://doi.org/10.1074/jbc.M411694200. PMID: 15961403.

[89] Ikeda Y, Aihara K, Yoshida S, Sato T, Yagi S, et al. Androgen-androgen receptor system protects against angiotensin II-induced vascular remodeling. Endocrinology June 2009;150(6):2857—64. https://doi.org/10.1210/en.2008-1254. PMID: 19196803.

[90] Lucas-Herald AK, Alves-Lopes R, Montezano AC, Ahmed SF, Touyz RM. Genomic and non-genomic effects of androgens in the cardiovascular system: clinical implications. Clin Sci (Lond) July 1, 2017;131(13):1405—18. https://doi.org/10.1042/CS20170090. PMID: 28645930.

[91] Carbajal-García A, Reyes-García J, Montaño LM. Androgen effects on the adrenergic system of the vascular, airway, and cardiac myocytes and their relevance in pathological processes. Int J Endocrinol November 12, 2020;2020:8849641. https://doi.org/10.1155/2020/8849641. PMID: 33273918.

[92] Clayton RN, Jones PW, Reulen RC, Stewart PM, Hassan-Smith ZK, Ntali G, et al. Mortality in patients with Cushing's disease more than 10 years after remission: a multicentre, multinational, retrospective cohort study. Lancet Diabetes Endocrinol 2016;4:569−76. https://doi.org/10.1016/S2213-8587(16)30005-5.

[93] Fardet L, Flahault A, Kettaneh A, Tiev KP, Généreau T, Tolédano C, et al. Corticosteroid-induced clinical adverse events: frequency, risk factors and patient's opinion. Br J Dermatol 2007;157:142−8.

[94] Neary NM, Booker OJ, Abel BS, Matta JR, Muldoon N, Sinaii N, et al. Hypercortisolism is associated with increased coronary arterial atherosclerosis: analysis of noninvasive coronary angiography using multidetector computerized tomography. J Clin Endocrinol Metab 2013;98(5):2045−52.

[95] Pivonello R, Isidori AM, De Martino MC, Newell-Price J, Biller BMK, Colao A. Complications of Cushing's syndrome: state of the art. Lancet Diabetes Endocrinol 2016;4:611−29. https://doi.org/10.1016/S2213-8587(16)00086-3.

[96] Faggiano A, Pivonello R, Spiezia S, De Martino MC, Filippella M, Di Somma C, et al. Cardiovascular risk factors and common carotid artery caliber and stiffness in patients with Cushing's disease during active disease and 1 year after disease remission. J Clin Endocrinol Metab 2003;88(6):2527−33.

[97] Kayser SC, Dekkers T, Groenewoud HJ, van der Wilt GJ, Carel Bakx J, van der Wel MC, et al. Study heterogeneity and estimation of prevalence of primary aldosteronism: a systematic review and meta-regression analysis. J Clin Endocrinol Metab 2016;101(7):2826−35.

[98] Monticone S, Burrello J, Tizzani D, Bertello C, Viola A, Buffolo F, et al. Prevalence and clinical manifestations of primary aldosteronism encountered in primary care practice. J Am Coll Cardiol 2017;69(14):1811−20.

[99] Carey RM, Calhoun DA, Bakris GL, Brook RD, Daugherty SL, Dennison-Himmelfarb CR, et al. Resistant hypertension: detection, evaluation, and management: a scientific statement from the American Heart Association. Hypertension 2018;72(5):e53−90.

[100] Funder JW, Carey RM, Mantero F, Murad MH, Reincke M, Shibata H, et al. The management of primary aldosteronism: case detection, diagnosis, and treatment: an endocrine society clinical practice guideline. J Clin Endocrinol Metab 2016;101(5):1889−916.

[101] Fernandes-Rosa FL, Boulkroun S, Zennaro MC. Genetic and genomic mechanisms of primary aldosteronism. Trends Mol Med September 2020;26(9):819−32. https://doi.org/10.1016/j.molmed.2020.05.005. PMID: 32563556.

[102] Diaz-Otero JM, Fisher C, Downs K, Moss ME, Jaffe IZ, Jackson WF, et al. Endothelial mineralocorticoid receptor mediates parenchymal arteriole and posterior cerebral artery remodeling during angiotensin II-induced hypertension. Hypertension 2017;70(6):1113−21.

[103] McCurley A, Pires PW, Bender SB, Aronovitz M, Zhao MJ, Metzger D, et al. Direct regulation of blood pressure by smooth muscle cell mineralocorticoid receptors. Nat Med 2012;18(9):1429−33.

[104] Tesch GH, Young MJ. Mineralocorticoid receptor signaling as a therapeutic target for renal and cardiac fibrosis. Front Pharmacol 2017;8:313.

[105] Matsumura K, Fujii K, Oniki H, Oka M, Iida M. Role of aldosterone in left ventricular hypertrophy in hypertension. Am J Hypertens 2006;19(1):13−8.

[106] Rossi GP, Sacchetto A, Pavan E, Palatini P, Graniero GR, Canali C, et al. Remodeling of the left ventricle in primary aldosteronism due to Conn's adenoma. Circulation 1997;95(6):1471−8.

[107] Cesari M, Letizia C, Angeli P, Sciomer S, Rosi S, Rossi GP. Cardiac remodeling in patients with primary and secondary aldosteronism: a tissue Doppler study. Circ Cardiovasc Imaging June 2016;9(6):e004815. https://doi.org/10.1161/CIRCIMAGING.116.004815. PMID: 27307552.

[108] Mulatero P, Monticone S, Bertello C, Viola A, Tizzani D, Iannaccone A, et al. Long-term cardio- and cerebrovascular events in patients with primary aldosteronism. J Clin Endocrinol Metab 2013;98(12):4826−33.

[109] Savard S, Amar L, Plouin PF, Steichen O. Cardiovascular complications associated with primary aldosteronism: a controlled cross-sectional study. Hypertension 2013;62(2):331−6.

[110] Hundemer GL, Curhan GC, Yozamp N, Wang M, Vaidya A. Incidence of atrial fibrillation and mineralocorticoid receptor activity in patients with medically and surgically treated primary aldosteronism. JAMA Cardiol 2018;3(8):768−74.

[111] Reincke M, Fischer E, Gerum S, Merkle K, Schulz S, Pallauf A, et al. Observational study mortality in treated primary aldosteronism: the German Conn's registry. Hypertension 2012;60(3):618−24.

[112] Hanslik G, Wallaschofski H, Dietz A, Riester A, Reincke M, Allolio B, et al. Increased prevalence of diabetes mellitus and the metabolic syndrome in patients with primary aldosteronism of the German Conn's Registry. Eur J Endocrinol 2015;173(5):665−75.

[113] Wu VC, Chueh SJ, Chen L, Chang CH, Hu YH, Lin YH, et al. Risk of new-onset diabetes mellitus in primary aldosteronism: a population study over 5 years. J Hypertens 2017;35(8):1698−708.

[114] Reil JC, Tauchnitz M, Tian Q, et al. Hyperaldosteronism induces left atrial systolic and diastolic dysfunction. Am J Physiol Heart Circ Physiol 2016;311(4):H1014−23. https://doi.org/10.1152/ajpheart.00261.2016.

[115] Seccia TM, Caroccia B, Adler GK, Maiolino G, Cesari M, Rossi GP. Arterial hypertension, atrial fibrillation, and hyperaldosteronism: the triple trouble. Hypertension 2017;69(4):545−50. https://doi.org/10.1161/HYPERTENSIONAHA.116.08956.

[116] Williams TA, Lenders JWM, Mulatero P, Burrello J, Rottenkolber M, Adolf C, et al. Outcomes after adrenalectomy for unilateral primary aldosteronism: an international consensus on outcome measures and analysis of remission rates in an international cohort. Lancet Diabetes Endocrinol 2017;5(9):689−99.

[117] Burrello J, Burrello A, Stowasser M, Nishikawa T, Quinkler M, Prejbisz A, et al. The primary aldosteronism surgical outcome score for the prediction of clinical outcomes after adrenalectomy for unilateral primary aldosteronism. Ann Surg 2020;272(6):1125−32. https://doi.org/10.1097/SLA.0000000000003200.

[118] Vorselaars W, Nell S, Postma EL, Zarnegar R, Drake FT, Duh QY, et al. Clinical outcomes after unilateral adrenalectomy for primary aldosteronism. JAMA Surg 2019:e185842.

[119] Morineau G, Sulmont V, Salomon R, Fiquet-Kempf B, Jeunemaître X, Nicod J, Ferrari P. Apparent mineralocorticoid excess: report of six new cases and extensive personal experience. J Am Soc Nephrol 2006;17(11):3176.

[120] Lavery GG, Ronconi V, Draper N, Rabbitt EH, Lyons V, Chapman KE, Walker EA, McTernan CL, Giacchetti G, Mantero F, Seckl JR, Edwards CR, Connell JM, Hewison M, Stewart PM. Late-onset apparent mineralocorticoid excess caused by novel compound heterozygous mutations in the HSD11B2 gene. Hypertension 2003;42(2):123.

[121] Moretti C, Lanzolla G, Moretti M, Gnessi L, Carmina E. Androgens and hypertension in men and women: a unifying view. Curr Hypertens Rep May 2017;19(5):44. https://doi.org/10.1007/s11906-017-0740-3. PMID: 28455674.

[122] Kirlangic OF, Yilmaz-Oral D, Kaya-Sezginer E, Toktanis G, Tezgelen AS, Sen E, Khanam A, Oztekin CV, Gur S. The effects of androgens on cardiometabolic syndrome: current therapeutic concepts. Sex Med June 2020;8(2):132–55. https://doi.org/10.1016/j.esxm.2020.02.006. PMID: 32201216.

[123] de Vries L, Lebenthal Y, Phillip M, Shalitin S, Tenenbaum A, Bello R. Obesity and cardiometabolic risk factors in children and young adults with non-classical 21-hydroxylase deficiency. Front Endocrinol October 11, 2019;10:698. https://doi.org/10.3389/fendo.2019.00698. PMID: 31681171.

[124] Usselman CW, Yarovinsky TO, Steele FE, Leone CA, Taylor HS, Bender JR, Stachenfeld NS. Androgens drive microvascular endothelial dysfunction in women with polycystic ovary syndrome: role of the endothelin B receptor. J Physiol June 2019;597(11):2853–65. https://doi.org/10.1113/JP277756. PMID: 30847930.

[125] Wenner MM, Taylor HS, Stachenfeld NS. Androgens influence microvascular dilation in PCOS through ET-A and ET-B receptors. Am J Physiol Endocrinol Metab October 1, 2013;305(7):E818–25. https://doi.org/10.1152/ajpendo.00343.2013. PMID: 23921139.

[126] Ye W, Xie T, Song Y, Zhou L. The role of androgen and its related signals in PCOS. J Cell Mol Med 2021;25(4):1825–37. https://doi.org/10.1111/jcmm.16205. PMID: 33369146.

[127] Boese AC, Kim SC, Yin KJ, Lee JP, Hamblin MH. Sex differences in vascular physiology and pathophysiology: estrogen and androgen signaling in health and disease. Am J Physiol Heart Circ Physiol September 1, 2017;313(3):H524–45. https://doi.org/10.1152/ajpheart.00217.2016. PMID: 28626075.

Chapter 4

Hypothalamic–pituitary–adrenal axis and blood pressure regulation

Joseph M. Pappachan[1], Cornelius J. Fernandez[2] and Constantine A. Stratakis[3]

[1]Department of Endocrinology and Metabolism, Lancashire Teaching Hospitals NHS Trust, Preston and Manchester Metropolitan University, Manchester, United Kingdom; [2]Department of Endocrinology and Metabolism, Pilgrim Hospital, United Lincolnshire Hospitals NHS Trust, Boston, United Kingdom; [3]Human Genetics and Precision Medicine, IMMB, FORTH & ELPEN Research Institute, Pikermi, Greece

Visit the *Endocrine Hypertension: From Basic Science to Clinical Practice, First Edition* companion web site at: https://www.elsevier.com/books-and-journals/book-companion/9780323961202.

Graphical Abstract

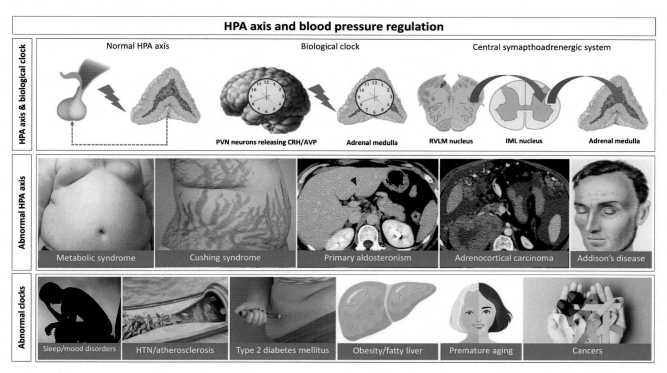

Endocrine Hypertension. **https://doi.org/10.1016/B978-0-323-96120-2.00018-2**

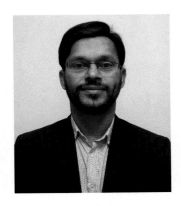

Joseph M Pappachan

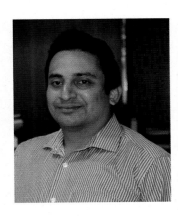

Cornelius J Fernandez

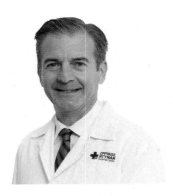

Constantine A Stratakins

Introduction

The hypothalamic—pituitary—adrenal (HPA) axis is an important neuroendocrine circuit that controls the adaptive stress response and metabolic homeostasis of the human body. The paraventricular nucleus (PVN) of hypothalamus has neurons that express angiotensin Type 1a receptors (PVN^{Agtr1a}) and is implicated in many neuroendocrine, as well as autonomic adaptive responses [1]. Arterial blood pressure regulation depends on many of the neuroendocrine and autonomic functions of the HPA axis. The blood pressure response to physiological and pathological stress and its relationship to the output of HPA axis neural circuitry had been an area of immense scientific research in the past few decades [2—4]. This chapter evaluates the relationship between HPA axis and blood pressure regulation in health and disease states, and presents the relevant up-to-date evidence.

Physiology of blood pressure regulation and HPA axis

POMC (pro-opiomelanocortin): its role in metabolism and energy balance

Pro-opiomelanocortin is a polypeptide prohormone synthesized by the corticotrophs and melanotrophs of the pituitary gland and from the neurons of the arcuate nucleus of hypothalamus [5]. POMC neurons play pivotal roles in the control of several physiological functions including feeding behavior and the regulation of energy balance to maintain metabolic homeostasis [6—8]. By fine-tuning the divergent metabolic pathways and behaviors necessary for survival, the POMC neuronal circuitry is thought to integrate appetite regulation and whole-body metabolic physiology, and thereby modulate the likelihood of obesity development [9]. Melanocortins, the peptide hormones derived from POMC (mainly adreno-corticotropin [ACTH] and different forms of melanocyte stimulating hormones [MSHs]) and neuropeptide-Y from the arcuate nucleus of hypothalamus exert opposing effects (anorexigenic and orexigenic, respectively) on feeding and metabolism through the hypothalamic neural pathways mediated by leptin [10,11]. Imbalance between the actions/functionality of these two molecules in the central nervous system may result in obesity as a consequence. Leptin, on the other hand, increases the electrical activity of anorexigenic POMC neurons and thereby prevents obesity [11]. Obesity as such is a risk factor for both essential hypertension and endocrine hypertension [12—14]. Animal models such as the ob/ob and db/db mice and Zucker fatty rats have, in addition, derangements of adipokine (e.g., leptin) signaling and/or nervous system networks (e.g., POMC—melanocortin signaling) that mediate sympathetic hyperactivity and hypertension in obesity, and may not exactly explain what happens in human obesity [15]. Indeed, more research is needed to elucidate the exact pathophysiological alterations in the POMC neural network that control energy homeostasis, and how obesity and hypertension link to each other in human beings.

CRH (corticotropin-releasing hormone) and AVP (arginine vasopressin) control the expression of POMC (pro-opiomelanocortin)

Human CRH is a peptide hormone encoded by the *CRH* gene and secreted by the hypothalamus in response to stressful stimuli [16]. Several molecules such as interleukin-1 (IL-1), IL-6, tumor necrosis factor-α (TNF-α), serotonin, acetylcholine, histamine, norepinephrine, epinephrine, arginine vasopressin (AVP), angiotensin II, neuropeptide Y (NPY), cholecystokinin, activin, encephalin, estrogens, γ-amino butyric acid, dynorphin, substance P (SP), somatostatin, galanin, and last but not least, glucocorticoids induce expression of *CRH* gene and therefore the CRH release [17]. Several pharmacological agents including psychotropic drugs cause CRH secretion. Most of these molecules are formed in the body as part of physical, physiologic, metabolic, and adaptive stress response to prepare the individual in combating such vulnerable situations.

CRH binds to the CRH receptors in various tissues including the pituitary gland and activates various biochemical pathways for additional hormone/neurotransmitter signaling [17]. Hypothalamic neurons produce CRH and AVP, which are transported by local vascular network to the anterior pituitary. Both these neuropeptides increase the *POMC* gene transcription and, thus, synthesis of the prohormone that gives rise to ACTH, MSH molecules, and β-lipotropin [5,18]. The neural signals mediated through CRH and AVP during normal physiological state and in various pathophysiological conditions as part of adaptive response modulate the HPA axis function in health and disease.

Pathophysiology of hypertension and HPA axis

Blood pressure (BP) control in the human body depends on a multitude of factors. Significant diurnal variations occur in the BP values in any individual during physical activity and rest to ensure normal perfusion of vital organs and tissues in the body. This inherently programmed vital function is maintained through rigorous fine-tuning during evolution to preserve homeostasis essential for normal life and well-being [19]. There is a circadian pattern of BP in healthy individuals with a morning surge upon waking that plateaus during the day, and a 10%—20% decrease ('dip') in BP during sleep such that average nocturnal BP is lower than the BP in the awake period during the day [20,21]. Around 30% of individuals show a nocturnal dip in BP that is less than 10%, and are considered nondippers. Although the main reason for circadian variations in BP is thought to be the activity of sympathetic nervous system, several other neurohormonal systems including dietary sodium intake, salt sensitivity, impaired sodium excretion capacity during daytime, and HPA axis function might play their roles [22].

Normal HPA axis function is highly influenced by the physical, environmental, neurohumoral, and emotional milieu of an individual, and any form of stress in these factors can have major impacts in its neurohormonal output. Stress, a state of disharmony in the physiological normality, is counteracted by various physiologic and behavioral responses to reestablish homeostasis termed as adaptive stress response mediated through complex neuroendocrine, cellular, and molecular mechanisms in the central and peripheral nervous systems [19,23]. The key components of the central neurochemical circuitry responsible for the stress system activation are hypothalamic CRH and AVP neurons in combination with the catecholaminergic locus coeruleus [LC] and norepinephrine [NE] neurons, whereas the peripheral limb of this complex circuit is formed by the sympathetic adrenomedullary system controlled by the HPA axis [24]. There are also multiple negative and positive feedback loops to maintain homeostasis in health. For example, NPY stimulates CRH neurons and inhibits the central sympathetic nervous system [25,26], and thereby influences the central stress system activity in opposite ways.

HPA axis is a key component of the central and peripheral limbs of the stress system, the integrity and precise regulation of the function of which are crucial for successful adaptive response to any form of stress [19,24]. Under normal conditions, the circadian control of HPA axis is maintained by pulsatile release of CRH and AVP [27]. This orchestrates the HPA axis function according to the sleep-wake cycle in tuning the biologic clock rhythm of a healthy individual. The HPA axis gets activated within minutes of stressful stimuli with the release of CRH from the hypothalamus that stimulates pituitary to release ACTH into the circulation [28]. ACTH stimulates adrenal cortex to secrete cortisol that elicits negative feedback on the pituitary to stop ACTH release. However, chronic stress can inhibit this negative feedback and contribute to poor health due to diseases and states that are associated with higher cortisol values [29]. Sometimes medications, addiction, trauma, or chronic stress can cause activation of HPA axis and high cortisol levels, leading to a condition that was previously termed "pseudo-Cushing's" syndrome, and now is better known as nonneoplastic Cushing's syndrome (NCS) [30—32]. Elevated blood pressure is almost always a feature of NCS, regardless of the degree of activation of the HPA axis or the peripheral cortisol levels. In classical Cushing's syndrome (CS), hypertension is one of the most common symptoms, typically more severe with higher cortisol levels, and with long-lasting consequences in cardiovascular morbidity even long after the surgical or medical cure of the underlying condition; in patients, with active CS, typically there is an abnormal circadian rhythm of blood pressure with lack of nocturnal dipping [33].

The stress system is closely connected to and communicates with the biological clock system that controls the circadian rhythm of the body and regulates multiple physiologic bodily functions [24,34]. There is a central master clock situated in the hypothalamus that orchestrates the functions of the peripheral clocks in multiple organs such as adrenal glands. The central clock system is closely linked to the HPA axis [35]. The circadian cortisol rhythm with morning surge and late evening nadir is maintained by the light-activated central clock system and the HPA axis activity via its central connections mediated through CRH/AVP-neurons [24,36]. Through the connections of the central autonomic nervous system to the adrenal medulla, the local adrenal clock is reset modulating the adrenal sensitivity to ACTH through epinephrine and NPY which also contributes to the circadian glucocorticoid rhythm [24,37]. Through these complex neurohormonal circuitries, HPA axis directly and indirectly contributes to the maintenance of blood pressure especially during stress.

HPA axis and autonomic nervous system (in relation to BP)

The PVN of the hypothalamus possesses several neuroendocrine and autonomic functions and contributes to the control and maintenance of blood pressure through its coordinated neural output [38]. Within the PVN, angiotensin-II (AT-II) is implicated in orchestrating the neuroendocrine and autonomic responses to stressful stimuli through activation of the AT-II type 1a receptors [39]. This in turn results in activation of the HPA axis and sympathetic outflow to augment cardiovascular reactivity as a part of the fight-or-flight response during any form of stress [40,41]. The coordinated activity and the novel cross-talks between the HPA axis (along with its neuroendocrine output) with the central autonomic nervous system and its peripheral limb in the splanchnic nervous system through its sympathoadrenal effector organs regulate the blood pressure to a great extent during rest and stressful stimuli. The catecholamines secreted from the peripheral autonomic nervous system controlled by the central autonomic pathways finally modulate the cardiovascular responses to maintain BP in health and during illness. The role of local factors in the vasculature and the effects of catecholamines on blood pressure regulation are detailed in Chapter 2.

A graphical representation of HPA axis and the central to peripheral sympathoadrenal axes are shown in Fig. 4.1.

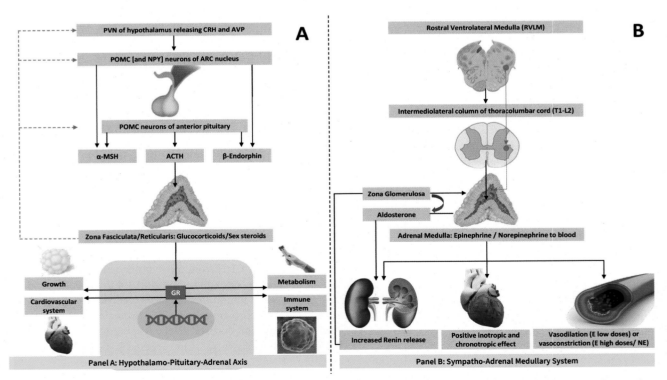

FIGURE 4.1 Panel A shows the graphical representation of hypothalamic–pituitary–adrenal (HPA) axis and panel B that of sympatho–adrenomedullary axis. *ACTH*, adrenocorticotropin; *AVP*, arginine vasopressin; *ARC*, arcuate; *CRH*, corticotropin releasing hormone; *E*, epinephrine; *MSH*, melanocyte stimulating hormone; *NE*, norepinephrine; *NPY*, neuropeptide Y; *POMC*, pro-opiomelanocortin; *PVN*, paraventricular nucleus.

HPA axis, adrenal hormones, and blood pressure

Adrenocortical hormones such as glucocorticoids and androgens are under the direct control of the HPA axis, unlike mineralocorticoids which are largely under the control of the renin—angiotensin—aldosterone system (RAAS) and plasma potassium levels. The principal mineralocorticoid in circulation is aldosterone, the main actions of which are salt and water balance and maintenance of blood pressure in normal levels. The details of blood pressure regulation by mineralocorticoids are given in the Chapters 3, 6 and 7 and therefore not elaborated here.

Cortisol is the main glucocorticoid in circulation that possesses protean effects in the body especially in the metabolic homeostasis. Cortisol mainly exerts its pressor effect in blood pressure control through the mineralocorticoid receptors (MRs) in the renal tubules, though at physiological plasma levels there is only negligible pressor effect, as this steroid hormone is inactivated by the enzyme 11β-hydroxysteroid-dehydrogenase type 2 (11β-HSD2) [1,42]. In pathological hypercortisolism states such as in CS, this enzyme is overwhelmed which results in overactivation of the MR and consequently the development of hypertension. Other mechanisms of BP abnormalities and hypertension in patients with CS are detailed in Chapters 13 and 14.

As sex steroids are mainly produced by the gonads, adrenal contribution to the circulating sex hormone pool is minimal. Adrenal androgens are vasoactive substances with testosterone possessing some vasoconstrictive effect [43] and estrogen causing vasodilatation [44]. Except in adrenal disorders of androgen overproduction, blood pressure is not affected by the adrenocortical androgens.

HPA axis and metabolic syndrome

As described in the previous sections, HPA axis and the central biological clock have influence on the feeding and emotional behavior of human beings, and therefore, abnormalities in this central neural circuitry can be associated with development of obesity and metabolic syndrome (MetS). Energy metabolism can be altered as a physiological response to stress and conversely the changes in energy availability can affect the physiological response to the stressor by activation of HPA axis and the sympathetic nervous system [45]. Stress during early life and the related activation of the HPA axis and central autonomic system has been shown to be associated with future risk of development of MetS and other cardiometabolic disorders in adult life [46,47]. Obesity and poorly controlled type 2 diabetes mellitus as consequences of MetS may result in further activation of the HPA axis as discussed earlier and re-establish the vicious circle of further worsening of the problems in the affected individual.

HPA axis, various hormonal disorders, and hypertension

Various hormonal disorders are associated with marked alterations in the physiological and neurohormonal output of the HPA axis. The most profound effects on HPA axis are from CS, either from pituitary pathology or from extrapituitary disease. Cushing's disease (CD) results from an autonomously functioning corticotroph adenoma that causes hypercortisolemia from chronic adrenal stimulation. CD accounts for ≈80% cases of endogenous CS, while adrenal CS accounts for ≈15—20% of cases, whereas ectopic ACTH production causes up to 1—2% of all cases of CS [48]. Suppression of pituitary production of ACTH with the disruption of HPA axis is classical of adrenal CS and exogenous hypercortisolism. Prolonged suppression of HPA axis for several months is usual following successful management of adrenal CS (see Chapter 14). Regardless of the etiology of CS, hypertension is common among patients and the pathophysiology is detailed in the Chapters 3, 13 and 14.

Primary aldosteronism (PA), the most common cause of endocrine hypertension, results from overproduction of mineralocorticoids from the adrenal glands and the common causes are adrenal hyperplasia and aldosterone-producing adenoma. Aldosterone production is partially controlled by ACTH, and therefore, HPA axis plays an important role in PA along with RAAS. ACTH stimulation test is useful to differentiate between some forms of PA. It is also useful during adrenal venous sampling to identify unilateral from bilateral aldosterone excess [49,50].

A subset of incidentally detected adrenal adenomas may turn out to become functional on follow-up with mild autonomous cortisol secretion (ACS; subclinical CS) with variable effects on the HPA axis function. The prevalence estimates of ACS vary widely (5—30%) because of the reporting bias [51—53]. An overnight dexamethasone (1 mg) suppression test is the preferred diagnostic screening test to check the integrity of HPA axis in patients with suspected ACS in such situations [54]. Metabolic complications of chronic steroid excess such as type 2 diabetes mellitus, hypertension, dyslipidemia, osteoporosis, and MetS are the anticipated long-term consequences of ACS, and therefore, excision of the adrenal adenoma may be considered although there is still no clear international consensus on this approach [53,54].

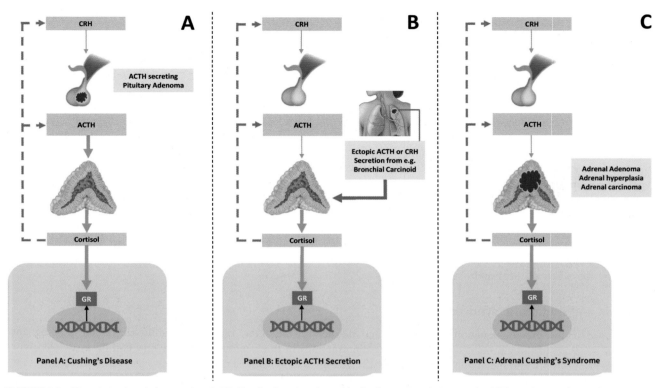

FIGURE 4.2 Hypothalamic—pituitary—adrenal (HPA) axis alterations in cushing's disease (panel A), ectopic ACTH (adrenocorticotropin) syndrome (panel B), and adrenal cushing's syndrome (panel C). *CRH*, corticotropin-releasing hormone; *GR*, glucocorticoid receptor.

Improvement of hypertension occurred in 66.7% of patients with ACS after surgery, while worsening of hypertension was observed in 80% of those followed up conservatively [55].

Sex steroid-producing adrenal tumors are often malignant and co-secrete glucocorticoids and therefore present with marked alterations in the HPA axis function and virilization or feminization [56−58]. They are rare and often present diagnostic and therapeutic challenges to the clinicians. Hypertension and metabolic complications such as diabetes mellitus are usual in these patients, but the classical features of CS are less common owing to the rapidity with which the clinical progression occurs [58,59]. Prognosis depends on the tumor invasiveness, operability, comorbidities including hypertension and cardiovascular disease, and the Ki67 index [58]. Because of the rarity of these tumors and marked variations in the clinicopathological features, the statistical figures of prognostic outcomes are not very reliable.

A pictorial representation of CS from different causes is shown in Fig. 4.2.

Adrenal insufficiency (AI) is another disease associated with marked alterations in the HPA axis function. Primary adrenal insufficiency occurs from various insults to both the adrenal glands such as autoimmune destruction, infectious diseases like tuberculosis, various systemic mycosis (histoplasmosis, blastomycosis, paracoccidioidomycosis, cryptococcosis, candidiasis, and coccidioidomycosis), human immunodeficiency virus infection, and rarely *Pneumocystis jirovecii* infection, bilateral adrenal hemorrhage (Waterhouse—Friderichsen syndrome) resulting from severe systemic sepsis, bilateral adrenalectomy for other indications, and adrenal involvement in primary and metastatic cancers [60,61]. Interruption of the negative feedback loop from lack of glucocorticoid production by the adrenal glands results in elevated production of CRH and ACTH as shown in Fig. 4.3. Increased stimulation of the melanocytes from excess MSH results in cutaneous hyperpigmentation especially in the skin creases, mucous membranes, and scars [60]. Patients often present with severe tiredness, low blood pressure with significant postural hypotension, hypoglycemia, hyperkalemia, hyponatremia, and in severe cases hemodynamic collapse and coma (adrenal crisis). A cosyntropin (synthetic ACTH/synacthen/tetracosactide) challenge test shows inadequate cortisol secretion response confirming AI in such patients (Fig. 4.4).

Secondary adrenal insufficiency occurs following various insults to the pituitary glands or the hypothalamus that results in lack of production of CRH/ACTH. These include pituitary apoplexy from large neoplasms, hypophysitis, pituitary/cranial irradiation, various genetic disorders, sarcoidosis, storage disorders such as hemochromatosis, and sudden withdrawal of long term exogenous glucocorticoid therapy [60,61]. Long-standing absence of stimulation from the trophic

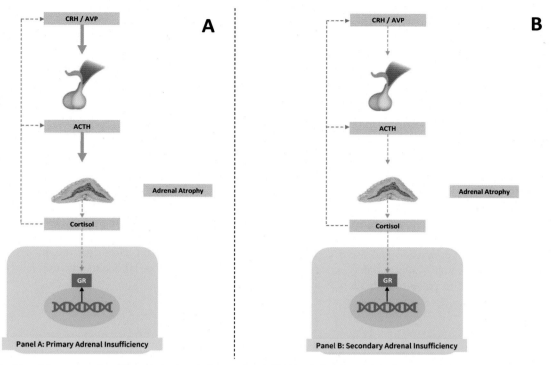

FIGURE 4.3 Pictorial representation of hypothalamic—pituitary—adrenal (HPA) axis in primary (panel A) and secondary adrenal insufficiency (panel B). *ACTH*, adrenocorticotropin; *AVP*, arginine vasopressin; *CRH*, corticotropin-releasing hormone; *GR*, glucocorticoid receptor.

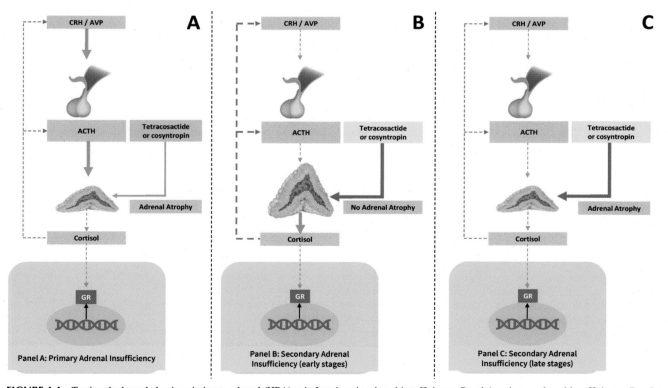

FIGURE 4.4 Testing the hypothalamic—pituitary—adrenal (HPA) axis functions in adrenal insufficiency. Panel A: primary adrenal insufficiency; Panel B: acute secondary adrenal insufficiency; Panel C: chronic secondary adrenal insufficiency. *ACTH*, adrenocorticotropin; *AVP*, arginine vasopressin; *CRH*, corticotropin-releasing hormone; *GR*, glucocorticoid receptor.

hormone (ACTH) results in bilateral adrenal atrophy and secondary AI. Hyperpigmentation does not occur, and electrolyte abnormalities are less common compared to those in primary AI as the RAAS may still be functional because of its control from factors other than stimulation by the ACTH (refer Chapters 3 and 5). Cosyntropin (synacthen) test may show optimal cortisol response in the early stages of secondary AI but becomes suboptimal 6 weeks later owing to the adrenal atrophy from lack of chronic ACTH stimulation as shown in Fig. 4.4. Chronic primary AI is distinguished from secondary AI by measuring ACTH levels which shall be high in primary and low in secondary [60].

Summary and conclusions

HPA axis is an extremely important biological system involved in the control and coordination of adaptive stress response, blood pressure regulation, and metabolic homeostasis. The endocrine and paracrine signals from the HPA axis and the central autonomic nervous system not only regulate the blood pressure, but also the biological clock mechanisms to ensure the bodily functions are appropriately orchestrated for well-being and survival. Marked variations in the HPA axis function occur in response to different stressors, and the ability to combat such adversities with the integrity of the HPA axis and other central mechanisms decides if the individual falls ill or remains healthy. Various hormonal disorders such as CS, PA, ACS from an adrenal incidentaloma or adrenocortical carcinomas, and primary or secondary AI can affect the HPA axis functions markedly, and hypertension and MetS as consequences of these conditions can affect the quality of life and prognosis of these patients unless appropriately managed. Thorough understanding of HPA axis function is important for appropriate endocrine care of patients with such disorders.

Learning points

- HPA axis is an important neuroendocrine electrical circuitry, the connections of which control many of the bodily functions including blood pressure regulation and metabolic homeostasis.
- HPA axis is closely integrated to the biological clock mechanism of human body involved in the maintenance of health and well-being.
- Abnormalities in the HPA axis function occur in various endocrine and metabolic disorders that may lead on to ill health.
- Hormonal abnormalities in CS, PA, autonomous hypercortisolemia from incidentally detected adrenal adenomas, adrenal carcinomas, and adrenal insufficiency can grossly disrupt the HPA axis function, and optimal treatment of the primary disease and consequent hypertension should be provided in such patients on time to ensure good prognosis.

References

[1] Stewart PM, Walker BR, Holder G, O'Halloran D, Shackleton CH. 11 beta-Hydroxysteroid dehydrogenase activity in Cushing's syndrome: explaining the mineralocorticoid excess state of the ectopic adrenocorticotropin syndrome. J Clin Endocrinol Metab December 1995;80(12):3617−20. https://doi.org/10.1210/jcem.80.12.8530609. PMID: 8530609.

[2] Tsigos C, Chrousos GP. Hypothalamic-pituitary-adrenal axis, neuroendocrine factors and stress. J Psychosom Res October 2002;53(4):865−71. https://doi.org/10.1016/s0022-3999(02)00429-4. PMID: 12377295.

[3] Singh A, Petrides JS, Gold PW, Chrousos GP, Deuster PA. Differential hypothalamic-pituitary-adrenal axis reactivity to psychological and physical stress. J Clin Endocrinol Metab June 1999;84(6):1944−8. https://doi.org/10.1210/jcem.84.6.5746. PMID: 10372691.

[4] Tsigos C, Chrousos GP. Physiology of the hypothalamic-pituitary-adrenal axis in health and dysregulation in psychiatric and autoimmune disorders. Endocrinol Metab Clin N Am September 1994;23(3):451−66. PMID: 7805648.

[5] Cawley NX, Li Z, Loh YP. 60 years OF POMC: biosynthesis, trafficking, and secretion of pro-opiomelanocortin-derived peptides. J Mol Endocrinol May 2016;56(4):T77−97. https://doi.org/10.1530/JME-15-0323. PMID: 26880796.

[6] King CM, Hentges ST. Relative number and distribution of murine hypothalamic proopiomelanocortin neurons innervating distinct target sites. PLoS One 2011;6(10):e25864. https://doi.org/10.1371/journal.pone.0025864. PMID: 21991375.

[7] Williams KW, Elmquist JK. From neuroanatomy to behavior: central integration of peripheral signals regulating feeding behavior. Nat Neurosci October 2012;15(10):1350−5. https://doi.org/10.1038/nn.3217. PMID: 23007190.

[8] Zhan C, Zhou J, Feng Q, Zhang JE, Lin S, Bao J, Wu P, Luo M. Acute and long-term suppression of feeding behavior by POMC neurons in the brainstem and hypothalamus, respectively. J Neurosci February 20, 2013;33(8):3624−32. https://doi.org/10.1523/JNEUROSCI.2742-12.2013. PMID: 23426689.

[9] Quarta C, Claret M, Zeltser LM, et al. POMC neuronal heterogeneity in energy balance and beyond: an integrated view. Nat Metab 2021;3:299−308. https://doi.org/10.1038/s42255-021-00345-3.

[10] Kalra SP, Dube MG, Pu S, Xu B, Horvath TL, Kalra PS. Interacting appetite-regulating pathways in the hypothalamic regulation of body weight. Endocr Rev 1999;20:68—100. https://doi.org/10.1210/edrv.20.1.0357. PMID: 10047974.

[11] Cowley M, Smart J, Rubinstein M, et al. Leptin activates anorexigenic POMC neurons through a neural network in the arcuate nucleus. Nature 2001;411:480—4. https://doi.org/10.1038/35078085.

[12] Marin JM, Agusti A, Villar I, Forner M, Nieto D, Carrizo SJ, et al. Association between treated and untreated obstructive sleep apnea and risk of hypertension. JAMA 2012;307(20):2169—76.

[13] Prejbisz A, Kołodziejczyk-Kruk S, Lenders JW, Januszewicz A. Primary aldosteronism and obstructive sleep apnea: is this a bidirectional relationship? Horm Metab Res 2017;49(12):969—76.

[14] Oduro-Donkor D, Barbar TM. Obesity, insulin resistance and obstructive sleep apnoea. In: Pappachan JM, Fernandes CJ, editors. Endocrine hypertension: from basic science to clinical practice; 2022.

[15] Hall JE, do Carmo JM, da Silva AA, Wang Z, Hall ME. Obesity, kidney dysfunction and hypertension: mechanistic links. Nat Rev Nephrol June 2019;15(6):367—85. https://doi.org/10.1038/s41581-019-0145-4. PMID: 31015582.

[16] Vale W, Spiess J, Rivier C, Rivier J. Characterization of a 41-residue ovine hypothalamic peptide that stimulates secretion of corticotropin and beta-endorphin. Science September 18, 1981;213(4514):1394—7. https://doi.org/10.1126/science.6267699. PMID: 6267699.

[17] Slominski AT, Zmijewski MA, Zbytek B, Tobin DJ, Theoharides TC, Rivier J. Key role of CRF in the skin stress response system. Endocr Rev December 2013;34(6):827—84. https://doi.org/10.1210/er.2012-1092. PMID: 23939821.

[18] Dinan TG, Scott LV. Anatomy of melancholia: focus on hypothalamic-pituitary-adrenal axis overactivity and the role of vasopressin. J Anat September 2005;207(3):259—64. https://doi.org/10.1111/j.1469-7580.2005.00443.x. PMID: 16185250.

[19] Chrousos GP. Stress and disorders of the stress system. Nat Rev Endocrinol 2009;5(7):374—81.

[20] Ivy JR, Bailey MA. Nondipping blood pressure: predictive or reactive failure of renal sodium handling? Physiology January 1, 2021;36(1):21—34. https://doi.org/10.1152/physiol.00024.2020. PMID: 33325814.

[21] Turner JR, Viera AJ, Shimbo D. Ambulatory blood pressure monitoring in clinical practice: a review. Am J Med January 2015;128(1):14—20. https://doi.org/10.1016/j.amjmed.2014.07.021. PMID: 25107387.

[22] Bankir L, Bochud M, Maillard M, Bovet P, Gabriel A, Burnier M. Nighttime blood pressure and nocturnal dipping are associated with daytime urinary sodium excretion in African subjects. Hypertension April 2008;51(4):891—8. https://doi.org/10.1161/HYPERTENSIONAHA.107.105510. PMID: 18316653.

[23] Chrousos GP, Gold PW. The concepts of stress and stress system disorders. Overview of physical and behavioral homeostasis. JAMA 1992;267:1244—52.

[24] Tsigos C, Kyrou I, Kassi E, Chrousos GP. Stress: endocrine physiology and pathophysiology. In: Feingold KR, Anawalt B, Boyce A, Chrousos G, de Herder WW, Dhatariya K, et al., editors. Endotext [internet]. South Dartmouth (MA: MDText.com, Inc.; October 17, 2020. 2000—. PMID: 25905226.

[25] Egawa M, Yoshimatsu H, Bray GA. Neuropeptide Y suppresses sympathetic activity to interscapular brown adipose tissue in rats. Am J Physiol 1991;260:R328—34.

[26] Oellerich WF, Schwartz DD, Malik KU. Neuropeptide Y inhibits adrenergic transmitter release in cultured rat superior cervical ganglion cells by restricting the availability of calcium through a pertussis toxin-sensitive mechanism. Neuroscience 1994;60:495—502.

[27] Engler D, Pham T, Fullerton MJ, Ooi G, Funder JW, Clarke IJ. Studies of the secretion of corticotropin-releasing factor and arginine vasopressin into the hypophysial-portal circulation of the conscious sheep. I. Effect of an audiovisual stimulus and insulin-induced hypoglycemia. Neuroendocrinology 1989;49:367—81.

[28] Yang HJ, Koh E, Kang Y. Susceptibility of women to cardiovascular disease and the prevention potential of mind-body intervention by changes in neural circuits and cardiovascular physiology. Biomolecules May 10, 2021;11(5):708. https://doi.org/10.3390/biom11050708. PMID: 34068722.

[29] Silverman MN, Sternberg EM. Glucocorticoid regulation of inflammation and its functional correlates: from HPA axis to glucocorticoid receptor dysfunction. Ann N Y Acad Sci July 2012;1261:55—63.

[30] Findling JW, Raff H. Diagnosis of endocrine disease: differentiation of pathologic/neoplastic hypercortisolism (Cushing's syndrome) from physiologic/non-neoplastic hypercortisolism (formerly known as pseudo-Cushing's syndrome). Eur J Endocrinol May 2017;176(5):R205—16. https://doi.org/10.1530/EJE-16-0946. PMID: 28179447.

[31] Gatta B, Chabre O, Cortet C, Martinie M, Corcuff JB, Roger P, Tabarin A. Reevaluation of the combined dexamethasone suppression-corticotropin-releasing hormone test for differentiation of mild Cushing's disease from pseudo-Cushing's syndrome. J Clin Endocrinol Metab November 2007;92(11):4290—3. https://doi.org/10.1210/jc.2006-2829. PMID: 17635947.

[32] Scaroni C, Albiger NM, Palmieri S, Iacuaniello D, Graziadio C, Damiani L, Zilio M, Stigliano A, Colao A, Pivonello R. Altogether to beat cushing's syndrome (ABC) study group. Approach to patients with pseudo-Cushing's states. Endocr Connect January 2020;9(1):R1—13. https://doi.org/10.1530/EC-19-0435. PMID: 31846432.

[33] Barbot M, Ceccato F, Scaroni C. The pathophysiology and treatment of hypertension in patients with cushing's syndrome. Front Endocrinol May 21, 2019;10:321. https://doi.org/10.3389/fendo.2019.00321. PMID: 31164868.

[34] Nicolaides NC, Charmandari E, Kino T, Chrousos GP. Stress-related and circadian secretion and target tissue actions of glucocorticoids: impact on health. Front Endocrinol 2017;8:70.

[35] Nader N, Chrousos GP, Kino T. Interactions of the circadian clock system and the HPA axis. Trends Endocrinol Metab 2010;21:277—86.

[36] Ishida A, Mutoh T, Ueyama T, Bando H, Masubuchi S, Nakahara D, Tsujimoto G, Okamura H. Light activates the adrenal gland: timing of gene expression and glucocorticoid release. Cell Metabol 2005;2:297—307.

[37] Ulrich-Lai YM, Arnhold MM, Engeland WC. Adrenal splanchnic innervation contributes to the diurnal rhythm of plasma corticosterone in rats by modulating adrenal sensitivity to ACTH. Am J Physiol Regul Integr Comp Physiol 2006;290:R1128–35.

[38] Sladek CD, Michelini LC, Stachenfeld NS, Stern JE, Urban JH. Endocrine-autonomic linkages. Compr Physiol 2015;5:1281–323. https://doi.org/10.1002/cphy.c140028.

[39] Saavedra JM, Ando H, Armando I, Baiardi G, Bregonzio C, Jezova M, Zhou J. Brain angiotensin II, an important stress hormone: regulatory sites and therapeutic opportunities. Ann NY Acad Sci 2004;1018:76–84. https://doi.org/10.1196/annals.1296.009.

[40] de Kloet AD, Wang L, Pitra S, Hiller H, Smith JA, Tan Y, Nguyen D, Cahill KM, Sumners C, Stern JE, Krause EG. A unique 'angiotensin-sensitive' neuronal population coordinates neuroendocrine, cardiovascular, and behavioral responses to stress. J Neurosci 2017;37:3478–90. https://doi.org/10.1523/JNEUROSCI.3674-16.2017.

[41] Elsaafien K, Kirchner MK, Mohammed M, Eikenberry SA, West C, Scott KA, de Kloet AD, Stern JE, Krause EG. Identification of novel cross-talk between the neuroendocrine and autonomic stress axes controlling blood pressure. J Neurosci 2021;41(21):4641–57. https://doi.org/10.1523/JNEUROSCI.0251-21.2021. PMID: 33858944.

[42] Ulick S, Wang JZ, Blumenfeld JD, Pickering TG. Cortisol inactivation overload: a mechanism of mineralocorticoid hypertension in the ectopic adrenocorticotropin syndrome. J Clin Endocrinol Metab May 1992;74(5):963–7. https://doi.org/10.1210/jcem.74.5.1569172. PMID: 1569172.

[43] Gonzales RJ, Krause DN, Duckles SP. Testosterone suppresses endothelium-dependent dilation of rat middle cerebral arteries. Am J Physiol Heart Circ Physiol 2004;286:H552–60.

[44] Somani YB, Pawelczyk JA, De Souza MJ, Kris-Etherton PM, Proctor DN. Aging women and their endothelium: probing the relative role of estrogen on vasodilator function. Am J Physiol Heart Circ Physiol August 1, 2019;317(2):H395–404. https://doi.org/10.1152/ajpheart.00430.2018. PMID: 31173499.

[45] Seal SV, Turner JD. The 'jekyll and hyde' of gluconeogenesis: early life adversity, later life stress, and metabolic disturbances. Int J Mol Sci March 25, 2021;22(7):3344. https://doi.org/10.3390/ijms22073344. PMID: 33805856.

[46] Delpierre C, Fantin R, Barboza-Solis C, Lepage B, Darnaudéry M, Kelly-Irving M. The early life nutritional environment and early life stress as potential pathways towards the metabolic syndrome in mid-life? A lifecourse analysis using the 1958 British Birth cohort. BMC Publ Health 2016;16:815.

[47] Chandan JS, Okoth K, Gokhale KM, Bandyopadhyay S, Taylor J, Nirantharakumar K. Increased cardiometabolic and mortality risk following childhood maltreatment in the United Kingdom. J Am Heart Assoc 2020;9:e015855. https://doi.org/10.1161/JAHA.119.015855.

[48] Fleseriu M, Auchus R, Bancos I, Ben-Shlomo A, Bertherat J, Biermasz NR, et al. Consensus on diagnosis and management of Cushing's disease: a guideline update. Lancet Diabetes Endocrinol December 2021;9(12):847–75. https://doi.org/10.1016/S2213-8587(21)00235-7. PMID: 34687601.

[49] Inoue K, Kitamoto T, Tsurutani Y, Saito J, Omura M, Nishikawa T. Cortisol Co-secretion and clinical usefulness of ACTH stimulation test in primary aldosteronism: a systematic review and biases in epidemiological studies. Front Endocrinol March 16, 2021;12:645488. https://doi.org/10.3389/fendo.2021.645488. PMID: 33796078.

[50] Funder JW. The potential of ACTH in the genesis of primary aldosteronism. Front Endocrinol 2016;7:40. https://doi.org/10.3389/fendo.2016.00040.

[51] Chiodini I. Clinical review: diagnosis and treatment of subclinical hypercortisolism. J Clin Endocrinol Metab 2011;96(5):1223–36. https://doi.org/10.1210/jc.2010-2722. PMID: 21367932.

[52] Chiodini I, Morelli V. Subclinical hypercortisolism: how to deal with it? Front Horm Res 2016;46:28–38. https://doi.org/10.1159/000443862.

[53] Ceccato F, Barbot M, Scaroni C, Boscaro M. Frequently asked questions and answers (if any) in patients with adrenal incidentaloma. J Endocrinol Invest December 2021;44(12):2749–63. https://doi.org/10.1007/s40618-021-01615-3. PMID: 34160793.

[54] Fassnacht M, Arlt W, Bancos I, et al. Management of adrenal incidentalomas: European society of endocrinology clinical practice guideline in collaboration with the European network for the study of adrenal tumors. Eur J Endocrinol 2016;175(2):G34. https://doi.org/10.1530/EJE-16-0467.

[55] Toniato A, Merante-Boschin I, Opocher G, Pelizzo MR, Schiavi F, Ballotta E. Surgical versus conservative management for subclinical Cushing syndrome in adrenal incidentalomas: a prospective randomized study. Ann Surg March 2009;249(3):388–91. https://doi.org/10.1097/SLA.0-b013e31819a47d2. PMID: 19247023.

[56] Hodgson A, Pakbaz S, Mete O. A diagnostic approach to adrenocortical tumors. Surg Pathol Clin 2019;12:967–95. https://doi.org/10.1016/j.path.2019.08.005.

[57] Moreno S, Guillermo M, Decoulx M, Dewailly D, Bresson R, Proye C. Feminizing adreno-cortical carcinomas in male adults. A dire prognosis. Three cases in a series of 801 adrenalectomies and review of the literature. Ann Endocrinol 2006;67:32–8. https://doi.org/10.1016/s0003-4266(06)72537-9.

[58] Mete O, Erickson LA, Juhlin CC, de Krijger RR, Sasano H, Volante M, Papotti MG. Overview of the 2022 WHO classification of adrenal cortical tumors. Endocr Pathol March 2022;33(1):155–96. https://doi.org/10.1007/s12022-022-09710-8. Epub 2022 Mar 14. PMID: 35288842.

[59] Stratakis CA. Cushing syndrome caused by adrenocortical tumors and hyperplasias (corticotropin-independent Cushing syndrome). Endocr Dev 2008;13:117–32. https://doi.org/10.1159/000134829.

[60] Vaidya A, Morris CA, Ross JJ. Interactive medical case. Stalking the diagnosis. N Engl J Med February 11, 2010;362(6):e16. https://doi.org/10.1056/NEJMimc0900128. PMID: 20175296.

[61] Mukhopadhyay P, Pandit K, Ghosh S. Adrenal disorders in the tropics. In: Feingold KR, Anawalt B, Boyce A, Chrousos G, de Herder WW, Dhatariya K, et al., editors. Endotext [internet]. South Dartmouth (MA: MDText.com, Inc.; May 22, 2021. 2000–. PMID: 34033308.

Chapter 5

Renin–angiotensin–aldosterone system and blood pressure regulation

Gino Seravalle[1] and Guido Grassi[2]

[1]*Cardiology Department, IRCCS Istituto Auxologico Italiano, and University Milano-Bicocca, Milano, Italy;* [2]*Clinica Medica, University Milano-Bicocca, Milano, Italy*

Visit the *Endocrine Hypertension: From Basic Science to Clinical Practice, First Edition* companion web site at: https://www.elsevier.com/books-and-journals/book-companion/9780323961202.

Graphical Abstract

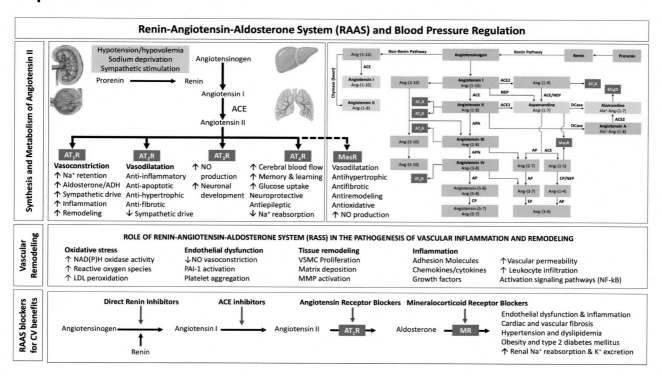

Endocrine Hypertension. **https://doi.org/10.1016/B978-0-323-96120-2.00002-9**

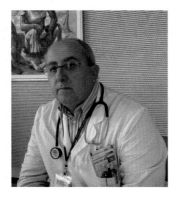

Gino Seravalle

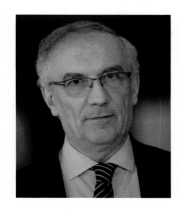

Guido Grassi

Introduction

Arterial hypertension is a highly prevalent condition characterized by increasing incidence rate in the global population (which is expected to rise to 30% by 2025) [1] and associated with important end-organ complications (heart diseases, cerebrovascular diseases, and renal diseases) [2,3]. The renin—angiotensin—aldosterone system (RAAS) plays a pivotal role in the pathogenesis of hypertension by regulating the systemic vascular resistance and circulatory volume through its effects on water and electrolyte balance. The renin agniotensin system is also involved in vascular inflammation and remodeling [4,5] (Fig. 5.1). The adverse effects of chronic exposure to high concentrations of angiotensin II (Ang II) and aldosterone are outlined in Table 5.1 [6—10]. Suppression of RAAS represents a key strategy in the treatment of

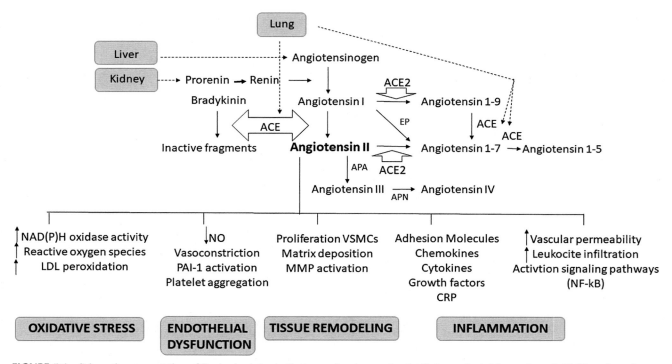

FIGURE 5.1 Schematic representation of Renin Angiotensin System and various molecular factors activated by angiotensin II. The role on hypertension, vascular inflammation, remodeling, and endothelial dysfunction is also depicted. *ACE*, angiotensin-converting enzyme; *AP*, aminopeptidase; *CRP*, C-reactive protein; *EP*, endopeptidase; *LDL*, low-density lipoprotein; *NAD(P)H*, nicotinamide dinucleotide phosphate; *MMP*, matrix metalloproteinase; *NF-κB*, nuclear factor kappa-light-chain-enhancer of activated B cells; *NO*, nitric oxide; *PAI-1*, plasminogen activator inhibitor type-1; *VSMC*, vascular smooth muscle cell.

TABLE 5.1 Harmful cardiovascular and renal effects of angiotensin II (Ang II) and aldosterone (Aldo).

Adverse effect	Direct effect of Ang II	Direct effect of Aldo
Myocardial remodeling (fibrosis, hypertrophy)	Yes	Yes
Vascular remodeling (fibrosis, hypertrophy)	Yes	Yes
Increase ROS	Yes	Yes
Proinflammatory	Yes	Yes
Arrhythmogenic	Yes	Yes
Vascular endothelial dysfunction	Yes	Yes
Systemic hypertension	Yes	Yes
Glomerular damage	Yes	Yes
Glomerular dysfunction (proteinuria)	Yes	Yes
Increased intraglomerular pressure	Vasoconstriction	Fluid retention and increase SNS activity
Tubulo-interstitial injury	Yes	Yes
Baroreceptor dysfunction	Yes	Yes
Sympathetic activation	Yes	Yes
Inotropy	Yes	No
Direct heart rate increase	Yes	No
Salt appetite	Yes	Yes
Increased thirst	Yes	No
Sodium and water retention	Yes	Yes
Potassium wasting	No	Yes

ROS, reactive oxygen species; *SNS*, sympathetic nervous system.

hypertension, cardiovascular disease, and chronic renal disease. The aim of this chapter is to elaborate the physiologic role of RAAS and to evaluate the effects of RAAS modifying therapeutic agents.

Physiological aspects of RAAS

Renin is synthetized as prorenin in the juxtaglomerular epithelioid cells and either released as prorenin or further processed to form active renin, which is stored as granules. These granules are then released in a controlled manner. Conversely, angiotensinogen (a renin substrate) is constitutively released from the liver and is usually present in excess. Increased renin synthesis and release occur during low systemic blood pressure, hypovolemia, sodium deprivation, and sympathetic stimulation. In the circulation, renin metabolizes angiotensinogen liberating angiotensin I (Ang I). Angiotensin-converting enzyme (ACE), which is released from endothelial cells (mainly of the pulmonary vasculature), converts Ang I to Ang II. Alternative pathways involving aminopeptidases and non-ACE enzymes can also take part in the transformation of Ang I into Ang II [11], and production of other angiotensin fragments such as angiotensin III and finally IV [11]. These fragments have strong effects on memory, cognition, renal vasodilatation, natriuresis, and extracellular matrix remodeling [12]. The main product of ACE and alternative pathways is Ang II which regulates the cardiovascular homeostasis by modulating its own effects through binding to specific receptors.

Four Ang II receptors (AT1R, AT2R, AT3R, and AT4R) have been identified to date [13]. The action at the AT1R leads to increased sodium retention, vasoconstriction—especially that of the efferent arteriole of the kidney, stimulation of the thirst mechanism and desire for salt, enhanced sympathetic activation, and enhanced aldosterone release from the adrenal gland. The interaction of Ang II and this receptor mediates much of the changes associated with chronic RAAS activation summarized in Table 5.1 including ventricular hypertrophy, inflammation, fibrosis, structural remodeling, and cardiac dysfunction. To counterbalance the adverse effects of chronic RAAS activation, natriuretic peptides (NPs) are released to facilitate salt and water excretion and to cause vasodilatation [14]. Neprilysin is a degrading enzyme for many of the NPs. Neprilysin inhibition alone is not sufficient to counterbalance the chronic RAAS activation that occurs in cardiovascular diseases like hypertension and heart failure. Hence, a combination of angiotensin receptor blocker and neprilysin inhibitor is used. Actions of AT2R stimulation are counterregulatory to those of the AT1R, leading to antiinflammatory, antifibrotic, and vasodilatory effects. The activation of AT3R leads to the production of nitric oxide (NO) and is responsible for neuronal development. The AT4R plays a role in regulating blood flow, inhibiting the reabsorption of sodium, in memory processes, and in vasodilatation.

Angiotensin I, II, III, and IV are also represented as Ang-(1−10), Ang-(1−8), Ang-(2−8), and Ang-(3−8), respectively [15]. The discovery of a new angiotensin-converting enzyme, ACE2, that has 42% homology to ACE and is expressed in the heart, kidney, testis, endothelium of coronary arteries, and intrarenal vessels, and renal tubular epithelium introduced more complexity to our understanding about the RAAS [16]. ACE2 acts as a counterregulatory molecule of the classical ACE effects, regulates the levels of Ang II, and limits its effects. The preferential substrate of ACE2 is Ang II, meaning that Ang II binds to ACE2 with a higher affinity than Ang I, leading to the formation of angiotensin 1-7 [Ang-(1−7)], also known as aspamandine [17]. The latter molecule has pleiotropic effects that are mediated by a specific receptor (MasR) known as Mas-1. By binding to this Mas-1 receptor, the Ang-(1−7) induces vasodilation, natriuresis, and diuresis [18,19], the effects that oppose that of Ang 1 through AT1R. The binding of Ang I to ACE2 results in the formation of angiotensin 1−9 [Ang-(1−9)], which in turn can be converted to Ang-(1−7), by the action of ACE [15]. The Ang-(1−7) or aspamandine can in turn be decarboxylated to form alamandine [20]. The latter binds to Mas-related G-protein-coupled receptor member D (MrgD). The AT2R, MasR, and MrgD form the protective arm of the RAAS as they protect the kidney and heart through their antihypertensive actions [20].

The terminal hormone of RAAS, aldosterone, exerts 90% of the mineralocorticoid activity of adrenal hormones and is a key regulator of sodium, potassium, and body fluid balance [7,8,21]. Ang II level and an increased extracellular K^+ concentration increase the expression of the *CYP11B2* gene which encodes aldosterone synthase [22]. Acting via the mineralocorticoid receptor (MR), aldosterone modulates the expression of ion channels [epithelial sodium channel (ENaC)], pumps, and exchangers in the epithelial tissues. This leads to an increase in the transepithelial Na^+ and water reabsorption, and K^+ excretion. MRs are present not only in the kidneys, colon, salivary, and sweats glands, but also in the nonepithelial tissues such as the retina, brain, myocardium, vascular smooth muscle cells, macrophages, fibroblasts, and adipocytes [23−25]. Since blood pressure is finely tuned by the RAAS, any imbalance in this system will produce arterial blood pressure alterations.

RAAS, inflammation, and remodeling

RAAS plays important roles in the initiation and maintenance of vascular inflammation and remodeling. Vascular inflammation leads to endothelial dysfunction. This facilitates migration of inflammatory cells into the vascular wall and stimulates smooth muscle cell proliferation and tissue injury, favoring atherosclerotic process. There is increasing evidence indicating a link between hypertension and atherosclerosis via Ang II-mediated inflammation. Animal and human studies show that Ang II has proinflammatory responses in the arteries, heart, and kidneys by regulating the expression of cytokines and chemokines. In human vascular smooth muscle cells, Ang II induces nuclear factor (NF)-κB (a proinflammatory factor downstream of tumor necrosis factor alpha—TNFα) activation and the expression of interleukin-6 (IL-6) [26], while in vivo, it causes increased expression of Vascular Cell Adhesion Molecule-1 that is inhibited by administration of the AT1R antagonist losartan [27]. Ang II plays a significant role in the initiation and progression of atherogenesis, an inflammation-mediated process. In injured arteries, Ang II favors recruitment of inflammatory cells inducing a feedback loop that produces more Ang II. It also induces the production of superoxide anions and activates the prooxidant NADH/NADPH signaling [28]. Ang II-mediated oxidative stress reduces the NO levels and activates the redox sensitive genes, particularly cytokines, adhesion molecules, and matrix metalloproteinases [29]. Ang II is also a profibrotic factor. In animal studies, chronic infusion of Ang II increases the blood pressure and favors the inflammatory cell infiltration into the myocardium and induces cardiac fibrosis, oxidative stress, and endothelial dysfunction [30−33]. The use of valsartan and fluvastatin, in atherosclerosis mouse model, can reduce the level of atherosclerotic lesions, superoxide anion, and the expression of Monocyte Chemoattractant Protein-1 and Intercellular Adhesion Molecule-1, indicating that blocking the inflammation and oxidative stress has beneficial effects on endothelium [34]. Clinical studies show a reduction in cardiovascular events beyond blood pressure lowering. Thus, positively altering the endothelium and vascular wall structures, in turn, mediates a reduction in cardiovascular disease burden. The increase in NO bioavailability, mediated by several RAAS inhibitors, induces vasodilation; inhibits platelet aggregation, leukocyte adhesion to endothelium, DNA synthesis, and vascular smooth muscle cell proliferation, thus counteracting the oxidative stress and hypertension [35,36].

The proinflammatory and profibrotic effects of the RAAS are also mediated by aldosterone [37]. In the vascular smooth muscle cells, aldosterone alters the insulin-like growth factor-1 receptor (IGF-1R) and modulates membrane structure via tyrosine kinase receptors. In the vascular endothelium, it decreases the synthesis of NO, and the formation of bone marrow-derived endothelial progenitor cells via oxidative stress and decreased levels of Vascular Endothelial Growth Factor Receptor 2 expression [38]. In endothelial cells, aldosterone increases the expression of sodium channels (like ENaC), known as endothelial sodium channels (EnNaCs). The combination of raised aldosterone levels associated with high salt (sodium) intake leads to raised plasma sodium levels, stiffening of the cell cortex of the endothelial cells, decrease in endothelial (NO synthase-mediated) NO release, stiff endothelial cell syndrome (SECS), and impaired vascular function [39,40]. Thus, high aldosterone in combination with high salt intake may result in endothelial dysfunction which may contribute to a rise in blood pressure independent of the renal effects of aldosterone. Several molecular pathways activated by the interaction of aldosterone with the VSMC-MR and contributing to vascular remodeling have been described [41,42]. Effects of aldosterone may be also mediated by G-protein-coupled estrogen receptor-1 [43]. The complexity of this system is due to the fact that other than systemic and local tissue RAAS, intracellular RAAS has been identified [44—46], and that several other molecules such as ERK1/2, NADPH, and NF-κB may participate to activate the system or be activated.

RAAS blocking agents and cardiovascular protection in hypertension

The European Society of Cardiology/European Society of Hypertension (ESC/ESH) 2018 guidelines [47] underline that blockade of RAAS should be part of the first therapeutic approach in combination with other antihypertensive drug classes for the management of patients with hypertension. The most widely used classes of drugs for this scope are as follows: (1) drugs inhibiting angiotensin-converting enzyme (ACEI), (2) antagonists of the AT1 receptors (ARBs), and (3) direct inhibitors of renin. Indirectly, we can also obtain the inhibition of renin release through β-blockers and α2-agonists. Last but not the least, the use of MR receptor antagonists blocking the actions of aldosterone on target tissues is also found to offer significant benefits in blood pressure control and cardiovascular protection.

ACE inhibitors

ACEIs are currently the most widely used agents for the treatment of hypertension; other cardiovascular diseases including heart failure and ischemic heart disease; and renal disease. These drugs act by inhibiting the ACE, thereby blocking the conversion of Ang I into Ang II. The antihypertensive activity of ACEI is the result of various effects: (a) the systemic and local tissue level inhibition of the effects of Ang II, with subsequent vasodilatation and reduction in plasma aldosterone levels, associated with increased natriuresis, diuresis, and reduction in left ventricular hypertrophy [48,49]; (b) increase in the circulating levels of bradykinin (with subsequent vasodilatation), prostacyclin and endothelium-derived hyper-polarizing factor, all of which induce vasodilation and inhibit vascular smooth muscle cells proliferation, and platelet adhesion [50,51]; (c) inhibitory effect on the release of antidiuretic hormone and reduction of both central and peripheral sympathetic activity [52]; and (d) antioxidant activity [53].

The evidence for the beneficial effects of ACEI on the cardiovascular outcomes was seen in several placebo-controlled studies (Fig. 5.2). The Captopril Prevention Project (CAPPP) trial [54] was a large-scale randomized controlled trial that compared the effects of ACEI and conventional therapy on the cardiovascular morbidity and mortality in patients with hypertension. More than 10,000 patients aged 25—66 years with a diastolic blood pressure >100 mmHg were randomized to captopril or diuretics and β-blockers. Both the treatment arms had similar reduction in blood pressure. For similar primary outcomes, captopril was associated with 25% reduced risk for stroke ($P = .04$). In the Antihypertensive and Lipid-Lowering treatment to Prevent Heart Attack Trial (ALLHAT) [55], more than 33,000 hypertensive subjects aged >55 years and at least one of other coronary heart disease risk factors were randomized to chlorthalidone, amlodipine, or lisinopril. Both amlodipine and chlortalidone arms achieved lower blood pressure than lisinopril arm with a high percentage of blood pressure goal <140/90 mmHg. After a 6-year follow-up, there was no difference in primary outcomes, while for the secondary outcomes the lisinopril arm showed a lower risk for combined cardiovascular risk, stroke, and heart failure. In a meta-analysis [56] of 20 major randomized controlled trials on RAAS inhibitors in hypertension, ACEIs were associated with 10% reduction in all-cause ($P = .004$), and 12% reduction in cardiovascular mortality ($P = .05$). The meta-analysis included three trials [57—59] that were not pure ACEI trials, and that accounted for the largest mortality reduction. Thus, the results should be interpreted with caution. Perindopril is an ACEI that is lipophilic and has a long duration of antihypertensive action [60,61]. In perindopril-based trials, compared to other compounds of the same class, in addition to reducing blood pressure, perindopril has been shown to have beneficial effect on endothelium [62], regress atherosclerosis, and reduce arterial stiffness in patients with mild-to-moderate essential hypertension [63].

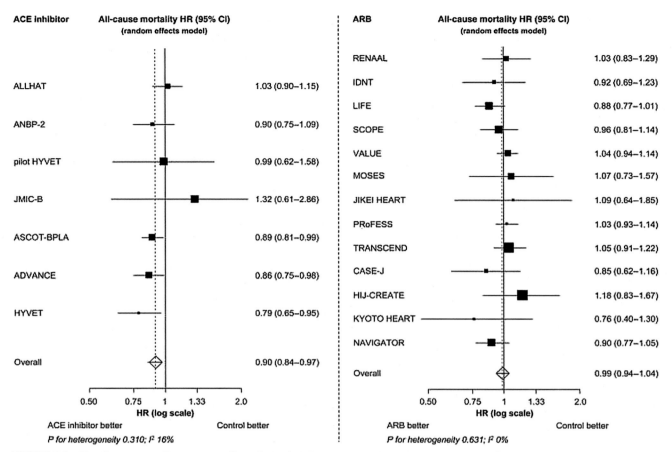

FIGURE 5.2 The all-cause mortality treatment effect of ACE inhibitor and ARB trials. HR, hazard ratio; CI, confidence interval; ACE, angiotensin-converting enzyme; ARB, angiotensin receptor blocker. $P = .004$ for the treatment effect of ACE inhibitor on all-cause mortality. $P = .683$ for the treatment effect of ARB on all-cause mortality. *From van Vark LC, Bertrand M, Akkerhuis KM, et al. Angiotensin-converting enzyme inhibitors reduce mortality in hypertension: a meta-analysis of randomized clinical trials of renin-angiotensin-aldosterone system inhibitors involving 158998 patients. Eur Heart J 2012;33:2088−97, with permission.*

ARBs

ARBs predominantly act by blocking the AT1R for Ang II and can be differentiated based on their affinity for this receptor. ARBs induce marked vasodilatation reducing both preload and afterload, thus, decreasing the systolic wall stress and left ventricular end-diastolic volume. The blockade of AT1R allows Ang II to exert its effect on AT2R which mediate the vasodilatation; improvement of vascular and cardiac function; and a reduction in cough from the absence of bradykinin increase. They also induce the activation of peroxisome proliferator-activated receptor-gamma and enhance the release of adiponectin from adipocytes which increase the insulin sensitivity, reduce the levels of circulating lipids, and promote antiinflammatory activity [64]. In vitro and in vivo studies demonstrate that antiinflammatory effect of ARBs is through the suppression of the inflammatory toll-like receptors 2 (TLR2) which is also known as cluster of differentiation 282 (CD282) and TLR4, that are implicated in the development and progression of cardiovascular disease [65]. In hypertensive patients, irbesartan has been shown to improve the endothelial function, vascular reactivity, and oxidative stress [66]. Use of valsartan prevents the formation of reactive oxygen species and suppresses the activity of NF-κB that regulates the expression of inflammatory cytokines and cell adhesion molecules that contribute to vascular inflammation and vascular events [67].

In hypertensive subjects, several trials have shown the efficacy of ARBs (Fig. 5.2). In the Valsartan Antihypertensive Long-term Use Evaluation (VALUE) trial [68], 15,245 patients with hypertension at high-risk for cardiovascular events aged >50 years were randomized to valsartan or amlodipine-based therapy. The mean BP reduction was 15/8 and 17/9 mmHg in the valsartan and amlodipine arms, respectively ($P < .0001$ between groups). After a mean follow-up of 4.2 years, there was no significant difference in the primary outcome of cardiac mortality and morbidity. A subsequent meta-analysis [69] found no increase in the risk of myocardial infarction while on treatment with ARBs. The Losartan

Intervention For Endpoint reduction in hypertension (LIFE) trial [70] evaluated 9193 hypertensive patients with left ventricular hypertrophy aged 55—80 years, treated with losartan or atenolol-based therapy. After a mean follow-up of 4.8 years, both treatments were associated with similar blood pressure reduction (−30/−17 mmHg), but the losartan group showed a 15% reduction in the primary outcome of cardiovascular mortality, stroke, and myocardial infarction ($P = .009$), indicating benefits beyond blood pressure reduction. However, despite a reduction in blood pressure values, ARBs were not so effective in cardiovascular risk reduction compared to placebo in several trials [71—73].

ARBs and ACEIs are recommended not only in the treatment of hypertension, but they have demonstrated to be effective in preventing the onset of microalbuminuria and to slow the progression toward renal failure [74—76]. Their use is also recommended by international guidelines for patients with heart failure in view of their favorable effects on cardiovascular morbidity and mortality [77]. With regards to the ischemic heart disease, some meta-analyses suggested that the ARBs are less effective than ACEIs, independent of blood pressure lowering effect, in preventing the myocardial infarction and all-cause mortality—the so called "ARB-MI Paradox" [78,79].

Direct renin inhibitors

Aliskiren is the first representative of the new class of orally active renin inhibitors [80]. Comparable antihypertensive effects to most other agents were observed with aliskiren [81]. The beneficial effects of aliskiren and its good tolerance in combinations with ARBs or a diuretic were confirmed in a meta-analysis on 12,000 patients with essential hypertension [82]. Based on the results of the Aliskiren Trial in Type 2 Diabetes Using Cardiorenal Endpoints (ALTITUDE) [83], with the increased incidence of adverse events (hyperkalemia and hypotension), co-administration of aliskiren with ACEIs or ARBs in patients with diabetes and moderate-to-advanced renal failure is not recommended. Recent analyses concerning renin inhibitors in their nephroprotection emphasize that double blockade of the RAAS can be considered in chronic nephropathy patients with albuminuria who are not fully controlled with conventional agents. In these patients, a strict monitoring of potassium levels and renal function should be stressed [84].

Dual RAAS inhibition

The combination of an ACEI and ARB was initially considered to be a way of obtaining a stronger suppression of RAAS, which would improve the beneficial effects beyond blood pressure lowering. A meta-analysis of randomized controlled trials found that this combination reduced the ambulatory blood pressure by 4.7/3.0 mmHg compared with ACEI alone, and 3.8/2.9 mmHg compared with ARB alone [85]. However, an increased risk of adverse events has been documented (worsening renal function, hyperkalemia, hypotension, and increased medical discontinuation due to side effects) [86]. The additive effects of the dual blockade on blood pressure control have been shown to be less than that attained by either drug combined with a diuretic or a calcium channel blocker [87]. The data from the ONTARGET study have shown that dual blockade of this type does not add any benefit in patients with high global cardiovascular risk and/or proteinuria, when compared to either agent used individually (monotherapy), and it increases the adverse events [88].

ACEI versus ARBs

The antihypertensive efficacy of ACEIs and ARBS appears to be equivalent [89,90]. Across studies, the difference in systolic or diastolic blood pressure generally did not exceed 4 mmHg. There are limited trials that compared the cardiovascular outcomes between ACEIs and ARBs in hypertension [91—112] (Fig. 5.3, [89]). Other than ONTARGET [88] previously described, there is another head-to-head comparison study known as the Diabetics Exposed to Telmisartan and Enalapril (DETAIL) study [113]. In the DETAIL study, 250 type 2 diabetic subjects with early nephropathy and mild to moderate hypertension were randomized to receive either telmisartan or enalapril. After 5 years, there were no significant differences in the primary outcome of renal function and cardiovascular events, all-cause mortality, heart failure, or myocardial infarction. In both trials, ARBs reduced the blood pressure more than respective ACEI, and this could be due to the comparison of a long-acting ARB versus a short-acting ACEI administered once daily. As previously described, only in patients with ischemic heart disease, it has been shown that ARBs appear to be less effective than ACEIs, in preventing myocardial infarction and all-cause mortality independent of blood pressure lowering effect [78,79].

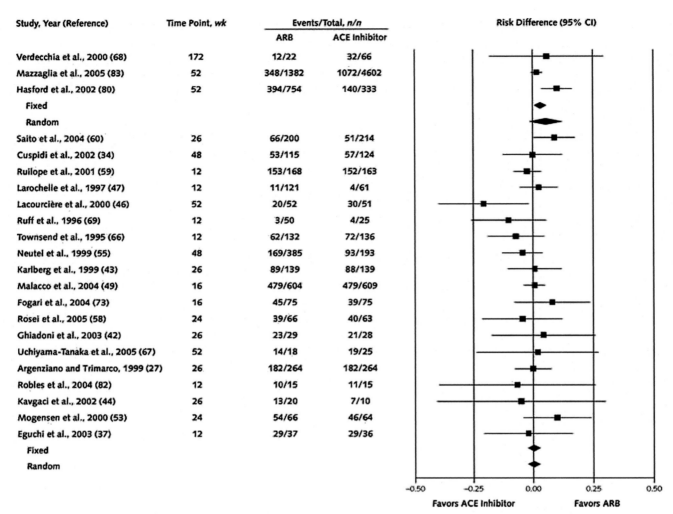

FIGURE 5.3 Successful monotherapy: angiotensin-converting enzyme (*ACE*) inhibitors versus angiotensin II receptor blockers (*ARBs*). *From Matchar DB, McCrory DC, Orlando LA, et al. Systematic review: comparative effectiveness of angiotensin-converting enzyme inhibitors and angiotensin II receptor blockers for treating essential hypertension. Ann Intern Med 2008;148:16—29, with permission.*

Mineralocorticoid receptor antagonists

The MR has been demonstrated in the connecting tubule and cortical collecting duct in the kidneys, in the heart, including cardiomyocytes, coronary endothelial and vascular smooth muscle cells, and inflammatory cells. Cardiac fibrosis and remodeling have been clearly shown in response to direct actions of aldosterone in the cardiovascular system rather than secondary to the well-known renal effects that include sodium retention at the expense of potassium wasting [114]. Animal and human studies have clearly shown that mineralocorticoid-dependent inflammation and oxidative stress responses in the vessel wall can be identified before the onset of fibrosis and are independent of blood pressure [115]. Inhibition of MR with spironolactone improves endothelium-dependent vasodilatation via inhibition of NAD(P)H oxidase pathway [116]. Moreover, blocking aldosterone signaling improves heart muscle cell proliferation and arterial wall remodeling, endothelial function, and NO synthesis [8].

Many clinical studies have shown that inhibition of MR decreases the incidence of heart attack, stroke, and mortality in addition to lowering blood pressure [117]. In subjects with primary aldosteronism, changes in blood pressure values and norepinephrine levels have been documented before (compared to after) removal of the aldosterone producing adenoma [118]. Other studies have shown a significant increase in adrenergic tone and an impairment in baroreflex responses in patients with primary aldosteronism and essential hypertension compared to nonhypertensive subjects and that adrenergic tone was decreased and baroreflex responses restored after surgical resolution of the disease [119,120]. The spironolactone-mediated inhibition of central sympathetic nervous system activity, associated to reduction in vascular stiffness and improvement of endothelial function, has been proposed as the principal mechanisms of blood pressure-lowering effects in resistant hypertension [121,122]. Clinical trials with the use of MR antagonists on top of standard therapy have clearly shown a significant reduction on morbidity and mortality in heart failure patients and in patients with renal diseases [123—126]. Hyperkalemia is a significant adverse event and one of the most common concerns associated with the use of MR antagonists that necessitates routine monitoring of serum electrolytes and renal function.

Conclusions

RAAS plays very important roles in the regulation of salt—water balance, blood pressure, and homeostasis of several body organs including the vasculature, heart, and kidney. Modulation of RAAS by ACEIs, ARBs, direct renin inhibitors, and MR antagonists has been proven to be effective blood pressure-lowering agents with comparable efficacy. The efficacy of RAAS blockers extends beyond blood pressure reduction. Guidelines suggest considering these drugs as the first-line agents not only in uncomplicated hypertensive patients but also in hypertension associated with heart failure, ischemic heart disease, and chronic kidney disease.

Learning points

- Arterial hypertension can be triggered by many factors, and molecules of the RAAS play important roles in the control of blood pressure.
- RAAS plays an important role in the initiation and maintenance of vascular inflammation, remodeling, and endothelial dysfunction favoring the atherosclerotic process and the cardiovascular continuum
- Agents capable of blocking the RAAS at different level of the cascade have shown to induce reduction in the primary outcome of cardiovascular mortality, stroke, and myocardial infarction, indicating benefits beyond blood pressure reduction.
- Different guidelines emphasize that blockade of RAAS should be part of the first therapeutic approach in combination with other antihypertensive drug classes for the management of patients with hypertension, heart failure, and renal diseases. This therapeutic approach is also useful in metabolic diseases such as obesity, metabolic syndrome, and type 2 diabetes.
- Due to the increased risk of adverse events (worsening renal function, hyperkalemia, hypotension, and increased medical discontinuation due to side effects), the combination of ACEIs and ARBs should be avoided, and a continuous monitoring strategy should be followed during treatment with mineralocorticoid antagonists co-administered with ACEI or ARB.

References

[1] Kearney PM, Whelton M, Reynolds K, et al. Global burden of hypertension: analysis of worldwide data. Lancet 2005;365:217—23.

[2] Wong ND, Dede J, Chow VH, et al. Global cardiovascular risk associated with hypertension and extent of treatment and control according to risk group. Am J Hypertens 2012;25:561—7.

[3] Bromfield MP. High blood pressure: the leading global burden of disease risk factor and the need for worldwide prevention programs. Curr Hypertens Rep 2013;15:134—6.

[4] Ferrario CM, Strawn WB. Role of the renin-angiotensin-aldosterone system and proinflammatory mediators in cardiovascular disease. Am J Cardiol 2006;98:121—8.

[5] Touyz RM, Schiffrin EL. Signal transduction mechanisms mediating the physiological and pathophysiological actions of angiotensin II in vascular smooth muscle cells. Pharmacol Rev 2000;52:639—72.

[6] Weber KT, Brilla CG. Pathological hypertrophy and cardiac interstitium. Fibrosis and renin-angiotensin-aldosterone system. Circulation 1991;83:1849—65.

[7] Schiffrin EL. Effects of aldosterone on the vasculature. Hypertension 2006;47:312—8.

[8] Martinez FA. Aldosterone inhibition and cardiovascular protection: more important than it once appeared. Cardiovasc Drugs Ther 2010;24:345—50.

[9] Riet L, van Esch JHM, Roks AJM, et al. Hypertension. Renin-angiotensin-aldosterone system alterations. Circ Res 2015;116:960—75.

[10] Munoz-Durango N, Fuentes CA, Castillo AE, et al. Role of the renin-angiotensin-aldosterone system beyond blood pressure regulation: molecular and cellular mechanisms involved in end-organ damage during arterial hypertension. Int J Mol Sci 2016;17:797.

[11] Lorenz JN. Chymase: the other ACE? Am J Physiol Ren Physiol 2010;298:F35—6.

[12] Romero CA, Orias M, Weir MR. Novel RAAS agonists and antagonists: clinical applications and controversies. Nat Rev Endocrinol 2015;11:242—52.

[13] Carey RM, Siragy HM. Newly recognized components of the renin-angiotensin system: potential roles in cardiovascular and renal regulation. Endocr Rev 2003;24:261−71.

[14] Sutanto H, Dobrev D, Heijman J. Angiotensin receptor-neprilysin inhibitor (ARNI) and cardiac arrhythmias. Int J Mol Sci 2021;22:8994.

[15] Guimond MO, Gallo-Payet N. The angiotensin II type 2 receptor in brain functions: an update. Int J Hypertens 2012;2012:351758.

[16] Donoghue M, Hsieh F, Baronas E, et al. A novel angiotensin-converting enzyme-related carboxypeptidase (ACE2) converts angiotensin I to angiotensin 1-9. Circ Res 2000;87:E1−9.

[17] Matsoukas J, Apostolopoulos V, Zulli A, et al. From angiotensin II to cyclic peptides and angiotensin receptor blockers (ARBs): perspectives of ARBs in COVID-19 therapy. Molecules 2021;26:618.

[18] Ferrao FM, Lara LS, Lowe J. Renin-angiotensin system in the kidney: what is new? World J Nephrol 2014;3:64−76.

[19] Etelvino GM, Peluso AA, Santos RA. New components of the renin-angiotensin system: alamandine and the MAS-related G protein-coupled receptor D. Curr Hypertens Rep 2014;16:433.

[20] Gong J, Luo M, Yong Y, et al. Alamandine alleviates hypertension and renal damage via oxidative-stress attenuation in Dahl rats. Cell Death Dis 2022;8:22.

[21] Hall JE, Guyton AC. Role of the kidneys in long-term control of arterial pressure and in hypertension: the integrated system for arterial pressure regulation. In: Guyton AC, Hall IE, editors. Textbook of medical physiology. Philadelphia, PA: Elsevier Health Sciences; 2010. p. 213−28.

[22] Beuschlein F. Regulation of aldosterone secretion: from physiology to disease. J Endocrinol 2013;168:R85−93.

[23] Jaisser F, Farman N. Emerging roles of the mineralocorticoid receptor in pathology: toward new paradigms in clinical pharmacology. Pharmacol Rev 2015;68:49−75.

[24] Gomez-Sanchez E, Gomez-Sanchez CE. The multifaceted mineralocorticoid receptor. Compr Physiol 2014;4:965−94.

[25] Fuller PJ, Yang J, Young MJ. 30 years of the mineralocorticoid receptor: coregulators as mediators of mineralocorticoid receptor signaling diversity. J Endocrinol 2017;234:T23−34.

[26] Kranzhofer R, Schmidt J, Pfeiffer A, et al. Angiotensin induces inflammatory activation of human vascular smooth muscle cells. Arterioscler Thromb Vasc Biol 1999;19:1623−9.

[27] Tummala PE, Chen XL, Sundell CL, et al. Angiotensin II induces vascular cell adhesion molecule-1 expression in rat vasculature: a potential link between the renin-angiotensin system and atherosclerosis. Circulation 1999;100:1223−9.

[28] Rajagopalan S, Kurz S, Munzel T, et al. Angiotensin II-mediated hypertension in the rat increases vascular superoxide production via membrane NADH/NADPH oxidase activation: contribution to alterations of vasomotor tone. J Clin Invest 1996;97:1916−23.

[29] Wassmann S, Nickenig G. Pathophysiological regulation of the AT1-receptor and implications for vascular disease. J Hypertens 2006;24:S15−21.

[30] Qi G, Jia L, Li Y, et al. Angiotensin II infusion-induced inflammation, monocytic fibroblast precursor infiltration, and cardiac fibrosis are pressure dependent. Cardiovasc Toxicol 2011;11:157−67.

[31] Gul R, Shawl AI, Kim SH, et al. Cooperative interaction between reactive oxygen species and Ca++ signals contributes to angiotensin II-induced hypertrophy in adult rat cardiomyocytes. Am J Physiol Heart Circ Physiol 2012;302:H901−9.

[32] Probstfield JL, O'Brien KD. Progression of cardiovascular damage: the role of renin-angiotensin system blockade. Am J Cardiol 2010;105 (1 Suppl):10A−20A.

[33] Tumbull F, Neal B, Pfeffer M, et al. Blood pressure lowering treatment trialists' collaboration. Blood pressure-dependent and independent effects of agents that inhibit the renin-angiotensin system. J Hypertens 2007;25:951−8.

[34] Li Z, Iwai M, Wu L, et al. Fluvastatin enhances the inhibitory effects of a selective AT1 receptor blocker, valsartan, on atherosclerosis. Hypertension 2004;44:758−63.

[35] Ritchie RH, Drummond GR, Sobey CG, et al. The opposing roles of NO and oxidative stress in cardiovascular disease. Pharmacol Res 2017;116:57−69.

[36] Masi S, Georgiopoulos G, Chiriacò M, et al. The importance of endothelial dysfunction in resistance artery remodelling and cardiovascular risk. Cardiovasc Res 2020;116:429−37.

[37] Ferreira NS, Tostes RC, Paradis P, et al. Aldosterone, inflammation, immune system, and hypertension. Am J Hypertens 2021;34:15−27.

[38] Marumo T, Uchimura H, Hayashi M, et al. Aldosterone impairs bone marrow-derived progenitor cell formation. Hypertension 2006;48:490−6.

[39] Oberleithner H, Riethmuller C, Schillers H, et al. Plasma sodium stiffens vascular endothelium and reduces nitric oxide release. Proc Natl Acad Sci USA 2007;104:16281−6.

[40] Korte S, Sträter AS, Drüppel V, et al. Feedforward activation of endothelial ENaC by high sodium. Faseb J 2014;28:4015−25.

[41] Galmiche G, Pizard A, Gueret A, et al. Smooth muscle cell mineralocorticoid receptors are mandatory for aldosterone-salt to induce vascular stiffness. Hypertension 2014;63:520−6.

[42] Montezano AC, Callera GE, Yogi A, et al. Aldosterone and angiotensin II synergistically stimulate migration in vascular smooth muscle cells through c-Src-regulated redox-sensitive RhoA pathways. Arterioscler Thromb Vasc Biol 2008;28:1511−8.

[43] Gros R, Ding Q, Liu B, et al. Aldosterone mediates its rapid effects in vascular endothelial cells through GPER activation. Am J Physiol Cell Physiol 2013;304:C532−40.

[44] Cook JL, Zhang Z, Re RN. In vitro evidence for an intracellular site of angiotensin action. Circ Res 2001;89:1138−46.

[45] Wang JM, Slembrouck D, Tan J, et al. Presence of cellular renin-angiotensin system in chromaffin cells of bovine adrenal medulla. Am J Physiol Heart Circ Physiol 2002;283:H1811−8.

[46] Patel S, Rauf A, Khan H, et al. Renin angiotensin aldosterone: the ubiquitous system for homeostasis and pathologies. Biomed Pharmacother 2017;94:317−25.

[47] Williams B, Mancia G, Spiering W, et al. 2018 ESC/ESH guidelines for the management of arterial hypertension: the task force for the management of arterial hypertension of the European Society of Cardiology and the European Society of Hypertension. J Hypertens 2018;36:1953−2041.

[48] Shahin Y, Khan JA, Samuel N, et al. Angiotensin converting enzyme inhibitors effect on endothelial dysfunction: a meta-analysis of randomized controlled trials. Atherosclerosis 2011;216:7−16.

[49] Schmieder RE, Martus P, Klingbeil A. Reversal of left ventricular hypertrophy in essential hypertension: a meta-analysis of randomized double-blind studies. JAMA 1996;275:1507−13.

[50] Mombouli JV, Illiano S, Nagao T, et al. Potentiation of endothelium-dependent relaxations to bradykinin by angiotensin I converting enzyme inhibitors in canine coronary artery involves both endothelium-derived relaxing and hyperpolarizing factors. Circ Res 1992;71:137−44.

[51] Barrow SE, Dollery CT, Heavey DJ, et al. Effect of vasoactive peptides on prostacyclin synthesis in man. Br J Pharmacol 1986;87:243−7.

[52] Grassi G, Turri C, Dell'Oro R, et al. Effects of chronic angiotensin converting enzyme inhibition on sympathetic nerve traffic and baroreflex control of the circulation in essential hypertension. J Hypertens 1998;16:1789−96.

[53] Bhuyan BJ, Mugesh G. Antioxidant activity of peptide-based angiotensin converting enzyme inhibitors. Org Biomol Chem 2012;10:2237−47.

[54] Hansson L, Lindholm LH, Niskanen L, et al. Effect of angiotensin-converting-enzyme inhibition compared with conventional therapy on cardiovascular morbidity and mortality in hypertension: the Captopril Prevention Project (CAPPP) randomized trial. Lancet 1999;353:611−6.

[55] Officers and Coordinators for the ALLHAT collaborative Research Group. Major outcomes in high-risk hypertensive patients randomized to angiotensin-converting enzyme inhibitor or calcium channel blocker vs diuretic: the Antihypertensive and Lipid-Lowering Treatment to Prevent Heart Attack Trial (ALLHAT). JAMA 2002;288:2981−97.

[56] van Vark LC, Bertrand M, Akkerhuis KM, et al. Angiotensin-converting enzyme inhibitors reduce mortality in hypertension: a meta-analysis of randomized clinical trials of renin-angiotensin-aldosterone system inhibitors involving 158998 patients. Eur Heart J 2012;33:2088−97.

[57] Dahlof B, Sever PS, Poulter NR, et al. Prevention of cardiovascular events with an antihypertensive regimen of amlodipine adding perindopril as required versus atenolol adding Bendroflumethiazide as required, in the Anglo-Scandinavian Cardiac Outcomes Trial-Blood Pressure Lowering Arm (ASCOT-BPLA): a multicentre randomized controlled trial. Lancet 2005;366:895−906.

[58] Patel A, Group AC, MacMahon S, et al. Effects of a fixed combination of perindopril and indapamide on macrovascular and microvascular outcomes in patients with type 2 diabetes mellitus (the ADVANCE trial): a randomized controlled trial. Lancet 2007;370:829−40.

[59] Beckett NS, Peters R, Fletcher AE, et al. Treatment of hypertension in patients 80 years of age and older. N Engl J Med 2008;358:1887−98.

[60] Julius S, Cohn JN, Neutel J, et al. Antihypertensive utility of perindopril in a large, general practice-based clinical trial. J Clin Hypertens (Greenwich). 2004;6:10−7.

[61] Dolan E, Stanton AV, Thom S, et al. Ambulatory blood pressure monitoring predicts cardiovascular events in treated hypertensive patients − an Anglo-Scandinavian cardiac outcomes trial substudy. J Hypertens 2009;27:876−85.

[62] Ferrari R, Fox K. Insight into the mode of action of ACE inhibition in coronary artery disease: the ultimate EUROPA study. Drugs 2009;69:265−77.

[63] Asmar R, Topouchian J, Pannier B, et al. Pulse wave velocity as endpoint in large-scale intervention trial. The Complior study. J Hypertens 2001;19:813−8.

[64] Nickenig G, Ostergren J, Struijker-Boudier H. Clinical evidence for the cardiovascular benefits of angiotensin receptor blockers. J Renin Angiotensin Aldosterone Syst 2006;7(Suppl. 1):S1−7.

[65] Bomfim GF, dos Santos RA, Oliveira MA, et al. Toll-like receptor 4 contributes to blood pressure regulation and vascular contraction in spontaneously hypertensive rats. Clin Sci 2012;122:535−43.

[66] Sola S, Mir MQS, Cheema FA, et al. Irbesartan and lipoic acid improve endothelial function and reduce markers of inflammation in the metabolic syndrome: results of the Irbesartan and Lipoic Acid in Endothelial Dysfunction (ISLAND) study. Circulation 2005;111:343−8.

[67] Dandona P, Kumar V, Aljada A, et al. Angiotensin II receptor blocker valsartan suppresses reactive oxygen species generation in leukocytes, nuclear factor-kB, in mononuclear cells of normal subjects: evidence of an anti-inflammatory action. J Clin Endocrinol Metab 2003;88:4496−501.

[68] Julius S, Kjeldsen SE, Weber M, et al. Outcomes in hypertensive patients at high cardiovascular risk treated with regimen based on valsartan or amlodipine: the VALUE randomized trial. Lancet 2004;363:2022−31.

[69] Bangalore S, Kumar S, Wetterslev J, et al. Angiotensin receptor blockers and risk of myocardial infarction: meta-analyses and trial sequential analyses of 147020 patients from randomized trials. BMJ 2011;342:d2234.

[70] Dahlof B, Devereux RB, Kjeldsen SE, et al. Cardiovascular morbidity and mortality in the Losartan Intervention for Endpoint reduction in hypertension study (LIFE): a randomized trial against atenolol. Lancet 2002;359:995−1003.

[71] Lithell H, Hansson L, Skoog I, et al. The Study on Cognition and Prognosis in the Elderly (SCOPE): principal results of a randomized double-blind intervention trial. J Hypertens 2003;21:875−86.

[72] Yusuf S, Diener HC, Sacco RL, et al. Telmisartan to prevent recurrent stroke and cardiovascular events. N Engl J Med 2008;359:1225−37.

[73] Group NS, McMurray JJ, Holman RR, et al. Effect of valsartan on the incidence of diabetes and cardiovascular events. N Engl J Med 2010;362:1477−90.

[74] Chen JY, Tsai IJ, Pan HC, et al. The impact of angiotensin-converting enzyme inhibitors or angiotensin II receptor blockers on clinical outcomes of acute kidney disease patients: a systematic review and meta-analysis. Front Pharmacol 2021;12:665250.

[75] Lambers Heerspink HJ, Weldegiorgis M, Inker LA, et al. Estimated GFR decline as surrogate end point for kidney failure: a post hoc analysis from the Reduction of End Points in Non-Insulin-Dependent Diabetes with the angiotensin II antagonist Losartan (RENAAL) study and Irbesartan Diabetic Nephropathy Trial (IDNT). Am J Kidney Dis 2014;63:244−50.

[76] Pugh D, Gallacher PJ, Dhaun N. Management of hypertension in chronic kidney disease. Drugs 2019;79:365—79.

[77] Seferovic PM, Ponikowski P, Anker SD, et al. Clinical practice update on heart failure 2019: pharmacotherapy, procedures, devices, and patient management. An expert consensus meeting report of the Heart Failure Association of the European Society of Cardiology. Eur J Heart Fail 2019;21:1169—86.

[78] Strauss MH, Hall AS. The divergent cardiovascular effects of angiotensin-converting enzyme inhibitors and angiotensin receptor blockers on myocardial infarction and death. Prog Cardiovasc Dis 2016;58:473—82.

[79] Ferrari R. RAAS inhibition and mortality in hypertension. Global Cardiol Sci Prac 2013;34.

[80] Wood JM, Maibaum J, Rahuel J, et al. Structure-based design of aliskiren, a novel orally effective renin inhibitor. Biochem Biophys Res Commun 2003;308:698—705.

[81] Chen Y, Meng L, Shao H, et al. Aliskiren vs other antihypertensive drugs in the treatment of hypertension: a meta-analysis. Hypertens Res 2013;36:252—61.

[82] White WB, Bresalier R, Kaplan AP, et al. Safety and tolerability of the direct renin inhibitor aliskiren in combination with angiotensin receptor blockers and thiazide diuretics: a pooled analysis of clinical experience of 12942 patients. J Clin Hypertens (Greenwich) 2011;13:506—16.

[83] Parving HH, Person F, Lewis JB, et al. Cardiorenal endpoints in a trial of aliskiren for type 2 diabetes. N Engl J Med 2012;367:2204—13.

[84] Tylicki L, Lizabowski S, Rutkowski B. Renin-angiotensin-aldosterone system blockade for nephroprotection: current evidence and future directions. J Nephrol 2012;25:900—10.

[85] Doulton TW, He FJ, MacGregor GA. Systematic review of combined angiotensin-converting enzyme inhibition and angiotensin receptor blockade in hypertension. Hypertension 2005;45:880—6.

[86] Makani H, Bangalore S, Desouza KA, et al. Efficacy and safety of dual blockade of the renin-angiotensin system: meta-analysis of randomized trials. BMJ 2013;346:f360.

[87] Nessbitt SD. Antihypertensive combination therapy: optimizing blood pressure control and cardiovascular risk reduction. J Clin Hypertens 2007;9:26—32.

[88] Yusuf S, Teo KK, et al. For the ONTARGET investigators. Telmisartan, ramipril, or both in patients at high risk for cardiovascular events. N Engl J Med 2008;358:1547—59.

[89] Matchar DB, McCrory DC, Orlando LA, et al. Systematic review: comparative effectiveness of angiotensin-converting enzyme inhibitors and angiotensin II receptor blockers for treating essential hypertension. Ann Intern Med 2008;148:16—29.

[90] Li ECK, Heran BS, Wright JM. Angiotensin converting enzyme (ACE) inhibitors versus angiotensin receptor blockers for primary hypertension. Cochrane Database Syst Rev 2014:CD009096.

[91] Verdecchia P, Schillaci G, Reboldi G, et al. Long-term effects of losartan and enalapril, alone or with a diuretic, on ambulatory blood pressure and cardiac performance in hypertension: a case—control study. Blood Pres Monit 2000;5:187—93.

[92] Mazzaglia G, Mantovani LG, Sturkenboom MC, et al. Patterns of persistence with antihypertensive medications in newly diagnosed hypertensive patients in Italy: a retrospective cohort study in primary care. J Hypertens 2005;23:2093—100.

[93] Hasford J, Mimran A, Simons WR. A population-based European cohort study of persistence in newly diagnosed hypertensive patients. J Hum Hypertens 2002;16:569—75.

[94] Saito S, Asayama K, Ohkubo T, , et alHOMED-BP Study Group. The second progress report on the Hypertension Objective treatment based on Measurement by Electrical Devices of Blood Pressure (HOMED-BP) study. Blood Pres Monit 2004;9:243—7.

[95] Cuspidi C, Muiesan ML, Valagussa L, et al. CATCH investigators. Comparative effects of candesartan and enalapril on left ventricular hypertrophy in patients with essential hypertension: the candesartan assessment in the treatment of cardiac hypertrophy (CATCH) study. J Hypertens 2002;20:2293—300.

[96] Ruilope L, Jäger B, Prichard B. Eprosartan versus enalapril in elderly patients with hypertension: a double-blind, randomized trial, vol 10. Blood Press; 2001. p. 223—9.

[97] Larochelle P, Flack JM, Marbury TC, et al. Effects and tolerability of irbesartan versus enalapril in patients with severe hypertension. Irbesartan Multicenter Investigators. Am J Cardiol 1997;80:1613—5.

[98] Lacourcière Y, Bélanger A, Godin C, et al. Long-term comparison of losartan and enalapril on kidney function in hypertensive type 2 diabetics with early nephropathy. Kidney Int 2000;58:762—9.

[99] Ruff D, Gazdick LP, Berman R, et al. Comparative effects of combination drug therapy regimens commencing with either losartan potassium, an angiotensin II receptor antagonist, or enalapril maleate for the treatment of severe hypertension. J Hypertens 1996;14:263—70.

[100] Townsend R, Haggert B, Liss C, et al. Efficacy and tolerability of losartan versus enalapril alone or in combination with hydrochlorothiazide in patients with essential hypertension. Clin Ther 1995;17:911—23.

[101] Neutel JM, Frishman WH, Oparil S, et al. Comparison of telmisartan with lisinopril in patients with mild-to-moderate hypertension. Am J Ther 1999;6:161—6.

[102] Karlberg BE, Lins LE, Hermansson K. Efficacy and safety of telmisartan, a selective AT1 receptor antagonist, compared with enalapril in elderly patients with primary hypertension. TEES Study Group. J Hypertens 1999;17:293—302.

[103] Malacco E, Santonastaso M, Vari NA, et al. Blood Pressure Reduction and Tolerability of Valsartan in Comparison with Lisinopril Study. Comparison of valsartan 160 mg with lisinopril 20 mg, given as monotherapy or in combination with a diuretic, for the treatment of hypertension: the Blood Pressure Reduction and Tolerability of Valsartan in Comparison with Lisinopril (PREVAIL) study. Clin Ther 2004;26:855—65.

[104] Fogari R, Mugellini A, Zoppi A, et al. Effects of valsartan compared with enalapril on blood pressure and cognitive function in elderly patients with essential hypertension. Eur J Clin Pharmacol 2004;59:863—8.

[105] Rosei EA, Rizzoni D, Muiesan ML, et al. CENTRO (CandEsartaN on aTherosclerotic Risk factors) Study Investigators. Effects of candesartan cilexetil and enalapril on inflammatory markers of atherosclerosis in hypertensive patients with non−insulin-dependent diabetes mellitus. J Hypertens 2005;23:435−44.

[106] Ghiadoni L, Magagna A, Versari D, et al. Different effect of antihypertensive drugs on conduit artery endothelial function. Hypertension 2003;41:1281−6.

[107] Uchiyama-Tanaka Y, Mori Y, Kishimoto N, et al. Comparison of the effects of quinapril and losartan on carotid artery intima-media thickness in patients with mild-to-moderate arterial hypertension. Kidney Blood Press Res 2005;28:111−6.

[108] Argenziano L, Trimarco B. Effect of eprosartan and enalapril in the treatment of elderly hypertensive patients: subgroup analysis of a 26-week, double-blind, multicentre study. Eprosartan Multinational Study Group. Curr Med Res Opin 1999;15:9−14.

[109] Robles NR, Angulo E, Grois J, et al. Comparative effects of fosinopril and irbesartan on hematopoiesis in essential hypertensives. Ren Fail 2004;26:399−404.

[110] Kavgaci H, Sahin A, Onder Ersoz H, et al. The effects of losartan and fosinopril in hypertensive type 2 diabetic patients. Diabetes Res Clin Pract 2002;58:19−25.

[111] Mogensen CE, Neldam S, Tikkanen I, et al. Randomised controlled trial of dual blockade of renin-angiotensin system in patients with hypertension, microalbuminuria, and non-insulin dependent diabetes: the candesartan and lisinopril microalbuminuria (CALM) study. BMJ 2000;321:1440−4.

[112] Eguchi K, Kario K, Shimada K. Comparison of candesartan with lisinopril on ambulatory blood pressure and morning surge in patients with systemic hypertension. Am J Cardiol 2003;92:621−4.

[113] Barnett AH, Bain SC, Bouter P, et al. Angiotensin receptor blockade versus converting enzyme inhibition in type 2 diabetes and nephropathy. N Engl J Med 2004;351:1952−61.

[114] Young MJ, Funder JW. The renin-angiotensin-aldosterone system in experimental mineralocorticoid-salt-induced cardiac fibrosis. Am J Physiol 1996;271:E883−8.

[115] Sun Y, Zhang J, Lu L, et al. Aldosterone-induced inflammation in the rat heart: role of oxidative stress. Am J Pathol 2002;161:1773−81.

[116] Haznedaroglu IC, Ozturk MA. Towards the understanding of the local hematopoietic bone marrow renin-angiotensin system. Int J Biochem Cell Biol 2003;35:867−80.

[117] McCurley A, Jaffe IZ. Mineralocorticoid receptors in vascular function and disease. Mol Cell Endocrinol 2012;350:256−65.

[118] Nicholls MG, Espiner EA, Ikram H, et al. Hormone and blood pressure relationships in primary aldosteronism. Clin Exp Hypertens 1984;6:1441−58.

[119] Kontak AC, Wang Z, Arbique D, et al. Reversible sympathetic overactivity in hypertensive patients with primary aldosteronism. J Clin Endocrinol Metab 2010;95:4756−61.

[120] Monahan KD, Leuenberger UA, Ray CA. Aldosterone impairs baroreflex sensitivity in healthy adults. Am J Physiol Heart Circ Physiol 2007;292:H190−7.

[121] De Souza F, Muxfeldt E, Fiszman R, et al. Efficacy of spironolactone therapy in patients with true resistant hypertension. Hypertension 2010;55:147−52.

[122] Raheja P, Price A, Wang Z, et al. Spironolactone prevents chlorthalidone-induced sympathetic activation and insulin resistance in hypertensive patients. Hypertension 2012;60:319−25.

[123] Pitt B, Zannad F, Remme W, et al. The effect of spironolactone on morbidity and mortality in patients with severe heart failure. Randomized Aldactone Evaluation Study Investigators. N Engl J Med 1999;341:709−17.

[124] Pitt B, Remme W, Zannad F, et al. Eplerenone post-acute myocardial infarction heart failure efficacy and survival study investigators. Eplerenone , a selective aldosterone blocker, in patients with left ventricular dysfunction after myocardial infarction. N Engl J Med 2003;348:1309−21.

[125] Zannad F, McMurray JJ, Krum H, et al. EMPHASIS-HF study group. Eplerenone in patients with systolic heart failure and mild symptoms. N Engl J Med 2011;364:11−21.

[126] Mavrakanas TA, Gariani K, Martin PY. Mineralocorticoid receptor blockade in addition to angiotensin converting enzyme inhibitor or angiotensin II receptor blocker treatment: an emerging paradigm in diabetic nephropathy: a systematic review. Eur J Intern Med 2014;25:173−6.

Chapter 6

Monogenic hypertension: an overview

Cornelius J. Fernandez[1], Joseph M. Pappachan[2,4] and Ute I. Scholl[3]

[1]Department of Endocrinology and Metabolism, Pilgrim Hospital, United Lincolnshire Hospitals NHS Trust, Boston, United Kingdom; [2]Department of Endocrinology and Metabolism, Lancashire Teaching Hospitals NHS Trust, Preston, United Kingdom; [3]Center of Functional Genomics, Berlin Institute of Health at Charité—Universitätsmedizin Berlin, Berlin, Germany; [4]Manchester Metropolitan University, and The University of Manchester, Manchester, United Kingdom

Visit the *Endocrine Hypertension: From Basic Science to Clinical Practice, First Edition* companion web site at: https://www.elsevier.com/books-and-journals/book-companion/9780323961202.

Graphical Abstract

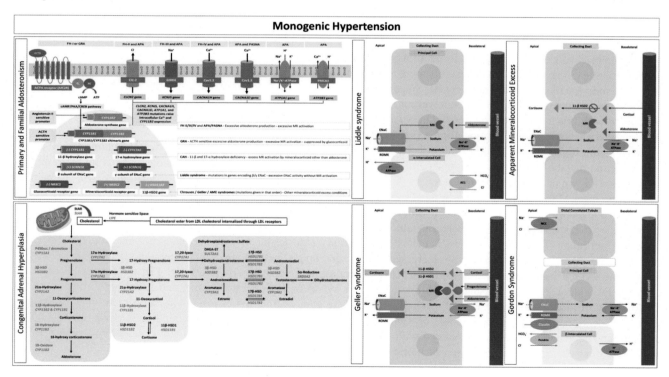

Endocrine Hypertension. https://doi.org/10.1016/B978-0-323-96120-2.00023-6

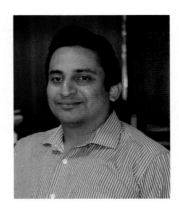

Cornelius J Fernandez

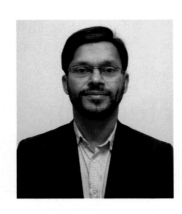

Joseph M Pappachan

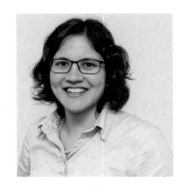

Ute I Scholl

Introduction

Primary hypertension, or hypertension without an identifiable secondary cause, is the most common form of arterial hypertension. Over 900 genetic variants have been associated with blood pressure as a polygenic trait [1]. In addition, environmental factors contribute to the development of primary hypertension. In contrast, rare forms of hypertension are monogenic, i.e., hypertension associated with single genetic alterations that follow a Mendelian pattern of inheritance. Patients with monogenic hypertension typically present with early-onset, severe, or resistant hypertension, potentially with a positive family history [2]. However, family studies have revealed incomplete penetrance in some cases, with carriers of disease variants showing milder phenotypes or even normotension [3]. Similarly, electrolyte abnormalities typically associated with some forms of monogenic hypertension may not be present in all mutation carriers.

The majority of known monogenic forms of hypertension directly or indirectly lead to increased renal salt reabsorption, plasma volume expansion, and, as a result, suppressed renin levels. Renin thus represents a suitable screening parameter in untreated individuals in whom monogenetic hypertension is suspected. Interpretation can, however, be complicated by antihypertensive medications raising or lowering renin levels. Exceptions with typically normal renin levels include hypertension with brachydactyly (previously known as autosomal dominant hypertension with brachydactyly or ADHB) and familial pheochromocytoma—paraganglioma (see below).

Monogenic hypertension with low renin levels is often associated with characteristic electrolyte abnormalities: either hyperkalemic metabolic acidosis or hypokalemic metabolic alkalosis, although their expression is variable. Gordon syndrome, also known as pseudohypoaldosteronism type II (PHAII) or familial hyperkalemic hypertension (FHHt), is the only monogenic form of hypertension characterized by hyperkalemic metabolic acidosis associated with low renin and normal aldosterone levels [4]. Subforms associated with hypokalemic alkalosis can again be subdivided into those with increased aldosterone levels and those with decreased aldosterone levels. Those with raised aldosterone levels include familial hyperaldosteronism (FH—I, FH-II, FH-III, FH-IV, and primary aldosteronism with seizures and neurological abnormalities). On the other hand, subforms with decreased aldosterone levels include apparent mineralocorticoid excess (AME), congenital adrenal hyperplasia (CAH) due to 11β-hydroxylase deficiency (11β-OHD) and 17α-hydroxylase deficiency (17α-OHD), glucocorticoid resistance syndrome (Chrousos syndrome), Geller syndrome, and Liddle syndrome.

Majority of monogenic hypertension syndromes are due to gain-of-function or loss-of-function mutations resulting in altered mineralocorticoid, glucocorticoid, or sympathetic pathways [5], or changes in renal salt reabsorption and its regulation. The genetic mutations associated with monogenetic hypertension identified kidneys and adrenal glands as the most important players in the regulation of blood pressure [6].

Monogenic hypertension should be considered in patients with otherwise unexplained childhood-onset hypertension and patients with a family history of early-onset or severe hypertension associated with either low or high potassium levels. Suppressed renin in such patients should trigger further investigations, including aldosterone levels. Associated syndromic features (such as brachydactyly) should similarly trigger genetic investigations. However, mild hypertension and absence of electrolyte abnormalities do not exclude monogenic hypertension, and therefore, hormonal studies should be coupled with genetic testing if monogenic hypertension is suspected. Fig. 6.1 provides an overview and classification of monogenic hypertension. Of note, response to certain medications is increasingly replaced by genetic testing for diagnosis.

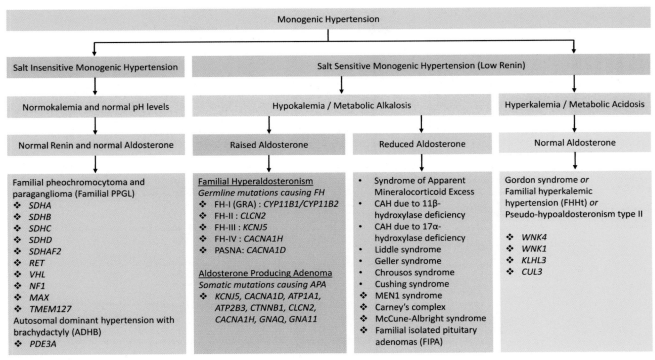

FIGURE 6.1   An overview and classification of monogenic hypertension. *APA*, aldosterone-producing adenoma; *CAH*, congenital adrenal hyperplasia; *FH*, familial hyperaldosteronism; *GRA*, glucocorticoid remediable aldosteronism; *MEN*, multiple endocrine neoplasia; *PASNA*, primary aldosteronism with seizures and neurological abnormalities; *PHA*, pseudohypoaldosteronism.

Genetics of monogenic hypertension

Monogenic hypertension with hypokalemic alkalosis, low renin, and raised aldosterone

Primary aldosteronism (PA) associated with autonomous aldosterone production by the adrenal gland is the most frequent cause of endocrine hypertension. It has a prevalence of around 6% among hypertensive patients in primary care and around 10% among those referred to hypertension centers [7,8]. The two major causes of PA are aldosterone-producing adenomas (APAs) that account for about 30% of cases and bilateral hyperaldosteronism that accounts for about 60% of cases [9]. Unilateral adrenal hyperplasia is less common, whereas adrenocortical carcinoma and familial hyperaldosteronism (FH) are both very rare. APAs are typically sporadic. Familial aggregation of APAs has been reported, but most instances are likely chance associations [10]. More than 95% of sporadic APAs are associated with heterozygous somatic mutations in known disease genes including *KCNJ5, CACNA1D, ATP1A1, ATP2B3, CLCN2, CACNA1H, CTNNB1, GNA11, and GNAQ* [11]. Many of these genes encode ion channels or pumps. The *KCNJ5* gene, mutated in approximately 40% of APAS, encodes an inwardly rectifying K$^+$ channel, GIRK4 [12]. *CACNA1D* encodes the voltage-dependent L-type calcium channel subunit alpha-1D (Ca$_v$1.3) [13]. *ATP1A1* encodes the Na$^+$/K$^+$-ATPase α1 subunit, and *ATP2B3* a plasma membrane calcium ATPase (PMCA3) [14]. *CLCN2* encodes the chloride voltage-gated channel 2 (ClC-2) [15], and *CACNA1H* encodes the voltage-dependent T-type calcium channel subunit alpha-1H (Ca$_v$3.2) [16]. *KCNJ5, CACNA1D, ATP1A1, ATP2B3, CLCN2,* and *CACNA1H* mutations directly or indirectly raise intracellular Ca^{2+} levels and thereby increase the expression of the aldosterone synthase gene *CYP11B2*, increasing aldosterone production [17].

CTNNB1 encodes β-catenin involved in the Wnt cell-differentiation pathway [18]. *GNA11* and *GNAQ* encode G-protein alpha subunits downstream of angiotensin II [19]. Somatic mutations in these genes confer gain of function.

A causative role of somatic mutations in *PRKACA* (encoding the cyclic adenosine monophosphate-dependent protein kinase catalytic subunit alpha mutated in cortisol-producing adenomas) [20] and germline mutations in *ARMC5* (encoding armadillo repeat containing 5) in APAs is still debated [21].

Evidence suggests that race and gender have an impact in the somatic mutation spectrum of APAs. Somatic mutations in the *KCNJ5* gene are more common in APAs from Asian populations, whereas those in the *CACNA1D* gene are more common in patients with recent African ancestry [21]. Similarly, *KCNJ5* and *CTNNB1* gene mutations are more frequent in women than in men, whereas *CACNA1D* and *ATP1A1* mutations are more frequent in men. Somatic mutations in genes

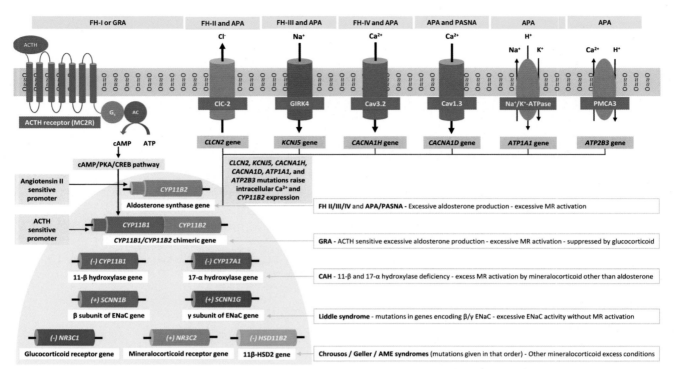

FIGURE 6.2 Various somatic and germline mutations involved in aldosterone-producing adenomas (APAs), familial hyperaldosteronism (FH), and other mineralocorticoid disorders associated with monogenic hypertension. *ACTH*, adrenocorticotropin; *AME*, apparent mineralocorticoid excess; *ATP*, adenosine triphosphate; Ca^{2+}, calcium; *cAMP*, cyclic adenosine monophosphate; Cl^-, chloride; *CREB*, cyclic AMP response element-binding protein; *ENaC*, epithelial sodium channel; *GRA*, glucocorticoid remediable aldosteronism; H^+, hydrogen ion; *HSD*, hydroxysteroid dehydrogenase; K^+, potassium; *MR*, mineralocorticoid receptor; Na^+, sodium; *PASNA*, primary aldosteronism with seizures and neurological abnormalities; *PKA*, protein kinase A.

overlapping with APA disease genes also contribute to the development of aldosterone-producing micronodules as a cause of unilateral or bilateral hyperaldosteronism. Such lesions also occur with advancing age in apparently healthy individuals [22,23].

Contrary to these somatic mutations in sporadic cases, germline mutations cause FH. FH type 1, also known as glucocorticoid-remediable aldosteronism, is an autosomal dominant disease associated with an unequal crossing-over event between *CYP11B1* (11-beta-hydroxylase involved in cortisol synthesis) and *CYP11B2* (aldosterone synthase), generating a chimeric gene [24]. The chimeric *CYP11B1/CYP11B2* gene leads to ectopic expression of *CYP11B2* in the zona fasciculata, with an inappropriate ACTH-dependent regulation of aldosterone biosynthesis. Unlike other genes associated with FH, the chimeric *CYP11B1/CYP11B2* gene is not detected in association with sporadic APA [25]. FH type 2 is an autosomal dominant disease associated with gain-of-function mutation in the *CLCN2* gene [26,27]. FH type 3 is an autosomal dominant disease associated with gain-of-function mutation in the *KCNJ5* gene [12]. FH type 4 is an autosomal dominant disease associated with gain-of-function mutation in the *CACNA1H* gene [28]. For a more detailed discussion of FH, see Chapter 8. Fig. 6.2 illustrates various somatic and germline mutations involved in APAs, FH, and other mineralocorticoid disorders associated with monogenic hypertension.

Monogenic hypertension with hypokalemic alkalosis, low renin, and reduced aldosterone

Liddle syndrome is an autosomal dominant disease associated with gain-of-function mutations in the genes for the β, γ, and rarely α subunits of the epithelial sodium channel (ENaC), namely *SCNN1B* [29], *SCNN1G* [30], and *SCNN1A* [31], respectively. In Liddle syndrome with *SCNN1B* and *SCNN1G* mutations, these gain-of-function mutations result in the inability to remove ENaC from the cell surface, leading to a constitutively active ENaC associated with excessive sodium transport from the tubular lumen into the interstitium through the sodium/potassium ATPase pump [32]. The excessive sodium flow thorough the ENaC and the sodium/potassium ATPase pump generates a negative transepithelial voltage, which leads to potassium diffusion through the renal outer medullary potassium (ROMK) channels from the apical membrane of the principal cells to the tubular lumen and facilitates active H^+ secretion from the apical membrane of the

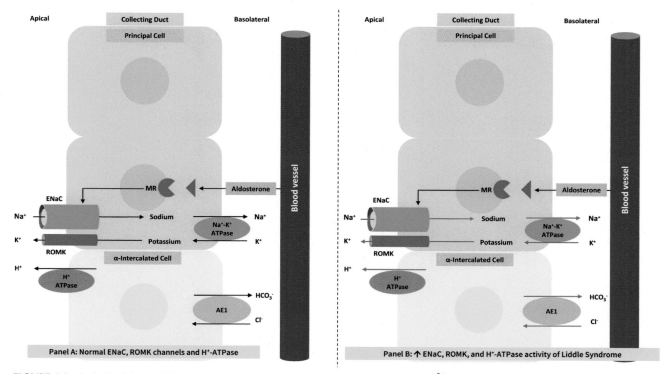

FIGURE 6.3 Pathophysiology of Liddle syndrome. *AE1*, anion exchanger 1; *ATPase*, pump; Ca^{2+}, calcium; Cl^-, chloride; *ENaC*, epithelial sodium channel; H^+, hydrogen ion; HCO_3, bicarbonate; K^+, potassium; *MR*, mineralocorticoid receptor; Na^+, sodium; *ROMK*, renal outer medullary potassium.

intercalated cells into the lumen with the help of the proton pump. This results in hypokalemic alkalosis. Patients with Liddle syndrome are treated with ENaC inhibitors (amiloride or triamterene). The pathogenesis of Liddle syndrome-mediated hypokalemic alkalosis is shown in Fig. 6.3.

For a better understanding of Figs. 6.3 and 6.5, the function of the collecting duct is explained in the following paragraph. Though most collecting duct cells are the principal cells (expressing ENaC), different types of intercalated cells including the α-, β-, and non-α/non-β-intercalated cells are also present and contribute to acid base homeostasis [33]. The acid-secreting α-intercalated cells express H^+-ATPase and the Cl^-/HCO3$^-$ anion exchanger (AE1) at the apical and basolateral membranes, respectively. In contrast, bicarbonate-secreting β-intercalated cells express the Cl^-/HCO3$^-$ anion exchanger (pendrin) and H^+-ATPase at the apical and basolateral membranes, respectively. Finally, the non-α, non-β intercalated cells have both pendrin and H^+-ATPase at the apical membrane. Pendrin transporters are involved in trans-cellular chloride reabsorption [34], whereas claudin channels are involved in paracellular chloride absorption [35].

Apparent mineralocorticoid excess is an autosomal recessive disease associated with inactivating mutations in the *HSD11B2* (hydroxysteroid 11-beta dehydrogenase 2) gene [36]. The encoded enzyme converts cortisol, which is more abundant than aldosterone and can bind to the mineralocorticoid receptor, to inactive cortisone. Loss of enzyme function results in abnormal mineralocorticoid receptor activation, hypertension, and hypokalemia. Unlike patients with Liddle syndrome, patients with AME respond to treatment with the mineralocorticoid receptor blockers spironolactone and eplerenone. CAH resulting from 11β-hydroxylase deficiency is an autosomal recessive disease associated with inactivating mutations in *CYP11B1* gene. CAH due to 17α-hydroxylase deficiency is an autosomal recessive disease associated with inactivating mutations in *CYP17A1* gene. Both are infrequent subforms of CAH associated with accumulation of mineralocorticoids, which cause hypertension. Glucocorticoid resistance syndrome (Fig. 6.4) is an autosomal recessive or dominant disease associated with inactivating mutations in the glucocorticoid receptor gene (*NR3C1*), associated with increased cortisol and mineralocorticoid levels. As these topics are discussed in detail in other chapters of this textbook, we are avoiding repetition in this chapter.

Geller syndrome (hypertension exacerbated by pregnancy) is an extremely rare autosomal dominant disease associated with gain-of-function mutation in the mineralocorticoid receptor gene (*NR3C2*) [37]. This mutation results in constitutive activation of the mineralocorticoid receptor and impaired specificity such that some steroid hormone antagonists including

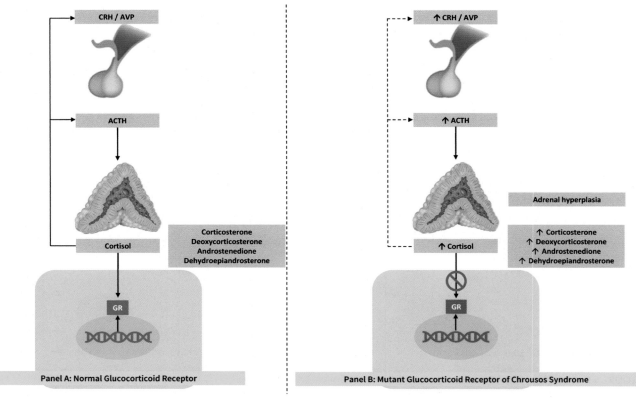

FIGURE 6.4 Pathophysiology of glucocorticoid resistance syndrome. *ACTH*, adrenocorticotropin; *AVP*, arginine vasopressin; *CRH*, corticotropin-releasing hormone; *GR*, glucocorticoid receptor.

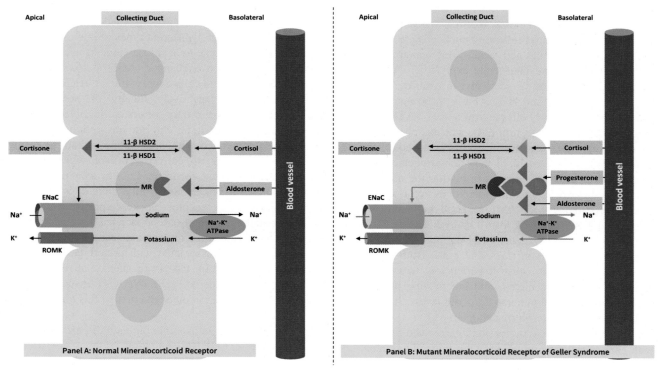

FIGURE 6.5 Pathophysiological aspects of Geller syndrome. *ATPase*, pump; *ENaC*, epithelial sodium channel; *HSD*, hydroxysteroid dehydrogenase; K^+, potassium; *MR*, mineralocorticoid receptor; Na^+, sodium; *ROMK*, renal outer medullary potassium.

progesterone and cortisone act as agonists to this mutated receptor resulting in increased ENaC and Na^+/K^+-ATPase expression and activity, thereby augmenting sodium reabsorption (Fig. 6.5) [5]. Pregnant women with Geller syndrome present with early-onset hypertension and hypokalemia exacerbated during pregnancy (likely due to the rise in progesterone). Hypertension is improved by delivery. In men and nonpregnant women, the early-onset severe hypertension of Geller syndrome is not likely to be mediated by progesterone, but by cortisone [38]. There is no specific treatment for hypertension in nonpregnant women and in men. Spironolactone increases blood pressure by activating the mutated mineralocorticoid receptors.

Monogenic hypertension with hyperkalemic acidosis, low renin, and variable aldosterone

Gordon syndrome (pseudohypoaldosteronism type II or familial hyperkalemic hypertension) is an autosomal dominant or autosomal recessive disease associated with mutations in the regulators of the thiazide-sensitive Na^+-Cl^- Co-transporter (NCC), including "With No lysine [K]" kinases (*WNK1* and *WNK4*, both autosomal dominant) [39], KeLcH-Like3 (*KLHL3*, autosomal dominant or recessive) and CULlin3 (*CUL3*, autosomal dominant) [40,41]. The pathogenesis of hyperkalemia and metabolic acidosis in Gordon syndrome is as follows [42,43].

Under physiological conditions, NCC is expressed in the apical membrane of the distal convoluted tubule where it is involved in reabsorption of 5%−10% of filtered NaCl. As discussed above, ROMK is an ATP-dependent K^+ channel involved in K^+ secretion in the principal cells of the collecting duct [42]. *WNK1* and *WNK4* increase the phosphorylation and expression of NCC on the apical membrane via oxidative stress-responsive gene 1 (OSR1)/Ste20-related proline−alanine-rich kinase (SPAK). This causes increased NaCl reabsorption in the DCT. The resulting decreased more distal NaCl reabsorption via ENaC also reduces potassium secretion via ROMK. Finally, the proteins encoded by *KLHL3* and *CUL3* genes and "really interesting new gene" *(RING)* form a cullin-RING ligase (CRL) complex that mediates ubiquitination and proteasomal degradation of WNK1 and WNK4 proteins.

Mutations in *CUL3*, *KLHL3*, or *WNK4* impair the CRL process or otherwise lead to increased WNK expression or activity [44−48]. Mutant *WNK4* cannot bind to and be ubiquitinated by the CRL complex or shows increased activity. Mutations in *CUL3* and *KLHL3* lead to increased WNK1 and WNK4 protein abundance due to the inability to form the CRL complex. Mutations in *WNK1* either increase the abundance of its long isoform (L-WNK1) in the DCT or impair the

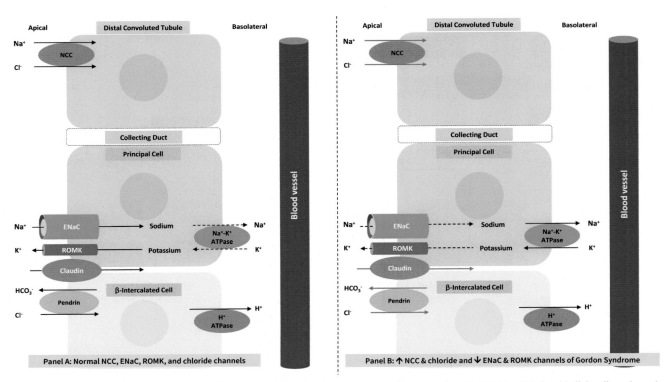

FIGURE 6.6 The pathogenesis of Gordon syndrome-mediated hyperkalemic acidosis. *ATPase*, pump; *Cl⁻*, chloride; *ENaC*, epithelial sodium channel; *H⁺*, hydrogen ion; *HCO₃*, bicarbonate; *K⁺*, potassium; *Na⁺*, sodium; *NCC*, sodium chloride cotransporter; *ROMK*, renal outer medullary potassium.

degradation of its shorter, kidney-specific isoform (KS-WNK1) by the CRL complex. The resultant increased WNK1 and WNK4 protein abundance leads to increased phosphorylation and increased expression of NCC along distal convoluted tubule. This causes excessive sodium and chloride reabsorption in the DCT via NCC [43]. Because less NaCl is delivered to the collecting duct, sodium reabsorption by ENaC in the cortical collecting duct decreases. This reduces the negative potential required for potassium secretion through ROMK. In addition to this mechanism, mutant WNK4 directly inhibits ENaC, accelerates the internalization of the secretory ROMK channel, thereby reducing potassium secretion in the collecting duct. Moreover, mutant WNK4 enhances chloride reabsorption via paracellular pathways (by increasing claudin channel permeability) and transcellular pathways (by enhancing the expression and activity of pendrin). The pathogenesis of Gordon syndrome-mediated hyperkalemic acidosis is shown in Fig. 6.6. Of note, some patients with Gordon syndrome have hyperkalemic acidosis, but are normotensive, specifically those with a subtype of *WNK1* mutations [49]. Patients with recessive *KLHL3* mutations and with dominant *CUL3* mutations tend to have more severe phenotypes [50]. Both hypertension and hyperkalemic acidosis respond to therapy with thiazide diuretics.

Monogenic hypertension with normokalemia and normal renin and aldosterone levels

Familial PPGL is described elsewhere in this textbook (Chapters 10, 11, and 12). Hence, we will focus on a rare condition previously known as autosomal dominant hypertension with brachydactyly (ADHB), currently known by the name hypertension with brachydactyly (HTNB). It is characterized by short stature, brachydactyly and severe age-dependent, but salt-independent hypertension [51,52]. It is an autosomal dominant condition caused by a gain-of-function mutation in the *PDE3A* gene (located at chromosome 12p12.2) that encodes a phosphodiesterase hydrolyzing the cyclic adenosine monophosphate (cAMP). The mutant *PDE3A* gene product (phosphodiesterase 3A enzyme with altered enzyme phosphorylation) results in lowered cAMP levels in vascular smooth muscle cells, allowing for excessive proliferation and contraction, vascular hypertrophy, decreased blood vessel lumen, increased peripheral vascular resistance, and raised blood pressure. The lowered cAMP levels also lower the levels of parathyroid hormone-related peptide (PTHrP)—a key moderator of chondrogenesis—resulting in brachydactyly. Animal studies suggest a potential benefit from increasing the cyclic guanosine monophosphate levels with a soluble guanylyl cyclase stimulator [53].

Several other syndromes can be associated with hypertension including neurofibromatosis type 1, Grange syndrome, monogenic causes of chronic kidney disease, etc., but are beyond the scope of this chapter.

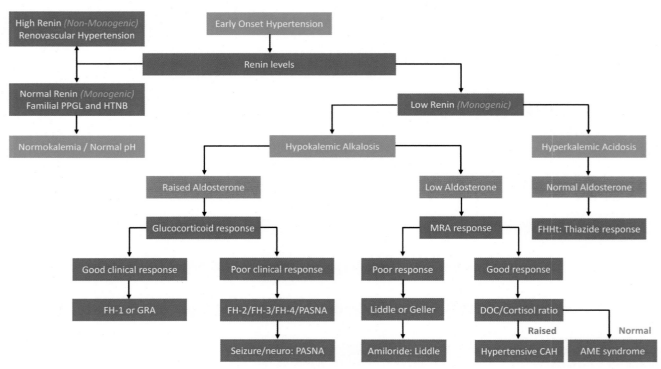

FIGURE 6.7 An algorithm for the diagnostic evaluation of monogenic hypertension. *AME*, apparent mineralocorticoid excess; *CAH*, congenital adrenal hyperplasia; *DOC*, deoxycorticosterone; *FH*, familial hyperaldosteronism; *FHHt*, familial hyperkalemic hypertension; *GRA*, glucocorticoid remediable aldosteronism; *HTNB*, hypertension and brachydactyly syndrome; *MRA*, mineralocorticoid receptor antagonist; *PASNA*, primary aldosteronism with seizures and neurological abnormalities; *PPGL*, pheochromocytoma paraganglioma.

An algorithm for the diagnostic evaluation of monogenic hypertension is given in Fig. 6.7.

Summary

Monogenic hypertension develops due to genetic mutations in single genes (either gain-of-function or loss-of-function). Most known monogenic forms of hypertension interfere with normal renal and/or adrenal regulation of blood pressure, by altering renal salt reabsorption, the mineralocorticoid, glucocorticoid, or sympathetic pathways. As some of them respond better to certain medications and treatment with those medications significantly improves morbidity and mortality, accurate diagnosis of monogenic hypertension is important. Establishing a genetic diagnosis has implications for potentially affected family members. Because monogenic forms of hypertension are very rare, establishing the correct diagnosis typically requires a high level of clinical suspicion, laboratory investigations, and genetic testing.

Learning points

- Monogenic hypertension is the term coined to describe familial hypertensive disorders that follow a Mendelian pattern of inheritance.
- Their phenotypic expression including the age of onset and disease severity varies depending on the underlying disease gene, type of mutation, and penetrance.
- Diagnostic evaluation involves clinical profiling coupled with measurement of plasma renin, aldosterone, and electrolyte levels and analysis of disease-associated genes, which is increasingly performed using panel sequencing.

References

[1] Evangelou E, Warren HR, Mosen-Ansorena D, Mifsud B, Pazoki R, Gao H, et al. Genetic analysis of over 1 million people identifies 535 new loci associated with blood pressure traits. Nat Genet 2018;50(10):1412–25.

[2] Garovic VD, Hilliard AA, Turner ST. Monogenic forms of low-renin hypertension. Nat Clin Pract Nephrol 2006;2(11):624–30.

[3] Lu YT, Fan P, Zhang D, Zhang Y, Meng X, Zhang QY, et al. Overview of monogenic forms of hypertension combined with hypokalemia. Front Pediatr 2021;8:543309. https://doi.org/10.3389/fped.2020.543309. PMID: 33569358; PMCID: PMC7868374.

[4] Levanovich PE, Diaczok A, Rossi NF. Clinical and molecular perspectives of monogenic hypertension. Curr Hypertens Rev 2020;16(2):91–107. https://doi.org/10.2174/1573402115666190409115330. PMID: 30963979.

[5] Burrello J, Monticone S, Buffolo F, Tetti M, Veglio F, Williams TA, et al. Is there a role for genomics in the management of hypertension? Int J Mol Sci 2017;18(6):1131. https://doi.org/10.3390/ijms18061131. PMID: 28587112.

[6] Ehret GB, Caulfield MJ. Genes for blood pressure: an opportunity to understand hypertension. Eur Heart J 2013;34(13):951–61. https://doi.org/10.1093/eurheartj/ehs455. PMID: 23303660; PMCID: PMC3612776.

[7] Monticone S, Burrello J, Tizzani D, Bertello C, Viola A, Buffolo F, et al. Prevalence and clinical manifestations of primary aldosteronism encountered in primary care practice. J Am Coll Cardiol 2017;69(14):1811–20. https://doi.org/10.1016/j.jacc.2017.01.052. PMID: 28385310.

[8] Hannemann A, Wallaschofski H. Prevalence of primary aldosteronism in patient's cohorts and in population-based studies–a review of the current literature. Horm Metab Res 2012;44(3):157–62. https://doi.org/10.1055/s-0031-1295438. PMID: 22135219.

[9] Funder JW, Carey RM, Mantero F, Murad MH, Reincke M, Shibata H, et al. The management of primary aldosteronism: case detection, diagnosis, and treatment: an endocrine society clinical practice guideline. J Clin Endocrinol Metab 2016;101(5):1889–916. https://doi.org/10.1210/jc.2015-4061. PMID: 26934393.

[10] Korah HE, Scholl UI. An update on familial hyperaldosteronism. Horm Metab Res 2015;47(13):941–6.

[11] Scholl UI. Genetics of primary aldosteronism. Hypertension 2022;79:887–897.. https://doi.org/10.1161/HYPERTENSIONAHA.121.16498.

[12] Choi M, Scholl UI, Yue P, Bjorklund P, Zhao B, Nelson-Williams C, et al. K^+ channel mutations in adrenal aldosterone-producing adenomas and hereditary hypertension. Science 2011;331(6018):768–72.

[13] Scholl UI, Goh G, Stolting G, de Oliveira RC, Choi M, Overton JD, et al. Somatic and germline CACNA1D calcium channel mutations in aldosterone-producing adenomas and primary aldosteronism. Nat Genet 2013;45(9):1050–4.

[14] Beuschlein F, Boulkroun S, Osswald A, Wieland T, Nielsen HN, Lichtenauer UD, et al. Somatic mutations in ATP1A1 and ATP2B3 lead to aldosterone-producing adenomas and secondary hypertension. Nat Genet 2013;45(4):440–4.

[15] Dutta RK, Arnesen T, Heie A, Walz M, Alesina P, Soderkvist P, et al. A somatic mutation in CLCN2 identified in a sporadic aldosterone-producing adenoma. Eur J Endocrinol 2019;181(5):K37–41.

[16] Nanba K, Blinder AR, Rege J, Hattangady NG, Else T, Liu CJ, et al. Somatic CACNA1H mutation as a cause of aldosterone-producing adenoma. Hypertension 2020;75(3):645–9.

[17] Fernandes-Rosa FL, Boulkroun S, Zennaro MC. Genetic and genomic mechanisms of primary aldosteronism. Trends Mol Med 2020;26(9):819–32. https://doi.org/10.1016/j.molmed.2020.05.005. PMID: 32563556.

[18] Tadjine M, Lampron A, Ouadi L, Bourdeau I. Frequent mutations of beta-catenin gene in sporadic secreting adrenocortical adenomas. Clin Endocrinol (Oxf) 2008;68(2):264−70.

[19] Zhou J, Azizan EAB, Cabrera CP, Fernandes-Rosa FL, Boulkroun S, Argentesi G, et al. Somatic mutations of GNA11 and GNAQ in CTNNB1-mutant aldosterone-producing adenomas presenting in puberty, pregnancy or menopause. Nat Genet 2021;53(9):1360−72.

[20] Rhayem Y, Perez-Rivas LG, Dietz A, Bathon K, Gebhard C, Riester A, et al. PRKACA somatic mutations are rare findings in aldosterone-producing adenomas. J Clin Endocrinol Metab 2016;101(8):3010−7.

[21] Nanba K, Rainey WE. Genetics in endocrinology: impact of race and sex on genetic causes of aldosterone-producing adenomas. Eur J Endocrinol 2021;185(1):R1−11.

[22] Nishimoto K, Tomlins SA, Kuick R, Cani AK, Giordano TJ, Hovelson DH, et al. Aldosterone-stimulating somatic gene mutations are common in normal adrenal glands. Proc Natl Acad Sci U S A 2015;112(33):E4591−9.

[23] Omata K, Satoh F, Morimoto R, Ito S, Yamazaki Y, Nakamura Y, et al. Cellular and genetic causes of idiopathic hyperaldosteronism. Hypertension 2018;72(4):874−80.

[24] Lifton RP, Dluhy RG, Powers M, Rich GM, Cook S, Ulick S, et al. A chimaeric 11 beta-hydroxylase/aldosterone synthase gene causes glucocorticoid-remediable aldosteronism and human hypertension. Nature 1992;355(6357):262−5. https://doi.org/10.1038/355262a0. PMID: 1731223.

[25] Carroll J, Dluhy R, Fallo F, Pistorello M, Bradwin G, Gomez-Sanchez CE, et al. Aldosterone-producing adenomas do not contain glucocorticoid-remediable aldosteronism chimeric gene duplications. J Clin Endocrinol Metab 1996;81(12):4310−2. https://doi.org/10.1210/jcem.81.12.8954032. PMID: 8954032.

[26] Stowasser M, Gordon RD, Tunny TJ, Klemm SA, Finn WL, Krek AL. Familial hyperaldosteronism type II: five families with a new variety of primary aldosteronism. Clin Exp Pharmacol Physiol May 1992;19(5):319−22. https://doi.org/10.1111/j.1440-1681.1992.tb00462.x. PMID: 1521363.

[27] Scholl UI, Stölting G, Schewe J, Thiel A, Tan H, Nelson-Williams C, et al. CLCN2 chloride channel mutations in familial hyperaldosteronism type II. Nat Genet 2018;50(3):349−54. https://doi.org/10.1038/s41588-018-0048-5. PMID: 29403011; PMCID: PMC5862758.

[28] Scholl UI, Stölting G, Nelson-Williams C, Vichot AA, Choi M, Loring E, et al. Recurrent gain of function mutation in calcium channel CACNA1H causes early-onset hypertension with primary aldosteronism. Elife 2015;4:e06315. https://doi.org/10.7554/eLife.06315. PMID: 25907736; PMCID: PMC4408447.

[29] Shimkets RA, Warnock DG, Bositis CM, Nelson-Williams C, Hansson JH, Schambelan M, et al. Liddle's syndrome: heritable human hypertension caused by mutations in the beta subunit of the epithelial sodium channel. Cell 1994;79(3):407−14.

[30] Hansson JH, Nelson-Williams C, Suzuki H, Schild L, Shimkets R, Lu Y, et al. Hypertension caused by a truncated epithelial sodium channel gamma subunit: genetic heterogeneity of Liddle syndrome. Nat Genet 1995;11(1):76−82.

[31] Salih M, Gautschi I, van Bemmelen MX, Di Benedetto M, Brooks AS, Lugtenberg D, et al. A missense mutation in the extracellular domain of alpha ENaC causes Liddle syndrome. J Am Soc Nephrol 2017;28(11):3291−9.

[32] Shibata S. 30 years of the mineralocorticoid receptor: mineralocorticoid receptor and NaCl transport mechanisms in the renal distal nephron. J Endocrinol 2017;234(1):T35−47. https://doi.org/10.1530/JOE-16-0669. PMID: 28341694.

[33] Roy A, Al-bataineh MM, Pastor-Soler NM. Collecting duct intercalated cell function and regulation. Clin J Am Soc Nephrol 2015;10(2):305−24. https://doi.org/10.2215/CJN.08880914. PMID: 25632105; PMCID: PMC4317747.

[34] Quentin F, Chambrey R, Trinh-Trang-Tan MM, Fysekidis M, Cambillau M, Paillard M, et al. The Cl-/HCO3- exchanger pendrin in the rat kidney is regulated in response to chronic alterations in chloride balance. Am J Physiol Renal Physiol 2004;287(6):F1179−88.

[35] Hou J, Renigunta A, Yang J, Waldegger S. Claudin-4 forms paracellular chloride channel in the kidney and requires claudin-8 for tight junction localization. Proc Natl Acad Sci U S A 2010;107(42):18010−5.

[36] Mune T, Rogerson FM, Nikkila H, Agarwal AK, White PC. Human hypertension caused by mutations in the kidney isozyme of 11 beta-hydroxysteroid dehydrogenase. Nat Genet 1995;10(4):394.

[37] Geller DS, Farhi A, Pinkerton N, Fradley M, Moritz M, Spitzer A, et al. Activating mineralocorticoid receptor mutation in hypertension exacerbated by pregnancy. Science 2000;289(5476):119−23. https://doi.org/10.1126/science.289.5476.119. PMID: 10884226.

[38] Rafestin-Oblin ME, Souque A, Bocchi B, Pinon G, Fagart J, Vandewalle A. The severe form of hypertension caused by the activating S810L mutation in the mineralocorticoid receptor is cortisone related. Endocrinology February 2003;144(2):528−33. https://doi.org/10.1210/en.2002-220708. PMID: 12538613.

[39] Wilson FH, Disse-Nicodeme S, Choate KA, Ishikawa K, Nelson-Williams C, Desitter I, et al. Human hypertension caused by mutations in WNK kinases. Science 2001;293(5532):1107−12.

[40] Boyden LM, Choi M, Choate KA, Nelson-Williams CJ, Farhi A, Toka HR, et al. Mutations in kelch-like 3 and cullin 3 cause hypertension and electrolyte abnormalities. Nature 2012;482(7383):98−102.

[41] Stowasser M, Pimenta E, Gordon RD. Familial or genetic primary aldosteronism and Gordon syndrome. Endocrinol Metab Clin North Am 2011;40:343−68.

[42] Mabillard H, Sayer JA. The molecular genetics of Gordon syndrome. Genes (Basel) 2019;10(12):986. https://doi.org/10.3390/genes10120986. PMID: 31795491; PMCID: PMC6947027.

[43] Ceccato F, Mantero F. Monogenic forms of hypertension. Endocrinol Metab Clin North Am 2019;48(4):795−810. https://doi.org/10.1016/j.ecl.2019.08.009. PMID: 31655777.

[44] Ferdaus MZ, McCormick JA. Mechanisms and controversies in mutant Cul3-mediated familial hyperkalemic hypertension. Am J Physiol Renal Physiol 2018;314(5):F915–20. https://doi.org/10.1152/ajprenal.00593.2017. PMID: 29361671; PMCID: PMC6031903.

[45] Golbang AP, Murthy M, Hamad A, Liu CH, Cope G, Van't Hoff W, et al. A new kindred with pseudohypoaldosteronism type II and a novel mutation (564D>H) in the acidic motif of the WNK4 gene. Hypertension August 2005;46(2):295–300. https://doi.org/10.1161/01.HYP.0000174326.96918.d6. PMID: 15998707.

[46] Wu G, Peng JB. Disease-causing mutations in KLHL3 impair its effect on WNK4 degradation. FEBS Lett 2013;587(12):1717–22. https://doi.org/10.1016/j.febslet.2013.04.032. PMID: 23665031; PMCCID: PMC3697765.

[47] Ohta A, Schumacher FR, Mehellou Y, Johnson C, Knebel A, Macartney TJ, et al. The CUL3-KLHL3 E3 ligase complex mutated in Gordon's hypertension syndrome interacts with and ubiquitylates WNK isoforms: disease-causing mutations in KLHL3 and WNK4 disrupt interaction. Biochem J 2013;451(1):111–22. https://doi.org/10.1042/BJ20121903. PMID: 23387299; PMCID: PMC3632089.

[48] Murillo-de-Ozores AR, Rodriguez-Gama A, Carbajal-Contreras H, Gamba G, Castaneda-Bueno M. WNK4 kinase: from structure to physiology. Am J Physiol Renal Physiol 2021;320(3):F378–403.

[49] Louis-Dit-Picard H, Kouranti I, Rafael C, Loisel-Ferreira I, Chavez-Canales M, Abdel-Khalek W, et al. Mutation affecting the conserved acidic WNK1 motif causes inherited hyperkalemic hyperchloremic acidosis. J Clin Invest 2020;130(12):6379–94.

[50] Hureaux M, Mazurkiewicz S, Boccio V, Vargas-Poussou R, Jeunemaitre X. The variety of genetic defects explains the phenotypic heterogeneity of Familial Hyperkalemic Hypertension. Kidney Int Rep 2021;6(10):2639–52.

[51] Maass PG, Aydin A, Luft FC, Schächterle C, Weise A, Stricker S, et al. PDE3A mutations cause autosomal dominant hypertension with brachydactyly. Nat Genet 2015;47(6):647–53. https://doi.org/10.1038/ng.3302. PMID: 25961942.

[52] Toka O, Tank J, Schächterle C, Aydin A, Maass PG, Elitok S, et al. Clinical effects of phosphodiesterase 3A mutations in inherited hypertension with brachydactyly. Hypertension 2015;66(4):800–8. https://doi.org/10.1161/HYPERTENSIONAHA.115.06000. PMID: 26283042.

[53] Ercu M, Marko L, Schachterle C, Tsvetkov D, Cui Y, Maghsodi S, et al. Phosphodiesterase 3A and arterial hypertension. Circulation 2020;142(2):133–49.

Chapter 7

Primary aldosteronism (Conn's syndrome)

Filippo Ceccato, Irene Tizianel, Giacomo Voltan and Franco Mantero
Endocrinology Unit, Department of Medicine DIMED, University Hospital of Padova, Padova, Italy

Visit the *Endocrine Hypertension: From Basic Science to Clinical Practice*, *First Edition* companion web site at: https://www.elsevier.com/books-and-journals/book-companion/9780323961202.

Graphical Abstract

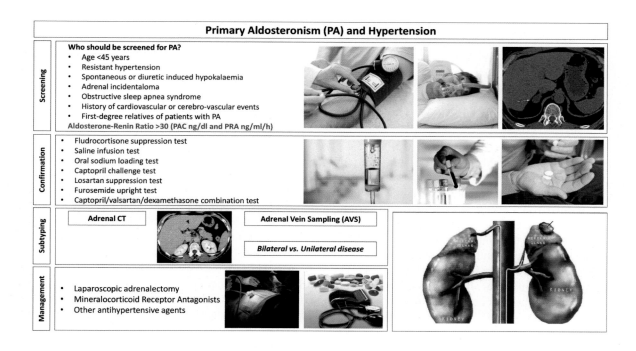

Endocrine Hypertension. https://doi.org/10.1016/B978-0-323-96120-2.00014-5

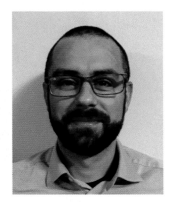

Filippo Ceccato

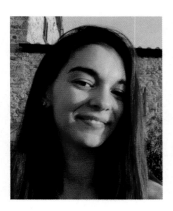

Irene Tizianel

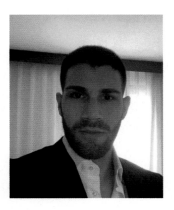

Giacomo Voltan

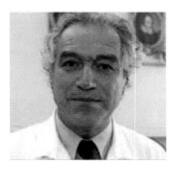

Franco Mantero

Introduction

Hypertension (HTN) is a highly prevalent condition in the general population (up to 30%−40% in large epidemiological studies, with more than 1 billion adults affected globally) [1,2], with persistently high incidence in central and eastern Europe, and from high-income countries to low-income countries [3]. The close relationship between blood pressure (BP) and cardiovascular (CV) events is continuous, thus complicating the distinction between normal BP levels and hypertension; nonetheless, level ≥140/90 mmHg is widely accepted as hypertension [1]. The most common form is essential hypertension [4,5]; on the contrary, at least 15%−20% of patients are affected by secondary hypertension (including endocrine and renal/renovascular forms), characterized by a specific and potentially reversible etiology that leads to increased BP levels. Endocrine forms of HTN are mainly secondary to uncontrolled cortisol, aldosterone, or catecholamine production [6−9]. All patients with early onset hypertension (not clearly evidence-based, albeit <40−45 years is widely accepted), resistant hypertension (defined as above-goal elevated blood pressure despite the use of three antihypertensive drugs, with at least one diuretic), or hypertension associated with electrolyte imbalance should be screened for secondary forms of HTN.

Primary aldosteronism (PA) is the most common form of endocrine hypertension; its prevalence is up to 10% among hypertensive patients and up to 20% of those with resistant hypertension [10,11]. PA is not a single disease, it should be considered as a group of disorders characterized by an inappropriately high aldosterone production for sodium status, not controlled by renin−angiotensin or potassium levels. Such inappropriate production of aldosterone causes sodium retention, hypertension, CV damage, and hypokalemia [6,12].

Common causes of PA are adrenal adenoma (also termed as Conn's disease/syndrome, first described by Jerome Conn in 1955 [13]), unilateral or bilateral adrenal hyperplasia, and in rare cases adrenal carcinoma or familial hyperaldosteronism. Patients with PA present an increased risk for cerebrovascular and CV events [14], due to target-organ damage, higher than in the matched group of patients with essential hypertension [6,10,12]. Moreover, glucose metabolism is also impaired in patients with PA, due to increased prevalence of diabetes and metabolic syndrome, with a further increase of the CV risk [14—18]. This chapter discusses the pathophysiology, clinical picture, diagnostic evaluation and management of PA.

The renin—angiotensin—aldosterone system

The differentiation of the adrenal cortex into distinct zones has important functional consequences and is thought to be dependent on the temporal expression of peculiar transcription factors.

Beneath the capsule, the zona glomerulosa layer comprises approximately 15% of the cortex (depending upon the sodium intake); aldosterone from this layer is the main mineralocorticoid in humans. Briefly, after cholesterol uptake into the mitochondria, it is cleaved by the cytochrome P450 enzyme for cholesterol side chain cleavage (steroidogenic acute regulatory protein) to pregnenolone. In the cytoplasm, pregnenolone is converted to progesterone and then 21-hydroxylase, derived from *CYP21A2* gene, performs 21-hydroxylation of progesterone to deoxycorticosterone (in the zona glomerulosa) or 17-OH-progesterone to 11-deoxycortisol (in the zona fasciculata). The final step is controlled by the enzyme CYP11B2 (aldosterone synthase), expressed only in the zona glomerulosa [19]. The adrenocortical steroidogenesis pathway is shown in Fig. 7.1.

Aldosterone production in the body is controlled by three principal factors: angiotensin II (the so-called renin—angiotensin—aldosterone system, RAAS), potassium, and to a lesser extent by adrenocorticotrophin (ACTH) [20]. Angiotensin II and potassium stimulate aldosterone secretion principally by increasing the transcription of *CYP11B2* through common intracellular signaling pathways, with cyclic adenosine monophosphate (cAMP), intracellular Ca^{2+}, and activation of calmodulin kinases. The potassium effect is mediated through membrane depolarization and opening of the calcium channels.

The effect of ACTH upon aldosterone secretion is modest and differs in time: an acute ACTH bolus will increase aldosterone secretion by stimulating the early pathways of adrenal steroidogenesis; on the contrary, chronic continual ACTH stimulation has either no effect, or even can reduce aldosterone production: this inhibitory effect is possibly secondary to receptor downregulation [21].

50%—70% of aldosterone circulates bound to either albumin or weakly to corticosteroid-binding globulin; 30%—50% of total plasma aldosterone is free, with a short half-life of 15—20 min. Aldosterone is inactivated to tetrahydroaldosterone in the liver. The classical functions of aldosterone are regulation of extracellular fluid volume and control of potassium homeostasis. These effects are mediated by binding of free aldosterone to the mineralocorticoid receptor in the cytosol of epithelial cells, principally in the kidney. Mineralocorticoid receptors have a tissue-specific expression, especially at distal nephron and colon. Aldosterone leads to modification of the apical sodium channel, resulting in increased sodium ion

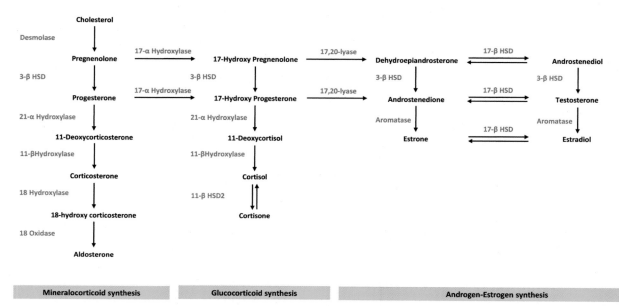

FIGURE 7.1 A schematic diagram of adrenocortical steroidogenesis pathway. *11β-HSD2*, 11β-hydroxysteroid dehydrogenase type 2; *HSD*, hydroxysteroid dehydrogenase.

transport across the cell membrane. Glucocorticoids and mineralocorticoids bind equally to the mineralocorticoid receptor: specificity is provided by the presence of a glucocorticoid-degrading enzyme, 11β-hydroxysteroid dehydrogenase type 2, which prevents glucocorticoids from interacting with the aldosterone receptor by converting cortisol to inactive cortisone.

Renin is a 340-aminoacid enzyme produced primarily in the juxtaglomerular apparatus of the kidney, controlled by the macula densa (a group of distal convoluted tubular cells that function as chemoreceptors for sodium) and juxtaglomerular cells (pressure transducers that sense stretch of the afferent arteriolar wall and thus renal perfusion pressure). Also the sympathetic nervous system and potassium levels control renin secretion [22]. Angiotensinogen, synthesized in the liver, is the substrate for renin and is broken down into angiotensin I. Angiotensin II is formed by cleavage of the two carboxy-terminal peptides of angiotensin I by angiotensin-converting enzyme (ACE), localized to cell membranes in the lung and intracellular granules [23]. Angiotensin II then stimulates aldosterone secretion.

Aldosterone has additional nonclassic effects primarily on nonepithelial cells. These actions, although probably genomic and therefore mediated by activation of the cytosolic mineralocorticoid receptor, do not include modification of sodium—potassium balance. Aldosterone-mediated actions include the expression of several collagen genes, growth factors, plasminogen activator inhibitor type 1, or genes mediating inflammation. These actions lead to microangiopathy and fibrosis in various tissues such as heart, blood vessels, and kidney. Increased levels of aldosterone are not necessary to cause this damage; an imbalance between the volume or sodium balance state and the level of aldosterone appears to be the critical factor [24].

For further reading on RAAS, please refer Chapter 5.

Who should be screened? (The epidemiology of primary aldosteronism)

The diagnostic pathway of PA consists of three main steps: screening tests, confirmatory tests, and identification of PA subtype [25]. The high-risk category of hypertensive patients that should be screened for PA, recommended by the Endocrine Society (ES) Clinical Practice Guideline [12] are those with: age <45 years, spontaneous or diuretic-induced hypokalaemia, adrenal incidentaloma, history of CV or cerebro-vascular events, first-degree relatives of patients with PA, resistant hypertension, and obstructive sleep apnea syndrome (OSAS).

In patients with resistant hypertension, the prevalence of PA varies from 11% to 30% [26,27]. The high prevalence of PA in patients with resistant hypertension reflects that the use of mineralocorticoid receptor antagonists (MRAs) would be particularly effective in such cases [28].

Prevalence of PA is also reported high in patients with hypertension and atrial fibrillation [29]. Elevated aldosterone levels predispose to atrial fibrillation [30]. The aldosterone-induced inflammation, myocardial necrosis, cardiac collagen deposition, and fibrosis can induce atrial arrhythmias [31]. Also diabetic patients are at high-risk for PA: in a recent study published in 2020, 99 out of 256 patients (39%) presented a positive screening test, and 49 (19%) were diagnosed with PA after a confirmatory captopril challenge test [32].

One of the novel high-risk conditions for PA is OSAS: it is a chronic condition characterized by frequent episodes of upper airway collapse resulting in hypoxemia while sleeping, and can lead to severe complications if left untreated. OSAS prevalence is 3%—7% in the general population, with some groups in the general population carrying a higher risk [33]. Aldosterone excess may play a pathophysiological part in the relationship between hypertension and OSAS, since higher plasma aldosterone concentrations (PACs) and OSAS were seen in patients with refractory hypertension [34], and the prevalence of OSAS was higher in subjects with PA than in patients with essential hypertension [35]. In 2004, Calhoun et al. studied the renin—aldosterone axis in more than 100 patients with OSAS: subjects at high risk of OSAS were almost twice as likely to have PA and tended to have lower renin levels [36].

For more detailed reading on the relationship between OSAS and PA, please refer Chapter 17.

Despite the high prevalence of PA in the hypertensive population, its occurrence among patients with an adrenal incidentaloma is relatively low, ranging from 1.5% to 7% only [37,38]. Obviously, adrenal lesions of patients investigated with abdominal imaging in search of the causes of secondary hypertension are not "incidentalomas" [8]. The question regarding the cost-effectiveness of exploring aldosterone secretion in all patients with adrenal incidentaloma or only in hypertensive subjects is a matter of ongoing debate [37,39—41]. Subclinical hyperaldosteronism can exist in an adrenal incidentaloma, especially in those with increased diastolic blood pressure levels [42].

Aldosterone—renin ratio as screening test

Aldosterone—renin ratio (ARR) is recommended as the initial test to screen for PA. ARR has been proposed as a screening test since early 1980s [43]. Its application is recommended in the current Endocrine Society guidelines [12] and leads to an increased detection of PA, especially among hypertensive normokalaemic patients. The routine use of ARR as a screening test led to a 5 to 15-fold increase in the PA identification [44]. A recent metaanalysis in 2021, in which the performance of ARR to detect PA in 4110 participants (ten studies) was evaluated, reported that the sensitivity of ARR ranged from 10% to 100% and the specificity ranged from 70% to 100%, and that no single ARR could be recommended for definitive diagnosis [45].

The concentrations of aldosterone and renin are affected by several drugs, especially those directed to RAAS, as well as by clinical conditions. Consequently, special attention should be paid about antihypertensive treatment and potassium levels of the patients with suspected PA. In Table 7.1 we describe drugs or other clinical conditions that could affect the measurement of aldosterone and renin.

The concentrations and units are different for aldosterone and renin (either direct renin concentration, DRC, or plasma renin activity, PRA), and this must be considered while calculating the ARR. In this regard, it was decided not to establish a rigid cut-off for ARR in consideration of the variability of the RIA assays for aldosterone and renin and the different criteria for entering the values of the two parameters in various centers. In fact, some believe it is appropriate to use the PAC absolute values when the PRA or DRC values are extremely low (cut-off for PAC values greater than 10 ng/dL or 280 pmol/L). A raised ARR value resulting from an extremely low PRA or DRC values in the presence of a PAC value that is low-normal is inconsistent with PA. Thus, ARR should be used when PRA is not lower than 0.2 ng/mL/h or DRC is not lower than 6 mU/L. One of the better combinations in diagnostic accuracy considering ARR cutoff, as the best in sensitivity and specificity, is 30 (PAC in ng/dL and PRA in ng/mL/h) or 3.7 (PAC in ng/dL and DRC in mU/L) [46].

Blood sample has to be collected in the morning, after the patient has been up (sitting, standing, or walking) for at least 2 h and seated for 5−15 min. It is advisable to correct potassium depletion and ask the patient not to limit sodium intake in the days before blood sampling. Medical wash-out period should be 4 weeks for MRAs (spironolactone, potassium canrenoate, and eplerenone), diuretics and liquorice; and ideally at least 2−3 weeks before the sampling for nonsteroidal antiinflammatory drugs, β-adrenergic blockers, ACE-i, ARBs, dihydropiridine calcium-channel antagonists, and renin inhibitors. Other antihypertensive agents that do not affect the RAAS such as slow-release verapamil, hydralazine, and the α1-selective adrenergic blockers are recommended for HTN control if needed [8,12].

If discontinuation of all the confounding agents is not possible (e.g., severe hypokalemia or uncontrolled hypertension), an ARR should be performed and the results interpreted in light of the potentially interrupting factors. However, careful attention must be paid not only to the ARR, but also to plasma renin and aldosterone concentrations. ARR is a ratio, and therefore, a very low denominator value (renin) leads to an increased ARR, despite normal or even low aldosterone levels. Consequently, a minimum aldosterone concentration is suggested (10−15 ng/dL or 280−420 pmol/L) to suspect PA biochemically [6].

Notably, the results of an ARR during interfering medications can still be informative: a suppressed renin during medical treatment that should increase renin (as ACE-i, ARBs, diuretics, or MRAs) is highly suggestive of PA. Moreover, ARR cutoffs are different if aldosterone is measured with liquid chromatography coupled with tandem mass spectrometry (LS-MS/MS) [47].

Confirmatory test after positive ARR

ARR is a screening test, with a high sensitivity (68%−94%), high negative predictive value (100%), but only a moderate specificity. Therefore, false-positive results (i.e., increased ARR in patients who do not have PA) are common, and a second-line confirmatory test is often suggested to confirm or exclude PA [25,48].

It is recommended that during the few days before the confirmatory test, patients have a normal sodium intake and also receive potassium supplementation in order to correct hypokalemia. Saline infusion test is the most widely used, followed by the captopril challenge test, which is simple and effective, and the oral sodium loading test which is less often used. Other tests including the losartan suppression test, the furosemide upright test, and the captopril/valsartan/dexamethasone combination test have also been described [49].

Indeed, fludrocortisone suppression test (oral 0.1 mg every 6 h over 4 days) is considered by some authors as the most effective method; unsuppressed aldosterone (>6 ng/dL; 167 pmol/L) is highly likely to suggest PA, especially in a case of suppressed renin. However, this test is cumbersome and requires hospitalization. A more feasible and commonly used suppression test (with an acute load of 2 L of isotonic saline over 4 h) is saline infusion test: aldosterone <5 ng/dL (140 pmol/L) after 4 h excludes PA, while >10 ng/dL (280 pmol/L) confirms PA, and levels between 5 and 10 ng/dL (140−280 pmol/L) are considered a "gray zone" and may be seen in patients with idiopathic adrenal hyperplasia [49]. The saline infusion test has a sensitivity of 88% using the aldosterone cut-off of <5 ng/dL to exclude PA. If a patient is at risk

TABLE 7.1 Drugs and other conditions that could interfere with endocrine assessment of patients with primary aldosteronism.

	Aldosterone	Renin	ARR
Drugs			
Beta-adrenergic blockers	↓	↓↓	↑
Central agonist (clonidine)	↓	↓↓	↑
NSAIDs	↓	↓↓	↑
K+-wasting diuretics	→↑	↑↑	↓
K+-sparing diuretics	↑	↑↑	↓
ACE inhibitors	↓	↑↑	↓
ARBs	↓	↑↑	↓
Renin inhibitors	↓	↓(PRA)↑(DRC)	↑↓
Ca^{2+} blockers (DHPs)	→↓	↑↑	↓
Ca^{2+} blockers (non DHPs)	→	→	→
Alpha1-adrenergic blockers	→	→	→
Antiepileptic drugs	→	→	→
Rifampin, rifapentine	→	→	→
Pioglitazone	→	→	→
Itraconazole, ritonavir, fluoxetine, cimetidine, aprepitant	→	→	→
Estrogens	↑	↑↑	↓
11β-HSD2 inhibitors (licorice)	↓→	↓→	↓→
Potassium status			
Hypokalemia	↓	↑	↓
Potassium loading	↑	→↓	↑
Dietary sodium			
Sodium restriction	↑	↑↑	↓
Sodium loading	↓	↓↓	↑
Advancing age	↓	↓↓	↑
Premenopausal women (vs. male)	→↑	↓	↑
Other conditions			
Renal impairment	→	↓	↑
Pregnancy	↑	↑↑	↓
Renovascular HTN	↑	↑↑	↓
Malignant HTN	↑	↑↑	↓

↑, levels increased; ↓, levels reduced; →, unaffected test; *11β-HSD2*, 11 beta hydroxysteroid dehydrogenase type 2; *ARR*, aldosterone to renin ratio; *ACE*, angiotensin-converting enzyme; *ARBs*, angiotensin II type 1 receptor blockers; *Ca^{2+}*, calcium; *DHPs*, dihydropyridines; *DRC*: direct renin concentration; *HTN*, hypertension; *K^{+}*, potassium; *NSAIDs*, nonsteroidal antiinflammatory drugs; *PRA*: plasma renin activity.

of volume overload, the captopril challenge test is preferred among confirmatory tests: 25—50 mg of captopril is administered orally, and aldosterone, plasma renin activity (or direct renin concentration) are measured after 2 h. After captopril challenge test, a decrease in PAC by <30% and suppressed renin confirms PA (other aldosterone cutoff thresholds between 246 and 390 pmol/L could be considered).

Actually, based on abundant retrospective data, solid evidence is emerging from several authors that in many cases, in which clinical and basic endocrine evaluation are strongly in favor of hyperaldosteronism without any dispute, confirmation tests can be avoided. Of course, this choice, albeit with some risk, could greatly simplify the diagnosis of this pathology. As a matter of fact, confirmatory tests might be redundant if the clinical likelihood of PA is high as in patients with resistant hypertension, low potassium levels, high aldosterone concentration, and suppressed renin.

Subtyping in primary aldosteronism: adrenal vein sampling or imaging?

The subtype diagnosis is pivotal in identifying patients who are suitable for unilateral adrenalectomy. The two subtypes of PA are unilateral or bilateral, although true unilateral PA without any contralateral hypersecretion is less common [50].

The first step of subtype detection is adrenal computed tomography (CT), which can identify unilateral or bilateral adenomas, micro- or macronodular adrenal hyperplasia, or the rare unilateral carcinoma. CT will not be able to identify the secretory nature of the nodules, neither with CT Hounsfield units (HU) measurement nor with contrast washout characteristics [51]. Except in selected cases (such as a single adrenal nodule in a young-onset PA), adrenal vein sampling (AVS) is a reasonable choice, especially in the modern concept of multidisciplinary approach to adrenal diseases [52].

Since the correct localization of adrenal vein is of utmost importance in the AVS interpretation, the interventional radiologist should be skilled and must examine the CT imaging for better planning of AVS. Moreover, incidentally discovered adrenal adenomas are more prevalent in older patients (peak incidence over 65 years); therefore, the accuracy of CT imaging in the diagnosis of subtyping in these patients is lower (i.e., the presence of an adrenal incidentaloma contralateral to the source of aldosterone secretion). On the contrary, due to the low prevalence of adrenal adenomas in the young population, finding a small unilateral adrenal adenoma in a young patient with PA is more likely to suggest ipsilateral disease [53,54]. Moreover, CT imaging is discordant with AVS in 40% of patients with PA [53,55]. Magnetic resonance (MR) is a second choice for imaging adrenal nodules because it's inferior to CT due to its lower spatial resolution [56].

AVS is considered the gold standard for subtyping of PA and it is recommended by all international guidelines. It is an essential investigation in order to provide appropriate treatment in patients with PA who have a high probability of unilateral aldosterone-producing adenoma and are willing to have a potential surgical cure [12,57].

AVS is not widely available because it is a challenging procedure, poorly standardized, and has to be performed by an interventional radiologist with great expertise. However, in experienced hands, the technical success rate can be near 90%. It is done by a percutaneous femoral approach and adrenal veins are catheterized simultaneously or sequentially [58]. Blood samples are obtained from both adrenal veins and from the inferior vena cava (IVC), and assayed for aldosterone and cortisol concentrations. The cortisol concentrations from the adrenal veins and IVC are used to confirm successful catheterization. Adrenal vein to IVC cortisol ratio should be at least 2:1. Dividing the right and left adrenal vein aldosterone concentration values by their respective cortisol concentration provides cortisol-corrected ratios. Then, divide the higher cortisol-corrected aldosterone ratio to the lower one provides the lateralization index. A lateralization index >4 indicates unilateral aldosterone excess, whereas a lateralization index <3 may suggest bilateral aldosterone excess; values between 3 and 4 are indeterminate and may be defined as in "gray zone" [56,58].

According to a recent study, 46% of centers use synthetic ACTH (cosyntropin; ATCH 1—24) infusion during AVS. The logic behind using ACTH is to minimize the stress-induced fluctuations in aldosterone secretion during nonsimultaneous AVS, to maximize cortisol gradient from adrenal vein to IVC and thus confirming accurate sampling, and to maximize the secretion of aldosterone from aldosterone-producing adenomas [59]. Complications of AVS are uncommon and these include groin hematoma, adrenal hemorrhage, and adrenal vein dissection [60]. It is noteworthy that AVS can be performed regardless of concomitant medications only if plasma renin activity remains suppressed [61]. In some patients with PA there is concomitant cortisol hypersecretion, but in most cases, this cortisol excess is mild. Steroid metabolome analysis reveals prevalent glucocorticoid excess in PA [62]. In these cases, a low-grade cortisol cosecretion has a limited impact on ACTH-stimulated AVS parameters in PA [63]. Recently, it has been reported that simultaneous androstenedione or metanephrine assays outperformed the cortisol correlation for ascertaining AVS success [64].

Regarding the role of imaging and AVS in the diagnosis of subtyping PA, one prospective randomized trial comparing AVS with CT-based decision on treatment (SPARTACUS trial) found no significant differences between the postoperative need for antihypertensive therapy and quality of life in 184 patients with PA [65]. On the contrary, another multicenter international retrospective nonrandomized study reported biochemical remission ratio in 80% (188 of 235) cases after a CT-based treatment decision vs 93% (491 of 526) after an AVS-based treatment decision. In conclusion, patients diagnosed by imaging study only are less likely to achieve complete biochemical remission compared with those diagnosed with AVS [66].

These data were confirmed by a recent multicenter international study on 1311 patients, which found that imaging alone did not provide an accurate diagnostic value in PA, especially in unilateral PA. In fact in this cohort, cross-sectional imaging did not identify a lateralized cause of disease in around 40% of PA patients and failed to identify the culprit adrenal in 28% of patients with unilateral PA [67]. Aldosterone-producing cell clusters (APCCs) are one of the main pitfalls of AVS. To describe this briefly, APCCs are group of cells positive for *CYP11B2* expression (aldosterone synthetase gene) focally in the subcapsular portion of the human adult adrenal cortex; they produce and secrete excessive aldosterone, but are too small that even modern imaging techniques are unable to localize them [68]. For further reading on adrenal imaging studies, please refer Chapter 20.

Laparoscopic surgery and peri-operative management

Surgical treatment of PA aims to remove the source of aldosterone excess and to treat hyperaldosteronism-related comorbidities such as hypertension, hypokalemia, CV, and kidney damages.

Unilateral adrenalectomy is the gold standard treatment for patients with unilateral PA. Laparoscopic adrenalectomy is the preferred surgical approach. However, this should be performed by an expert adrenal surgeon. The duration of hospitalization and the rate of clinical and surgical complications are lower compared with open adrenalectomy [69]. Adrenalectomy of the entire gland is the treatment of choice. Adrenal sparing approach (cortical sparing partial adrenalectomy) should be avoided as additional aldosterone producing micronodules or APCC clusters, even in case of AVS lateralization, could be present unilaterally. Moreover AVS is usually able to identify which adrenal is responsible for overproduction of aldosterone, but not which part of the gland; hence, nodulectomy of the single lesion alone might not be always curative [70].

In the recent years, the improvement of surgical techniques, especially with close collaboration between surgeons and endocrinologists, allowed the reduction of perioperative complications. According to the Endocrine Society's guidelines, blood pressure and potassium levels should be normalized in patients with PA before surgery [12]. The experience of surgical team and anesthetic support is fundamental, since during surgery a 20 mmHg blood pressure increase and 0.5—1 mEq/L plasma potassium level drop may be observed [71]. During the first day after surgery, the blood pressure and potassium levels must be strictly monitored. Withdrawal of MRAs and potassium supplementation should be considered in order to avoid postsurgical hypotension and hyperkalemia [52].

The improvement of blood pressure occurs in a time lapse of 1—6 months after surgery; thus, the concomitant antihypertensive drugs must be downtitrated. An evidence-based approach is not available, so potassium levels and blood pressure should be determined within 3 months after surgery to identify whether to reduce or discontinue the antihypertensive drugs and to optimize potassium supplementation if necessary [52]. After surgery, the reasonable endpoints are the reduction (47%) or withdrawal (37%) of antihypertensive therapy, and the normalization of serum potassium and ARR (94%) [65,72].

During the first few weeks after surgery, hypoaldosteronism must be anticipated due to chronic suppression of the contralateral adrenal gland, and therefore, a large sodium intake is suggested. Physicians should also pay attention to the development of hyperkalemia, which is reported in 16% of patients; postoperative increased creatinine and microalbuminuria are significant predictors of postsurgical hyperkalemia [73]. It should be remembered that a minor proportion of patients (close to 5%) who underwent unilateral adrenalectomy could present with persistent hypoaldosteronism requiring further mineralocorticoid replacement therapy [74], probably due to long-term renin suppression.

In some cases, signs of postsurgical adrenal insufficiency are due to cosecretion of cortisol by aldosterone producing adenomas. In these cases, adrenalectomy could unmask a glucocorticoid insufficiency of the contralateral adrenal gland [62]; therefore, glucocorticoid substitution treatment should be considered after adrenalectomy.

Medical therapy of primary aldosteronism

The goals of medical treatment of PA are the normalization of blood pressure and potassium levels and the reduction of CV risk. Medical therapy is usually recommended in patients with bilateral adrenal hyperplasia, bilateral aldosterone producing adenomas, and genetic forms of hyperaldosteronism; it is also the treatment of choice in patients with unilateral PA who refuse surgery or in whom surgery is contraindicated [75].

MRAs are effective in controlling blood pressure and the systemic effects of aldosterone excess. Nowadays, there are two classes of MRAs available in the market, viz. spironolactone and eplerenone.

Spironolactone is a potassium-sparing diuretic which exerts a competitive inhibition on the mineralocorticoid receptor. After oral administration, it's converted to other active metabolites with long half-lives, such as canrenoate, which are responsible for the majority of pharmacological effects [76].

The starting dose of spironolactone should be 12.5–25 mg/day; and the dose might be gradually uptitrated until the lowest effective dose is reached, with a maximum ideal dose suggested at 100 mg/day [12]. Doses between 25 and 50 mg/day had been reported effective in lowering systolic blood pressure by 15 mmHg and diastolic by 8 mmHg, and half of the patients had a blood pressure lower than 140/90 mmHg with spironolactone monotherapy. However, the onset of action of the drug is slow, and it requires many weeks to reach the maximum effects in blood pressure reduction [77]. Spironolactone often causes some dose-related side effects including gynecomastia and impotence in males and spotting/menstrual irregularities in females. In males, gynecomastia was reported in 10% of cases at a dose of 25 mg/day, while at a dose greater than 150 mg/day its incidence increased to about 52%. The incidence of menstrual irregularities, instead, is not well known. Monitoring potassium levels is suggested though hyperkalemia during spironolactone therapy is rare in patients with PA.

Eplerenone is a newer steroid-selective MRA without significant antiandrogen and progesterone agonist effects. Eplerenone has a 3–6 h half-life and it requires twice daily administration. Due to its receptor selectivity, the side effects are lower compared with spironolactone; however, it has only 50% of the antagonist potency of spironolactone. The main indication of eplerenone is left ventricular dysfunction after myocardial infarction, while its use for PA and hypertension is not approved in every country. Despite its better tolerability, the efficacy in controlling blood pressure could be lower and eplerenone is much more expensive than spironolactone [78].

Third-generation MRAs (as selective as eplerenone, as potent as spironolactone, and with a nonsteroidal chemical structure) are in development: finerenone has a balanced distribution between the heart and the kidney, equinatriuretic doses of finerenone show more potent antiinflammatory and antifibrotic effects on the kidney in rodent models than

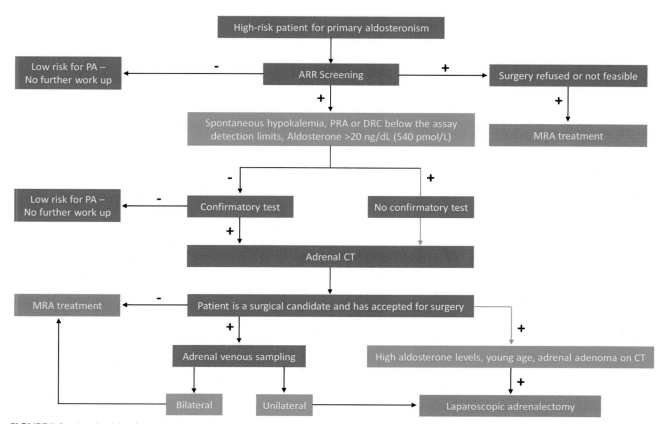

FIGURE 7.2 An algorithm for evaluation and management of patients with sporadic primary aldosteronism. *ARR*, aldosterone renin ratio; *CT*, computed tomography; *DRC*, direct renin concentration; *MRA*, mineralocorticoid receptor antagonist; *PA*, primary aldosteronism; *PRA*, plasma renin activity.

spironolactone. Overall, nonsteroidal MRAs appear to demonstrate a better benefit—risk ratio than steroidal MRAs where risk is measured as the propensity for hyperkalaemia. Finerenone reduced chronic kidney disease progression, kidney failure, or kidney death when added to the standard of care, especially in diabetic patients [79].

MRA treatment can be complimented with other drugs like amiloride, calcium channel blockers, or thiazide diuretics. The use of ACE-i or ARBs could be considered because aldosterone in some adenomas and especially in bilateral hyperplasia is angiotensin responsive; furthermore, after an effective blockade of MR receptor, renin levels are no longer suppressed reexposing RAAS to pharmacological inhibition [25].

Surgical treatment of PA seems to be more effective than therapy with MRAs not only in controlling blood pressure and reducing the number of antihypertensive drugs, but also in lowering the risk of atrial fibrillation, kidney diseases, and in reversing left ventricular hypertrophy. Moreover, adrenalectomy appears to be superior in reducing long-term mortality than the treatment with mineralocorticoid receptor blockade [80,81].

Fig. 7.2 summarizes the evaluation and management of patients with sporadic PA.

For additional reading on PA, please refer Chapter 21.

Familial forms of primary aldosteronism

Familial hyperaldosteronism (FH, summarized in Table 7.2) is a rare form of PA and all the known subtypes are characterized by an autosomal dominant pattern of inheritance.

The first discovered form is FH-I, also known as GRA (Glucocorticoid-Remediable Aldosteronism), and it was described for the first time in 1966 studying a father and a son with hypertension at a young age and hypokalemia [82]. The phenotype consists of an early-onset hypertension with a positive family history; also cerebral hemorrhages and ruptured intracranial aneurysms are common. The historical diagnosis was based on the attenuation of phenotype and decrease of aldosterone levels after dexamethasone administration [83].

FH-I is caused by a recombination, through an unequal crossing-over, between the genes *CYP11B1*, encoding 11 beta-hydroxylase (involved in cortisol synthesis and controlled by ACTH), and *CYP11B2* encoding aldosterone synthase. The consequence is the ectopic expression of *CYP11B2* in the zona fasciculata, which leads to increased aldosterone production under the control of ACTH. Hybrid steroids like 18-oxocortisol and 18-hydroxycortisol are also produced in excess and this is a marker of abnormal colocalization of enzymes involved in aldosterone and cortisol synthesis [84]. Treatment is based on the administration of glucocorticoids (dexamethasone or prednisone) in order to suppress pituitary ACTH; MR antagonists could be added to achieve a better blood pressure and potassium level control. In adults, the starting doses of dexamethasone and prednisone are 0.125—0.25 mg/day and 2.5—5 mg/day respectively, administered at bedtime [12].

FH-II denotes individuals with a germline mutation of *CLCN2* gene, encoding the chloride channel ClC-2 which regulates net outflow of chloride in the zona glomerulosa. Mutations of this channel lead to an increased chloride efflux with consequent cell depolarization, voltage-dependent calcium channel opening, calcium influx, and increased aldosterone production. FH-II patients typically show early-onset hypertension, usually with an age at diagnosis before 20 years. As in FH-I, incomplete penetrance with variable phenotypical expression has been reported. These forms are usually well controlled using MR antagonists alone, or in combination with other antihypertensive drugs [85].

TABLE 7.2 Familial hyperaldosteronism (FH) subtypes, gene abnormalities, classical features, and treatment options.

Subtype	Gene mutation	Distinctive features	Therapy
FH-I	CYP11B1/CYP11B2	Responsive to glucocorticoids	Dexamethasone/prednisone, MRA
FH-II	CLCN2		MRA
FH-III	KCNJ5	Possible adrenal hyperplasia	MRA, bilateral adrenalectomy
FH-IV	CACNA1H		MRA
PASNA Syndrome	CACNA1D	Seizures, neurological abnormalities, heart defects	MRA

MRA, mineralcorticoid receptor antagonist; *PASNA*, primary aldosteronism, seizures, and neurologic abnormalities.

FH-III refers to patients who present with germline mutations of *KCNJ5* gene, encoding for an inward rectifier potassium channel. Mutations lead to a massive sodium influx with cell depolarization and activation of the calcium channel; the final result is an overproduction of aldosterone. Several types of mutation are described associated with different disease severity; for example, T158A shows a severe phenotype characterized by bilateral enlargement of adrenal glands and intractable PA. Mutation G151R also leads to adrenal hyperplasia, while patients G151E mutation present normal adrenal glands and a good response to medical therapy [86,87].

FH-IV is secondary to germline mutations in *CACNA1H* gene encoding for a T-type calcium channel. Those mutations induce gain of function activity of the channel, leading to an increased calcium influx and aldosterone overproduction [88].

Another rare complex disorder is PASNA syndrome, characterized by PA, seizures, and neurological abnormalities have been associated with germline gain of function mutations in *CACNA1D*, encoding an L-type calcium channel. Epilepsy, autism, heart defects, and hypoglycemia are described as associated symptoms [89,90].

Several somatic mutations recently reported (*KCNJ5, ATP1A1, ATP2B3, CACNA1D, CLCN2,* or *CTNNB1*) were identified and recognized in a large number of adrenal adenomas of patients with PA, which are able to activate calcium signaling and activate *CYP11B2* gene transcription in the adrenal cells. Furthermore, DNA methylation analysis revealed that promoter region of *CYP11B2* was entirely hypomethylated in PA [68].

The most useful drug to manage hypertension in patients with familial hyperaldosteronism is MRAs. However, for patients with GRA, the treatment of choice is glucocorticoid drugs, in order to partially suppress ACTH secretion by the pituitary gland. Synthetic glucocorticoids with a long half-life such as dexamethasone or prednisone are preferred to hydrocortisone; they should be taken at bedtime to suppress the morning ACTH surge [91]. In order to avoid glucocorticoid overtreatment which could lead to iatrogenic Cushing's syndrome, physician must use the lowest possible dose of glucocorticoid for normalizing the blood pressure and controlling the potassium levels. Assessment of plasma renin activity or direct renin concentration could be useful to titrate medical treatment and to prevent overtreatment [92]. Glucocorticoid treatment might not be enough to normalize the blood pressure. Hence, MRAs could be added, preferring eplerenone to spironolactone in children affected because of the lack of antiandrogenic effects [12].

For more details on inherited forms of PA and monogenic HTN, please refer Chapters 6, 8, and 10.

Conclusions

PA is the most common form of endocrine hypertension; an effort from the endocrine community should be to spread the knowledge to all the other physicians who treat hypertension, in order to achieve a prompt, timely, and correct diagnosis. With a correct diagnosis, achieving long-term remission is often possible with surgery or with appropriate medical treatment.

In order to reduce health-related costs, and to optimize diagnostic evaluation, recent efforts have been taken to reduce the number of second-line tests and the suggestion of AVS only to the patients with high likelihood of remission after surgery.

Learning points

- PA is the most common disorder resulting in endocrine hypertension with an estimated prevalence of approximately 10% in the hypertensive population.
- ARR measurement is the proposed screening test with special attention to be paid about antihypertensive treatment and potassium levels before blood collection. Its diagnostic accuracy is not great, and no single ARR could be recommended for definitive diagnosis.
- The diagnosis of subtype is essential for the appropriate management: adrenalectomy in case of unilateral disease and medical treatment for bilateral forms. CT can identify unilateral or bilateral adenomas; however, the highest accuracy for identifying the lateralization is the AVS.
- The goals of medical treatment of PA are the normalization of blood pressure and potassium levels and the reduction of CV risk. MRAs are effective in controlling blood pressure and most systemic effects of aldosterone excess.
- Familial hyperaldosteronism is a rare form of PA characterized by an autosomal dominant pattern of inheritance and several somatic mutations in aldosterone producing adenomas are also reported and recognized.

References

[1] Mancia G, Fagard R, Narkiewicz K, et al. 2013 ESH/ESC guidelines for the management of arterial hypertension: the task force for the management of arterial hypertension of the European Society of Hypertension (ESH) and of the European Society of Cardiology (ESC). Eur Heart J 2013;34(28):2159–219. https://doi.org/10.1093/eurheartj/eht151.

[2] Mills KT, Bundy JD, Kelly TN, et al. Global disparities of hypertension prevalence and control. Circulation 2016;134(6):441–50. https://doi.org/10.1161/CIRCULATIONAHA.115.018912.

[3] Zhou B, Bentham J, Di Cesare M, et al. Worldwide trends in blood pressure from 1975 to 2015: a pooled analysis of 1479 population-based measurement studies with 19·1 million participants. Lancet 2017;389(10064):37–55. https://doi.org/10.1016/S0140-6736(16)31919-5.

[4] Rimoldi SF, Scherrer U, Messerli FH. Secondary arterial hypertension: when, who, and how to screen? Eur Heart J 2014;35(19):1245–54. https://doi.org/10.1093/eurheartj/eht534.

[5] Manosroi W, Williams GH. Genetics of human primary hypertension: focus on hormonal mechanisms. Endocr Rev 2019;40(3):825–56. https://doi.org/10.1210/er.2018-00071.

[6] Cicala MV, Mantero F. Primary Aldosteronism: what consensus for the diagnosis. Best Pract Res Clin Endocrinol Metab 2010;24(6):915–21. https://doi.org/10.1016/j.beem.2010.10.007.

[7] Cicala MV, Mantero F. Hypertension in Cushing's syndrome: from pathogenesis to treatment. Neuroendocrinology 2010;92(1):44–9. https://doi.org/10.1159/000314315.

[8] Grasso M, Boscaro M, Scaroni C, Ceccato F. Secondary arterial hypertension: from routine clinical practice to evidence in patients with adrenal tumor. High Blood Pres Cardiovasc Prev 2018;25(4):345–54. https://doi.org/10.1007/s40292-018-0288-6.

[9] Ceccato F, Mantero F. Monogenic forms of hypertension. Endocrinol Metab Clin North Am 2019;48(4):795–810. https://doi.org/10.1016/j.ecl.2019.08.009.

[10] Sabbadin C, Fallo F. Hyperaldosteronism: screening and diagnostic tests. High Blood Pres Cardiovasc Prev 2016;23(2):69–72. https://doi.org/10.1007/s40292-016-0136-5.

[11] Williams TA, Reincke M. Management of endocrine disease: diagnosis and management of primary aldosteronism: the endocrine society guideline 2016 revisited. Eur J Endocrinol 2018;179(1):R19–29. https://doi.org/10.1530/EJE-17-0990.

[12] Funder JW, Carey RM, Mantero F, et al. The management of primary aldosteronism: case detection, diagnosis, and treatment: an endocrine society clinical practice guideline. J Clin Endocrinol Metab 2016;101(5):1889–916. https://doi.org/10.1210/jc.2015-4061.

[13] CONN JW. Presidential address. I. Painting background. II. Primary aldosteronism, a new clinical syndrome. J Lab Clin Med 1955;45(1):3–17. http://www.ncbi.nlm.nih.gov/pubmed/13233623.

[14] Monticone S, D'Ascenzo F, Moretti C, et al. Cardiovascular events and target organ damage in primary aldosteronism compared with essential hypertension: a systematic review and meta-analysis. Lancet Diabetes Endocrinol 2018;6(1):41–50. https://doi.org/10.1016/S2213-8587(17)30319-4.

[15] Fallo F, Veglio F, Bertello C, et al. Prevalence and characteristics of the metabolic syndrome in primary aldosteronism. J Clin Endocrinol Metab 2006;91(2):454–9. https://doi.org/10.1210/jc.2005-1733.

[16] Fischer E, Adolf C, Pallauf A, et al. Aldosterone excess impairs first phase insulin secretion in primary aldosteronism. J Clin Endocrinol Metab 2013;98(6):2513–20. https://doi.org/10.1210/jc.2012-3934.

[17] Hanslik G, Wallaschofski H, Dietz A, et al. Increased prevalence of diabetes mellitus and the metabolic syndrome in patients with primary aldosteronism of the German Conn's Registry. Eur J Endocrinol 2015;173(5):665–75. https://doi.org/10.1530/EJE-15-0450.

[18] Beuschlein F, Mulatero P, Asbach E, et al. The SPARTACUS trial: controversies and unresolved issues. Horm Metab Res 2017;49(12):936–42. https://doi.org/10.1055/s-0043-120524.

[19] Miller WL, Auchus RJ. The molecular biology, biochemistry, and physiology of human steroidogenesis and its disorders. Endocr Rev 2011;32(1):81–151. https://doi.org/10.1210/er.2010-0013.

[20] El Ghorayeb N, Bourdeau I, Lacroix A. Role of ACTH and other hormones in the regulation of aldosterone production in primary aldosteronism. Front Endocrinol (Lausanne) 2016;7:1–10. https://doi.org/10.3389/fendo.2016.00072. June.

[21] Ceccato F, Scaroni C, Boscaro M. The adrenal glands. 2016. p. 1–35. https://doi.org/10.1007/978-3-319-27318-1_16-1.

[22] Zaman MA, Oparil S, Calhoun DA. Drugs targeting the renin–angiotensin–aldosterone system. Nat Rev Drug Discov 2002;1(8):621–36. https://doi.org/10.1038/nrd873.

[23] De Mello WC. Intracellular angiotensin II as a regulator of muscle tone in vascular resistance vessels. Pathophysiological implications. Peptides 2016;78:87–90. https://doi.org/10.1016/j.peptides.2016.02.006.

[24] Gao J, Zhang K, Chen J, et al. Roles of aldosterone in vascular calcification: an update. Eur J Pharmacol 2016;786:186–93. https://doi.org/10.1016/j.ejphar.2016.05.030.

[25] Reincke M, Bancos I, Mulatero P, Scholl UI, Stowasser M, Williams TA. Diagnosis and treatment of primary aldosteronism. Lancet Diabetes Endocrinol 2021;9(12):876–92. https://doi.org/10.1016/S2213-8587(21)00210-2.

[26] Brown JM, Siddiqui M, Calhoun DA, et al. The unrecognized prevalence of primary aldosteronism. Ann Intern Med 2020;173(1):10–20. https://doi.org/10.7326/M20-0065.

[27] Parasiliti-Caprino M, Lopez C, Prencipe N, et al. Prevalence of primary aldosteronism and association with cardiovascular complications in patients with resistant and refractory hypertension. J Hypertens 2020;38(9):1841–8. https://doi.org/10.1097/HJH.0000000000002441.

[28] Acelajado MC, Hughes ZH, Oparil S, Calhoun DA. Treatment of resistant and refractory hypertension. Circ Res 2019;124(7):1061–70. https://doi.org/10.1161/CIRCRESAHA.118.312156.

[29] Seccia TM, Letizia C, Muiesan ML, et al. Atrial fibrillation as presenting sign of primary aldosteronism: results of the Prospective Appraisal on the Prevalence of Primary Aldosteronism in Hypertensive (PAPPHY) study. J Hypertens 2020;38(2):332−9. https://doi.org/10.1097/HJH.0000000000002250.

[30] Tsai C-H, Chen Y-L, Pan C-T, et al. New-onset atrial fibrillation in patients with primary aldosteronism receiving different treatment strategies: systematic review and pooled analysis of three studies. Front Endocrinol (Lausanne) 2021;12. https://doi.org/10.3389/fendo.2021.646933.

[31] Seccia TM, Caroccia B, Adler GK, Maiolino G, Cesari M, Rossi GP. Arterial hypertension, atrial fibrillation, and hyperaldosteronism: the triple trouble. Hypertension (Dallas, Tex 1979) 2017;69(4):545−50. https://doi.org/10.1161/HYPERTENSIONAHA.116.08956.

[32] Hu Y, Zhang J, Liu W, Su X. Determining the prevalence of primary aldosteronism in patients with new-onset type 2 diabetes and hypertension. J Clin Endocrinol Metab 2020;105(4):1079−85. https://doi.org/10.1210/clinem/dgz293.

[33] Ceccato F, Bernkopf E, Scaroni C. Sleep apnea syndrome in endocrine clinics. J Endocrinol Invest 2015;38(8). https://doi.org/10.1007/s40618-015-0338-z.

[34] Pratt-Ubunama MN, Nishizaka MK, Boedefeld RL, Cofield SS, Harding SM, Calhoun DA. Plasma aldosterone is related to severity of obstructive sleep apnea in subjects with resistant hypertension. Chest 2007;131(2):453−9. https://doi.org/10.1378/chest.06-1442.

[35] Gonzaga CC, Gaddam KK, Ahmed MI, et al. Severity of obstructive sleep apnea is related to aldosterone status in subjects with resistant hypertension. J Clin Sleep Med 2010;6(4):363−8. http://www.ncbi.nlm.nih.gov/pubmed/20726285.

[36] Calhoun DA, Nishizaka MK, Zaman MA, Harding SM. Aldosterone excretion among subjects with resistant hypertension and symptoms of sleep apnea. Chest 2004;125(1):112−7. https://doi.org/10.1378/chest.125.1.112.

[37] Terzolo M, Stigliano A, Chiodini I, et al. AME position statement on adrenal incidentaloma. Eur J Endocrinol 2011;164(6):851−70. https://doi.org/10.1530/EJE-10-1147.

[38] Young WF. Clinical practice. The incidentally discovered adrenal mass. N Engl J Med 2007;356(6):601−10. https://doi.org/10.1056/NEJMcp065470.

[39] Zeiger MA, Thompson GB, Duh Q-Y, et al. American Association of Clinical Endocrinologists and American Association of Endocrine Surgeons medical guidelines for the management of adrenal incidentalomas: executive summary of recommendations. Endocr Pract 2009;15(5):450−3. https://doi.org/10.4158/EP.15.5.450.

[40] Médeau V, Moreau F, Trinquart L, et al. Clinical and biochemical characteristics of normotensive patients with primary aldosteronism: a comparison with hypertensive cases. Clin Endocrinol (Oxf). 2008;69(1):20−8. https://doi.org/10.1111/j.1365-2265.2008.03213.x.

[41] Ito Y, Takeda R, Karashima S, Yamamoto Y, Yoneda T, Takeda Y. Prevalence of primary aldosteronism among prehypertensive and stage 1 hypertensive subjects. Hypertens Res 2011;34(1):98−102. https://doi.org/10.1038/hr.2010.166.

[42] Piaditis GP, Kaltsas GA, Androulakis II, et al. High prevalence of autonomous cortisol and aldosterone secretion from adrenal adenomas. Clin Endocrinol (Oxf). 2009;71(6):772−8. https://doi.org/10.1111/j.1365-2265.2009.03551.x.

[43] Hiramatsu K, Yamada T, Yukimura Y, et al. A screening test to identify aldosterone-producing adenoma by measuring plasma renin activity. Results in hypertensive patients. Arch Intern Med 1981;141(12):1589−93. http://www.ncbi.nlm.nih.gov/pubmed/7030245.

[44] Mulatero P, Stowasser M, Loh K-C, et al. Increased diagnosis of primary aldosteronism, including surgically correctable forms, in centers from five continents. J Clin Endocrinol Metab 2004;89(3):1045−50. https://doi.org/10.1210/jc.2003-031337.

[45] Hung A, Ahmed S, Gupta A, et al. Performance of the aldosterone to renin ratio as a screening test for primary aldosteronism. J Clin Endocrinol Metab 2021;106(8):2423−35. https://doi.org/10.1210/clinem/dgab348.

[46] Mantero F, Ceccato F. Novità nelle linee guida dell'iperaldosteronismo primario. L'Endocrinologo. 2019;20(6):370−3. https://doi.org/10.1007/s40619-019-00642-w.

[47] Eisenhofer G, Kurlbaum M, Peitzsch M, et al. The saline infusion test for primary aldosteronism: implications of immunoassay inaccuracy. J Clin Endocrinol Metab 2022;107(5):e2027−36. https://doi.org/10.1210/clinem/dgab924.

[48] te Riet L, van Esch JHM, Roks AJM, van den Meiracker AH, Danser AHJ. Hypertension. Circ Res 2015;116(6):960−75. https://doi.org/10.1161/CIRCRESAHA.116.303587.

[49] Morera J, Reznik Y. Management of endocrine disease: the role of confirmatory tests in the diagnosis of primary aldosteronism. Eur J Endocrinol 2019;180(2):R45−58. https://doi.org/10.1530/EJE-18-0704.

[50] Yamazaki Y, Nakamura Y, Omata K, et al. Histopathological classification of cross-sectional image negative hyperaldosteronism. J Clin Endocrinol Metab 2017;102(4):1182−92. https://doi.org/10.1210/jc.2016-2986.

[51] Blake MA, Cronin CG, Boland GW. Adrenal imaging. AJR Am J Roentgenol 2010;194(6):1450−60. https://doi.org/10.2214/AJR.10.4547.

[52] Voltan G, Boscaro M, Armanini D, Scaroni C, Ceccato F. A multidisciplinary approach to the management of adrenal incidentaloma. Expert Rev Endocrinol Metab 2021;16(4):201−12. https://doi.org/10.1080/17446651.2021.1948327.

[53] Lim V, Guo Q, Grant CS, et al. Accuracy of adrenal imaging and adrenal venous sampling in predicting surgical cure of primary aldosteronism. J Clin Endocrinol Metab 2014;99(8):2712−9. https://doi.org/10.1210/jc.2013-4146.

[54] Umakoshi H, Ogasawara T, Takeda Y, et al. Accuracy of adrenal computed tomography in predicting the unilateral subtype in young patients with hypokalaemia and elevation of aldosterone in primary aldosteronism. Clin Endocrinol (Oxf) 2018;88(5):645−51. https://doi.org/10.1111/cen.13582.

[55] Kempers MJE, Lenders JWM, van Outheusden L, et al. Systematic review: diagnostic procedures to differentiate unilateral from bilateral adrenal abnormality in primary aldosteronism. Ann Intern Med 2009;151(5):329−37. https://doi.org/10.7326/0003-4819-151-5-200909010-00007.

[56] Mulatero P, Sechi LA, Williams TA, et al. Subtype diagnosis, treatment, complications and outcomes of primary aldosteronism and future direction of research: a position statement and consensus of the Working Group on Endocrine Hypertension of the European Society of Hypertension. J Hypertens 2020;38(10):1929−36. https://doi.org/10.1097/HJH.0000000000002520.

[57] Mulatero P, Monticone S, Deinum J, et al. Genetics, prevalence, screening and confirmation of primary aldosteronism: a position statement and consensus of the Working Group on Endocrine Hypertension of the European Society of Hypertension. J Hypertens 2020;38(10):1919−28. https://doi.org/10.1097/HJH.0000000000002510.

[58] Rossi GP, Auchus RJ, Brown M, et al. An expert consensus statement on use of adrenal vein sampling for the subtyping of primary aldosteronism. Hypertension 2014;63(1):151−60. https://doi.org/10.1161/HYPERTENSIONAHA.113.02097.

[59] Rossi GP, Barisa M, Allolio B, et al. The Adrenal Vein Sampling International Study (AVIS) for identifying the major subtypes of primary aldosteronism. J Clin Endocrinol Metab 2012;97(5):1606−14. https://doi.org/10.1210/jc.2011-2830.

[60] Monticone S, Satoh F, Dietz AS, et al. Clinical management and outcomes of adrenal hemorrhage following adrenal vein sampling in primary aldosteronism. Hypertension 2016;67(1):146−52. https://doi.org/10.1161/HYPERTENSIONAHA.115.06305.

[61] Nanba AT, Wannachalee T, Shields JJ, et al. Adrenal vein sampling lateralization despite mineralocorticoid receptor antagonists exposure in primary aldosteronism. J Clin Endocrinol Metab 2019;104(2):487−92. https://doi.org/10.1210/jc.2018-01299.

[62] Arlt W, Lang K, Sitch AJ, et al. Steroid metabolome analysis reveals prevalent glucocorticoid excess in primary aldosteronism. JCI Insight 2017;2(8). https://doi.org/10.1172/jci.insight.93136.

[63] O'Toole SM, Sze W-CC, Chung T-T, et al. Low-grade cortisol cosecretion has limited impact on ACTH-stimulated AVS parameters in primary aldosteronism. J Clin Endocrinol Metab 2020;105(10):e3776−84. https://doi.org/10.1210/clinem/dgaa519.

[64] Ceolotto G, Antonelli G, Caroccia B, et al. Comparison of cortisol, androstenedione and metanephrines to assess selectivity and lateralization of adrenal vein sampling in primary aldosteronism. J Clin Med 2021;10(20):4755. https://doi.org/10.3390/jcm10204755.

[65] Dekkers T, Prejbisz A, Kool LJS, et al. Adrenal vein sampling versus CT scan to determine treatment in primary aldosteronism: an outcome-based randomised diagnostic trial. Lancet Diabetes Endocrinol 2016;4(9):739−46. https://doi.org/10.1016/S2213-8587(16)30100-0.

[66] Williams TA, Burrello J, Sechi LA, et al. Computed tomography and adrenal venous sampling in the diagnosis of unilateral primary aldosteronism. Hypertension 2018;72(3):641−9. https://doi.org/10.1161/HYPERTENSIONAHA.118.11382.

[67] Rossi GP, Crimì F, Rossitto G, et al. Identification of surgically curable primary aldosteronism by imaging in a large, multiethnic international study. J Clin Endocrinol Metab 2021;106(11):e4340−9. https://doi.org/10.1210/clinem/dgab482.

[68] Oki K, Gomez-Sanchez CE. The landscape of molecular mechanism for aldosterone production in aldosterone-producing adenoma. Endocr J 2020;67(10):989−95. https://doi.org/10.1507/endocrj.EJ20-0478.

[69] Jacobsen N-EB, Campbell JB, Hobart MG. Laparoscopic versus open adrenalectomy for surgical adrenal disease. Can J Urol 2003;10(5):1995−9. http://www.ncbi.nlm.nih.gov/pubmed/14633327.

[70] Ishidoya S, Ito A, Sakai K, et al. Laparoscopic partial versus total adrenalectomy for aldosterone producing adenoma. J Urol 2005;174(1):40−3. https://doi.org/10.1097/01.ju.0000162045.68387.c3.

[71] Choi SH, Kwon TG, Kim T-H. Active potassium supplementation might be mandatory during laparoscopic adrenalectomy for primary hyperaldosteronism. J Endourol 2012;26(6):666−9. https://doi.org/10.1089/end.2011.0566.

[72] Williams TA, Lenders JWM, Mulatero P, Burrello J, Rottenkolber M, Adolf C, et al. Primary Aldosteronism Surgery Outcome (PASO) investigators. Outcomes after adrenalectomy for unilateral primary aldosteronism: an international consensus on outcome measures and analysis of remission rates in an international cohort. Lancet Diabetes Endocrinol September 2017;5(9):689−99. https://doi.org/10.1016/S2213-8587(17)30135-3.

[73] Mattsson C, Young WF. Primary aldosteronism: diagnostic and treatment strategies. Nat Clin Pract Nephrol 2006;2(4):198−208. https://doi.org/10.1038/ncpneph0151. quiz, 1 pp. following 230.

[74] Fischer E, Hanslik G, Pallauf A, et al. Prolonged zona glomerulosa insufficiency causing hyperkalemia in primary aldosteronism after adrenalectomy. J Clin Endocrinol Metab 2012;97(11):3965−73. https://doi.org/10.1210/jc.2012-2234.

[75] Mancia G, De Backer G, Dominiczak A, et al. 2007 ESH-ESC practice guidelines for the management of arterial hypertension: ESH-ESC task force on the management of arterial hypertension. J Hypertens 2007;25(9):1751−62. https://doi.org/10.1097/HJH.0b013e3282f0580f.

[76] Overdiek HW, Merkus FW. The metabolism and biopharmaceutics of spironolactone in man. Rev Drug Metab Drug Interact 1987;5(4):273−302. https://doi.org/10.1515/dmdi.1987.5.4.273.

[77] Lim PO, Jung RT, MacDonald TM. Raised aldosterone to renin ratio predicts antihypertensive efficacy of spironolactone: a prospective cohort follow-up study. Br J Clin Pharmacol 1999;48(5):756−60. https://doi.org/10.1046/j.1365-2125.1999.00070.x.

[78] Pitt B, Remme W, Zannad F, et al. Eplerenone, a selective aldosterone blocker, in patients with left ventricular dysfunction after myocardial infarction. N Engl J Med 2003;348(14):1309−21. https://doi.org/10.1056/NEJMoa030207.

[79] Agarwal R, Kolkhof P, Bakris G, et al. Steroidal and non-steroidal mineralocorticoid receptor antagonists in cardiorenal medicine. Eur Heart J 2021;42(2):152−61. https://doi.org/10.1093/eurheartj/ehaa736.

[80] Katabami T, Fukuda H, Tsukiyama H, et al. Clinical and biochemical outcomes after adrenalectomy and medical treatment in patients with unilateral primary aldosteronism. J Hypertens 2019;37(7):1513−20. https://doi.org/10.1097/HJH.0000000000002070.

[81] Chen Y-Y, Lin Y-HH, Huang W-C, et al. Adrenalectomy improves the long-term risk of end-stage renal disease and mortality of primary aldosteronism. J Endocr Soc 2019;3(6):1110−26. https://doi.org/10.1210/js.2019-00019.

[82] Sutherland DJ, Ruse JL, Laidlaw JC. Hypertension, increased aldosterone secretion and low plasma renin activity relieved by dexamethasone. Can Med Assoc J 1966;95(22):1109−19. http://www.ncbi.nlm.nih.gov/pubmed/4288576.

[83] Litchfield WR, Anderson BF, Weiss RJ, Lifton RP, Dluhy RG. Intracranial aneurysm and hemorrhagic stroke in glucocorticoid-remediable aldosteronism. Hypertension (Dallas, Tex 1979) 1998;31(1 Pt 2):445−50. https://doi.org/10.1161/01.hyp.31.1.445.

[84] Lifton RP, Dluhy RG, Powers M, et al. A chimaeric llβ-hydroxylase/aldosterone synthase gene causes glucocorticoid-remediable aldosteronism and human hypertension. Nature 1992;355(6357):262−5. https://doi.org/10.1038/355262a0.

[85] Scholl UI, Stölting G, Schewe J, et al. CLCN2 chloride channel mutations in familial hyperaldosteronism type II. Nat Genet 2018;50(3):349−54. https://doi.org/10.1038/s41588-018-0048-5.

[86] Geller DS, Zhang J, Wisgerhof MV, Shackleton C, Kashgarian M, Lifton RP. A novel form of human mendelian hypertension featuring nonglucocorticoid-remediable aldosteronism. J Clin Endocrinol Metab 2008;93(8):3117−23. https://doi.org/10.1210/jc.2008-0594.

[87] Scholl UI, Nelson-Williams C, Yue P, et al. Hypertension with or without adrenal hyperplasia due to different inherited mutations in the potassium channel KCNJ5. Proc Natl Acad Sci 2012;109(7):2533−8. https://doi.org/10.1073/pnas.1121407109.

[88] Scholl UI, Stölting G, Nelson-Williams C, et al. Recurrent gain of function mutation in calcium channel CACNA1H causes early-onset hypertension with primary aldosteronism. Elife 2015;4. https://doi.org/10.7554/eLife.06315.

[89] Scholl UI, Goh G, Stölting G, et al. Somatic and germline CACNA1D calcium channel mutations in aldosterone-producing adenomas and primary aldosteronism. Nat Genet 2013;45(9):1050−4. https://doi.org/10.1038/ng.2695.

[90] Pinggera A, Lieb A, Benedetti B, et al. CACNA1D de novo mutations in autism spectrum disorders activate Cav1.3 L-type calcium channels. Biol Psychiatr 2015;77(9):816−22. https://doi.org/10.1016/j.biopsych.2014.11.020.

[91] Dluhy RG, Anderson B, Harlin B, Ingelfinger J, Lifton R. Glucocorticoid-remediable aldosteronism is associated with severe hypertension in early childhood. J Pediatr 2001;138(5):715−20. https://doi.org/10.1067/mpd.2001.112648.

[92] Stowasser M, Gordon RD. Familial hyperaldosteronism. J Steroid Biochem Mol Biol 2001;78(3):215−29. https://doi.org/10.1016/S0960-0760(01)00097-8.

Chapter 8

Familial hyperaldosteronism

Joseph M. Pappachan[1], Cornelius J. Fernandez[2] and David S. Geller[3]

[1]*Department of Endocrinology & Metabolism, Lancashire Teaching Hospitals NHS Trust, Preston & Manchester Metropolitan University, Manchester, United Kingdom;* [2]*Department of Endocrinology & Metabolism, Pilgrim Hospital, United Lincolnshire Hospitals NHS Trust, Boston, United Kingdom;* [3]*Department of Nephrology, West Haven VA Hospital, West Haven and Yale University School of Medicine, New Haven, CT, United States*

Visit the *Endocrine Hypertension: From Basic Science to Clinical Practice*, *First Edition* companion web site at: https://www.elsevier.com/books-and-journals/book-companion/9780323961202.

Graphical Abstract

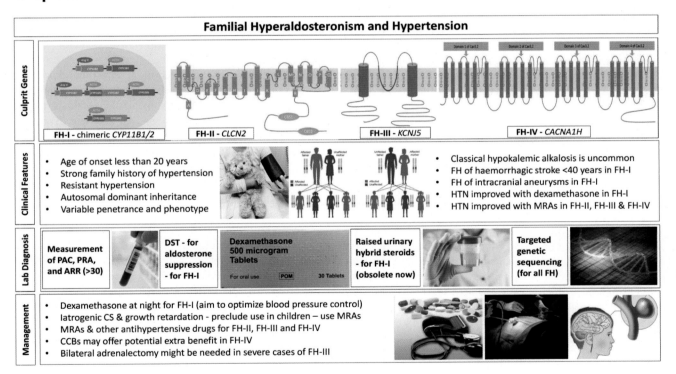

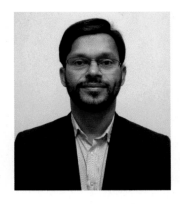

Joseph M. Pappachan

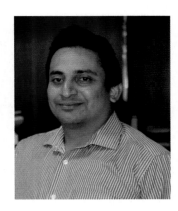

Cornelius J. Fernandez

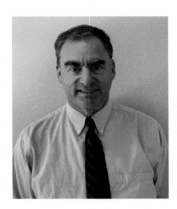

David S. Geller

Introduction

Primary aldosteronism (PA), the most common cause of endocrine hypertension, is characterized by autonomous over-production of aldosterone from the adrenal gland(s). Of the several subtypes of PA, bilateral adrenal hyperplasia or idiopathic hyperaldosteronism accounts for ~60% of cases and aldosterone-producing adenomas (APAs) ~30% of cases, with unilateral hyperplasia (less common), malignancy, and familial hyperaldosteronism (FH; both rare) forming the remainder [1,2]. The genetic landscape of PA has been well characterized in recent years, and somatic mutations have been identified in more than 90% of APAs [2,3]. Germline mutations are also described in sporadic PA with bilateral adrenal hyperplasia making our understanding of the disease more complex.

FH is a group of rare disorders causing monogenic hypertension, and all these are inherited in an autosomal dominant manner [4–6]. Although genotypically distinct often with a positive family history, FH is characterized by a mineralo-corticoid excess state (as in sporadic PA) with early-onset refractory hypertension, hypokalemia, metabolic alkalosis, raised aldosterone–renin ratio (ARR), and probable hypertension-related cardiovascular complications. An accurate diagnosis requires genetic testing, as clinically and biochemically these disorders are often indistinguishable from sporadic PA [4–6]. This chapter is to equip the readers with the current evidence-based scientific knowledge on these rare genetic disorders causing endocrine hypertension.

Pathophysiology of familial hyperaldosteronism

Depending on the genetic characteristics, molecular features, and pathophysiological aspects, FH is classified into four major subcategories (FH-I, II, III, and IV). In addition, a complex syndrome of familial PA with neurological abnormalities such as cerebral palsy and seizures known as PASNA (primary aldosteronism, seizures, and neurological abnormalities) syndrome has also been described [2,7]. Genetic testing for FH is recommended in an individual with biochemically proven mineralocorticoid excess when there is a family history of PA with early onset of hypertension [2]. A detailed review of the pathophysiological aspects, clinical profiles, and management options of individual disorders is discussed under the subtypes of FH below.

Subtypes of familial hyperaldosteronism
Familial hyperaldosteronism type 1

Pathophysiology: FH-I, also known as glucocorticoid-remediable aldosteronism (GRA), is the most common form of monogenic hypertension [3]. FH-I was first identified in 1966 by Sutherland et al. in a father and son presenting with hypertension, elevated aldosterone, suppressed renin, and metabolic alkalosis that improved with dexamethasone treatment [8]. This genetic disorder occurs as a result of an unequal cross-over between the neighboring and highly homologous *CYP11B1* and *CYP11B2* genes on chromosome 8q24.3, generating a chimeric variant gene [9]. The *CYP11B1* gene encodes 11β-hydroxylase. It is expressed under the control of ACTH in the adrenal zona fasciculata. The *CYP11B2* encodes aldosterone synthase, which differs from 11β-hydroxylase in that it possesses an 18-hydroxylase activity in addition to the

11β-hydroxylase activity. Its expression is triggered by both angiotensin II and hyperkalemia and is confined normally to the zona glomerulosa. The unequal cross-over event results in an enzyme with aldosterone synthase activity but expressed under the control of ACTH in the zona fasciculata. The ectopic expression of an enzyme with 18-hydroxylase activity in the zona fasciculata results in the synthesis of aldosterone and other hybrid steroids such as 18-oxocortisol and 18-hydroxycortisol. The conversion of cortisol to 18-oxocortisol and 18-hydroxycortisol leads to decreased cortisol secretion, triggering further ACTH production, and as such, mineralocorticoid levels are often grossly elevated in FH-I cases [3,10,11]. FH-I shows an autosomal dominant inheritance pattern with variable penetrance that results in milder forms of the disease in a proportion of patients [2,10,11]. Fig. 8.1 shows the schematic representation of the pathophysiological aspects of FH-I.

Clinical features: Classical clinical picture of patients with FH-I is early-onset hypertension with a strong family history and refractory hypertension not amenable to the standard antihypertensive medications [12]. In a large retrospective study reviewing 376 patients from an international registry of FH-I, 18% had cerebrovascular accidents (CVAs) [13]. This cohort included 27 genetically proven FH-I pedigrees in whom the incidence of CVA was 48%. Of these, 70% were hemorrhagic strokes with an overall case fatality rate of 61%. Intracranial aneurysms were the cause of brain hemorrhage, the prevalence of which appeared to be comparable to that in adult polycystic kidney disease [13]. Variable degree of penetrance of the genetic defect may result in phenotypic variations with mild hypertension or even normotension in some individuals with FH-I [14–16]. There is an increased risk of preeclampsia in pregnant women with FH-I [17].

Diagnostic evaluation: Patients with onset of PA before the age of 20 years with a family history of PA or stroke at an age below 40 years should be tested for FH-I as per the current guidelines of the Endocrine Society [1,11,18]. The initial diagnosis is based on the biochemical confirmation of PA. Although hypertension with hypokalemic alkalosis is the classical description of PA, plasma potassium levels are often normal with hypokalemia an infrequent feature ($\approx 20\%$) except when diuretics are used. Initial screening is with estimation of plasma aldosterone concentration coupled with plasma renin activity as per the standard testing protocol to obtain ARR [1,18]. An ARR cut off >30 in a patient with clinical suspicion of the disease has a high sensitivity for PA. Biochemical confirmation of PA is as per the standard

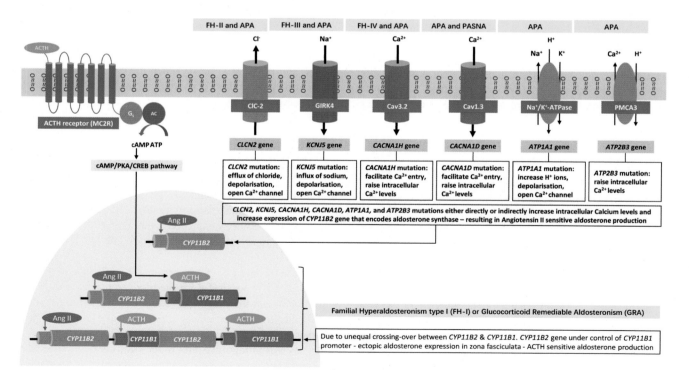

FIGURE 8.1 A graphical summary of various germline and somatic mutations associated with familial hyperaldosteronism. *ACTH*, adrenocorticotrophin; *APA*, aldosterone producing adenoma; *FH (I–IV)*, familial hyperaldosteronism; Ca^{2+}, calcium ion; H^+, hydrogen ion; Cl^-, chloride ion; K^+, potassium ion; *CIC2, GIRK4, Cav3.2, Cav1.3, Na$^+$/K$^+$-ATPase, and PMCA3*, various ion channels; *cAMP*, cyclic adenosine monophosphate; *ATP*, adenosine triphosphate; *PKA*, protein kinase A; *CREB*, cAMP response element binding protein; *Ang II*, angiotensin II (genes' names are given in italics).

recommendations with special precautions taken to avoid fluid overload or hypertension-related complications and is described in Chapters 7, 10, and 21.

Once the diagnosis of PA is established, genetic testing for the chimeric *CYP11B1/2* gene can be performed for confirmation of FH-I. A low-dose dexamethasone suppression test (DST) for suppression of plasma aldosterone levels to <4 ng/dL (<110 pmol/L) and/or >80% suppression from baseline after oral dexamethasone 0.75–2 mg daily for 2 days has very high sensitivity and specificity for biochemical evidence of FH-I that also confirms the ACTH control of aldosterone overproduction in these patients and has a high correlation with genetic testing [19]. Patients with FH-I also excrete large amounts of urinary hybrid steroids including 18-hydroxycortisol and 18-oxocortisol that were used for the diagnostic screening in the past along with their suppression following DST [20]. However, these biochemical screening tests are largely obsolete now with the advent of targeted genetic sequencing methods for the culprit gene in the recent years, coupled with the finding that the hybrid steroids are also observed in other familial forms of aldosteronism [21].

Management: Usual antihypertensive agents are less likely to be effective in patients with FH-I. Low doses of oral steroids to optimally suppress the ACTH to keep the levels of aldosterone and hybrid steroids normal usually help to control hypertension in these patients. Dexamethasone 0.125–0.250 mg administered at night to suppress the normal early morning surge of ACTH will usually control the disease in patients with FH-I [1,3]. Dexamethasone is preferred because of its least mineralocorticoid activity among the oral corticosteroids and a less preferred alternative is prednisolone at the dose of 2.5–5 mg daily. Iatrogenic Cushing's syndrome and growth retardation may preclude the use of steroids among children in whom mineralocorticoid receptor (MR) antagonists such as spironolactone or eplerenone can be effective alternatives to control hypertension [1,3,11,22]. The target of treating patients with FH-I should be the optimal control of blood pressure rather than the normalization of elevated mineralocorticoids to avoid undesirable side effects of long-term steroids in these patients [22].

Familial hyperaldosteronism type 2

Pathophysiology: FH-II was first described by Stowasser et al. among 13 patients from 5 families in whom FH was not suppressible with dexamethasone and these cases also had a high tendency for APA formation [23]. The culprit gene associated with FH-II is a gain-of-function mutation in *CLCN2* gene with variable penetrance that encodes a chloride channel ClC2 as demonstrated by Scholl et al. in 2018 [24]. The mutation was identified from the DNA analysis by exome sequencing of three patients from one of the families with FH-II originally described by Stowasser et al. in 1992. The mutant variant p.Arg172Gln was also shown in five other family members of the original cohort [24]. *CLCN2* gene is located on chromosome 3q27 and the voltage-gated chloride channel (ClC2) is widely expressed in mammalian tissues such as the brain, heart, gastrointestinal tract, kidney, adrenal glands, and the liver [11,25]. When the ClC2 opens (with a higher tendency among *CLCN2* mutant genes), it depolarizes adrenal zona glomerulosa cells inducing aldosterone synthase (the rate-limiting enzyme for aldosterone synthesis) expression, resulting in overproduction of aldosterone [24]. The mineralocorticoid excess state, as a consequence, results in hypertension that is indistinguishable from other sporadic forms of PA biochemically. *CLCN2* somatic mutations are also described in APAs and bilateral adrenal hyperplasia, though FH-II almost always presents in childhood or adolescence with germline mutations in these patients. Fig. 8.1 demonstrates the pathophysiology of FH-II.

Clinical features: FH-II is clinically indistinguishable from the sporadic forms of PA except for the early age of onset as mentioned above. As in FH-I, the disease severity can vary depending on the penetrance of the genetic mutation [2,24]. Early-onset hypertension with typical age at diagnosis before 20 years is characteristic. Classical clinical presentation "hypokalemic metabolic alkalosis" is uncommon. Although this form of FH has been considered the most common type in the past, recent identification of the culprit gene has changed this notion as many of the case with a diagnosis FH-II would have been cases with sporadic PA [11].

Diagnostic evaluation: Once PA diagnosis is established in a child or adolescent with hypertension as described above, genetic testing is recommended in patients with a family history of PA. DST is not useful for the biochemical identification of the disease. Targeted gene sequencing for *CLCN2* would help to establish the diagnosis [24,26,27]. Screening among first-degree relatives with hypertension should be considered as per the Endocrine Society guidelines as we are still unaware of the exact prevalence of the disease and the degree of penetrance of the genetic defect [1].

Management: Hypertension in patients with FH-II may respond to MR antagonists and other antihypertensive agents [2]. However, there is inadequate global expertise on the long-term outcome of such a strategy owing to inadequate experience in managing such patients.

Familial hyperaldosteronism type 3

Pathophysiology: In 2008, Geller and colleagues described a new variant form of FH in a father and 2 daughters with severe refractory hypertension diagnosed at the age of 7 years [21]. These patients had high levels of hybrid steroids 18-oxocortisol and 18-hydroxycortisol, along with hyporeninemic hyperaldosteronism without suppression of aldosterone, cortisol, and hypertension on DST as expected in patients with FH-I. This autosomal dominant disease without any abnormalities in the aldosterone synthase gene and the abnormal biochemical profile implied a global defect the adrenal steroidogenesis pathway. Patients had to undergo bilateral adrenalectomy for the cure of severe and resistant hypertension [21]. The adrenal gland specimens of these cases revealed massive hyperplasia with a disorganized zonation pattern, and an enlargement of the zona fasciculata and transitional zone, with an atrophic zona glomerulosa layer. This disorganized zonation characteristic with the presence of cells that coexpress enzymes which are usually expressed in the distinct individual zones of the adrenal cortex, such as CYP11B1 and CYP11B2, and also CYP17A1, might explain abnormally exaggerated steroidogenesis including that of hybrid mineralocorticoids like 18-oxocortisol and 18-hydroxycortisol [12,28,29].

The culprit gene, later sequenced by Choi et al. in 2011 on chromosome 11q24, is a heterogenous gain-of-function mutation in *KCNJ5* that encodes a G-protein-coupled potassium channel 4 (Kir3.4) [11,30]. Kir3.4 with other Kir proteins controls the polarization of the zona glomerulosa cell membranes. The mutations described by Choi in *KCNJ5* result in a loss of channel specificity, allowing sodium to pass through this potassium channel from which it is normally excluded. Sodium current through the channel results in depolarization of the cell, triggering a voltage-sensitive calcium current which leads to overproduction of aldosterone [31]. Several mutations in the *KCNJ5* gene were described subsequently and only those familial cases with germline mutations are categorized as FH-III [2,3,11,12]. Somatic mutations of *KCNJ5* gene are also commonly seen in patients with APAs and bilateral adrenal hyperplasia associated with PA [2,32−34]. The pathophysiological aspects of FH-III are shown in Fig. 8.1.

Clinical presentation of FH-III: The disease is rare accounting for <1% of cases with PA [35]. The phenotype of FH-III patients varies widely with the mutation. The family described by Geller et al. harboring the T158A allele had severe disease requiring bilateral adrenalectomy [36]. A similar phenotype was reported for patients harboring a G151R allele [37]. In contrast, Scholl et al. reported that patients with a G151E mutation (a mutation not seen in APAs) had mild, easily controlled disease. Interestingly, the G151E mutation had a greater effect on loss of channel specificity; the relatively free flow of sodium into the cell leads to cell lethality, with the inference that this lethality limits adrenal cell mass and thus aldosterone production. It is a striking example of how small amino acid changes can result in markedly different phenotypes.

Diagnostic evaluation: Clinical picture and biochemical features of PA described earlier with a very early onset of hypertension in childhood may alert clinicians for a diagnostic evaluation with genetic testing. DST does not suppress the mineralocorticoid excess and improve hypertension. There may be a paradoxical rise in blood pressure and mineralocorticoid levels to DST as observed by Geller et al. in their cases [21]. The Endocrine Society suggests genetic testing for FH-III in patients with very early onset of hypertension with positive family history in PA [1].

Management: Mild forms of the disease may be managed with MR antagonists such as spironolactone or eplerenone [2,11]. However, severe cases may need bilateral adrenalectomy for control of the disease and hypertension [2,11,21,38]. Bilateral adrenalectomy is curative in severe cases, but triggers the need for lifelong steroid replacement therapy; early adrenalectomy presumably reduces the risk of cardiovascular sequelae of the aldosteronism, such as left ventricular hypertrophy, which was present in the young women described by Geller et al. [21].

Familial hyperaldosteronism type 4

Pathophysiology: FH-IV was first reported by Scholl et al. among five unrelated patients with early onset PA (≤10 years of age) in a cohort of 40 patients without any known PA genes [39]. By genome sequencing they found a gain-of-function mutation (p.Met1549Val) in the *CACNA1H* gene that encodes a T-type calcium channel subunit (Ca$_v$3.2) detected on chromosome 16p13 to cause the genetic anomaly. This abnormal Ca^{2+} channel causes increased calcium influx in the adrenal cortical cells, perhaps secondary to altered sodium conductivity of the mutant channel, but ultimately resulting in aldosterone overproduction [2,39−41]. *CACNA1H* is the second most expressed gene in the zona glomerulosa cell layer of adrenal gland for the synthesis of calcium channels [7,30]. Several other mutations have been subsequently described in this gene accounting for somatic and germline defects associated with PA [2,11]. Only those with germline mutations and heritability are classified as FH-IV, while the others with somatic gene defects may present with APAs. A schematic diagram explaining the pathophysiology of FH-IV is demonstrated in Fig. 8.1.

Clinical profile: Although FH-IV is an autosomal dominant genetic disorder, because of variable penetrance the clinical spectrum may range from mild disease expression (mild hypertension or even normotension) to severe and treatment resistant hypertension from early life [39]. In the patients described by Scholl et al., all children had clinical presentations suggestive of hyperaldosteronism, but adult carriers did not, suggesting decreased disease penetrance by age. The reasons for this are not clear.

Diagnostic evaluation: Patients presenting with PA in childhood and a family history of the disease should be tested for FH-IV as per the current Endocrine Society recommendations [1].

Management: MR antagonists such as spironolactone and eplerenone are useful for the management of hypertension in patients with FH-IV [2,11]. Calcium channel blockers have been found to inhibit Ca^{2+} currents through CACNA1H and thus may be of use as well, but there is not much experience with these agents because of the rarity and discovery of the disorder only in the recent years [2]. The long-term prognosis of the condition remains elusive for the same reasons.

PASNA syndrome

A rare and complex disorder comprising PA, seizures, and neurological abnormalities (PASNA) was described with de novo heterozygous gain-of-function mutations in the *CACNA1D* gene encoding an abnormal calcium channel (Ca_v1.3—a high voltage gated Ca^{2+} channel) among two individuals with cerebral palsy in 2013 [7]. However, expression of this channel in other organs such as the brain, heart, and pancreas without PA was identified later, and as such, this genetic defect is not considered as a classical form of FH [2,11]. Other *CACNA1D* mutations without PA also have been described [42].

Emerging research questions/future research

Genetic studies of PA are still evolving with newer genes identified in several somatic and germline defects identified in the recent years. More familial disorders causing PA are likely to emerge in the coming years. Germline mutations in the *ARMC5*, a tumor suppressor gene, have been found to be associated with PA recently [43]. It is not clear whether these would fall into the category of Familial PA in future with more cases and heritability of this entity described with evolving research. Rare germline variants of the phosphodiesterase 2A (*PDE2A*) and 3B (*PDE3B*) genes were identified from the unilateral adrenalectomy specimens in three patients with early onset hypertension and PA from bilateral adrenal hyperplasia [44]. We are unsure about the familial nature of these cases also, and future research should shed more light on the genetic landscape of PA for our better understanding of the disease.

Summary and conclusions

FH is associated with early-onset monogenic hypertension with a strong family history and accounts for only a small proportion of patients with PA. The disease severity may vary depending on the degree of penetrance of the FH causing gene disorder. GRA is the most common form of monogenic hypertension. Diagnostic work up of FH involves biochemical confirmation of PA followed by appropriate molecular genetic analysis to identify the culprit gene causing the disease. Newer genes associated with both familial and sporadic PA are still being discovered improving our understanding of these uncommon genetic disorders.

Learning points

- FH is a group of genetic disorders associated with childhood-onset monogenic hypertension and with a strong family history.
- FH-I or GRA is caused by an unequal cross-over between the *CYP11B1* and *CYP11B2* genes on chromosome 8q24.3, generating a chimeric gene that results in ACTH-dependent aldosterone production in other layers of adrenal cortex apart from zona glomerulosa. The disease therefore can be controlled by ACTH suppression with glucocorticoids.
- Phenotypic variations can occur in the disease severity in patients with FH depending on the gene penetrance in the affected individuals. On occasions, bilateral adrenalectomy may be necessary to control hypertension in severe forms of FH-III.

References

[1] Funder JW, Carey RM, Mantero F, Murad MH, Reincke M, Shibata H, Stowasser M, Young Jr WF. The management of primary aldosteronism: case detection, diagnosis, and treatment: an endocrine society clinical practice guideline. J Clin Endocrinol Metab 2016;101:1889—916. https://doi.org/10.1210/jc.2015-4061.

[2] Scholl UI. Genetics of primary aldosteronism. Hypertension 2022;79(5):887—97. https://doi.org/10.1161/HYPERTENSIONAHA.121.16498. PMID: 35139664; PMCID: PMC8997684.

[3] Monticone S, Buffolo F, Tetti M, Veglio F, Pasini B, Mulatero P. Genetics in endocrinology: the expanding genetic horizon of primary aldosteronism. Eur J Endocrinol 2018;178(3):R101—11. https://doi.org/10.1530/EJE-17-0946. PMID: 29348113.

[4] Lu YT, Fan P, Zhang D, Zhang Y, Meng X, Zhang QY, et al. Overview of monogenic forms of hypertension combined with hypokalemia. Front Pediatr 2021;8:543309. https://doi.org/10.3389/fped.2020.543309. PMID: 33569358.

[5] Raina R, Krishnappa V, Das A, Amin H, Radhakrishnan Y, Nair NR, et al. Overview of monogenic or mendelian forms of hypertension. Front Pediatr 2019;7:263. https://doi.org/10.3389/fped.2019.00263. PMID: 31312622.

[6] Burrello J, Monticone S, Buffolo F, Tetti M, Veglio F, Williams TA, et al. Is there a role for genomics in the management of hypertension? Int J Mol Sci 2017;18(6):1131. https://doi.org/10.3390/ijms18061131. PMID: 28587112.

[7] Scholl UI, Goh G, Stölting G, de Oliveira RC, Choi M, Overton JD, et al. Somatic and germline CACNA1D calcium channel mutations in aldosterone-producing adenomas and primary aldosteronism. Nat Genet September 2013;45(9):1050—4. https://doi.org/10.1038/ng.2695. PMID: 23913001.

[8] Sutherland DJ, Ruse JL, Laidlaw JC. Hypertension, increased aldosterone secretion and low plasma renin activity relieved by dexamethasone. Can Med Assoc J 1966;95(22):1109—19. PMID: 4288576.

[9] Lifton RP, Dluhy RG, Powers M, Rich GM, Cook S, Ulick S, Lalouel JM. A chimaeric 11 beta-hydroxylase/aldosterone synthase gene causes glucocorticoid-remediable aldosteronism and human hypertension. Nature January 16, 1992;355(6357):262—5. https://doi.org/10.1038/355262a0. PMID: 1731223.

[10] Halperin F, Dluhy RG. Glucocorticoid-remediable aldosteronism. viii Endocrinol Metab Clin North Am 2011;40(2):333—41. https://doi.org/10.1016/j.ecl.2011.01.012. PMID: 21565670.

[11] Perez-Rivas LG, Williams TA, Reincke M. Inherited forms of primary hyperaldosteronism: new genes, new phenotypes and proposition of a new classification. Exp Clin Endocrinol Diabetes 2019;127(2-03):93—9. https://doi.org/10.1055/a-0713-0629. PMID: 30199917.

[12] Levanovich PE, Diaczok A, Rossi NF. Clinical and molecular perspectives of monogenic hypertension. Curr Hypertens Rev 2020;16(2):91—107. https://doi.org/10.2174/1573402115666190409115330. PMID: 30963979.

[13] Litchfield WR, Anderson BF, Weiss RJ, Lifton RP, Dluhy RG. Intracranial aneurysm and hemorrhagic stroke in glucocorticoid-remediable aldosteronism. Hypertension January 1998;31(1 Pt 2):445—50. https://doi.org/10.1161/01.hyp.31.1.445. PMID: 9453343.

[14] Fallo F, Pilon C, Williams TA, Sonino N, Morra Di Cella S, Veglio F, De Iasio R, Montanari P, Mulatero P. Coexistence of different phenotypes in a family with glucocorticoid-remediable aldosteronism. J Hum Hypertens January 2004;18(1):47—51. https://doi.org/10.1038/sj.jhh.1001636. PMID: 14688810.

[15] Mulatero P, di Cella SM, Williams TA, Milan A, Mengozzi G, Chiandussi L, Gomez-Sanchez CE, Veglio F. Glucocorticoid remediable aldosteronism: low morbidity and mortality in a four-generation Italian pedigree. J Clin Endocrinol Metab July 2002;87(7):3187—91. https://doi.org/10.1210/jcem.87.7.8647. PMID: 12107222.

[16] Stowasser M, Huggard PR, Rossetti TR, Bachmann AW, Gordon RD. Biochemical evidence of aldosterone overproduction and abnormal regulation in normotensive individuals with familial hyperaldosteronism type I. J Clin Endocrinol Metab November 1999;84(11):4031—6. https://doi.org/10.1210/jcem.84.11.6159. PMID: 10566645.

[17] Wyckoff JA, Seely EW, Hurwitz S, Anderson BF, Lifton RP, Dluhy RG. Glucocorticoid-remediable aldosteronism and pregnancy. Hypertension 2000;35(2):668—72. https://doi.org/10.1161/01.hyp.35.2.668. PMID: 10679515.

[18] Mulatero P, Monticone S, Deinum J, Amar L, Prejbisz A, Zennaro MC, et al. Genetics, prevalence, screening and confirmation of primary aldosteronism: a position statement and consensus of the Working Group on Endocrine Hypertension of the European Society of Hypertension. J Hypertens 2020;38(10):1919—28. https://doi.org/10.1097/HJH.0000000000002510. PMID: 32890264.

[19] Litchfield WR, New MI, Coolidge C, Lifton RP, Dluhy RG. Evaluation of the dexamethasone suppression test for the diagnosis of glucocorticoid-remediable aldosteronism. J Clin Endocrinol Metab November 1997;82(11):3570—3. https://doi.org/10.1210/jcem.82.11.4381. PMID: 9360508.

[20] Mosso L, Gomez-Sanchez CE, Foecking MF, Fardella C. Serum 18-hydroxycortisol in primary aldosteronism, hypertension, and normotensives. Hypertension 2001;38:688—91.

[21] Geller DS, Zhang J, Wisgerhof MV, Shackleton C, Kashgarian M, Lifton RP. A novel form of human mendelian hypertension featuring nonglucocorticoid-remediable aldosteronism. J Clin Endocrinol Metab August 2008;93(8):3117—23. https://doi.org/10.1210/jc.2008-0594. PMID: 18505761.

[22] Stowasser M, Bachmann AW, Huggard PR, Rossetti TR, Gordon RD. Treatment of familial hyperaldosteronism type I: only partial suppression of adrenocorticotropin required to correct hypertension. J Clin Endocrinol Metab 2000;85:3313—8.

[23] Stowasser M, Gordon RD, Tunny TJ, Klemm SA, Finn WL, Krek AL. Familial hyperaldosteronism type II: five families with a new variety of primary aldosteronism. Clin Exp Pharmacol Physiol 1992;19(5):319—22. https://doi.org/10.1111/j.1440-1681.1992.tb00462.x. PMID: 1521363.

[24] Scholl UI, Stölting G, Schewe J, Thiel A, Tan H, Nelson-Williams C, et al. CLCN2 chloride channel mutations in familial hyperaldosteronism type II. Nat Genet March 2018;50(3):349—54. https://doi.org/10.1038/s41588-018-0048-5. PMID: 29403011.

[25] Thiemann A, Günder S, Pusch M, Jentsch TJ. A chloride channel widely expressed in epithelial and non-epithelial cells. Nature March 5, 1992;356(6364):57−60. https://doi.org/10.1038/356057a0. PMID: 1311421.

[26] Fernandes-Rosa FL, Daniil G, Orozco IJ, Göppner C, El Zein R, Jain V, et al. A gain-of-function mutation in the CLCN2 chloride channel gene causes primary aldosteronism. Nat Genet March 2018;50(3):355−61. https://doi.org/10.1038/s41588-018-0053-8. PMID: 29403012.

[27] Mourtzi N, Sertedaki A, Markou A, Piaditis GP, Charmandari E. Unravelling the genetic basis of primary aldosteronism. Nutrients 2021;13(3):875. https://doi.org/10.3390/nu13030875. PMID: 33800142.

[28] Lenders JWM, Williams TA, Reincke M, Gomez-Sanchez CE. Diagnosis of endocrine disease: 18-oxocortisol and 18-hydroxycortisol: is there clinical utility of these steroids? Eur J Endocrinol 2018;178(1):R1−9. https://doi.org/10.1530/EJE-17-0563. PMID: 28904009.

[29] Gomez-Sanchez CE, Qi X, Gomez-Sanchez EP, Sasano H, Bohlen MO, Wisgerhof M. Disordered zonal and cellular CYP11B2 enzyme expression in familial hyperaldosteronism type 3. Mol Cell Endocrinol 2017;439:74−80. https://doi.org/10.1016/j.mce.2016.10.025. PMID: 27793677.

[30] Choi M, Scholl UI, Yue P, Björklund P, Zhao B, Nelson-Williams C, et al. K+ channel mutations in adrenal aldosterone-producing adenomas and hereditary hypertension. Science 2011;331(6018):768−72. https://doi.org/10.1126/science.1198785. PMID: 21311022.

[31] Velarde-Miranda C, Gomez-Sanchez EP, Gomez-Sanchez CE. Regulation of aldosterone biosynthesis by the Kir3.4 (KCNJ5) potassium channel. Clin Exp Pharmacol Physiol 2013;40(12):895−901. https://doi.org/10.1111/1440-1681.12151. PMID: 23829355.

[32] Oki K, Plonczynski MW, Luis Lam M, Gomez-Sanchez EP, Gomez-Sanchez CE. Potassium channel mutant KCNJ5 T158A expression in HAC-15 cells increases aldosterone synthesis. Endocrinology 2012;153(4):1774−82. https://doi.org/10.1210/en.2011-1733. PMID: 22315453.

[33] Lee BC, Kang VJ, Pan CT, Huang JZ, Lin YL, Chang YY, et al. KCNJ5 somatic mutation is associated with higher aortic wall thickness and less calcification in patients with aldosterone-producing adenoma. Front Endocrinol (Lausanne) March 2, 2022;13:830130. https://doi.org/10.3389/fendo.2022.830130. PMID: 35311227.

[34] Peng KY, Liao HW, Chueh JS, Pan CY, Lin YH, Chen YM, Chen PY, Huang CL, Wu VC. Pathophysiological and pharmacological characteristics of KCNJ5 157-159delITE somatic mutation in aldosterone-producing adenomas. Biomedicines August 17, 2021;9(8):1026. https://doi.org/10.3390/biomedicines9081026. PMID: 34440230.

[35] Maria AG, Suzuki M, Berthon A, Kamilaris C, Demidowich A, Lack J, et al. Mosaicism for KCNJ5 causing early-onset primary aldosteronism due to bilateral adrenocortical hyperplasia. Am J Hypertens 2020;33(2):124−30. https://doi.org/10.1093/ajh/hpz172. PMID: 31637427.

[36] Monticone S, Else T, Mulatero P, Williams TA, Rainey WE. Understanding primary aldosteronism: impact of next generation sequencing and expression profiling. Mol Cell Endocrinol 2015;399:311−20. https://doi.org/10.1016/j.mce.2014.09.015. PMID: 25240470.

[37] Scholl UI, Nelson-Williams C, Yue P, Grekin R, Wyatt RJ, Dillon MJ, et al. Hypertension with or without adrenal hyperplasia due to different inherited mutations in the potassium channel KCNJ5. Proc Natl Acad Sci U S A February 14, 2012;109(7):2533−8. https://doi.org/10.1073/pnas.1121407109. PMID: 22308486; PMCID: PMC3289329.

[38] Monticone S, Tetti M, Burrello J, Buffolo F, De Giovanni R, Veglio F, et al. Familial hyperaldosteronism type III. J Hum Hypertens 2017;31(12):776−81. https://doi.org/10.1038/jhh.2017.34. PMID: 28447626.

[39] Scholl UI, Stölting G, Nelson-Williams C, Vichot AA, Choi M, Loring E, et al. Recurrent gain of function mutation in calcium channel CACNA1H causes early-onset hypertension with primary aldosteronism. Elife 2015;4:e06315. https://doi.org/10.7554/eLife.06315. PMID: 25907736.

[40] Gürtler F, Jordan K, Tegtmeier I, Herold J, Stindl J, Warth R, Bandulik S. Cellular pathophysiology of mutant voltage-dependent Ca2+ channel CACNA1H in primary aldosteronism. Endocrinology October 1, 2020;161(10):bqaa135. https://doi.org/10.1210/endocr/bqaa135. PMID: 32785697.

[41] Reimer EN, Walenda G, Seidel E, Scholl UI. CACNA1H(M1549V) mutant calcium channel causes autonomous aldosterone production in HAC15 cells and is inhibited by mibefradil. Endocrinology August 2016;157(8):3016−22. https://doi.org/10.1210/en.2016-1170. PMID: 27258646.

[42] Pinggera A, Mackenroth L, Rump A, Schallner J, Beleggia F, Wollnik B, Striessnig J. New gain-of-function mutation shows CACNA1D as recurrently mutated gene in autism spectrum disorders and epilepsy. Hum Mol Genet 2017;26(15):2923−32. https://doi.org/10.1093/hmg/ddx175. PMID: 28472301.

[43] Zilbermint M, Xekouki P, Faucz FR, Berthon A, Gkourogianni A, Schernthaner-Reiter MH, et al. Primary aldosteronism and ARMC5 variants. J Clin Endocrinol Metab 2015;100(6):E900−9. https://doi.org/10.1210/jc.2014-4167. PMID: 25822102.

[44] Rassi-Cruz M, Maria AG, Faucz FR, London E, Vilela LAP, Santana LS, et al. Phosphodiesterase 2A and 3B variants are associated with primary aldosteronism. Endocr Relat Cancer 2021;28(1):1−13. https://doi.org/10.1530/ERC-20-0384. PMID: 33112806.

Chapter 9

Congenital adrenal hyperplasia and hypertension

Busra Gurpinar Tosun and Tulay Guran

Department of Pediatric Endocrinology and Diabetes, Marmara University, School of Medicine, Istanbul, Turkey

Visit the *Endocrine Hypertension: From Basic Science to Clinical Practice, First Edition* companion web site at: https://www.elsevier.com/books-and-journals/book-companion/9780323961202.

Graphical Abstract

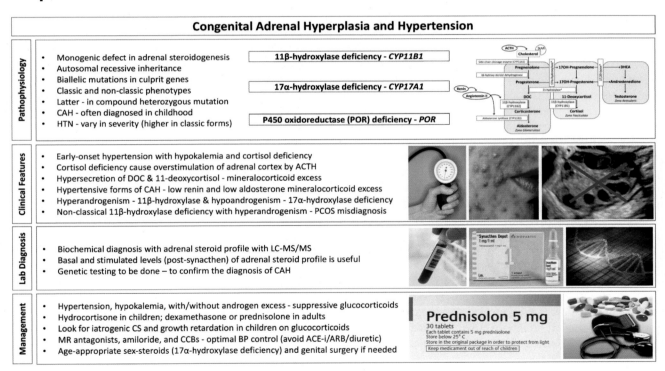

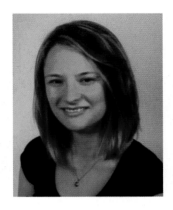

Busra Gurpinar Tosun

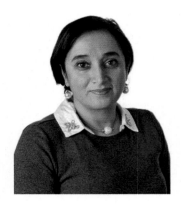

Tulay Guran

Introduction

Congenital adrenal hyperplasia (CAH) is a group of autosomal recessive disorders caused by variations in the genes encoding enzymes and cofactor proteins which are involved in the adrenal steroidogenesis [1]. These disorders are often diagnosed in childhood. CAH due to 21-hydroxylase deficiency, the most common type that constitutes ~95% of all cases, is not associated with hypertension [2−4]. On the other hand, 11β-hydroxylase deficiency (the second common type that constitutes ~5% of all CAH), and 17α-hydroxylase deficiency (a rare form of CAH) are associated with hypertension due to hypersecretion of DOC (deoxycorticosterone) [5]. These two disorders are characterized by early-onset hypertension associated with hypokalemia, mediated by hypersecretion of mineralocorticoids. Those with partial enzyme defects can present with hypertension in adult life. The mineralocorticoid excess state is associated with a reduction in the renin and aldosterone secretion. Cytochrome P450 oxidoreductase (POR) deficiency is a rare form of CAH, which may also present with hypertension, similar to 17α-hydroxylase deficiency [6,7]. Other rare forms of CAH that are not associated with hypertension and hypokalemia include 3β-hydroxysteroid dehydrogenase type 2 deficiency, congenital lipoid adrenal hyperplasia (due to a defect in the transport protein namely steroidogenic acute regulatory protein or StAR), and cholesterol side-chain cleavage enzyme deficiency [8]. The CAH subtypes, in the order in which they are mentioned above, are associated with mutations in the following genes: *CYP21A2, CYP11B1, CYP17A1, POR, HSD3B2, StAR,* and *CYP11A1,* respectively. The incidence of CAH due to 21-hydroxylase deficiency is ~ 1 in 10,000; that due to 11β-hydroxylase deficiency is ~ 1 in 100,000; and that due to 17α-hydroxylase deficiency is ~ 1 in 1,000,000 [9].

Genetic defects in CAH reduce the activity of the enzymes necessary for cortisol production, leading to chronic overstimulation of the adrenal cortex. Thus, except for StAR and cholesterol side-chain cleavage enzyme deficiency, cases with CAH show the clinical features of both deficient steroids distal to and excessive steroids proximal to the enzyme block [8]. Impaired enzyme function at each step of adrenal steroidogenesis creates a unique steroid profile as a combination of elevated precursors and deficient products, which facilitates biochemical diagnosis [10]. Once a biochemical diagnosis of CAH has been established, we should confirm it by molecular genetic analysis. Increasing data on genotype−phenotype correlations reinforces the knowledge that genotyping should be performed early as part of routine clinical care. This provides information on the severity of clinical disease expression and shines a light on possible future discussions about antenatal diagnosis, treatment, and family planning [11].

Genetics of CAH (in general—all forms)

All forms of CAH are monogenic with autosomal recessive inheritance pattern. Most patients have compound heterozygote mutations. The clinical presentation is consistent with the allele that results in a more functional enzyme, and there is usually a genotype-phenotype correlation [12]. The genetic studies of CAH have provided insight into the pathophysiology and subtle clinical aspects of the disease and may provide prognostic information on disease severity. Furthermore, genotyping is essential in confirming carrier status and is useful for genetic counseling because biochemical methods typically cannot distinguish heterozygotes from the normal population, and assess the disease severity [3]. The genes for

TABLE 9.1 Genetic causes of congenital adrenal hyperplasia and relation to hypertension.

	Gene (OMIM number)	Chromosome	Affected organs	Hypertension
21-hydroxylase deficiency	CYP21A2 (#201910)	6p21.1	Adrenal glands	No
11β-hydroxylase deficiency	CYP11B1 (#202010)	8q21	Adrenal glands	Yes
17α-hydroxylase/17,20 lyase deficiency	CYP17A1 (#202110)	10q24.3	Adrenal glands and gonads	Yes
3β-hydroxysteroid dehydrogenase type 2 deficiency	HSD3B2 (#201810)	1p13.1	Adrenal glands and gonads	No
P450 oxidoreductase deficiency	POR (#201750)	7q11.2	Adrenal glands, gonads, liver, skeletal structures	Yes
Lipoid adrenal hyperplasia	StAR (#600617)	8p11.2	Adrenal glands and gonads	No
Cholesterol side-chain cleavage enzyme deficiency	CYP11A1 (#118485)	15q23-q24	Adrenal glands and gonads	No

OMIM, Online Mendelian Inheritance in Man; POR, P450 oxidoreductase; StAR, steroidogenic acute regulatory protein.

different variants of CAH are well characterized, and the mutation analysis is widely available. Genetic causes of CAH are illustrated in Table 9.1.

Although biochemical differential diagnosis and genetic diagnosis in rare forms of CAH are not compelling, the diagnosis of 21-hydroxylase deficiency, the most common type can be complicated due to different and misleading clinical presentation, relevant gene region, and mutations. 21-hydroxylase deficiency is caused by inactivating biallelic mutations in the CYP21A2 gene that encodes the microsomal P450 enzyme, 21-hydroxylase (CYP21A2, P450c21). The CYP21A2 are located on chromosome 6p21.3, approximately 30 kilobases (kb) apart from the nonfunctional CYP21A1P pseudogene. CYP21A2 and CYP21A1P both consist of 10 exons and share high nucleotide homology of about 98% and 96% in exons and introns, respectively [13,14]. To date, more than 300 mutations in the CYP21A2 gene have been identified. Over 90% of mutations causing 21-hydroxylase deficiency are the result of intergenic recombinations in the HLA region within the 30 kb tandem repeat [2,15,16]. Most of the studies conducted to date show that there is a genotype—phenotype relationship, especially in severe salt-wasting and mild nonclassic forms [2,4,16].

The 11β-hydroxylase enzyme has two isoenzymes encoded by the CYP11B1 and CYP11B2 genes on chromosome 8q21-q22. Both are located in the inner membrane of mitochondria. CYP11B1 gene mutations result in 11β-hydroxylase deficiency and expression of 11β-hydroxylase enzyme is induced by adrenocorticotropic hormone (ACTH) in the zona fasciculata and zona glomerulosa, whereas CYP11B2 is primarily expressed in zona glomerulosa and is controlled mainly by angiotensin II and potassium levels. Biallelic mutations of CYP11B1 cause 11β-hydroxylase deficiency and more than 100 mutations have been identified [17—20]). Mutations with a founder effect in the CYP11B1 gene have been described in some ethnic groups, for example, the p.Q356X and p.G379V mutations in Tunisians, the p.R448H mutation in Moroccan Jews, the p.N394Rfs*37 and p.L299P mutations in Turks [18,21—23]. The genotype—phenotype relationship has been reported in many studies [21,23—25]. As in 21-hydroxylase deficiency, 11β-hydroxylase deficiency may present as classic or nonclassic forms depending on the degree of clinical severity and the percentage of enzyme activity. In the literature, less than 20 mutations associated with the nonclassic form have been described [18,26,27]. Milder clinical presentation was observed in compound heterozygous mutations when one of the two alleles was milder than when both were severe, as in 21 hydroxylase deficiency [18].

Biallelic mutations of CYP17A1 encoding 17α-hydroxylase and 17,20-lyase cause a lack of 17α-hydroxylation in progesterone and pregnenolone, followed by impaired formation of the sex steroids, dehydroepiandrosterone (DHEA), and androstenedione [28]. CYP17A1 is located on chromosome 10q24.3 and more than 100 mutations have been described to date. Since this gene is expressed in both the adrenal and gonads, its mutations also result in a deficiency in sex steroids which causes sexual infantilism and puberty failure. The majority of identified mutations are associated with the classical phenotype of combined 17α-hydroxylase/17,20-lyase deficiency. Fewer *CYP17A1* missense variants have been reported to exhibit partial impairment of 17α-hydroxylase/17,20-lyase activity in 46,XY individuals with mild or absent hypertension and ambiguous genitalia [29−33]. Hypertension was not observed in a small number of individuals defined as isolated 17,20-lyase deficiency [34−37].

Cytochrome P450 oxidoreductase enzyme deficiency, caused by mutations in the *POR* gene, was first described in 2004 [38−40]. More than 130 cases have been documented. The clinical phenotype in POR deficiency depends on how much and which enzyme function the POR mutation affects [41]. A287P is the predominant mutation in patients of European ancestry that severely disrupts the 17α-hydroxylase activity and presents with hypertension [42].

Pathophysiology of hypertension in CAH

The adrenal cortex has three embryonic regions: The zona glomerulosa synthesizes aldosterone, the most important mineralocorticoid which regulates electrolyte excretion and intravascular volume mainly by its effects on the renal distal tubules and cortical collecting ducts. The zona reticularis and zona fasciculata share the same enzyme pathways to produce cortisol and weak androgens, DHEA, and androstenedione under the control of hypothalamic−pituitary−adrenal axis through ACTH. During the production of cortisol, there are several intermediate precursors, especially DOC and 11-deoxycortisol, that have mineralocorticoid effects [12,20,43]. Simplified adrenal steroidogenesis pathway is shown in Fig. 9.1.

Aldosterone is primarily regulated by the renin−angiotensin system. Hyperkalemia and ACTH are less effective on aldosterone release. Angiotensin II is the major stimulant for the release of aldosterone, and as a potent vasoconstrictor, its level increase when there is a decrease in effective blood volume. Aldosterone exerts its effect by increasing the sodium reabsorption and potassium excretion by the kidney [44]. Consequently, the net effect is to increase the plasma and extracellular volume and to reduce the renin and aldosterone secretion [45]. Excessive secretion of aldosterone or other mineralocorticoids suppresses the renin−angiotensin system, resulting in extracellular fluid volume expansion, hypertension, and consequently low renin and low aldosterone concentrations, hypokalemia, metabolic alkalosis (by the feedback mechanism), but the ability to produce aldosterone remains [20,28]. Renin−angiotensin system suppression may not occur in the neonatal period due to renal mineralocorticoid resistance present in the first few months of life [12]. Of the CAH subtypes, 11β-hydroxylase, 17α-hydroxylase/17,20-lyase, and POR deficiency are associated with hypertension due to the excessive production of DOC.

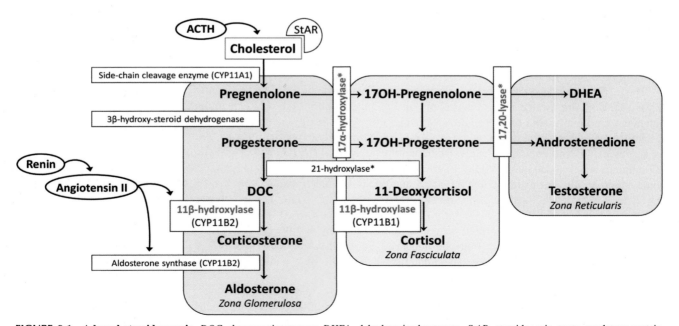

FIGURE 9.1 Adrenal steroidogenesis. *DOC*, deoxycorticosterone; *DHEA*, dehydroepiandrosterone, *StAR*, steroidogenic acute regulatory protein. Enzymes whose deficiency is associated with hypertension are illustrated in red. *17-hydroxylase, 17,20 lyase, and 21-hydroxylase depend on P450 oxidoreductase (POR) for their catalytic activities.

11β-hydroxylase converts DOC to corticosterone in the zona glomerulosa and 11-deoxycortisol to cortisol in the zona fasciculata. Patients with 11β-hydroxylase deficiency lack the cortisol production, leading to chronic overstimulation of the adrenal cortex by ACTH and accumulation of precursors with mainly mineralocorticoid effects (Fig. 9.2). However, some authors suggest a role for 18-hydroxy and 19-nor metabolites of DOC to have a stronger mineralocorticoid effect and are the main causes of hypertension in 11β-hydroxylase deficiency [19,46]. This hypothesis was established based on the facts that DOC having only weak mineralocorticoid activity when administered to humans or other animals, and DOC levels and blood pressure are not well correlated [47,48]. Hypokalemia, which is a result of excessive mineralocorticoid activity, is also not correlated with hypertension [49] although these steroids have not been documented to be elevated in 11β-hydroxylase deficiency, presumably requiring hydroxylations mediated mainly by 11β-hydroxylase during their synthesis [50]. Glucocorticoid treatment can normalize DOC and renin levels leading to reduction of excessive mineralocorticoid activity, but control of hypertension may require additional antihypertensive drugs [18,26,51,52].

17α-hydroxylase converts pregnenolone to 17-hydroxypregnenolone and progesterone to 17-hydroxyprogesterone. 17,20-lyase then converts 17-hydroxypregnenolone to DHEA and 17-hydroxyprogesterone to androstenedione, which are the major precursors to the sex steroids (testosterone and estrogen). The lack of cortisol production and therefore chronic overstimulation of the adrenal cortex in 17α-hydroxylase deficiency leads to accumulation of the common steroidogenic precursor progesterone, which then shunts toward the zona glomerulosa pathway to make DOC, corticosterone, and aldosterone (Fig. 9.3). Although these steroids are usually produced in response to renin/angiotensin II in healthy subjects in zona glomerulosa, these steroids are found in excessive amounts in zona fasciculata in 17α-hydroxylase deficiency, and several studies have shown that the production of mineralocorticoids from zona fasciculata is increased by ACTH but not by angiotensin II or postural stimulation [53,54]. Moreover, treatment with glucocorticoids (for ACTH suppression) rapidly reduces DOC and corticosterone levels, confirming the primary effect of ACTH on their formation [55].

In 17α-hydroxylase deficiency, it seems to be paradoxical that the immediate precursors of aldosterone are elevated, but aldosterone tends to be low. Initially, the second defect in aldosterone synthase was suggested. However, treatment of 17α-hydroxylase deficiency with glucocorticoids allowed aldosterone levels to become normal, indicating an intact aldosterone synthase [56]. It is assumed that DOC inhibits renin and thus aldosterone synthase, causing sodium retention and volume expansion [57].

POR plays a role in electron transport in the endoplasmic reticulum, and many enzymes including 17-hydroxylase, 21-hydroxylase and P450 aromatase depend on POR for their catalytic activity. In general, POR deficiency is not manifested with mineralocorticoid deficiency. But mild mineralocorticoid excess can be present and causes arterial hypertension due to particularly 17α-hydroxylase disruption that increases the production of mineralocorticoid intermediates, usually presenting in young adulthood [6,7,58].

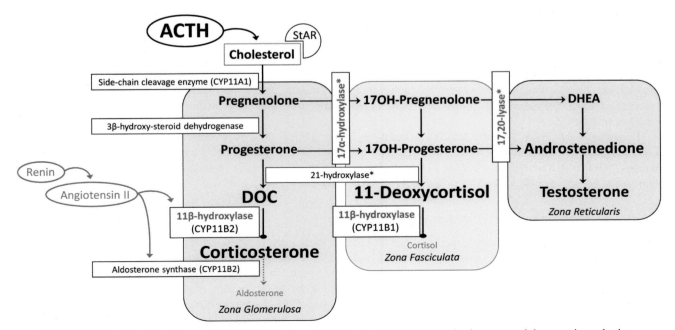

FIGURE 9.2 **Adrenal steroidogenesis in 11β-hydroxylase deficiency.** Font size shows relative increases and decreases in production.

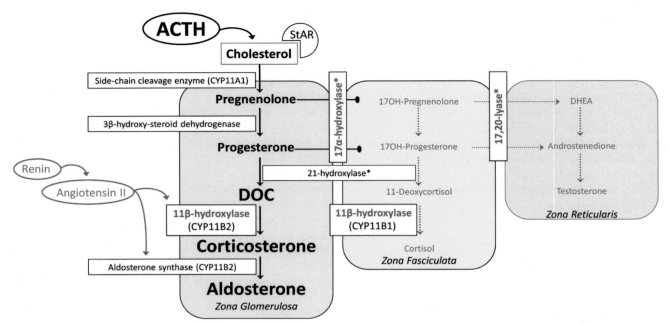

FIGURE 9.3 Adrenal steroidogenesis in 17-alpha hydroxylase deficiency.

The mainstay of treatment in classical forms of CAH is glucocorticoid therapy. Hydrocortisone, the most commonly used agent in the treatment, has dose-dependent mineralocorticoid activity. Hypertension as a side effect has been reported with high-dose treatment in patients with CAH [59].

11β-hydroxylase deficiency

Clinical presentations

Impaired 11-hydroxylation results in decreased corticosterone and cortisol synthesis, followed by an increase in ACTH, DOC, and 11-deoxycortisol, and the substrate mass effect results in excess production of androgens. This clinically presents as pre- and postnatal virilization of varying severity depending on the degree of enzyme deficiency in both sexes and with hypertension. In the reported series, 66%–80% of girls presented with ambiguous genitalia at birth with enlarged clitoral folds [18,60]. Affected boys appear normal at birth, but premature penile enlargement develops as the first symptom. Patients generally present during infancy and early childhood. Other features include precocious puberty, excessive linear growth, advanced epiphyseal maturation, short adult stature, masculine body habitus, hirsutism, menstrual irregularities, cystic acne, male pattern baldness, increased muscle mass, and hyperpigmentation [12,20]. In the nonclassical form, patients have milder degree of hyperandrogenism and may be misdiagnosed as polycystic ovary syndrome [52,54].

Hypertension of varying severity (mild to moderate) is found in 30%–66% of patients, and is usually diagnosed later in childhood [48,60–62]. It can be severe and can lead to retinopathy, left ventricular hypertrophy, and cerebrovascular disease [20,63–65]. Two-thirds of classic 11β-hydroxylase deficiency cases have hypertension at the time of diagnosis, in contrast the ones with nonclassical form are often normotensive at diagnosis [26].

Diagnostic approach for 11β-hydroxylase deficiency

Initial screening tests in clinically suspected patients include measurement of blood levels of DOC, 11-deoxycortisol, DHEA, androstenedione, and testosterone. Cortisol, renin, aldosterone, and corticosterone are low. Hypokalemia is relatively uncommon and is usually not found in infants. For the given low level of cortisol, ACTH remains elevated [60]. Although the level of 11-deoxycortisol is very high, it cannot compensate for the lack of cortisol due to low bioactivity. In mild cases (late-onset or nonclassical form) corticotropin-stimulated 11-deoxycortisol and DOC measurements may be helpful (11-deoxycortisol >3 times the upper limit of normal, several times higher for classic) [12]. Like 21-hydroxylase deficiency, both 3β-hydroxysteroid dehydrogenase type 2 and 11β-hydroxylase deficiencies that are presenting with hyperandrogenemia may have moderate 17OH-progesterone levels. Elevated 17OH-progesterone levels can mislead to the diagnosis of 21-hydroxylase deficiency when used in neonatal screening programs [66]. Differential diagnosis is made with the 11-deoxycortisol, DOC, and 17-hydroxypregnenolone values [26]. In recent years, analysis of the adrenal steroid profile with liquid chromatography-tandem mass spectrometry (LC-MS/MS) has been supportive in the differential diagnosis [17,67]. With the neonatal screening programs that include 11-deoxycortisol in the second stage, it is now possible to diagnose and treat cases of 11β-hydroxylase deficiency earlier [68]. Along with the hormonal evaluation, further genetic testing for the *CYP11B1* gene and functional characterization of mutations should be specifically performed to confirm the diagnosis [69].

Management algorithm

The goals of treatment are to control hypertension, androgen excess, and hypokalemia [70]. This is achieved by glucocorticoid administration, mostly in the form of hydrocortisone (10–15 mg/m^2/day in 2–3 divided doses), similar to 21-hydroxylase deficiency [59,69]. In adults, long-acting glucocorticoids such as prednisolone or dexamethasone (2.5–7.5 mg/day and 0.25–0.5 mg/day, respectively) may be preferred [69]. Glucocorticoid doses should be adjusted to minimize the risk of iatrogenic Cushing's syndrome [64]. Stress doses of glucocorticoids are required in acute illness even if the risk of adrenal crisis is less than that in 21-hydroxylase deficiency [26,52].

If the blood pressure remains high despite optimal glucocorticoid therapy, an antihypertensive medication should be added. Spironolactone or amiloride can be used as a single agent or in combination with a calcium channel blocker. Angiotensin-converting enzyme inhibitors and angiotensin receptor II blockers should be avoided, as the renin—angiotensin system is suppressed. Thiazide diuretics should also be avoided or used in combination with a potassium-sparing diuretic, as they may exacerbate or precipitate hypokalemia [71].

Adult short stature is an important complication on long-term follow-up. If the bone age continues to progress especially in children in their adolescence despite the use of optimal glucocorticoid therapy, aromatase inhibitors are an option [72]. The peripheral onset of precocious puberty can be centralized, and in this case, gonadotropin-releasing hormone analogue may be started [26].

Other considerations including individualized treatment plans to modulate patients' sexual development and surgical correction of genital malformations may be required in females [73].

Therapeutic targets

The efficacy of treatment is monitored by regular clinical evaluation documenting the degree of virilization, control of hypertension, growth rate, and bone maturation in children. On long-term follow-up, blood pressure should be normalized, normokalemia should be maintained, and DOC levels should decrease even if it is not within the normal range [49,70]. Serum androstenedione and testosterone levels should be evaluated according to age and gender. Higher levels in the postpubertal period are of adrenal origin and indicate inadequate treatment. A measurable renin level indicates adequate suppression of mineralocorticoids but can only occur months after treatment [49].

17α-hydroxylase deficiency

Clinical presentation

Impaired 17-hydroxylation results in decreased cortisol synthesis, followed by an increase in ACTH, DOC, and corticosterone [74]. Glucocorticoid deficiency is generally not symptomatic due to the overproduction of corticosterone that has glucocorticoid activity [37]. In the complete deficiency, due to the deficiency of both 17α-hydroxylase and 17,20-lyase, the adrenal and gonadal sex steroids synthesis is impaired. Patients typically have a female phenotype in most cases, regardless of karyotype and usually present during puberty as girls without secondary sexual characteristics, with hypergonadotropic hypogonadism, and low-renin hypertension [54,73]. Small uterus and ovaries can be detected in 46,XX individuals in childhood, and large cysts in the ovaries due to high gonadotropin levels in adolescence. In partial deficiency, 46,XY individuals usually present with ambiguous genitalia with intraabdominal or inguinal testis during infancy because sufficient androgen cannot be synthesized for external genitalia development [75,76]. Since there is no deficiency of anti-Mullerian Hormone, internal genital development is normal in 46,XY individuals, and Mullerian structures (uterus/cervix) are absent [2,30,54]. In the literature, 46,XX individuals misdiagnosed as gonadal dysgenesis and 46,XY individuals misdiagnosed with androgen insensitivity were reported [77,78]. Although patients tend to be taller due to the lack of epiphyseal closure caused by deficient sex steroids, short stature has also been reported in those who are less severely affected with point mutations [79].

Hypokalemia and hypertension are quite common and usually present from late childhood to adolescence, but their absence does not exclude the disease [53,80]. Even within the same family with the same mutation, varying degrees of hypertension have been reported previously and are thought to be due to factors other than 11β-hydroxylase enzyme activity, such as circulating DOC levels, diet, and environmental factors [81].

Diagnostic approach

Biochemical diagnosis of 17α-hydroxylase deficiency is established by elevated levels of DOC, corticosterone, ACTH, and gonadotropins with suppressed levels of renin, androgens, and estrogen [82]. Progesterone is also elevated as in 21-hydroxylase and 11β-hydroxylase deficiency, but 17α-hydroxylase deficiency leads to the absence of sex steroid-dependent puberty development rather than virilization [83]. Unlike 11β-hydroxylase deficiency, 17-hydroxyprogesterone levels are low and do not rise with the corticotropin stimulation test. Since basal values may be normal in patients with partial deficiency, a corticotropin stimulation test can be performed. The test reveals elevated DOC, pregnenolone, and progesterone [84]. The progesterone level is high in POR deficiency, but low 17-hydroxyprogesterone and very high DOC distinguish 17α-hydroxylase from POR deficiency. Genetic testing establishes the diagnosis with the identification of the related mutations [28].

Management algorithm

The goals of the treatment are to prevent glucocorticoid deficiency, to reduce the effects of mineralocorticoid excess and hypertension, and to provide age-appropriate development of secondary sex characters [74]. When treated with suppressive doses of glucocorticoids, DOC is suppressed and renin and aldosterone levels return to normal range [85]. The addition of mineralocorticoid receptor antagonists such as spironolactone or eplerenone may be necessary in some cases to treat hypertension. Patients should be treated with age-appropriate sex steroids and genital abnormalities due to virilization should be managed with appropriate surgical procedures [86].

Therapeutic targets

Blood pressure and serum potassium should be the two main parameters for titration therapy, especially in the first few months. Plasma renin activity can be used as an indicator of mineralocorticoid receptor antagonism but can only be used in the chronic phase as renin may not rise for months or years following chronic suppression [81].

Overtreatment of CAH

The main treatment option in the classic forms of CAH is chronic glucocorticoid supplements and mostly additional mineralocorticoid therapy. While long-acting glucocorticoid therapy is avoided in children due to its growth-suppressing effects, it is sometimes used in adults. Glucocorticoid therapy aims to prevent adrenal crisis and virilization, allowing nearly normal growth and development during childhood. In general, supraphysiological doses of glucocorticoids are needed to achieve adequate suppression of hormone excesses (10–15 mg/m^2 per day). Management of classic CAH is a difficult balance between hyperandrogenism and hypercortisolism. Laboratory results may be indicative but not always ensure optimal management. Therefore, regular clinical evaluation should always be performed. Overtreatment often leads to Cushingoid side effects such as in linear growth retardation, obesity, osteoporosis, and hypertension [2,12,87].

In patients with classic 21-hydroxylase deficiency, mineralocorticoid therapy allows the use of lower doses of glucocorticoids, thus optimizing growth. The only oral mineralocorticoid preparation available is fludrocortisone (9α-fluorocortisol). Hydrocortisone can also activate mineralocorticoid receptors. Approximately 20 mg of hydrocortisone is equivalent to the mineralocorticoid effect of about 0.1 mg of fludrocortisone [88]. Therefore, when stress doses of hydrocortisone are administered, fludrocortisone treatment is not required [89].

In infancy, however, mineralocorticoid susceptibility is naturally greater during the first year of life, and they often need higher doses of fludrocortisone therapy than in adults. In this period, finding the appropriate fludrocortisone dose without causing hypertension is the challenge of treatment, especially in the first few years of life, when higher doses and salt supplementation are often needed. In a prospective study, 57.6% of 33 infants with classic CAH, diagnosed by new-born screening, had hypertension in the first 18 months of life [90].

The majority of studies investigating hypertension in CAH patients, by ambulatory or 24-hour blood pressure measurement, have documented increased systolic and/or diastolic blood pressure values [87,91−99]. Moreover, even in CAH children without overt hypertension, a reduction in the physiological nocturnal drop response in blood pressure (nocturnal dip) was observed [93,95,98].

Subbarayan et al. reported that a large cohort of CAH children, regardless of gender, had significantly higher systolic hypertension (20.9%) compared to the reference population [87]. However, the prevalence of hypertension was lower than in previous studies, possibly due to the use of lower doses of glucocorticoids and mineralocorticoids in the recent years. Blood pressure was negatively associated with age, possibly due to reduction in fludrocortisone dose [87].

In a multicenter study, there was a relationship between fludrocortisone dose and blood pressure in 716 patients (2−18 years) diagnosed with 21-hydroxylase deficiency, and hypertension was less common in children who have regular PRA during follow-up. Blood pressure values were significantly correlated to body mass index, age, and the fludrocortisone dose [94].

Current findings indicate a higher prevalence of hypertension in children and adolescents with classic forms of CAH. In addition to obesity, an overtreatment of glucocorticoids and mineralocorticoids also plays an important pathogenic role.

When to suspect of CAH in patients with hypertension

Clinicians should screen children, adolescents, and young adults who present with hypertension, hypokalemia, and low aldosterone and renin levels. In addition, hyperpigmentation, muscle weakness, delayed or precocious puberty, growth failure, ambiguous genitalia, and virilization are important additional clues. Suspicion for 11β-hydroxylase deficiency should be highest in females with hyperandrogenemia signs such as hirsutism, clitoromegaly, menstrual irregularities, cystic acne, male pattern baldness, increased muscle mass, masculine body habitus, and in males with pseudoprecocious puberty. 17α-hydroxylase deficiency has the highest suspicion in females phenotype without secondary sexual characteristics, with hypergonadotropic hypogonadism. Clinical approaches to CAH-associated hypertension are illustrated in Fig. 9.4.

Future research

Despite a decrease in glucocorticoid doses over the past decade, many children with CAH are still obese and hypertensive. The development of new therapies is needed to address chronic glucocorticoid overexposure, lack of circadian rhythm in glucocorticoid replacement, and ineffective glucocorticoid delivery with attendant episodes of hyperandrogenism.

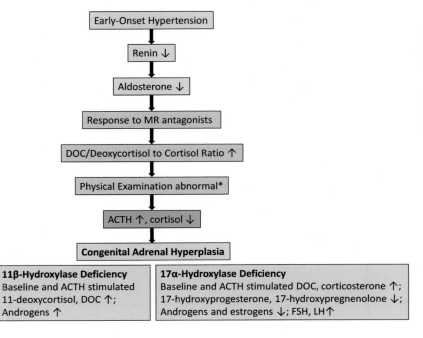

FIGURE 9.4 Clinical approach to congenital adrenal hyperplasia-associated hypertension. (* ambiguous genitalia, premature penile enlargement, precocious or delayed puberty, excessive linear growth, advanced epiphyseal maturation, short adult stature, masculine body habitus, hirsutism, menstrual irregularities, cystic acne, male pattern baldness and increased muscle mass, hyperpigmentation, polycystic ovary syndrome, hypergonadotropic hypogonadism).

Summary and conclusions

Disorders of steroidogenesis must remain on the differential diagnosis of mineralocorticoid hypertension especially in children and younger adults. While making the correct differential diagnosis of CAH, family history, physical examination, and measurement of potassium, renin and aldosterone blood levels are guiding. The initial diagnosis is made by evaluating the steroid hormone profile in suspected cases. Definitive genetic diagnosis is essential, allowing for individualized treatment options and in providing appropriate genetic counseling. Early recognition and specific management may improve prognosis and prevent long-term sequelae of severe hypertension.

Learning points

- CAH due to 11β-hydroxylase deficiency, 17α-hydroxylase deficiency, and POR deficiency can cause hypertension.
- Hypertension in CAH is often accompanied by hypokalemia and low aldosterone and renin levels.
- Regular blood pressure monitoring is essential in the diagnosis and follow-up of the patients with CAH.
- 17α-hydroxylase deficiency and 11β-hydroxylase deficiency may be diagnosed in adulthood, thus must remain on the differential diagnosis of hypertension in children, adolescents, and young adults.
- Women with symptoms of hyperandrogenemia and men with pseudoprecocious puberty should be evaluated for 11β-hydroxylase deficiency.
- 17α-hydroxylase deficiency can present in the female phenotype without secondary sexual characteristics and with hypergonadotropic hypogonadism.
- If blood pressure remains high despite optimal glucocorticoid therapy, an antihypertensive medication such as spironolactone or amiloride should be added.
- Since the prevalence of hypertension is also higher in children and adolescents with classical forms of CAH, treatment and clinical follow-up should include regular evaluation of blood pressure.

References

[1] Lu YT, Fan P, Zhang D, Zhang Y, Meng X, Zhang QY, et al. Overview of monogenic forms of hypertension combined with hypokalemia. Front Pediatr 2020;8:543309.

[2] Claahsen-van der Grinten HL, Speiser PW, Ahmed SF, Arlt W, Auchus RJ, Falhammar H, et al. Congenital adrenal hyperplasia-current insights in pathophysiology, diagnostics, and management. Endocr Rev 2022;43(1):91−159.

[3] Hannah-Shmouni F, Chen W, Merke DP. Genetics of congenital adrenal hyperplasia. Endocrinol Metab Clin North Am 2017;46(2):435−58.

[4] Speiser PW, Arlt W, Auchus RJ, Baskin LS, Conway GS, Merke DP, et al. Congenital adrenal hyperplasia due to steroid 21-hydroxylase deficiency: an endocrine society clinical practice guideline. J Clin Endocrinol Metab 2018;103(11):4043−88.

[5] Burrello J, Monticone S, Buffolo F, Tetti M, Veglio F, Williams TA, et al. Is there a role for genomics in the management of hypertension? Int J Mol Sci 2017;18(6):1131.

[6] Flück CE, Tajima T, Pandey AV, Arlt W, Okuhara K, Verge CF, et al. Mutant P450 oxidoreductase causes disordered steroidogenesis with and without Antley-Bixler syndrome. Nat Genet 2004;36(3):228−30.

[7] Krone N, Reisch N, Idkowiak J, Dhir V, Ivison HE, Hughes BA, et al. Genotype-phenotype analysis in congenital adrenal hyperplasia due to P450 oxidoreductase deficiency. J Clin Endocrinol Metab 2012;97(2):E257−67.

[8] Miller WL. Disorders in the initial steps of steroid hormone synthesis. J Steroid Biochem Mol Biol 2017;165(Pt A):18−37.

[9] Antal Z, Zhou P. Congenital adrenal hyperplasia: diagnosis, evaluation, and management. Pediatr Rev 2009;30(7):e49−57.

[10] Kirkgoz T, Guran T. Primary adrenal insufficiency in children: diagnosis and management. Best Pract Res Clin Endocrinol Metab 2018;32(4):397−424.

[11] Webb EA, Krone N. Current and novel approaches to children and young people with congenital adrenal hyperplasia and adrenal insufficiency. Best Pract Res Clin Endocrinol Metab 2015;29(3):449−68.

[12] El-Maouche D, Arlt W, Merke DP. Congenital adrenal hyperplasia. Lancet 2017;390(10108):2194−210.

[13] White PC, New MI, Dupont B. Structure of human steroid 21-hydroxylase genes. Proc Natl Acad Sci U S A 1986;83(14):5111−5.

[14] Higashi Y, Yoshioka H, Yamane M, Gotoh O, Fujii-Kuriyama Y. Complete nucleotide sequence of two steroid 21-hydroxylase genes tandemly arranged in human chromosome: a pseudogene and a genuine gene. Proc Natl Acad Sci U S A 1986;83(9):2841−5.

[15] Tusié-Luna MT, White PC. Gene conversions and unequal crossovers between CYP21 (steroid 21-hydroxylase gene) and CYP21P involve different mechanisms. Proc Natl Acad Sci U S A 1995;92(23):10796−800.

[16] Carvalho B, Marques CJ, Santos-Silva R, Fontoura M, Carvalho D, Carvalho F. Congenital adrenal hyperplasia due to 21-hydroxylase deficiency: an update on genetic analysis of CYP21A2 gene. Exp Clin Endocrinol Diabetes 2021;129(7):477−81.

[17] Karlekar MP, Sarathi V, Lila A, Rai K, Arya S, Bhandare VV, et al. Expanding genetic spectrum and discriminatory role of steroid profiling by LC-MS/MS in 11β-hydroxylase deficiency. Clin Endocrinol 2021;94(4):533−43.

[18] Yildiz M, Isik E, Abali ZY, Keskin M, Ozbek MN, Bas F, et al. Clinical and hormonal profiles correlate with molecular characteristics in patients with 11β-hydroxylase deficiency. J Clin Endocrinol Metab 2021;106(9):e3714−24.

[19] White PC, Curnow KM, Pascoe L. Disorders of steroid 11 beta-hydroxylase isozymes. Endocr Rev 1994;15(4):421−38.

[20] White PC. Inherited forms of mineralocorticoid hypertension. Hypertension 1996;28(6):927−36.

[21] Kharrat M, Trabelsi S, Chaabouni M, Maazoul F, Kraoua L, Ben Jemaa L, et al. Only two mutations detected in 15 Tunisian patients with 11β-hydroxylase deficiency: the p.Q356X and the novel p.G379V. Clin Genet 2010;78(4):398−401.

[22] Ben Charfeddine I, Riepe FG, Kahloul N, Kulle AE, Adala L, Mamaï O, et al. Two novel CYP11B1 mutations in congenital adrenal hyperplasia due to steroid 11β hydroxylase deficiency in a Tunisian family. Gen Comp Endocrinol 2012;175(3):514−8.

[23] Paperna T, Gershoni-Baruch R, Badarneh K, Kasinetz L, Hochberg Z. Mutations in CYP11B1 and congenital adrenal hyperplasia in Moroccan Jews. J Clin Endocrinol Metab 2005;90(9):5463−5.

[24] Chabraoui L, Abid F, Menassa R, Gaouzi A, El Hessni A, Morel Y. Three novel CYP11B1 mutations in congenital adrenal hyperplasia due to steroid 11Beta-hydroxylase deficiency in a moroccan population. Horm Res Paediatr 2010;74(3):182−9.

[25] Soardi FC, Penachioni JY, Justo GZ, Bachega TA, Inácio M, Mendonça BB, et al. Novel mutations in CYP11B1 gene leading to 11 beta-hydroxylase deficiency in Brazilian patients. J Clin Endocrinol Metab 2009;94(9):3481−5.

[26] Bulsari K, Falhammar H. Clinical perspectives in congenital adrenal hyperplasia due to 11β-hydroxylase deficiency. Endocrine 2017;55(1):19−36.

[27] Mooij CF, Parajes S, Rose IT, Taylor AE, Bayraktaroglu T, Wass JA, et al. Characterization of the molecular genetic pathology in patients with 11β-hydroxylase deficiency. Clin Endocrinol 2015;83(5):629−35.

[28] Khandelwal P, Deinum J. Monogenic forms of low-renin hypertension: clinical and molecular insights. Pediatr Nephrol 2021;37:1495−509.

[29] Rubtsov P, Nizhnik A, Dedov I, Kalinchenko N, Petrov V, Orekhova A, et al. Partial deficiency of 17α-hydroxylase/17,20-lyase caused by a novel missense mutation in the canonical cytochrome heme-interacting motif. Eur J Endocrinol 2015;172(5):K19−25.

[30] Yanase T, Simpson ER, Waterman MR. 17 alpha-hydroxylase/17,20-lyase deficiency: from clinical investigation to molecular definition. Endocr Rev 1991;12(1):91−108.

[31] Taniyama M, Tanabe M, Saito H, Ban Y, Nawata H, Yanase T. Subtle 17alpha-hydroxylase/17,20-lyase deficiency with homozygous Y201N mutation in an infertile woman. J Clin Endocrinol Metab 2005;90(5):2508−11.

[32] Yanase T, Kagimoto M, Suzuki S, Hashiba K, Simpson ER, Waterman MR. Deletion of a phenylalanine in the N-terminal region of human cytochrome P-450(17 alpha) results in partial combined 17 alpha-hydroxylase/17,20-lyase deficiency. J Biol Chem 1989;264(30):18076−82.

[33] Yao F, Huang S, Kang X, Zhang W, Wang P, Tian Q. CYP17A1 mutations identified in 17 Chinese patients with 17α-hydroxylase/17,20-lyase deficiency. Gynecol Endocrinol 2013;29(1):10−5.

[34] Sherbet DP, Tiosano D, Kwist KM, Hochberg Z, Auchus RJ. CYP17 mutation E305G causes isolated 17,20-lyase deficiency by selectively altering substrate binding. J Biol Chem 2003;278(49):48563−9.

[35] Van Den Akker EL, Koper JW, Boehmer AL, Themmen AP, Verhoef-Post M, Timmerman MA, et al. Differential inhibition of 17alpha-hydroxylase and 17,20-lyase activities by three novel missense CYP17 mutations identified in patients with P450c17 deficiency. J Clin Endocrinol Metab 2002;87(12):5714−21.

[36] Geller DH, Auchus RJ, Mendonça BB, Miller WL. The genetic and functional basis of isolated 17,20-lyase deficiency. Nat Genet 1997;17(2):201−5.

[37] Sun M, Mueller JW, Gilligan LC, Taylor AE, Shaheen F, Noczyńska A, et al. The broad phenotypic spectrum of 17α-hydroxylase/17,20-lyase (CYP17A1) deficiency: a case series. Eur J Endocrinol 2021;185(5):729−41.

[38] Pandey AV, Flück CE, Huang N, Tajima T, Fujieda K, Miller WL. P450 oxidoreductase deficiency: a new disorder of steroidogenesis affecting all microsomal P450 enzymes. Endocr Res 2004;30(4):881−8.

[39] Adachi M, Tachibana K, Asakura Y, Yamamoto T, Hanaki K, Oka A. Compound heterozygous mutations of cytochrome P450 oxidoreductase gene (POR) in two patients with Antley-Bixler syndrome. Am J Med Genet 2004;128a(4):333−9.

[40] Arlt W, Walker EA, Draper N, Ivison HE, Ride JP, Hammer F, et al. Congenital adrenal hyperplasia caused by mutant P450 oxidoreductase and human androgen synthesis: analytical study. Lancet 2004;363(9427):2128−35.

[41] Scott RR, Miller WL. Genetic and clinical features of p450 oxidoreductase deficiency. Horm Res 2008;69(5):266−75.

[42] Tomalik-Scharte D, Maiter D, Kirchheiner J, Ivison HE, Fuhr U, Arlt W. Impaired hepatic drug and steroid metabolism in congenital adrenal hyperplasia due to P450 oxidoreductase deficiency. Eur J Endocrinol 2010;163(6):919−24.

[43] Rodd CJ, Sockalosky JJ. Endocrine causes of hypertension in children. Pediatr Clin North Am 1993;40(1):149−64.

[44] Levanovich PE, Diaczok A, Rossi NF. Clinical and molecular perspectives of monogenic hypertension. Curr Hypertens Rev 2020;16(2):91−107.

[45] Ardhanari S, Kannuswamy R, Chaudhary K, Lockette W, Whaley-Connell A. Mineralocorticoid and apparent mineralocorticoid syndromes of secondary hypertension. Adv Chronic Kidney Dis 2015;22(3):185−95.

[46] Griffing GT, Dale SL, Holbrook MM, Melby JC. 19-nor-deoxycorticosterone excretion in primary aldosteronism and low renin hypertension. J Clin Endocrinol Metab 1983;56(2):218−21.

[47] Hassan-Smith Z, Stewart PM. Inherited forms of mineralocorticoid hypertension. Curr Opin Endocrinol Diabetes Obes 2011;18(3):177−85.

[48] New M. Hypertension in congenital adrenal hyperplasia and apparent mineralocorticoid excess. Ann N Y Acad Sci 2002;970:145−54.

[49] Rösler A, Leiberman E, Sack J, Landau H, Benderly A, Moses SW, et al. Clinical variability of congenital adrenal hyperplasia due to 11 beta-hydroxylase deficiency. Horm Res 1982;16(3):133−41.

[50] Ohta M, Fujii S, Ohnishi T, Okamoto M. Production of 19-oic-11-deoxycorticosterone from 19-oxo-11-deoxycorticosterone by cytochrome P-450(11)beta and nonenzymatic production of 19-nor-11-deoxycorticosterone from 19-oic-11-deoxycorticosterone. J Steroid Biochem 1988;29(6):699—707.

[51] Biglieri EG. Rare causes of adrenocortical hypertension. Cardiology 1985;72(Suppl. 1):70—5.

[52] Peter M. Congenital adrenal hyperplasia: 11beta-hydroxylase deficiency. Semin Reprod Med 2002;20(3):249—54.

[53] Kater CE, Biglieri EG. Disorders of steroid 17 alpha-hydroxylase deficiency. Endocrinol Metab Clin North Am 1994;23(2):341—57.

[54] Hinz L, Pacaud D, Kline G. Congenital adrenal hyperplasia causing hypertension: an illustrative review. J Hum Hypertens 2018;32(2):150—7.

[55] Kater CE, Biglieri EG, Brust N, Chang B, Hirai J. The unique patterns of plasma aldosterone and 18-hydroxycorticosterone concentrations in the 17 alpha-hydroxylase deficiency syndrome. J Clin Endocrinol Metab 1982;55(2):295—302.

[56] Saruta T, Kondo K, Saito I, Nagahama S, Suzuki H, Konishi K, et al. Control of aldosterone in 17 alpha-hydroxylase deficiency. Horm Res 1980;13(2):98—108.

[57] Bassett MH, White PC, Rainey WE. The regulation of aldosterone synthase expression. Mol Cell Endocrinol 2004;217(1—2):67—74.

[58] Aljabri A, Alnaim F, Alsaleh Y. Combined homozygous 21 hydroxylase with heterozygous P450 oxidoreductase mutation in a Saudi boy presented with hypertension. BMJ Case Rep 2020;13(9).

[59] Ng SM, Stepien KM, Krishan A. Glucocorticoid replacement regimens for treating congenital adrenal hyperplasia. Cochrane Database Syst Rev 2020;3(3):Cd012517.

[60] Khattab A, Haider S, Kumar A, Dhawan S, Alam D, Romero R, et al. Clinical, genetic, and structural basis of congenital adrenal hyperplasia due to 11β-hydroxylase deficiency. Proc Natl Acad Sci U S A 2017;114(10):E1933—e40.

[61] Zennaro MC, Boulkroun S, Fernandes-Rosa F. Inherited forms of mineralocorticoid hypertension. Best Pract Res Clin Endocrinol Metab 2015;29(4):633—45.

[62] Chemaitilly W, Wilson RC, New MI. Hypertension and adrenal disorders. Curr Hypertens Rep 2003;5(6):498—504.

[63] Kacem M, Moussa A, Khochtali I, Nabouli R, Morel Y, Zakhama A. Bilateral adrenalectomy for severe hypertension in congenital adrenal hyperplasia due to 11beta-hydroxylase deficiency: long term follow-up. Ann Endocrinol (Paris) 2009;70(2):113—8.

[64] Mooij CF, Kroese JM, Sweep FC, Hermus AR, Tack CJ. Adult patients with congenital adrenal hyperplasia have elevated blood pressure but otherwise a normal cardiovascular risk profile. PLoS One 2011;6(9):e24204.

[65] Marra AM, Improda N, Capalbo D, Salzano A, Arcopinto M, De Paulis A, et al. Cardiovascular abnormalities and impaired exercise performance in adolescents with congenital adrenal hyperplasia. J Clin Endocrinol Metab 2015;100(2):644—52.

[66] Güran T, Tezel B, Gürbüz F, Selver Eklioğlu B, Hatipoğlu N, Kara C, et al. Neonatal screening for congenital adrenal hyperplasia in Turkey: a pilot study with 38,935 infants. J Clin Res Pediatr Endocrinol 2019;11(1):13—23.

[67] Engels M, Pijnenburg-Kleizen KJ, Utari A, Faradz SMH, Oude-Alink S, van Herwaarden AE, et al. Glucocorticoid activity of adrenal steroid precursors in untreated patients with congenital adrenal hyperplasia. J Clin Endocrinol Metab 2019;104(11):5065—72.

[68] Güran T, Tezel B, Çakōr M, Akōncō A, Orbak Z, Keskin M, et al. Neonatal screening for congenital adrenal hyperplasia in Turkey: outcomes of extended pilot study in 241,083 infants. J Clin Res Pediatr Endocrinol 2020;12(3):287—94.

[69] Ceccato F, Mantero F. Monogenic forms of hypertension. Endocrinol Metab Clin North Am 2019;48(4):795—810.

[70] Nimkarn S, New MI. Steroid 11beta- hydroxylase deficiency congenital adrenal hyperplasia. Trends Endocrinol Metab 2008;19(3):96—9.

[71] White PC. Steroid 11 beta-hydroxylase deficiency and related disorders. Endocrinol Metab Clin North Am 2001;30(1):61—79. vi.

[72] Atay Z, Turan S, Buğdaycō O, Guran T, Bereket A. Restoration of height after 11 Years of letrozole treatment in 11β-hydroxylase deficiency. Horm Res Paediatr 2019;92(3):203—8.

[73] Raina R, Krishnappa V, Das A, Amin H, Radhakrishnan Y, Nair NR, et al. Overview of monogenic or Mendelian forms of hypertension. Front Pediatr 2019;7:263.

[74] Young Jr WF, Calhoun DA, Lenders JWM, Stowasser M, Textor SC. Screening for endocrine hypertension: an endocrine society scientific statement. Endocr Rev 2017;38(2):103—22.

[75] Qiao J, Chen X, Zuo CL, Gu YY, Liu BL, Liang J, et al. Identification of steroid biosynthetic defects in genotype-proven heterozygous individuals for 17alpha-hydroxylase/17,20-lyase deficiency. Clin Endocrinol (Oxf) 2010;72(3):312—9.

[76] Tiosano D, Knopf C, Koren I, Levanon N, Hartmann MF, Hochberg Z, et al. Metabolic evidence for impaired 17alpha-hydroxylase activity in a kindred bearing the E305G mutation for isolate 17,20-lyase activity. Eur J Endocrinol 2008;158(3):385—92.

[77] Sills IN, MacGillivray MH, Amrhein JA, Migeon CJ, Peterson RE. 17 alpha-hydroxylase deficiency in a genetic male and female sibling pair. Int J Gynaecol Obstet 1981;19(6):473—9.

[78] D'Armiento M, Reda G, Kater C, Shackleton CH, Biglieri EG. 17 alpha-hydroxylase deficiency: mineralocorticoid hormone profiles in an affected family. J Clin Endocrinol Metab 1983;56(4):697—701.

[79] Kardelen AD, Toksoy G, Baş F, Yavaş Abalō Z, Gençay G, Poyrazoğlu Ş, et al. A rare cause of congenital adrenal hyperplasia: clinical and genetic findings and follow-up characteristics of six patients with 17-hydroxylase deficiency including two novel mutations. J Clin Res Pediatr Endocrinol 2018;10(3):206—15.

[80] Asirvatham AR, Balachandran K, Jerome P, Venkatesan V, Koshy T, Mahadevan S. Clinical, biochemical and genetic characteristics of children with congenital adrenal hyperplasia due to 17α-hydroxylase deficiency. J Pediatr Endocrinol Metab 2020;33:1051—6.

[81] Auchus RJ. Steroid 17-hydroxylase and 17,20-lyase deficiencies, genetic and pharmacologic. J Steroid Biochem Mol Biol 2017;165(Pt A):71—8.

[82] Kurnaz E, Kartal Baykan E, Türkyōlmaz A, Yaralō O, Yavaş Abalō Z, Turan S, et al. Genotypic sex and severity of the disease determine the time of clinical presentation in steroid 17α-hydroxylase/17,20-lyase deficiency. Horm Res Paediatr 2020;93(9—10):558—66.

[83] Benetti-Pinto CL, Vale D, Garmes H, Bedone A. 17-Hydroxyprogesterone deficiency as a cause of sexual infantilism and arterial hypertension: laboratory and molecular diagnosis–a case report. Gynecol Endocrinol 2007;23(2):94–8.

[84] Martin RM, Lin CJ, Costa EM, de Oliveira ML, Carrilho A, Villar H, et al. P450c17 deficiency in Brazilian patients: biochemical diagnosis through progesterone levels confirmed by CYP17 genotyping. J Clin Endocrinol Metab 2003;88(12):5739–46.

[85] Scaroni C, Opocher G, Mantero F. Renin-angiotensin-aldosterone system: a long-term follow-up study in 17 alpha-hydroxylase deficiency syndrome (17OHDS). Clin Exp Hypertens 1986;8(4–5):773–80.

[86] Pappachan JM, Buch HN. Endocrine hypertension: a practical approach. Adv Exp Med Biol 2017;956:215–37.

[87] Subbarayan A, Dattani MT, Peters CJ, Hindmarsh PC. Cardiovascular risk factors in children and adolescents with congenital adrenal hyperplasia due to 21-hydroxylase deficiency. Clin Endocrinol 2014;80(4):471–7.

[88] Miller WL, Flück CE, Breault DT, Feldman BJ. The adrenal cortex and its disorders. In: Sperling pediatric endocrinology. Elsevier; 2021. p. 425–90.

[89] Arriza JL, Weinberger C, Cerelli G, Glaser TM, Handelin BL, Housman DE, et al. Cloning of human mineralocorticoid receptor complementary DNA: structural and functional kinship with the glucocorticoid receptor. Science 1987;237(4812):268–75.

[90] Bonfig W, Schwarz HP. Blood pressure, fludrocortisone dose and plasma renin activity in children with classic congenital adrenal hyperplasia due to 21-hydroxylase deficiency followed from birth to 4 years of age. Clin Endocrinol 2014;81(6):871–5.

[91] Tamhane S, Rodriguez-Gutierrez R, Iqbal AM, Prokop LJ, Bancos I, Speiser PW, et al. Cardiovascular and metabolic outcomes in congenital adrenal hyperplasia: a systematic review and meta-analysis. J Clin Endocrinol Metab 2018;103(11):4097–103.

[92] Finkielstain GP, Kim MS, Sinaii N, Nishitani M, Van Ryzin C, Hill SC, et al. Clinical characteristics of a cohort of 244 patients with congenital adrenal hyperplasia. J Clin Endocrinol Metab 2012;97(12):4429–38.

[93] Roche EF, Charmandari E, Dattani MT, Hindmarsh PC. Blood pressure in children and adolescents with congenital adrenal hyperplasia (21-hydroxylase deficiency): a preliminary report. Clin Endocrinol 2003;58(5):589–96.

[94] Bonfig W, Roehl FW, Riedl S, Dörr HG, Bettendorf M, Brämswig J, et al. Blood pressure in a large cohort of children and adolescents with classic adrenal hyperplasia (CAH) due to 21-hydroxylase deficiency. Am J Hypertens 2016;29(2):266–72.

[95] Mooij CF, van Herwaarden AE, Sweep F, Roeleveld N, de Korte CL, Kapusta L, et al. Cardiovascular and metabolic risk in pediatric patients with congenital adrenal hyperplasia due to 21 hydroxylase deficiency. J Pediatr Endocrinol Metab 2017;30(9):957–66.

[96] Akyürek N, Atabek ME, Eklioğlu BS, Alp H. Ambulatory blood pressure and subclinical cardiovascular disease in patients with congenital adrenal hyperplasia: a preliminary report. J Clin Res Pediatr Endocrinol 2015;7(1):13–8.

[97] Nebesio TD, Eugster EA. Observation of hypertension in children with 21-hydroxylase deficiency: a preliminary report. Endocrine 2006;30(3):279–82.

[98] Völkl TM, Simm D, Dötsch J, Rascher W, Dörr HG. Altered 24-hour blood pressure profiles in children and adolescents with classical congenital adrenal hyperplasia due to 21-hydroxylase deficiency. J Clin Endocrinol Metab 2006;91(12):4888–95.

[99] Hoepffner W, Herrmann A, Willgerodt H, Keller E. Blood pressure in patients with congenital adrenal hyperplasia due to 21-hydroxylase deficiency. J Pediatr Endocrinol Metab 2006;19(5):705–11.

Chapter 10

Endocrine hypertension: discovering the inherited causes

Farahnak Assadi[1], Nakysa Hooman[2], Mojgan Mazaheri[3] and Fatemeh Ghane Sharbaf[4]

[1]Rush University of Medical Center, Department of Pediatrics, Division of Nephrology, Chicago, IL, United States; [2]Aliasghar Clinical Research Development Center, Iran University of Medical Sciences, Pediatric Nephrology, Tehran, Iran; [3]Semnan University of Medical Sciences, Pediatric Nephrology, Semnan, Iran; [4]Pediatric Nephrology, Mashhad University of Medical Sciences, Mashhad, Iran

Visit the *Endocrine Hypertension: From Basic Science to Clinical Practice, First Edition* companion web site at: https://www.elsevier.com/books-and-journals/book-companion/9780323961202.

Graphical Abstract

Endocrine Hypertension: Discovering the Inherited Causes

Disease entities and the main organs involved

Adrenal cortex, kidney, and cardiovascular — FH-1, FH-2, FH-3 & FH-4, CAH, AME, JGCT

Kidney — Liddle, Gordon, Geller, Chrousos; Cardiovascular

Adrenal medulla — Familial pheochromocytoma; Autonomic paraganglia; Cardiovascular — Familial paragangliomas

Inheritance and Laboratory tests

Autosomal recessive
- **CAH** – increased blood DOC levels on ACTH challenge
  - 11-β-hydroxylase deficiency; *CYP11B1* abnormal
  - 17-α-hydroxylase deficiency; *CYP17A1* - abnormal
- **AME** - ↑plasma cortisol and urine cortisone; *HSD11B2* gene abnormal

Autosomal Dominant
- **Liddle** – ↓K$^+$, alkalosis, ↓PRA & ↓PAC; abnormal *SCNN1A, SCNN1B or SCNN1G*
- **Geller** – ↓K$^+$, alkalosis, ↓PRA & ↓PAC; abnormal *NR3C2* gene
- **FH-1 to 4** – ↓K$^+$, alkalosis, ↓PRA & ↑PAC; abnormal FH genes
- **Chrousos** – ↓K$^+$, alkalosis, →PRA & →PAC; abnormal *NR3C1* gene
- **Carney** – ↓K$^+$, alkalosis, →PRA & →PAC; CT/ MRI scans; abnormal *PRKAR1A*
- **PPGLs** – ↑metanephrines; →PRA & →PAC; CT/ MRI scans; anormal PPGL genes
- **Gordon** – ↑ K$^+$, acidosis, ↓PRA & →PAC; abnormal *WNK1,3,4, KLHL3/CUL3*

Polygenic (unclear on inheritance)
JGCT - ↓K$^+$, alkalosis, ↑ PRA and PAC; CT angiography to locate tumor

Management

- **FH-1**: glucocorticoids; MRA
- **FH-2**: MRA
- **FH-3**: MRA; adrenalectomy (in severe)
- **FH-4**: MRA

- **Liddle** : MRA and other antihypertensives
- **Geller** : Salt restriction +/- Amiloride
- **Chrousos** : Mineralocorticoid-sparing glucocorticoids
- **Carney** : Surgery for tumors +/- antihypertensives
- **PPGL** : Surgery for tumors +/- antihypertensives
- **Gordon** : Salt restriction & Thiazide diuretics
- **JGCT** : Surgery for tumor/ nephrectomy +/- antihypertensives

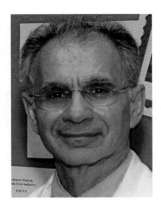

Farahnak Assadi

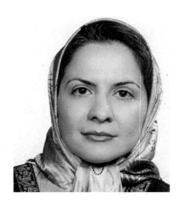

Nakysa Hooman

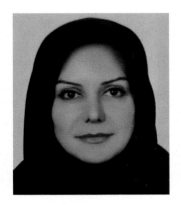

Mojgan Mazaheri

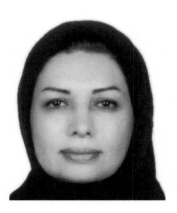

Ghane Sharbaf

Introduction

Hypertension (HTN) is a significant cause of cardiovascular and cerebrovascular morbidity and mortality in both children and adults. The prevalence and etiology of secondary HTN vary by age [1]. Approximately 5%−10% of adults and 75% −85% of children with HTN may have secondary HTN with an underlying and potentially curable cause. Secondary HTN should be suspected in patients with early-onset HTN (<6 years old). The most common secondary causes of HTN in children are renovascular HTN and renal parenchymal disease, followed by coarctation of the aorta [1]. Endocrine diseases account for approximately 10% of secondary HTN in children [1]. Monogenic forms of endocrine HTN should be suspected in children with a family history of the disease coupled with either hypokalemia or hyperkalemia in presence of suppressed renin secretion and metabolic alkalosis or acidosis. Thus, hormonal studies and genetic testing are warranted if a secondary or monogenetic cause is suspected.

Most of the monogenic causes of endocrine HTN resulting from single-gene mutations such as Liddle's syndrome, congenital adrenal hyperplasia (CAH) subtypes, apparent mineralocorticoid excess (AME), familial hyperaldosteronism (FH) subtypes including glucocorticoid-remediable aldosteronism (GRA), and familial primary generalized glucocorticoid resistance (Chrousos syndrome) increase the reabsorption of sodium in exchange with potassium leading to hypokalemic alkalosis, volume expansion and HTN with low plasma renin activity (PRA) [2−9]. Pseudo-hypoaldosteronism type II (Gordon syndrome) is the only monogenic HTN that manifests with hyperkalemia, metabolic acidosis, suppressed PRA and HTN due to increased sodium chloride reabsorption in the distal nephron and loss-of-function mutations in the *WNK4* and *CUL3* genes [10,11].

This chapter will revisit the diagnosis and management of the known causes of monogenic HTN.

Inherited disorders of endocrine hypertension

Under physiological conditions, sodium transport in the renal epithelial cells of the cortical collecting duct is regulated by the mineralocorticoid hormone aldosterone, which acts as the physiologic agonist of the mineralocorticoid receptor (MR) [7]. Even though cortisol and aldosterone have a nearly equal affinity toward the mineralocorticoid receptor in vitro, it is only the aldosterone that acts as the mineralocorticoid receptor agonist in vivo, despite the circulating cortisol levels being three times higher than the aldosterone levels. This is mediated by the enzyme 11β-hydroxysteroid dehydrogenase type 2 *(11βHSD2)* that inactivates the 11-hydroxysteroids including cortisol to their inactive keto-forms, thus protecting the mineralocorticoid receptor from activation by glucocorticoids. Excessive secretion of mineralocorticoids or abnormal sensitivity to mineralocorticoid hormones may result in volume expansion and HTN. Fig. 10.1 provides an overview of the adrenal steroid synthesis pathway.

HTN secondary to mineralocorticoid excess includes a spectrum of clinical disorders ranging from overproduction of aldosterone (primary hyperaldosteronism), overactivity of the renin-angiotensin-aldosterone system (RAAS) such as renin-secreting tumors, nonaldosterone mineralocorticoid causes including CAH, AME syndrome [4], Liddle syndrome [5,8,12], the various forms of Cushing syndrome, Pseudohypoaldosteronism type II (Gordon syndrome) [6], GRA, glucocorticoid receptor resistance syndrome (Chrousos syndrome) [10,11], and Geller syndrome [13].

Early-onset of HTN in a young individual resistant to standard antihypertensive medications indicates that all causes of inherited disorders of endocrine HTN have to be considered [14]. In these disorders, HTN is usually associated with hypokalemia, metabolic alkalosis, and low PRA secondary to renal sodium retention (Table 10.1) [4,14,15]. Severe hypokalemia, in addition to lowering the renal tubular cell pH, can also impair distal chloride reabsorption leading to increased urine chloride excretion (>15 mEq/L), and increased bicarbonate reabsorption [4,14].

Genetic forms of endocrine HTN result from activating or inactivating mutations within the mineralocorticoid, glucocorticoid, or sympathetic pathways. HTN results from excessive sodium reabsorption by hyperactive channels, hyperstimulation of MR due to increased glucocorticoid synthesis, or excessive mineralocorticoid synthesis.

It is helpful to approach patients with resistant HTN and hypokalemic alkalosis by obtaining plasma aldosterone concentration (PAC) and PRA as an initial step. This helps to separate patients into one of the three categories: (1) Those with suppressed PAC and PRA; (2) those with a high PAC and low PRA; (3) those with elevated PAC and PRA. Fig. 10.2 shows the diagnostic evaluation for monogenic HTN associated with hypokalemic alkalosis.

The ratio of PAC to PRA (Aldosterone renin ratio; ARR) is considered to be the best initial screening test for differentiating primary from secondary causes of hyperaldosteronism [9]. An ARR of at least 35 has 100% sensitivity and 92.3% specificity in diagnosing primary aldosteronism when baseline plasma aldosterone level is elevated above

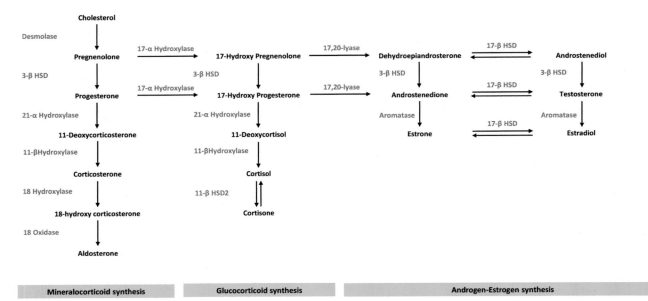

FIGURE 10.1   An overview of the glucocorticoid, mineralocorticoid, androgen, and estrogen synthesis pathways that occur in the adrenal cortex. *3β-HSD*, 3 beta-hydroxysteroid dehydrogenase; *11β-HSD1*, 11 beta-hydroxysteroid dehydrogenase type 1; *11β-HSD2*, 11 beta-hydroxysteroid dehydrogenase type 2; *DHT*, dihydrotestosterone; *DOC*, deoxycorticosterone; *DHEA*, dehydroepiandrosterone. Adrenal enzymes are highlighted in red.

TABLE 10.1 Common laboratory features of inherited conditions causing endocrine hypertension.

PRA and PAC levels	Medical condition	Hypokalemic alkalosis	Hyperkalemic acidosis
Low-PRA Low-PAC	Liddle's syndrome	+	−
	CAH	+	−
	AME	+	−
	Geller syndrome	+	−
	Chrousos syndrome	+	−
	Carney syndrome	+	−
Low-PRA High-PAC	Primary aldosteronism	+	−
	FH-1 to FH-4	+	−
High-PRA High-PAC	JGCT	+	−
Normal-PRA Normal-PAC	Pheochromocytoma	−	−
	Paragangliomas	−	−
Low-PRA Normal-PAC	Gordon syndrome	−	+

AME, apparent mineralocorticoid excess; *CAH*, congenital adrenal hyperplasia; *FH-1*, familial hyperaldosteronism type 1; *JGCT*, Juxta glomerular cell tumor; *PAC*, plasma aldosterone concentration; *PRA*, plasma renin activity.

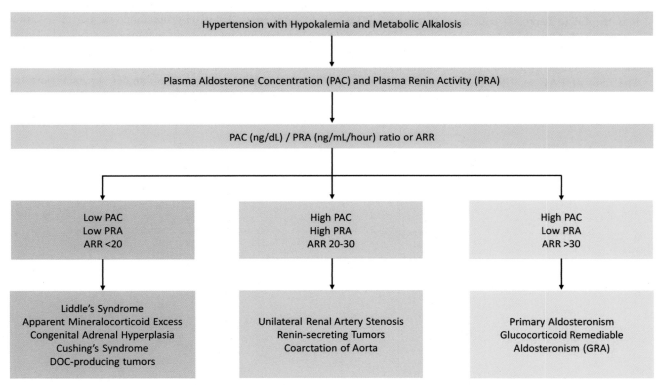

FIGURE 10.2 Diagnostic approach to hypertensive patients presenting with hypokalemic alkalosis. *ARR*, aldosterone renin ratio.

550 pmol/L (20 ng/mL). However, normal PAC and ARR values have been reported in hypertensive patients with primary hyperaldosteronism [16], Thus, in hypertensive patients with normal PAC and high ARR, dynamic confirmatory testing is required to exclude false-positive results. Confirmatory tests include aldosterone suppression by saline loading,

fludrocortisone administration, or converting enzyme inhibition by captopril or renin stimulation by furosemide administration [17].

The ARR should be measured in the context of an unrestricted sodium intake and values obtained in the upright position are more sensitive than supine test results.

Monogenic hypertension associated with suppressed PAC and PRA

Liddle syndrome

Epidemiology

The disease prevalence has not yet been established. Less than 80 patients have been formally diagnosed worldwide with an estimated prevalence of 1.5% documented with genetic testing among patients with early-onset HTN in a study of the Chinese population [18]. One study from the US among hypertensives with hypokalemia or high serum bicarbonate has shown that there was approximately a 6% prevalence of symptomatic Liddle syndrome.

The disease can be clinically heterogeneous, ranging from mild to severe cases. A lack of family history of early-onset HTN does not preclude the diagnosis of Liddle syndrome [5,19].

Pathophysiology

Liddle syndrome has an autosomal dominant inheritance and is caused by a mutation that increases the activity of the epithelial sodium channel (ENaC) in the aldosterone-sensitive cortical collecting duct that increases the sodium reabsorption [5,8,20,21]. The increased sodium reabsorption in this syndrome is independent of aldosterone and is the cause of suppressed PAC and PRA. HTN is associated with hypokalemic alkalosis, as the increased sodium reabsorption increases the net negative potential of the collecting duct lumen, causing an increase in urinary hydrogen ion and potassium excretion.

Genetics

Liddle syndrome is associated with gain-of-function mutations in the genes *SCNN1A*, *SCNN1B*, or *SCNN1G*, encoding the α, β, and γ-subunits of the (ENaC) [22−25] of which *SCNN1B* and *SCNN1G* are the most commonly affected [5,8]. These genes are located on different chromosomes: *SCNN1A* is situated on chromosome 12p13.31, *SCNN1B* and *SCNN1G* are on chromosome 16p12.2 [26]. These mutations cause the kidney to increase sodium reabsorption in exchange for potassium excretion, independent of aldosterone regulation (Table 10.2) [5,6,8].

Clinical features

The onset of HTN is typically at a young age, between late childhood and adolescence [22]. The youngest patient reported in the literature with Liddle syndrome was a 10-week-old girl who manifested with HTN [2]. The typical clinical presentations include HTN, resistance to conventional therapy associated with hypokalemic alkalosis, low levels of PAC and PRA, and a family history of early-onset HTN (Table 10.1) [2,5,8].

Investigations

Liddle syndrome must be distinguished from other forms of monogenetic endocrine HTN associated with hypokalemic alkalosis. The suppressed PAC and PRA along with an ARR less than 30 and differential response to potassium-sparing diuretics separates Liddle syndrome from primary hyperaldosteronism [22−24]. A urine steroid profile and genetic testing can distinguish it from AME and GRA (Table 10.3) [22].

The lack of therapeutic response to spironolactone and a good response to amiloride or triamterene strongly favors the diagnosis of Liddle syndrome (Table 10.4) [27,28].

Management

Treatment is based on blocking the ENaC with the administration of potassium-sparing diuretics such as amiloride or triamterene. This results in the correction of hypokalemic alkalosis and improvement of HTN. A low sodium diet is also helpful in controlling elevated blood pressure [5,22,24]. Spironolactone is not effective as the genetically altered ENaC is independent of aldosterone regulation [5,22].

TABLE 10.2 Inherited disorders of endocrine hypertension.

Medical condition	Inheritance	Pathophysiology	Prevalence
Liddle syndrome	AD	Mutations in *SCNN1A, SCNN1B,* or *SCNN1G* that encode the α, β, and γ subunits of the ENaC gene result in volume expansion and hypertension	Unknown
CAH	AR	Mutations in *CYP11B1 and CYP17A1 encoding* 11β-hydroxylase and 17-α hydroxylase cause an accumulation of intermediate steroids with MR activity	1/10,000
AME	AR	Inactivating mutations in *11βHSD2* gene that encodes 11β-hydroxysteroid dehydrogenase type 2 allows excess cortisol to activate the MR	Unknown
Geller syndrome	AD	Gain-of-function mutations in MR gene *NR3C2* allow atypical stimulation by other steroids	Unknown
Gordon syndrome	AD	Mutations in *WNK1,3,4, KLHL3,* and *CUL3* genes that modulate the thiazide-sensitive Na$^+$-Cl$^-$ co-transporter channel (NCC) allow unchecked activity, causing volume expansion and hypertension	Unknown
FH-1 (GRA)	AD	Unequal crossing over between the *CYP11B1* and *CYP11B2* genes generates a metabolite that is ACTH sensitive but produces aldosterone	Unknown
FH-2	AD	Activating mutations in *CLCN2* gene that encodes a chloride channel resulting in excess aldosterone production independent of ACTH	Unknown
FH-3	AD	Activating mutations in *KCNJ5* gene that encodes a potassium channel, stimulating aldosterone synthase activity independent of ACTH	Unknown
FH-4	AD	Activating mutations in *CACNA1H* gene that encodes calcium channels in the zona glomerulosa, enhancing aldosterone synthase activity independent of ACTH	Unknown
Familial PPGL	AD	Multiple gene mutations including *RET, VHL, NF1, SDHB, SDHD, SDHAF2, SDHC, MAX,* and *TMEM127* produce catecholamine-secreting tumors	Unknown
Chrousos syndrome	AD	Inactivating mutations on *NR3C1* gene that encodes the glucocorticoid receptor leads to generalized resistance to glucocorticoids in almost all tissues, excessive ACTH secretion and hypertension	Unknown

AD, autosomal dominant; *AR*, autosomal recessive; *AME*, apparent mineralocorticoid excess; *CAH*, congenital adrenal hyperplasia; *FH-1-4*, familial hyperaldosteronism type 1—4; *GRA*, glucocorticoid remediable aldosteronism; *JGCT*, Juxta glomerular cell tumor; *MR*, Mineralocorticoid receptor; *UK*, unknown.

TABLE 10.3 Laboratory evaluation of monogenic endocrine hypertension.

Medical condition	Blood test	Urine test	Genetic test
Liddle syndrome	–	–	Available
CAH	Increased 11-deoxycorticosterone and 11-deoxycortisol following ACTH challenge	–	Available
AME	Plasma-free cortisol > plasma-free cortisone	Urinary free cortisol > free cortisone; urinary metabolites of cortisol (tetrahydrocortisol and 5α-tetrahydrocortisol) > urinary metabolites of cortisone (tetrahydrocortisone) (THF + allo-THF/THE)	Available
Geller syndrome	–	–	Available
Gordon syndrome	Normal PAC	–	Available
FH-1 (GRA)	–	High urine 18-oxocortisol and 18-hydroxycortisol	Available
FH-2	–	Normal urine 18-oxocortisol and 18-hydroxycortisol levels	Available
FH-3	–	High urine 18-oxocortisol and 18-hydroxycortisol	Available
PPGL	High plasma-free metanephrine levels	High urinary fractionated metanephrine levels	Available
Chrousos syndrome	Elevated cortisol and ACTH levels	High 24-h free cortisol excretion	Available
JGCT	Elevated PAC and PRA levels	–	–

AME, apparent mineralocorticoid excess; CAH, congenital adrenal hyperplasia; FH-1-4, familial hyperaldosteronism type 1–4; PAC, plasma aldosterone concentration; PRA, plasma renin activity.

TABLE 10.4 Management of monogenic endocrine hypertension.

Medical condition	Response to MRA	Response to glucocorticoids	Response to BP-lowering agents
Liddle syndrome	−	−	ENaC blockers like amiloride or triamterene
CAH	+	+	−
AME	+	+	−
Geller syndrome	−	−	−
Gordon syndrome	−	−	Salt restriction/thiazide diuretics
FH-1 (GRA)	+	+	−
FH-2 to FH-4	+	−	−
PPGL	−	−	Alpha and beta-adrenergic blockers
Chrousos syndrome	−	−	High doses of mineralocorticoid-sparing synthetic glucocorticoids
JGCT	−	−	Surgical resection of tumor
Carney syndrome	−	−	Surgical resection of tumor

AME, apparent mineralocorticoid excess; *CAH*, congenital adrenal hyperplasia; *FH-1-4*, familial hyperaldosteronism type 1-4; *MRA*, mineralocorticoid receptor antagonist; *PAC*, plasma aldosterone concentration; *PRA*, plasma renin activity.

Genetic testing is available to confirm the diagnosis [24]. With proper treatment, the risk of cardiovascular and renal complications can be minimized.

Congenital adrenal hyperplasia (CAH)

Epidemiology

The overall estimated prevalence of CAH is 1/10,000 and annual incidence ranges between 1/5000 and 1/15,000. 11β-hydroxylase and 17α-hydroxylase deficiencies are associated with HTN and account for 5%−15% of CAH cases [29−32].

Pathophysiology

Both 11β-hydroxylase and 17α-hydroxylase deficiencies are inherited in an autosomal recessive fashion and are caused by loss-of-function mutations in several genes that control the cortisol and aldosterone production. CAH is characterized by adrenal insufficiency and variable degree of hyper or hypo androgenic manifestations depending on the type of enzyme deficiencies and the severity of the disease [29−32].

Genetics

The most common form of CAH (90%−95%) is caused by inactivating gene mutations in the *CYP21A2* located on chromosome 6 [6p21.31] (encoding 21α-hydroxylase) that controls cortisol and aldosterone production, followed by *CYP11B1* on chromosome 8 [8q22] (encoding 11β-hydroxylase) and *CYP17A1* on chromosome 10 [10q24.3] (encoding 17α-hydroxylase), which regulate different steps in steroid synthesis (Table 10.2). The latter two subtypes of CAH (11β-hydroxylase and 17α-hydroxylase deficiencies) are known to cause monogenic HTN [29−32].

Both subtypes of CAH, 11β-hydroxylase, and 17α-hydroxylase deficiencies, cause elevation of deoxycortisol and deoxycorticosterone levels with increased activity at the MR leading to significant mineralocorticoid activity independent of aldosterone regulation.

Clinical features

11β-hydroxylase deficiency (CAH type IV) prevents the conversion of deoxycorticosterone and deoxycortisol into corticosterone and cortisol. Reduction in cortisol and corticosterone syntheses with overproduction of 11-deoxycorticosterone and 11-deoxycortisol (DOC) leads to significant mineralocorticoid activity and subsequent sodium retention, hypokalemic alkalosis, HTN, reduced PRA and PAC (Table 10.1) [7,30].

Patients with 11β-hydroxylase deficiency, like other CAH subtypes, can present with disorders of sexual development. Newborn girls, due to androgen excess may present with ambiguous genitalia at birth. They have a normal uterus but abnormal vaginal development. Androgen excess can cause precocious puberty and short stature in both sexes [33].

The 21-hydroxylase deficiency can have a severe salt-wasting form and a mild non-classic form. The non-classic form from 21-hydroxylase deficiency is often not diagnosed until adolescence when the first symptoms appear. Affected females manifest acne, menstrual irregularities, anovulation, and hirsutism [7,34]. The salt-wasting forms can lead to severe dehydration and hypotension during the first few days of life.

Investigation

Diagnosis of 21α-hydroxylase deficiency is established by measuring 17-hydroxy-progesterone levels. Genetic testing confirms the diagnosis.

Diagnosis of 11β-hydroxylase is established by high levels of 11-deoxycorticosterone, 11-deoxycortisol and androgens, mainly androstenedione and dehydroepiandrosterone (DHEA) (Fig. 10.1) following adrenocorticotropic hormone (ACTH) challenging test (Table 10.3) [7]. Patients with an 11β-hydroxylase deficiency often exhibit signs of androgen excess similar to 21α-hydroxylase deficiency. HTN coupled with high levels of androgens can differentiate 11β-hydroxylase deficiencies from other causes of CAH and monogenic HTN [34,35].

Affected females are born with a degree of masculinization of their external genitalia and even ambiguous genitalia. Male patients may have premature sexual development.

17α-hydroxylase deficiency (CAH type V) causes decreased cortisol production associated with the accumulation of corticosterone and deoxycorticosterone, a mineralocorticoid precursor, leading to HTN, hypokalemia, and delayed puberty in both sexes. Because the production of cortisol is blocked so early in the pathway, there is little production of sex hormones (Table 10.1).

Male patients may exhibit ambiguous external genitalia and may even have a female phenotype, while females present with primary amenorrhea [36—38]. Steroid analysis following ACTH-stimulation would lead to a correct diagnosis, showing atypically elevated levels of pregnenolone and progesterone relative to 17α-pregnenolone and 17α-progesterone, respectively.

In 17α-hydroxylase deficiency, levels of androgens and estrogens are low and do not rise with ACTH challenge. A definitive diagnosis is available with genetic testing for the mutation (Table 10.3) [35].

Management

Treatment of both 11β-hydroxylase and 17α-hydroxylase deficiencies consists of administration of glucocorticoids to suppress the ACTH secretion and deoxycorticosterone synthesis, thereby inhibiting the MR stimulation. Spironolactone, amiloride, and calcium channel blockers may be further used to treat HTN [38]. Hydrocortisone can regulate the menstrual cycle and promote fertility in adult females. Fludrocortisone is usually given as a mineralocorticoid replacement [30,34,35,37]. Vaginoplasty is recommended during the first year of life. Patients with a 17α-hydroxylase deficiency should be treated with glucocorticoids with the addition of sex hormone therapy when clinically indicated [30,33,34].

Apparent mineralocorticoid excess (AME)

Epidemiology

The prevalence varies between populations depending on the level of consanguinity. Less than 100 cases have been reported in the literature [34,39—41].

Pathophysiology

Normally, the isozyme 11β hydroxysteroid dehydrogenase type 2 (11βHSD2) inactivates circulating cortisol to the less-active metabolite - cortisone [39,40,42]. In the absence of 11βHSD2, excess cortisol can bind and activate the mineralocorticoid receptors in the aldosterone-sensitive principal cells of the cortical collecting duct due to nonselectivity of the receptor. However, the defect in the AME, unlike primary aldosteronism, is at the level of the MR itself rather than downstream at the ENaC channel. Unregulated mineralocorticoid receptor activation results in aldosterone-like effects in the kidney causing hypernatremia, hypokalemia, volume expansion, and HTN (Fig. 10.3) [34,41].

Genetics

AME is a rare autosomal recessive disorder resulting from mutations in the *HSD11B2* gene, located on the long arm of chromosome 16 (16q22), which encodes the kidney isozyme of 11βHSD2 [36,39,42]. Mutations primarily involve exons 3−5 of the *HSD11B2* gene and more than 40 causative mutations in the *HSD11B2* gene have already been identified (Table 10.2) [42,43].

Clinical features

Depending on whether the affected individuals are homozygous or heterozygous for mutations, these individuals might present with early or late onset of HTN. Patients often present with severe HTN resistant to standard antihypertensive medications associated with polyuria, failure to thrive along with hypokalemic alkalosis, and suppressed PAC and PRA [34,41]. Hypercalciuria and nephrocalcinosis also have been reported in some cases [34,40]. Symptoms vary from one patient to another, and from a classic to nonclassic AME. The nonclassic form of AME is due to incomplete or partial 11βHSD2 deficiency with accompanying genetic disparity and epigenetic moderations [40].

Table 10.1 lists the common clinical features of patients with the syndrome of AME.

Investigation

Diagnosis of AME is currently based on the detection of elevated urinary cortisol to cortisone ratio in a 24-hour urine collection [44−46]. It is important to rule out chronic ingestion of licorice or carbenoxolone, as these cause similar symptoms due to inhibition of the 11βHSD2 and manifest as acquired AME syndrome. Genetic testing will confirm the

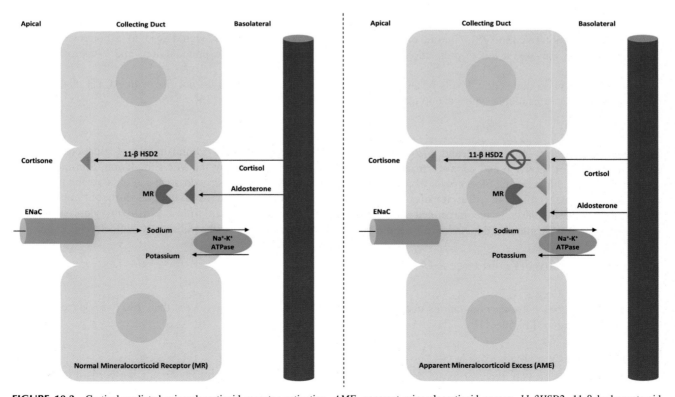

FIGURE 10.3 Cortisol-mediated mineralocorticoid receptor activation. *AME*, apparent mineralocorticoid excess; *11-βHSD2*, 11-β hydroxysteroid dehydrogenase type 2; *MR*, mineralocorticoid receptor.

diagnosis (Table 10.3) [36,38,39]. Prenatal diagnosis should be considered for families with a life-threatening case in a previous child.

Management

Patients with AME are usually treated with a mineralocorticoid receptor antagonist (MRA) such as Spironolactone (2−10 mg/kg/day), combined with a thiazide diuretic, potassium supplements, and dietary sodium restriction to help control the elevated blood pressure and reduce hypercalciuria and nephrocalcinosis [37,47]. The excess cortisol may call for glucocorticoid therapy to suppress the ACTH-stimulated cortisol production and mineralocorticoid receptor activation [41]. With adequate treatment, the prognosis is good and may prevent cardiovascular and renal complications (Table 10.4).

Geller syndrome

Epidemiology

The prevalence of the disease is not yet established

Pathophysiology

Activating mutation within the MR gene increases the susceptibility of the mineralocorticoid receptors to the activation by the atypical steroid hormones such as progesterone. The high circulating progesterone levels as in pregnancy causes activation of MR independent of RAAS leading to HTN with suppressed PAC and PRA [22,48].

Genetics

Geller syndrome is an autosomal dominant disorder resulting from a gain-of-function mutation in the MR gene (*NR3C2*) on chromosome 4 (4q31), resulting from the substitution of leucine for serine at amino acid position 810, which is in the hormone-binding domain, allowing atypical stimulation by other steroids, especially progesterone (Table 10.2) [23,48].

Clinical features

The syndrome is characterized by severe HTN associated with low PRA and PAC that usually starts before adolescence and can be exacerbated during pregnancy due to elevated progesterone levels (Table 10.1) [49].

Investigation

Genetic testing for the gene mutations in the mineralocorticoid receptor is available (Table 10.3) [22,48].

Management

Currently, there is no specific management for this syndrome. Salt restriction and the use of amiloride may improve electrolytes abnormalities and control elevated blood pressure. Spironolactone is contraindicated and will enhance the mutant receptor sensitivity (Table 10.4) [49,50].

Monogenic hypertension associated with normal PAC and low PRA

Pseudohypoaldosteronism type II (Gordon syndrome)

Epidemiology

The disease prevalence has not been established.

Pathophysiology

Gordon syndrome is the result of mutations in the *WNK* genes. Especially, loss-of-function mutation in the *WNK4* gene located on chromosome 17 (17q21.2), directly inhibits the thiazide-sensitive Na^+-Cl^- Cotransporter (NCC) activity by reducing its expression on the extracellular membrane. Moreover, gain-of-function mutation in the *WNK1* inhibits the *WNK4* to reduce the inhibition of NCC expression on the apical membrane [50−52]. Both *WNK4* loss-of-function and *WNK1* gain-of-function result in the genesis of Gordon syndrome [53].

Genetics

Gordon syndrome is a rare autosomal dominant genetic disorder caused by mutations of the *WNK1, WNK3, WNK4, KLHL3* and *CUL3* genes in the distal collecting duct of the kidney causing overactive NCC, leading to excessive sodium and chloride reabsorption in the distal convoluted tubule with intravascular volume expansion and HTN [53]. The resulting decrease in distal sodium delivery reduces normal sodium reabsorption by ENaC in the cortical collecting duct where ROMK (renal outer medullary K^+ channel) mediated potassium excretion and H^+- K^+ exchange is suppressed [11].

Clinical features

Gordon Syndrome is characterized by HTN, hyperkalemia, normal anion gap metabolic acidosis, low PRA and normal or mildly elevated levels of PAC (Table 10.1) [49,50].

Investigation

Molecular genetic testing is ideal for diagnosis, due to variation in phenotype presentation (Table 10.2) [8,54].

Management

Hypertension, hyperkalemia, and metabolic acidosis are managed with dietary salt restriction and a low dose of a thiazide diuretic, which directly inhibit NCC hyperactivity (Table 10.4) [49,50].

Monogenic hypertension associated with high PAC and low PRA

Familial hyperaldosteronism type 1 (FH-1) or glucocorticoid suppressible aldosteronism

Epidemiology

Familial hyperaldosteronism type 1 (FH-1) or Glucocorticoid-Remediable Aldosteronism (GRA) is the most common monogenic cause of HTN affecting up to 3.1% of the hypertensive pediatric population. Patient with this disorder present with severe HTN during early childhood. The exact prevalence has not been established. Most patients with FH-1 manifest severe HTN in early childhood or even infancy and suffer from a high incidence of intracranial hemorrhage with an increased mortality rate of up to 61% at an early age [29,55—58].

Pathophysiology

Normally, *CYP11B1 and CYP11B2* genes produce 11β-hydroxylase and aldosterone synthase and are responsive to ACTH and renin respectively. In FH-1, these genes are fused together to form a chimeric gene having ACTH responsive elements of *CYP11B1* and aldosterone synthase elements of *CYP11B2,* causing overproduction of aldosterone synthase ectopically from the zona fasciculata of the adrenal cortex following ACTH stimulation rather than renin stimulation [59]. This overproduction of aldosterone leads to overstimulation of MR resulting in excessive sodium reabsorption, intravascular volume expansion and HTN [29,55—58].

Genetics

FH-1 is an autosomal dominant disorder caused by activating mutations in the *CYP11B1* and *CYP11B2* genes, which are located on chromosome 8q24.3. In FH-1, these genes are abnormally fused together leading to ectopic aldosterone synthase activity in the cortisol-producing zona fasciculata of the adrenal cortex under the ACTH regulation [29,56].

Over-production of aldosterone leads to HTN, hypokalemia and metabolic alkalosis in the setting of suppressed PRA (Table 10.2) [56].

Clinical features

The disease is characterized by HTN, increased PAC, and suppressed PRA. HTN has its onset early in life, with 80% of children developing HTN by 13 years of age. Hypokalemic alkalosis is uncommon despite hyperaldosteronism. Aldosterone secretion is primarily regulated by ACTH and is suppressible by exogenous glucocorticoid therapy (Table 10.2) [60,61]. These patients also suffer from a high incidence of intracerebral hemorrhage with an associated excess mortality rate (61%) at an early age.

Investigation

Aldosterone suppression to <2 ng/dL by dexamethasone (0.5 mg every 6 h for 4 days) has been the traditional diagnostic test. The ARR is usually >30.

Elevated urinary levels of hybrid steroids (18-hydroxycortisol and 18-oxocortisol) are also used along with aldosterone suppression to differentiate GRA from primary aldosteronism (Table 10.3) [55]. Adrenal imaging and adrenal vein sampling may help in distinguishing GRA from other forms of hyperaldosteronism [61,62]. Identification of *CYP11B1/ CYP11B2* chimeric gene is recommended to confirm the diagnosis [29,63].

Management

Treatment includes glucocorticoids to reduce ACTH secretion (Table 10.4) [57,60]. Suppression of ACTH secretion with a long-acting glucocorticoid like dexamethasone or prednisone is the first-line therapy and should be administered at night to suppress the early morning peak of ACTH. The goal is to use the lowest possible dose to avoid adverse consequences of iatrogenic Cushing's syndrome, normalize blood pressure, and correction of hypokalemic alkalosis. Glucocorticoid therapy should be avoided in children with growth failure. The second line of therapy includes MRA such as spironolactone, or ENaC blockers such as triamterene to control resistant HTN and to prevent the cardiovascular effects of HTN due to partial suppression of ACTH.

Familial hyperaldosteronism type 2 (FH-2)

Epidemiology

The prevalence has not been established.

Pathophysiology

Familial hyperaldosteronism type 2 (FH-2) is characterized by primary hyperaldosteronism that is not suppressible by glucocorticoids and is often associated with an adrenocortical adenoma. The ACTH does not control the aldosterone synthase gene unlike in patients with FH-1 [62].

Genetics

FH-2 is a rare autosomal dominant disorder caused by activating mutations in the *CLCN2* gene on chromosome 3 (3q27) that encodes a chloride channel (ClC-2) leading to increased aldosterone production independent of ACTH regulation (Table 10.2) [62,64−66].

Clinical features and investigation

The disease is characterized by bilateral adrenal adenomas associated with HTN, hypokalemic alkalosis, increased PAC, and suppressed PRA (Table 10.1). Urinary 18-oxocortisol and 18-hydroxycortisol levels are normal or mildly elevated (Table 10.3) [62,66]. FH-2 is clinically and biochemically indistinguishable from noninherited primary aldosteronism. Genetic testing for *CLCN2* will establish the diagnosis.

Management

The mainstay of management is mineralocorticoid receptor antagonist with potential surgical resection.

In patients with FH-2, blood pressure does not respond to glucocorticoid challenge and the aldosterone suppression is usually absent. Therapy includes administration of MRA such as potassium-sparing diuretics or unilateral adrenalectomy (Table 10.4) [62,66].

Familial hyperaldosteronism type 3 (FH-3)

Epidemiology

Prevalence is not yet reported in the literature

Pathophysiology

FH-3 is an autosomal dominant form of hyperaldosteronism caused by activating mutations in the *KCNJ5* gene on chromosome 12 (12q24) leading to increased production of aldosterone independent of ACTH [66,67].

Genetics

Activating mutations of *KCNJ5* gene encodes a potassium channel enhancing the expression of aldosterone synthase and subsequently causing increased sodium reabsorption and HTN (Table 10.2) [66,67].

Investigation

Urinary 18-oxocortisol and 18-hydroxycortisol levels are very high and there is no suppression of aldosterone with exogenous dexamethasone (Table 10.3) [66,67].

Clinical features

FH-3 is characterized by early onset of severe HTN resistance to treatment, associated with profound hypokalemia that is unresponsive to dexamethasone suppression test (Table 10.1) [66,67].

Management

Medical management includes MRA with unilateral adrenalectomy depending on the severity of HTN (Table 10.4) [62,66].

Familial hyperaldosteronism type 4 (FH-4)

FH-4 is also an autosomal dominant disorder caused by activating mutations in the *CACNA1H* gene on chromosome 7 (7p22) that encodes a transient opening calcium channel located in the adrenal zona glomerulosa. These mutations allow for a greater influx of calcium resulting in the activation of aldosterone synthase (Table 10.2).

Treatment is similar to FH-2 and FH-3 (Table 10.4) [62,66].

Monogenic hypertension associated with elevated PAC and PRA

Renin-secreting juxtaglomerular cell tumors (JGCT)

Epidemiology

Hyperplasia and hypertrophy of the juxtaglomerular cells are extremely rare familial, or sporadic conditions. Its prevalence or incidence is unknown [68,69].

Genetics

Mutations with conditional deletions of *p53* and *Rb* on the 9th, 11th, and 'X' chromosomes in the renal and pancreatic renin-producing tumors have been reported to be associated with overactivity of RASS mechanism and increased PRA (Table 10.2) [68,70].

Pathophysiology

JGCT is a tumor of the smooth muscle cells in the afferent arteriole in the juxtaglomerular apparatus. RAAS-dependent HTN can lead to secondary aldosterone production, and hypokalemic alkalosis, associated with high PRA and PAC [68,69].

Clinical features

JGCT generally affects adolescents and young adults. It is more common in females. The classic presentation includes headache, polyuria, severe HTN, hypokalemia, and metabolic alkalosis in the setting of increased PRA and PAC (Table 10.1) [69,71].

Investigations

Renal vein lateralization for renin assay can be useful, with a sensitivity of around 60%. Contrast-enhanced CT represents the most useful radiological examination to visualize the tumor, with a sensitivity close to 100%, whereas laparoscopic ultrasonography is the most cost-effective investigation. The diagnosis, however, may be overlooked by noncontrast CT due to the hypodensity of the lesion. In this case, magnetic resonance imaging (MRI) of the kidney should be done [72].

Selective angiography can be associated with a high false-negative rate (40%), and therefore it is not recommended. Adrenal carcinoma, B-cell leukemia, hepatoblastoma, and Wilms' tumor are also renin-producing conditions that should be included in the differential diagnosis for JGCT [47]. Electron microscopic examination of tumor remains the gold standard for diagnosis of JGCT [68,69].

Management

Surgical resection is the best option for management. Conservative surgery (laparoscopic nephron-sparing surgery or partial nephrectomy) is also justified because these tumors are usually benign [69]. Aliskiren, a renin antagonist, could be useful to stop symptoms before the surgical procedure [70].

Monogenic hypertension associated with normal PAC and PRA

Familial pheochromocytoma and paragangliomas

Epidemiology

Approximately 75% of pheochromocytomas are considered to be associated with somatic or germline mutations, and 25% are sporadic [73–76].

Genetics and pathophysiology

Familial Pheochromocytoma and paragangliomas are rare catecholamine-producing tumors due to multiple gene mutations, including *RET, VHL, NF1, SDHB, SDHD, SDHAF2, SDHC, MAX, and TMEM127* (Table 10.2) [77,78]. Pheochromocytoma can be inherited alone or as a part of several syndromes including Von Hippel-Lindau disease (VHL), type 2 multiple endocrine neoplasia syndrome (MEN 2), and neurofibromatosis type 1 [73].

Multiple endocrine neoplasia type 2 (MEN2) is an autosomal-dominant syndrome caused by activating germline mutations in the *RET* proto-oncogene and has two subtypes MEN2A and MEN2B [76]. MEN2A is characterized by pheochromocytoma, medullary carcinoma of the thyroid, and hyperparathyroidism. MEN2B is associated with pheochromocytoma, medullary carcinoma of the thyroid, and mucosal neuromas [74]. The pheochromocytomas are usually of adrenal in localization, benign in nature and are bilateral.

Von Hippel-Lindau disease (VHL) is also an autosomal-dominant syndrome caused by heterozygous germline mutations in the *VHL* tumor suppressor gene on chromosome 3 (3p25-26). Among patients with VHL, the catecholamine-producing tumors are usually associated with bilateral pheochromocytomas, retinal and cerebellar hemangioblastomas, renal and pancreatic cysts, and renal cell carcinoma [73].

Pheochromocytoma has also been associated with neurofibromatosis type 1, caused by mutations in the *NF1* gene [77,78].

Clinical features

Patients with pheochromocytoma usually present with headache, tachycardia, sweating, and severe paroxysmal hypertension, associated with orthostatic hypotension.

Investigation

Measurement of plasma-free metanephrines and urinary fractionated metanephrines allow for successful screening and monitoring of the treatment response (Table 10.3) [74,79,80]. Magnetic Resonance Imaging (MRI) is preferred anatomical imaging in patients with suspected metastatic disease.

Functional imaging with ^{123}I-Metaiodobenzylguanidine (MIBG) scintigraphy is recommended to confirm the diagnosis and exclude the possibility of multisite disease in cases of paragangliomas (Table 10.3) [74,79,80]. Genetic testing is recommended to confirm the diagnosis, follow-up management, prognostication, and family screening [76,80].

Management

Hypertension can be managed prior to surgery with alpha-adrenergic antagonists such as phenoxybenzamine as first-line therapy. Other antihypertensive medications including dihydropyridine calcium channel blockers and beta-adrenergic blockers (labetalol) may be used prior to and following tumor resection (Table 10.4) [74,80].

Paragangliomas are autosomal dominant syndromes caused by inactivating mutations encoding *SDHA, SAHB, SAHC and SAHD* genes causing catecholamine-secreting tumors, characterized by sympathetic extraadrenal paragangliomas, intrarenal pheochromocytoma, and parasympathetic head and neck paragangliomas (Table 10.2) [79].

Primary generalized glucocorticoid resistance (Chrousos syndrome)

Epidemiology

Chrousos syndrome is a rare genetic condition of generalized end-organ insensitivity to glucocorticoids. Its prevalence or incidence is unknown [81–89].

Pathophysiology

Because of generalized glucocorticoid resistance, the glucocorticoid negative feedback inhibition at multiple levels along the hypothalamic-pituitary-adrenal (HPA) axis is decreased, leading to increased secretion of corticotropin-releasing hormone (CRH), arginine-vasopressin (AVP), and ACTH in the systemic circulation. The excess secretion of ACTH results in adrenocortical hyperplasia and increased secretion of cortisol, deoxycorticosterone (DOC), corticosterone, and androgenic hormones (androstenedione and dehydroepiandrosterone) without clinical features of Cushing syndrome [83,85,88].

Genetics

Chrousos syndrome is a rare autosomal dominant disorder caused by inactivating mutations in the *NR3C1* gene, which is located on chromosome 5 (5q31.3), and contains 10 exons [83] that encode the glucocorticoid receptor and are characterized by resistance to glucocorticoids in almost all tissues (Table 10.2) [6,81,82,84–87,89].

Clinical features

The clinical presentation includes HTN, hypokalemic metabolic alkalosis, normal PAC and PRA, ambiguous genitalia in female newborns, signs of hyperandrogenism in adult females, and oligospermia in adult males. See (Table 10.1) [83,85,88].

Investigation

The plasma cortisol and free cortisol excretion in a 24-hour urine collection are elevated (Table 10.3) [83,85,88].

Management

Treatment involves the administration of high doses of mineralocorticoid-sparing synthetic glucocorticoids (dexamethasone), which suppress the ACTH secretion (Table 10.4) [84]. To avoid the development of an ACTH-secreting adenoma, the dose of dexamethasone in affected patients should be strictly titrated, based on the clinical manifestations and biochemical findings of the patients [88].

Carney complex

Epidemiology

Carney complex is a rare genetic disease characterized by multiple endocrine and nonendocrine neoplasia including cortisol-producing adrenocortical adenomas due to inactivating mutations of *PRKAR1A* gene. The inactivating defects in *PRKAR1A* gene are found in 37% of patients with sporadic Carney complex and more than 70% in patients with familial Carney complex [90–93].

Approximately less than 700 affected individuals have been identified since the disorder was first described in the medical literature in 1985. It is estimated that up to 75% of cases of Carney complex are familial and the remaining 25% of cases appear to be sporadic. The prevalence or incidence of this disorder is unknown [94–96].

Pathophysiology

Carney complex is characterized by multiple skin abnormalities and a variety of endocrine and nonendocrine tumors. Primary Pigmented Nodular Adrenocortical Disease (PPNAD) is the most common manifestation of the Carney complex that is associated with bilateral pigmented adrenocortical nodules leading to ACTH-independent Cushing syndrome [94–98].

Genetics

Carney complex is inherited in an autosomal dominant pattern and is due to inactivating mutations in the *PRKAR1A* gene, located on the long arm of chromosome 17 (17q24.2-24.3) and encodes the regulatory subunit type 1α of protein kinase A (PKA). Inactivating defects of the *PRKAR1A* gene leads to activation of the cyclic AMP-PKA pathway causing increased PKA activity and early development of tumors including cortisol-producing adrenocortical adenomas [90–93].

More than 80% of patients with Carney complex have inactivating mutations of *PRKAR1A* leading to aberrant cyclic-AMP-protein kinase A signaling. Mutations in the *PRKAR1A* gene result in production of an abnormal type 1α protein kinase A (PKA), which in turn leads to the unregulated growth of cells in many organs including the adrenal gland causing Cushing's syndrome (Table 10.2). To date, more than 130 different *PRKAR1A* mutations have been identified [94–96].

Clinical features

Approximately 25%–60% of patients with Carney complex present with PPNAD. Symptoms of PPNAD occur more commonly in women than men, with 71% of patients being women of 30 years or older at diagnosis, and are often characterized by ACTH-independent Cushing syndrome associated with HTN and hypokalemic alkalosis in a setting of normal PRA and PAC levels [90].

Pigmented skin and mucosal lesions on the lips, conjunctivae, and genital area, and cardiac myxomas with multiple endocrine tumors involving adrenal, pituitary, and thyroid glands may occur (Table 10.1). Cancers associated with the Carney complex include ovarian, testicular, thyroid, liver, and pancreatic cancers [94–96].

Other endocrine manifestations of the Carney complex include growth hormone secreting pituitary adenoma (acromegaly), gonadal, and thyroid tumors. Nonendocrine tumors associated with the Carney complex include myxomas of the heart, breast ductal adenomas, osteochondromyxomas, and a number of malignancies arising from adrenal, thyroid, pancreas, and liver.

Investigation

High levels of plasma and urinary-free cortisol after the dexamethasone test establish the diagnosis. Lack of suppression of cortisol in 24-hour urine collection following low-dose dexamethasone (1 mg) has been reported in over 60% of patients with PPNAD [99]. Further, in patients with PPNAD, a high-resolution computed tomography of the adrenal glands may detect bilateral microadenomas in the majority of cases [99–102]. Genetic testing of *PRKAR1A* is recommended in all patients presenting with bilateral adrenal hyperplasia [95].

Management

There is no effective medical treatment. Bilateral adrenalectomy is the most effective treatment for patients with PPNAD and Cushing syndrome [103]. Surgical excision of myxomas, pituitary and thyroid tumors may be necessary in some selected cases [94].

Summary and conclusions

The differential diagnosis for a patient presenting with resistant HTN and hypokalemic alkalosis is broad and includes primary aldosteronism, Liddle syndrome, CAH, AME, Chrousos syndrome, and Geller syndrome.

Primary aldosteronism due to either an adrenal adenoma or adrenal hyperplasia manifests as HTN, hypokalemic alkalosis, increased PAC and suppressed PRA.

Liddle syndrome is due to a gain-of-function mutation in the *SCNN1A*, *SCNN1B*, or *SCNN1G* genes that encode the α, β, and γ-subunits of the ENaC leading to increased sodium absorption, volume expansion, resistant HTN, hyporeninemia and suppressed aldosterone secretion that often appears early in life.

CAH due to 11β-hydroxylase deficiency causes an excess of 11-deoxycortisol and DOC levels due to reduced conversion to cortisol and corticosterone, respectively. Similarly, deficiency of 17α-hydroxylase increases the DOC and corticosterone levels. As a result, these CAH subtypes manifest as HTN, hypokalemic alkalosis, low PRA, and low PAC.

Chrousos syndrome is a rare autosomal dominant disorder characterized by end-organ insensitivity to glucocorticoids due to inactivation mutations of the *NR3C1* gene leading to increased ACTH secretion and overproduction of DOC and eventually HTN and hypokalemic alkalosis. These patients might develop biochemical glucocorticoid excess, and mineralocorticoid excess with or without androgen excess, but without clinical features of Cushing syndrome.

AME is an autosomal recessive disorder associated with inactivating mutations in *HSD11B2* gene that encodes the 11βHSD2 enzyme, which normally inhibits the conversion of cortisol to cortisone. As a result, elevated cortisol levels activate the mineralocorticoid receptor, causing sodium retention, hypokalemic alkalosis, and HTN. Depending on whether the individual is homozygous or heterozygous for mutations, these individuals might present with early-onset or late onset of hypertension.

Geller syndrome is an autosomal dominant disease associated with a gain-of-function mutation in mineralocorticoid receptor gene *(NR3C2)*. The affected individuals present with hypokalemic alkalosis, low PRA, low PAC and HTN that is exacerbated during pregnancy.

GRA is an autosomal dominant disorder caused by mutations in the *CYP11B1* (11β-hydroxylase) and *CYP11B2* (aldosterone synthase) genes that disrupt the regulation of aldosterone synthesis by RAAS. In this syndrome the aldosterone production is under the ACTH control causing HTN, hypokalemic alkalosis, increased PAC and suppressed PRA.

JGCT is a rare form of high renin HTN. Deletion of *p53* and *Rb* in the renin-expressing compartment of the kidney and the pancreas is shown to increase renin secretion. JGCT generally affects adolescents and young adults. Affected individuals manifest severe refractory hypertension, hypokalemic alkalosis and elevated PAC and PRA.

Carney complex is a rare autosomal dominant disorder caused by inactivating mutations in *PRKAR1A* gene leading to adrenal hyperplasia, and Cushing's Syndrome and is characterized by multiple endocrine tumors including adrenal, pituitary, and thyroid carcinomas.

Familial pheochromocytomas and paragangliomas are rare catecholamine-producing tumors due to multiple gene mutations, including *RET, VHL, NF1, SDHB, SDHD, SDHA, SDHC, MAX,* and *TMEM127.* The disease is characterized by severe HTN refractory to standard antihypertensive medications and normal PAC and PRA.

Learning points

ARR remains the most sensitive test to differentiate primary hyperaldosteronism from secondary causes of mineralocorticoid excess

In the evaluation of a patient with HTN, hypokalemia, and metabolic alkalosis, an elevated ARR >35 suggests primary aldosteronism

Both MRAs and RAAS antagonists can only partially block the deleterious effect of aldosterone excess

Highly selective aldosterone synthase inhibitors (ASI) can block the production of aldosterone directly and are presently being evaluated as an alternative to MR and RAAS antagonists

Prenatal diagnosis of monogenetic endocrine HTN is important to prevent future cardiovascular and cerebrovascular complications when there is a strong family history of the disease.

References

[1] Kaelber DC, Baker-Smith CM, Blowey D, Carroll AE, Daniels SR, De Ferranti SD, Dionne JM, Falkner B, Flinn SK, Gidding SS, Goodwin C, Leu MG, Powers ME, Rea C, Samuels J, Simase M, Thaker VV, Urbina EM, Simasek M, Okechukwu K. Clinical practice guideline for screening and management of high blood pressure in children and adolescents. Pediatrics 2017;140(3). https://doi.org/10.1542/peds.2017-1904.

[2] Assadi FK, Kimura RE, Subramanian U, Patel S. Liddle syndrome in a newborn infant. Pediatr Nephrol 2002;17(8):609−11. https://doi.org/10.1007/s00467-002-0897-z.

[3] Assadi F. A practical approach to metabolic alkalosis. Springer Science and Business Media LLC; 2012a. p. 2677−82. https://doi.org/10.1007/978-3-642-02202-9_286.

[4] Bailey MA, Paterson JM, Hadoke PWF, Wrobel N, Bellamy COC, Brownstein DG, Seckl JR, Mullins JJ. A switch in the mechanism of hypertension in the syndrome of apparent mineralocorticoid excess. J Am Soc Nephrol 2008;19(1):47−58. https://doi.org/10.1681/ASN.2007040401.

[5] Cui Y, Tong A, Jiang J, Wang F, Li C. Liddle syndrome: clinical and genetic profiles. J Clin Hypertens 2017;19(5):524−9. https://doi.org/10.1111/jch.12949.

[6] Nicolaides NC, Charmandari E. Novel insights into the molecular mechanisms underlying generalized glucocorticoid resistance and hypersensitivity syndromes. Hormones (Basel) 2017;16(2):124−38. https://doi.org/10.14310/horm.2002.1728.

[7] Prentice P. Guideline review: congenital adrenal hyperplasia clinical practice guideline 2018. Arch Dis Childhood Educ Pract Edition 2020;106(6). https://doi.org/10.1136/archdischild-2019-317573. edpract-2019-317573.

[8] Vehaskari VM. Heritable forms of hypertension. Pediatr Nephrol 2009;24(10):1929–37. https://doi.org/10.1007/s00467-007-0537-8.

[9] Weiner ID. Endocrine and hypertensive disorders of potassium regulation: primary aldosteronism. Semin Nephrol 2013;33(3):265–76. https://doi.org/10.1016/j.semnephrol.2013.04.007.

[10] Charmandari E, Kino T, Chrousos GP. Primary generalized familial and sporadic glucocorticoid resistance (Chrousos syndrome) and hypersensitivity. Endocr Dev 2013;24:67–85. https://doi.org/10.1159/000342505.

[11] Pathare G, Hoenderop J, Bindels R, San-Cristobal P. A molecular update on pseudohypoaldosteronism type II. Am J Physiol Renal Physiol 2013;305:1513–20.

[12] Assadi F. Clinical disorders associated with altered potassium metabolism. Springer Science and Business Media LLC; 2012b. p. 2663–70. https://doi.org/10.1007/978-3-642-02202-9_284.

[13] Geller DS, Farhi A, Pinkerton N, Fradley M, Moritz M, Spitzer A, Meinke G, Tsai FTF, Sigler PB, Lifton RP. Activating mineralocorticoid receptor mutation in hypertension exacerbated by pregnancy. Science 2000;289(5476):119–23. https://doi.org/10.1126/science.289.5476.119.

[14] Patel RS, Masi S, Taddei S. Understanding the role of genetics in hypertension. Eur Heart J 2017;38(29):2309–12. https://doi.org/10.1093/eurheartj/ehx273.

[15] Fuller PJ, Young MJ. Mechanisms of mineralocorticoid action. Hypertension 2005;46(6):1227–35. https://doi.org/10.1161/01.HYP.0000193502.77417.17.

[16] Tanabe A, Naruse M, Takagi S, Tsuchiya K, Imaki T, Takano K. Variability in the renin/aldosterone profile under random and standardized sampling conditions in primary aldosteronism. J Clin Endocrinol Metab 2003;88(6):2489–94. https://doi.org/10.1210/jc.2002-021476.

[17] Reznik Y, Amar L, Tabarin A. SFE/SFHTA/AFCE consensus on primary aldosteronism, part 3: confirmatory testing. Ann Endocrinol 2016;77(3):202–7. https://doi.org/10.1016/j.ando.2016.01.007.

[18] Enslow BT, Stockand JD, Berman JM. Liddle's syndrome mechanisms, diagnosis and management. Integrated Blood Pres Control 2019;12:13–22. https://doi.org/10.2147/IBPC.S188869.

[19] Yang KQ, Xiao Y, Tian T, Gao LG, Zhou XL. Molecular genetics of Liddle's syndrome. Clin Chim Acta 2014;436:202–6. https://doi.org/10.1016/j.cca.2014.05.015.

[20] Fan P, Pan XC, Zhang D, Yang KQ, Zhang Y, Tian T, Luo F, Ma WJ, Liu YX, Wang LP, Zhang HM, Song L, Cai J, Zhou XL. Pediatric liddle syndrome caused by a novel SCNN1G variant in a Chinese family and characterized by early-onset hypertension. Am J Hypertens 2020;33(7):670–5. https://doi.org/10.1093/ajh/hpaa037.

[21] Kozina AA, Trofimova TA, Okuneva EG, Baryshnikova NV, Obuhova VA, Krasnenko AY, Tsukanov KY, Klimchuk OI, Surkova EI, Shatalov PA, Ilinsky VV. Liddle syndrome due to a novel mutation in the γsubunit of the epithelial sodium channel (ENaC) in family from Russia: a case report. BMC Nephrol 2019;20(1). https://doi.org/10.1186/s12882-019-1579-4.

[22] Melcescu E, Phillips J, Moll G, Subauste J, Koch CA. 11beta-hydroxylase deficiency and other syndromes of mineralocorticoid excess as a rare cause of endocrine hypertension. Horm Metab Res 2012;44(12):867–78. https://doi.org/10.1055/s-0032-1321851.

[23] Tapolyai M, Uysal A, Dossabhoy NR, Zsom L, Szarvas T, Lengvárszky Z, Fülöp T. High prevalence of Liddle syndrome phenotype among hypertensive US veterans in northwest Louisiana. J Clin Hypertens 2010;12(11):856–60. https://doi.org/10.1111/j.1751-7176.2010.00359.x.

[24] Wang LP, Yang KQ, Jiang XJ, Wu HY, Zhang HM, Zou YB, Song L, Bian J, Hui RT, Liu YX, Zhou XL. Prevalence of Liddle syndrome among young hypertension patients of undetermined cause in a Chinese population. J Clin Hypertens 2015;17(11):902–7. https://doi.org/10.1111/jch.12598.

[25] Yang KQ, Lu CX, Fan P, Zhang Y, Meng X, Dong XQ, Luo F, Liu YX, Zhang HM, Wu HY, Cai J, Zhang X, Zhou XL. Genetic screening of SCNN1B and SCNN1G genes in early-onset hypertensive patients helps to identify Liddle syndrome. Clin Exp Hypertens 2018;40(2):107–11. https://doi.org/10.1080/10641963.2017.1334799.

[26] Hanukoglu I, Hanukoglu A. Epithelial sodium channel (ENaC) family: phylogeny, structure-function, tissue distribution, and associated inherited diseases. Gene 2016;579(2):95–132. https://doi.org/10.1016/j.gene.2015.12.061.

[27] Kumar B, Swee M. Aldosterone-renin ratio in the assessment of primary aldosteronism. JAMA J Am Med Assoc 2014;312(2):184–5. https://doi.org/10.1001/jama.2014.64.

[28] Manolopoulou J, Fischer E, Dietz A, Diederich S, Holmes D, Junnila R, Grimminger P, Reincke M, Morganti A, Bidlingmaier M. Clinical validation for the aldosterone-to-renin ratio and aldosterone suppression testing using simultaneous fully automated chemiluminescence immunoassays. J Hypertens 2015;33(12):2500–11. https://doi.org/10.1097/HJH.0000000000000727.

[29] Ehret GB, Caulfield MJ. Genes for blood pressure: an opportunity to understand hypertension. Eur Heart J 2013;34(13):951–61. https://doi.org/10.1093/eurheartj/ehs455.

[30] Izzo JL, Sica DA, Black HR. Hypertension primer: the essentials of high blood pressure: basic science, population science, and clinical management. Lippincott William & Wilkins LTD; 2007.

[31] Martinez-Aguayo A, Fardella C. Genetics of hypertensive syndrome. Horm Res 2009;71(5):253–9. https://doi.org/10.1159/000208798.

[32] White PC. Disorders of steroid 11 beta-hydroxylase isozymes. Endocr Rev 1994;15(4):421–38. https://doi.org/10.1210/er.15.4.421.

[33] Burrello J, Monticone S, Buffolo F, Tetti M, Veglio F, Williams TA, Mulatero P. Is there a role for genomics in the management of hypertension? Int J Mol Sci 2017;18(6). https://doi.org/10.3390/ijms18061131.

[34] Zennaro MC, Boulkroun S, Fernandes-Rosa F. Inherited forms of mineralocorticoid hypertension. Best Pract Res Clin Endocrinol Metabol 2015;29(4):633–45. https://doi.org/10.1016/j.beem.2015.04.010.

[35] Aggarwal A, Rodriguez-Buritica D. Monogenic hypertension in children: a review with emphasis on genetics. Adv Chron Kidney Dis 2017;24(6):372–9. https://doi.org/10.1053/j.ackd.2017.09.006.

[36] Kim SM, Rhee JH. A case of 17 alpha-hydroxylase deficiency. Clin Exp Reprod Med 2015;42(2):72–6. https://doi.org/10.5653/cerm.2015.42.2.72.

[37] Sahay M, Sahay R. Low renin hypertension. Indian J Endocrinol Metab 2012;16(5):728. https://doi.org/10.4103/2230-8210.100665.

[38] Simonetti GD, Mohaupt MG, Bianchetti MG. Monogenic forms of hypertension. Eur J Pediatr 2012;171(10):1433–9. https://doi.org/10.1007/s00431-011-1440-7.

[39] Adamidis A, Cantas-Orsdemir S, Tsirka A, Abbott MA, Visintainer P, Tonyushkina K. Apparent mineralocorticoid excess in the pediatric population: report of a novel pathogenic variant of the 11β-HSD2 gene and systematic review of the literature. Pediatr Endocrinol Rev 2019;16(3):335–58. https://doi.org/10.17458/per.vol16.2019.act.mineralocorticoid.

[40] Bertulli C, Hureaux M, De Mutiis C, Pasini A, Bockenhauer D, Vargas-Poussou R, La Scola C. A rare cause of chronic hypokalemia with metabolic alkalosis: case report and differential diagnosis. Children 2020;7(11). https://doi.org/10.3390/children7110212.

[41] Morineau G, Sulmont V, Salomon R, Fiquet-Kempf B, Jeunemaître X, Nicod J, Ferrari P. Apparent mineralocorticoid excess: report of six new cases and extensive personal experience. J Am Soc Nephrol 2006;17(11):3176–84. https://doi.org/10.1681/ASN.2006060570.

[42] Carvaja CA, Tapia-Castillo A, Vecchiola A, Baudrand R, Fardella CE. Classic and nonclassic apparent mineralocorticoid excess syndrome. J Clin Endocrinol Metab 2020;105(4):E924–36. https://doi.org/10.1210/clinem/dgz315.

[43] New MI, Geller DS, Fallo F, Wilson RC. Monogenic low renin hypertension. Trends Endocrinol Metab 2005;16(3):92–7. https://doi.org/10.1016/j.tem.2005.02.011.

[44] De Santis D, Castagna A, Danese E, Udali S, Martinelli N, Morandini F, Veneri M, Bertolone L, Olivieri O, Friso S, Pizzolo F. Detection of urinary exosomal HSD11B2 mRNA expression: a useful novel tool for the diagnostic approach of dysfunctional 11β-HSD2-related hypertension. Front Endocrinol 2021;12. https://doi.org/10.3389/fendo.2021.681974.

[45] Luft FC. Monogenic hypertension: lessons from the genome. Kidney Int 2001;60(1):381–90. https://doi.org/10.1046/j.1523-1755.2001.00810.x.

[46] Williams SS. Advances in genetic hypertension. Curr Opin Pediatr 2007;19(2):192–8. https://doi.org/10.1097/MOP.0b013e32801e217c.

[47] Palermo M, Quinkler M, Stewart PM. Apparent mineralocorticoid excess syndrome: an overview. Arq Bras Endocrinol Metabol 2004;48(5):687–96. https://doi.org/10.1590/s0004-27302004000500015.

[48] Garovic VD, Hilliard AA, Turner ST. Monogenic forms of low-renin hypertension. Nat Clin Pract Nephrol 2006;2(11):624–30. https://doi.org/10.1038/ncpneph0309.

[49] Garg AK, Parajuli P, Mamillapalli CK. Pregnancy complicated by hypertension and hypokalemia. Am J Kidney Dis 2020;76(4):A21–2. https://doi.org/10.1053/j.ajkd.2020.04.012.

[50] Pintavorn P, Munie S. A case report of recurrent hypokalemia during pregnancies associated with nonaldosterone-mediated renal potassium loss. Can J Kidney Health Dis 2021;8. https://doi.org/10.1177/20543581211017424.

[51] Padmanabhan S, Caulfield M, Dominiczak AF. Genetic and molecular aspects of hypertension. Circ Res 2015;116(6):937–59. https://doi.org/10.1161/CIRCRESAHA.116.303647.

[52] Riepe FG. Clinical and molecular features of type 1 pseudohypoaldosteronism. Horm Res 2009;72(1):1–9. https://doi.org/10.1159/000224334.

[53] Mabillard H, Sayer JA. The molecular genetics of Gordon syndrome. Genes 2019;10(12). https://doi.org/10.3390/genes10120986.

[54] Boyden LM, Choi M, Choate KA, Nelson-Williams CJ, Farhi A, Toka HR, Tikhonova IR, Bjornson R, Mane SM, Colussi G, Lebel M, Gordon RD, Semmekrot BA, Poujol A, Välimäki MJ, De Ferrari ME, Sanjad SA, Gutkin M, Karet FE, Lifton RP. Mutations in kelch-like 3 and cullin 3 cause hypertension and electrolyte abnormalities. Nature 2012;482(7383):98–102. https://doi.org/10.1038/nature10814.

[55] Gates LJ, Benjamin N, Haites NE, MacConnachie AA, McLay JS. Is random screening of value in detecting glucocorticoid-remediable aldosteronism within a hypertensive population? J Hum Hypertens 2001;15(3):173–6. https://doi.org/10.1038/sj.jhh.1001152.

[56] Pascoe L, Curnow KM, Slutsker L, Connell JMC, Speiser PW, New MI, White PC. Glucocorticoid-suppressible hyperaldosteronism results from hybrid genes created by unequal crossovers between CYP11B1 and CYP11B2. Proc Natl Acad Sci U S A 1992;89(17):8327–31. https://doi.org/10.1073/pnas.89.17.8327.

[57] Stowasser M, Bachmann AW, Huggard PR, Rossetti TR, Gordon RD. Treatment of familial hyperaldosteronism type I: only partial suppression of adrenocorticotropin required to correct hypertension. J Clin Endocrinol Metab 2000;85(9):3313–8. https://doi.org/10.1210/jcem.85.9.6834.

[58] Sutherland DJ, Ruse JL, Laidlaw JC. Hypertension, increased aldosterone secretion and low plasma renin activity relieved by dexamethasone. Can Med Assoc J 1966;95(22):1109–19.

[59] Liu X, Jin L, Zhang H, Ma W, Song L, Zhou X, Cai J. A Chinese pedigree with glucocorticoid remediable aldosteronism. Hypertens Res 2021;44(11):1428–33. https://doi.org/10.1038/s41440-021-00685-3.

[60] Lee IS, Kim SY, Jang HW, Kim MK, Lee JH, Lee YH, Jo YS. Genetic analyses of the chimeric CYP11B1/CYP11B2 gene in a Korean family with glucocorticoid-remediable aldosteronism. J Kor Med Sci 2010;25(9):1379–83. https://doi.org/10.3346/jkms.2010.25.9.1379.

[61] Rahmi Oklu R, Deipolyi A. Adrenal vein sampling in the diagnosis of aldosteronism. J Vasc Diagn 2015;17. https://doi.org/10.2147/JVD.S79302.

[62] Torpy DJ, Gordon RD, Lin JP, Huggard PR, Taymans SE, Stowasser M, Chrousos GP, Stratakis CA. Familial hyperaldosteronism type II: description of a large kindred and exclusion of the aldosterone synthase (CYP11B2) gene. J Clin Endocrinol Metab 1998;83(9):3214–8. https://doi.org/10.1210/jc.83.9.3214.

[63] Brian Byrd J, Turcu AF, Auchus RJ. Primary aldosteronism: practical approach to diagnosis and management. Circulation 2018;138(8):823–35. https://doi.org/10.1161/CIRCULATIONAHA.118.033597.

[64] Fardella CE, Rodriguez H, Montero J, Zhang G, Vignolo P, Rojas A, Villarroel L, Miller WL. Genetic variation in P450c11AS in Chilean patients with low renin hypertension. J Clin Endocrinol Metab 1996;81(12):4347–51. https://doi.org/10.1210/jc.81.12.4347.

[65] Scholl UI, Stölting G, Schewe J, Thiel A, Tan H, Nelson-Williams C, Vichot AA, Jin SC, Loring E, Untiet V, Yoo T, Choi J, Xu S, Wu A, Kirchner M, Mertins P, Rump LC, Onder AM, Gamble C, Lifton RP. CLCN2 chloride channel mutations in familial hyperaldosteronism type II. Nat Genet 2018;50(3):349–54. https://doi.org/10.1038/s41588-018-0048-5.

[66] Stowasser M, Wolley M, Wu A, Gordon RD, Schewe J, Stölting G, Scholl UI. Pathogenesis of familial hyperaldosteronism type II: new concepts involving anion channels. Curr Hypertens Rep 2019;21(4). https://doi.org/10.1007/s11906-019-0934-y.

[67] Young WF. Primary aldosteronism: renaissance of a syndrome. Clin Endocrinol 2007;66(5):607–18. https://doi.org/10.1111/j.1365-2265.2007.02775.x.

[68] Glenn ST, Jones CA, Sexton S, LeVea CM, Caraker SM, Hajduczok G, Gross KW. Conditional deletion of p53 and Rb in the renin-expressing compartment of the pancreas leads to a highly penetrant metastatic pancreatic neuroendocrine carcinoma. Oncogene 2014;33(50):5706–15. https://doi.org/10.1038/onc.2013.514.

[69] Pearlman B, Lodebo BT. Renin secreting tumour: a rare cause of secondary hypertension. Lancet 2021;398(10305):1074. https://doi.org/10.1016/S0140-6736(21)01696-2.

[70] Inam R, Gandhi J, Joshi G, Smith NL, Khan SA. Juxtaglomerular cell tumor: reviewing a cryptic cause of surgically correctable hypertension. Curr Urol 2019;13(1):7–12. https://doi.org/10.1159/000499301.

[71] Gu WJ, Zhang LX, Jin N, Ba JM, Dong J, Wang DJ, Li J, Wang XL, Yang GQ, Lu ZH, Dou JT, Lu JM, Mu YM. Rare and curable renin-mediated hypertension: a series of six cases and a literature review. J Pediatr Endocrinol Metab 2016;29(2):209–16. https://doi.org/10.1515/jpem-2015-0025.

[72] Faucon AL, Bourillon C, Grataloup C, Baron S, Bernadet-Monrozies P, Vidal-Petiot E, Azizi M, Amar L. Usefulness of magnetic resonance imaging in the diagnosis of juxtaglomerular cell tumors: a report of 10 cases and review of the literature. Am J Kidney Dis 2019;73(4):566–71. https://doi.org/10.1053/j.ajkd.2018.09.005.

[73] Assadi F, Brackbill E. Bilateral pheochromocytoma and congenital anomalies associated with a de novo germline mutation in the von Hippel-Lindau gene. Am J Kidney Dis 2003;41(1). https://doi.org/10.1953/ajkd.2003.50021.

[74] Liu Z, Ma J, Jimenez C, Zhang M. Pheochromocytoma: a clinicopathologic and molecular study of 390 cases from a single center. Am J Surg Pathol 2021;45(9):1155–65. https://doi.org/10.1097/PAS.0000000000001768.

[75] Martins RG, Carvalho IP. Genetic testing for pheochromocytoma and paraganglioma: SDHx carriers' experiences. J Genet Counsel 2021;30(3):872–84. https://doi.org/10.1002/jgc4.1390.

[76] Welander J, Larsson C, Bäckdahl M, Hareni N, Sivlér T, Brauckhoff M, Söderkvist P, Gimm O. Integrative genomics reveals frequent somatic NF1 mutations in sporadic pheochromocytomas. Hum Mol Genet 2012;21(26):5406–16. https://doi.org/10.1093/hmg/dds402.

[77] Lefebvre M, Foulkes WD. Pheochromocytoma and paraganglioma syndromes: genetics and management update. Curr Oncol 2014;21(1):e8–17. https://doi.org/10.3747/co.21.1579.

[78] Nölting S, Bechmann N, Taieb D, Beuschlein F, Fassnacht M, Kroiss M, Eisenhofer G, Grossman A, Pacak K. Personalized management of pheochromocytoma and paraganglioma. Endocr Rev 2021. https://doi.org/10.1210/endrev/bnab019.

[79] Lenders JWM, Duh QY, Eisenhofer G, Gimenez-Roqueplo AP, Grebe SKG, Murad MH, Naruse M, Pacak K, Young WF. Pheochromocytoma and paraganglioma: an endocrine society clinical practice guideline. J Clin Endocrinol Metab 2014;99(6):1915–42. https://doi.org/10.1210/jc.2014-1498.

[80] Soares NA, Ferreira Pacheco MTP, de Sousa MJRFR, Matos ML, Ferreira SAL. Pheochromocytoma: a retrospective study from a single center. Endocr Regul 2021;55(1):16–21. https://doi.org/10.2478/enr-2021-0003.

[81] Al Argan R, Saskin A, Yang JW, D'Agostino MD, Rivera J. Glucocorticoid resistance syndrome caused by a novel NR3C1 point mutation. Endocr J 2018;65(11):1139–46. https://doi.org/10.1507/endocrj.EJ18-0135.

[82] Kaziales A, Rührnößl F, Richter K. Glucocorticoid resistance conferring mutation in the C-terminus of GR alters the receptor conformational dynamics. Sci Rep 2021;11(1). https://doi.org/10.1038/s41598-021-92039-9.

[83] Molnár Á, Patócs A, Likó I, Nyírő G, Rácz K, Tóth M, Sármán B. An unexpected, mild phenotype of glucocorticoid resistance associated with glucocorticoid receptor gene mutation case report and review of the literature. BMC Med Genet 2018;19(1). https://doi.org/10.1186/s12881-018-0552-6.

[84] Nicolaides NC, Geer EB, Vlachakis D, Roberts ML, Psarra AMG, Moutsatsou P, Sertedaki A, Kossida S, Charmandari E. A novel mutation of the hGR gene causing Chrousos syndrome. Eur J Clin Invest 2015;45(8):782–91. https://doi.org/10.1111/eci.12470.

[85] Nicolaides NC, Lamprokostopoulou A, Sertedaki A, Charmandari E. Recent advances in the molecular mechanisms causing primary generalized glucocorticoid resistance. Hormones (Basel) 2016;15(1):23–34. https://doi.org/10.14310/horm.2002.1660.

[86] Nicolaides NC, Skyrla E, Vlachakis D, Psarra AMG, Moutsatsou P, Sertedaki A, Kossida S, Charmandari E. Functional characterization of the hGRαT556I causing Chrousos syndrome. Eur J Clin Invest 2016;46(1):42–9. https://doi.org/10.1111/eci.12563.

[87] Nicolaides NC, Charmandari E. Chrousos syndrome: from molecular pathogenesis to therapeutic management. Eur J Clin Invest 2015;45(5):504–14. https://doi.org/10.1111/eci.12426.

[88] Nicolaides NC, Charmandari E. Glucocorticoid resistance. Experientia Suppl 2019;111:85–102. https://doi.org/10.1007/978-3-030-25905-1_6.

[89] Paragliola RM, Costella A, Corsello A, Urbani A, Concolino P. A novel pathogenic variant in the N-terminal domain of the glucocorticoid receptor, causing glucocorticoid resistance. Mol Diagn Ther 2020;24(4):473–85. https://doi.org/10.1007/s40291-020-00480-9.

[90] Bertherat J, Horvath A, Groussin L, Grabar S, Boikos S, Cazabat L, Libe R, René-Corail F, Stergiopoulos S, Bourdeau I, Bei T, Clauser E, Calender A, Kirschner LS, Bertagna X, Carney JA, Stratakis CA. Mutations in regulatory subunit type 1A of cyclic adenosine 5'-monophosphate-

dependent protein kinase (PRKAR1A): phenotype analysis in 353 patients and 80 different genotypes. J Clin Endocrinol Metab 2009;94(6):2085−91. https://doi.org/10.1210/jc.2008-2333.

[91] Cazabat L, Ragazzon B, Groussin L, Bertherat J. PRKAR1A mutations in primary pigmented nodular adrenocortical disease. Pituitary 2006;9(3):211−9. https://doi.org/10.1007/s11102-006-0266-1.

[92] Kamilaris CDC, Faucz FR, Voutetakis A, Stratakis CA. Carney complex. Exp Clin Endocrinol Diabetes 2019;127(2−3):156−64. https://doi.org/10.1055/a-0753-4943.

[93] Kirschner LS, Carney JA, Pack SD, Taymans SE, Giatzakis C, Cho YS, Cho-Chung YS, Stratakis CA. Mutations of the gene encoding the protein kinase A type I-α regulatory subunit in patients with the Carney complex. Nat Genet 2000;26(1):89−92. https://doi.org/10.1038/79238.

[94] Bouys L, Bertherat J. Management of endocrine disease: Carney complex: clinical and genetic update 20 years after the identification of the CNC1 (PRKAR1A) gene. Eur J Endocrinol 2021;184(3):R99−109. https://doi.org/10.1530/eje-20-1120.

[95] Correa R, Salpea P, Stratakis CA. Carney complex: an update. Eur J Endocrinol 2015;173(4):M85−97. https://doi.org/10.1530/EJE-15-0209. BioScientifica Ltd.

[96] Horvath A, Bertherat J, Groussin L, Guillaud-Bataille M, Tsang K, Cazabat L, Libé R, Remmers E, René-Corail F, Faucz FR, Clauser E, Calender A, Bertagna X, Carney JA, Stratakis CA. Mutations and polymorphisms in the gene encoding regulatory subunit type 1-alpha of protein kinase a (PRKAR1A): an update. Hum Mutat 2010;31(4):369−79. https://doi.org/10.1002/humu.21178.

[97] Espiard S, Bertherat J. Carney complex. Front Horm Res 2013;41:50−62. https://doi.org/10.1159/000345669.

[98] Stratakis CA, Kirschner LS, Carney JA. Clinical and molecular features of the carney complex: diagnostic criteria and recommendations for patient evaluation. J Clin Endocrinol Metab 2001;86(9):4041−6. https://doi.org/10.1210/jcem.86.9.7903.

[99] Louiset E, Stratakis CA, Perraudin V, Griffin KJ, Libé R, Cabrol S, Fève B, Young J, Groussin L, Bertherat J, Lefebvre H. The paradoxical increase in cortisol secretion induced by dexamethasone in primary pigmented nodular adrenocortical disease involves a glucocorticoid receptor-mediated effect of dexamethasone on protein kinase A catalytic subunits. J Clin Endocrinol Metab 2009;94(7):2406−13. https://doi.org/10.1210/jc.2009-0031.

[100] Bourdeau I, Lacroix A, Schürch W, Caron P, Antakly T, Stratakis CA. Primary pigmented nodular adrenocortical disease: paradoxical responses of cortisol secretion to dexamethasone occur in vitro and are associated with increased expression of the glucocorticoid receptor. J Clin Endocrinol Metab 2003;88(8):3931−7. https://doi.org/10.1210/jc.2002-022001.

[101] Courcoutsakis NA, Tatsi C, Patronas NJ, Lee CCR, Prassopoulos PK, Stratakis CA. The complex of myxomas, spotty skin pigmentation and endocrine overactivity (Carney complex): imaging findings with clinical and pathological correlation. Insights into Imaging 2013;4(1):119−33. https://doi.org/10.1007/s13244-012-0208-6.

[102] Stratakis CA, Sarlis N, Kirschner LS, Carney JA, Doppman JL, Nieman LK, Chrousos GP, Papanicolaou DA. Paradoxical response to dexamethasone in the diagnosis of primary pigmented nodular adrenocortical disease. Ann Intern Med 1999;131(8):585−91. https://doi.org/10.7326/0003-4819-131-8-199910190-00006.

[103] Lowe KM, Young WF, Lyssikatos C, Stratakis CA, Carney JA. Cushing syndrome in carney complex: clinical, pathologic, and molecular genetic findings in the 17 affected mayo clinic patients. Am J Surg Pathol 2017;41(2):171−81. https://doi.org/10.1097/PAS.0000000000000748.

Chapter 11

Pheochromocytomas and hypertension

Iuri Martin Goemann[1,2] and Ana Luiza Maia[1]

[1]*Universidade Federal do Rio Grande do Sul, Endocrinology, Porto Alegre, Brazil;* [2]*Universidade do Vale do Rio dos Sinos, Porto Alegre, Brazil*

Visit the *Endocrine Hypertension: From Basic Science to Clinical Practice, First Edition* companion web site at: https://www.elsevier.com/books-and-journals/book-companion/9780323961202.

Graphical Abstract

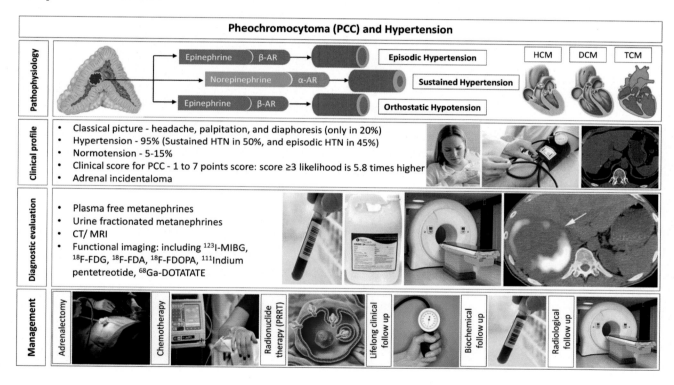

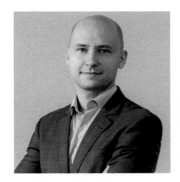

Iuri Martin Goemann

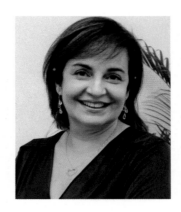

Ana Luiza Maia

Introduction

Pheochromocytomas (PCCs) are rare neuroendocrine tumors that arise from the adrenal medulla and typically secrete catecholamines. When these tumors arise from the extraadrenal sympathetic or parasympathetic ganglia, they are called paragangliomas (PGLs). Pheochromocytoma (PCC) and paraganglioma (PGL) are together referred to as PPGLs, as they belong to the same family of neural crest-derived neoplasms. The estimated prevalence of PCC among patients with hypertension attending general outpatient clinics is low (0.1%–0.6%) [1–3]. The annual incidence is approximately 2–8 per million [4] in the general population. However, PCC is found in 5%–7% of patients with incidentally discovered adrenal masses [5], which justifies the need to rule out PCC in patients with incidentally discovered adrenal tumors [6].

Although the classical clinical picture of episodic hypertension associated with postural hypotension, palpitations, sweating, and headache may suggest the possibility of a PCC, this type of presentation is rather uncommon [7]. The nature of the genetic mechanisms involved in the tumorigenesis, pathophysiology, molecular aspects, and the clinical profile of PCCs are complex. These often pose significant challenges to clinicians and laboratory scientists in the diagnostic workup, genetic evaluation, and the development of management algorithms, and in planning follow-up for these uncommon endocrine tumors. This chapter elucidates the pathobiological aspects, diagnostic evaluation, and management of PCCs and endocrine hypertension with the most up-to-date evidence.

Molecular and genetic aspects of PCCs

Understanding the genetic abnormalities and the consequent molecular alterations of PCC is essential for adequate diagnostic workup, treatment, and surveillance of patients and their families [8]. Up to 70% of PPGLs are genetically determined by either germline (up to 40%) or somatic (30%–40%) mutations in one of the known susceptibility genes [9,10]. Mutations in the von Hippel Lindau (*VHL*), *RET*, and Neurofibromin 1 (*NF1*) genes occur predominately in PCCs and are rare in PGLs. In contrast, mutations in succinate dehydrogenase genes (*SDHx* group), especially *SDHB* and *SDHD,* are common in PGLs but uncommon in PCCs. PPGLs can be classified into three major molecular clusters according to their underlying driver mutations [11].

Tumor clusters

Cluster 1 tumors are defined by a pseudohypoxic molecular signature and accelerated angiogenesis. Pseudohypoxic PPGL can be further classified into Krebs cycle-related PPGL (Cluster 1A) and VHL/Endothelial PAS domain-containing protein 1 (*VHL/EPAS1*) related PPGL (Cluster 1B). The cluster 1A tumors are associated with mutations in succinate dehydrogenase subunits (*SDHx* or *SDHA/SDHB/SDHC/SDHD*), succinate dehydrogenase complex assembly factor-2 (*SDHAF2*), fumarate hydratase (*FH*), malate dehydrogenase 2 (*MDH2*), glutamic-oxaloacetic transaminase (*GOT2*), 2-oxoglutarate-malate carrier *(SLC25A11),* dihydrolipoamide S-succinyltransferase (*DLST*), and isocitrate dehydrogenase 1 *(IDH1).* In contrast, the cluster 1B tumors are associated with mutations in *VHL*, hypoxia-induced factor 2α (*HIF2A*), Egl-9 prolyl hydroxylase-1 and -2 *(EGLN1/2* encoding PHD1/2*),* and iron regulatory protein 1 *(IRP1)* [12]. The pseudohypoxic molecular signature is partially explained by the capacity of *SDHx* (cluster 1A) and *VHL* (cluster 1B) mutated cells to enhance the expression and decrease the degradation of hypoxia-inducible factors (HIFs). Moreover, an important consequence of

SDHx inactivation is the accumulation of succinate and consequent chronic hypoxic stimulation. Thus, in summary, activation of the hypoxic pathway in *VHL* and *SDH*-related PPGLs results in enhanced expression and stabilization of HIFs (especially HIF2α), which in turn regulate/promote angiogenesis, energy metabolism, tumor progression, migration, invasion, and metastasis [13].

The signature of the second cluster involves the upregulation of kinase signaling pathways, including the phosphatidylinositol 3-kinase (PI3K)/protein kinase B (AKT) signaling pathway, the Ras/Raf/mitogen-activated protein kinase/extracellular-signal-regulated (ERK) kinase (MEK)/ERK cascade, and the mammalian target of rapamycin (mTOR) pathway, promoting cell growth and survival. These tumors develop due to gain-of-function mutations in *RET* or mutations in genes such as *NF1*, transmembrane protein 127 *(TMEM127)*, myc-associated factor X *(MAX)*, MET receptor tyrosine kinase *(MET)*, MER Proto-Oncogene Tyrosine Kinase *(MERTK)*, Fibroblast Growth Factor Receptor 1 (*FGFR1*), and Harvey rat sarcoma viral oncogene homolog (*HRAS*) [11]. The third cluster is less explored, comprising genes leading to activation of the Wnt/beta-catenin pathway resulting in increased angiogenesis, cell proliferation, and invasion. Sporadic PPGLs with somatic variants in cold shock domain-containing E1 (*CSDE1*) and mastermind-like transcriptional coactivator 3 (*MAML3*) fusion genes were also reported in this cluster.

Clinical and biochemical characteristics of PCC: genotype-phenotype correlations

The catecholamines epinephrine and norepinephrine are synthesized by chromaffin cells in the adrenal medulla in response to acetylcholine (ACh) released by the preganglionic neurons of the sympathetic system. Most hormonally active PCCs produce a combination of norepinephrine and epinephrine, some cases exclusively norepinephrine (noradrenergic phenotype), and a much smaller proportion exclusively epinephrine. These differences in catecholamine production reflect differences in the expression of phenylethanolamine-N-methyltransferase (PNMT), the enzyme in the catecholamine biosynthetic cascade that converts norepinephrine to epinephrine [14,15].

The biochemical phenotype of PCCs can indicate specific molecular alterations [16]. PCCs in MEN2 and NF1 patients express PNMT and secrete epinephrine, with an increase in plasma or urine metanephrines. In contrast, those PCCs related to VHL syndrome do not express PNMT and consequently do not produce epinephrine, but produce norepinephrine, as reflected by the solitary increases in plasma or urine levels of normetanephrines [17,18]. Similarly, tumors associated with the *SDHx* syndromes also do not express PNMT or produce epinephrine. They are characterized by norepinephrine production, but can also produce dopamine, manifested by increased normetanephrine and 3-methoxytyramine (3MT) levels [17]. A dopaminergic phenotype (with increased 3MT levels) suggests a deficiency in the enzyme dopamine-beta-hydroxylase, which converts dopamine to norepinephrine. Tumors that produce predominantly or exclusively dopamine are rare and are usually found as extra-adrenal paragangliomas [19]. These patients tend to be normotensive, which poses a substantial diagnostic challenge.

Genotype-phenotype correlations might impact the disease presentation, including catecholamine production. They have important implications for how genetic testing may be directed, or the results of testing interpreted, mainly if the conventional molecular testing is performed. When a PCC clinical presentation strongly suggests mutation in a specific gene (e.g., *RET* or *VHL*), then targeted genetic testing for a germline mutation might still be appropriate [20].

PCCs diagnosed at young ages suggest the presence of a germline pathogenic variant. Large tumors at diagnosis, extra-adrenal localization, and noradrenergic phenotype point toward germline *SDHx* gene variants (cluster 1), while adrenal localization and adrenergic phenotype point toward cluster 2 genetic abnormalities [21]. Moreover, cluster 2 tumors exhibit high symptom scores (see below) and episodic symptoms that indicate epinephrine secretion. Cluster 1 tumors and probably cluster 3 tumors exhibit aggressive phenotype with higher metastatic risk [22] (Table 11.1).

Pathophysiology

Catecholamines (dopamine, norepinephrine, and epinephrine) are synthesized in and secreted from the chromaffin cells in the adrenal medulla and the sympathetic ganglia. The PNMT is not expressed by the sympathetic ganglia, meaning that most of the epinephrine in circulation is produced by the adrenal glands. Catecholamines act through the G-protein coupled adrenoceptors to regulate broad physiological processes [23]. Norepinephrine signals through the α_1, α_2, and β_1 adrenoceptors, whereas epinephrine primarily stimulates the β_1 and β_2 adrenoceptors. Dopamine, on the other hand, has minimal effect on the adrenoceptors at physiological concentrations, but can stimulate both α and β adrenoceptors if the levels are increased as in dopamine secreting PPGL, leading to vasoconstriction and increased heart rate [24].

α_1-adrenoceptors are found on peripheral arteries and veins, causing vasoconstriction upon stimulation. Their stimulation increases the systemic blood pressure and reduces organ perfusion. It also induces positive inotropic effects in the

TABLE 11.1 Most frequent mutations associated with pheochromocytoma (PCC) and their metastatic risk.

Mutation	Association with PCC	Metastatic risk	Biochemical phenotype	Cluster
RET	Almost exclusively located adrenally (unilateral or bilateral)	<5%	Adrenergic	Cluster 2
NF1	Almost exclusively located adrenally (often unilateral)	2%–12%	Adrenergic	Cluster 2
TMEM127	Almost exclusively located adrenally (unilateral or bilateral)	Low	Adrenergic	Cluster 2
MAX	Almost exclusively located adrenally (bilateral)	10%	Adrenergic and noradrenergic	Cluster 2
SDHB	Less common (often unilateral)	35%–75%	Noradrenergic and/or dopaminergic	Cluster 1
SDHA	Very rare	30%–66%		Cluster 1
SDHC	Less common	Low	Noradrenergic	Cluster 1
SDHD	Less common (unilateral or bilateral)	15%–29%	Noradrenergic and/or dopaminergic	Cluster 1
HIF2A/ EPAS1	Common	>30%	Noradrenergic	Cluster 1
VHL	Very common (unilateral or bilateral)	5%–8%		Cluster 1

EPAS1, Endothelial PAS Domain Protein 1; *HIF2A*, hypoxia-induced factor 2alpha; *MAX*, myc-associated factor X; *NF1*, Neurofibromin 1; *SDHB*, succinate dehydrogenase complex, subunit B; *SDHA*, succinate dehydrogenase complex, subunit A; *SDHC*, succinate dehydrogenase complex, subunit C; *SDHD*, succinate dehydrogenase complex, subunit D; *TMEM127*, transmembrane protein 127; *VHL*, von Hippel Lindau.

cardiomyocytes. Stimulation of the α_2-adrenoceptors on smooth muscle cells results in peripheral arterial vasodilation and coronary vasoconstriction. β_1-adrenoceptors are stimulated by both norepinephrine and epinephrine and have a positive inotropic effect in the cardiomyocytes. β_2-adrenergic receptors respond mainly to epinephrine and induce vasodilation of muscular arteries [24]. Therefore, the concentration and type of catecholamine define the cardiovascular response. Acutely, catecholamines increase the heart rate, vascular resistance, and myocardial contractility. However, sustained catecholamine excess states would result in desensitization of the adrenoceptors. Several patients with PCC-related catecholamine excess are asymptomatic, and studies on the human and animal models report significant desensitization of both the α and β adrenoceptors [25].

Clinically, several cardiovascular complications arise from excessive catecholamine production. Catecholamine excess states can lead to an acute increase in arterial stiffness and tachyarrhythmias. Chronic catecholamine excess states can cause myocardial ischemia and hypertension. PCCs can also contribute to the development of chronic (hypertrophic, dilated, obstructive), or acute (ischemic, takotsubo) cardiomyopathies [23]. Moreover, catecholamine overproduction can lead to hypertensive encephalopathy, while paroxysmal hypertension can cause hemorrhagic or ischemic stroke. Vasoconstriction can also lead to renal failure as well as muscle ischemia and consequent rhabdomyolysis [24]. For further reading on catecholamines and blood pressure regulation, please refer to Chapter 2.

Metastatic risk

All PCCs have the potential to metastasize. Since no reliable biomarker has yet been identified that can accurately predict the metastatic potential of the disease, PCC-related malignancy is defined by the presence of distant metastasis in places where no chromaffin cells are physiologically found. Therefore, the term "malignant" has been replaced by "metastatic" PCC [12,26]. The presence of *SDHx* mutations, tumor size greater than 5 cm, multifocality, and the noradrenergic or dopaminergic biochemical phenotypes are the common risk factors for the development of metastatic disease [10].

Several relevant biomarkers have been suggested as surrogates of the metastatic potential of PCCs and can contribute to generating various grading scores, such as the Pheochromocytoma of the Adrenal Gland Scaled Score (PASS) grading system, the Grading of Adrenal Pheochromocytoma and Paraganglioma (GAPP), and the Composite Pheochromocytoma/paraganglioma Prognostic Score (COPPS) [27−29].

Both PASS and GAPP scoring systems have been used globally to evaluate the malignant potential of patients with PCCs. PASS score of four or more has a high sensitivity for malignant behavior (sensitivity of 100% and specificity of 75%) [29]. A tumor with GAPP score of less than 3 has a metastatic rate of 3% and 5-year survival of 100% [30]. This reflects the ability of both scores to "rule out" the metastatic or malignant behavior of PCCs.

Clinical presentation

The classic triad of symptoms associated with PCCs is headache, palpitation, and diaphoresis [7], which occur with a much higher frequency than other symptoms [31,32]. However, the complete triad is only found in about 20% of patients [33]. The most common sign associated with the disease is hypertension, found in up to 95% of patients [34]. The clinical presentation of hypertension can be (i) sustained hypertension, found in about 50% of patients, (ii) paroxysmal hypertension, found in 45% of patients, and (iii) normotension in about 5%−15% of patients [6,35]. Recently, based on the clinical signs and symptoms, a scoring system has been proposed (Table 11.2) in order to establish the pretest likelihood of the disease (symptom score ≥ or < 3). Higher scores were associated with higher biochemical indices of catecholamine excess, but not with tumor size [31]. Cluster 2 tumors are more likely to be related to episodic "flares" and paroxysmal symptoms, while tumors related to cluster 1 tend to present with sustained hypertension. Cluster 2 patients are more likely to present with pallor, tremor, and anxiety or panic attacks. Notably, clinically advanced PCC and PGL are now recognized as the commonest nonthyroid endocrine malignancies [36].

Diagnostic workup

Biochemical testing

Initial evaluation of suspected PCCs should be performed with plasma free metanephrines or urinary fractionated metanephrines, as per the current clinical guidelines [10,37]. Considering appropriate preanalytical precautions (e.g., at least 20 min of supine rest, avoidance of potentially interfering medications sufficiently prior to testing), plasma free and urine fractionated metanephrines have a high diagnostic sensitivity for PCC/PGL. There is no clear benefit of measuring metabolites in plasma as opposed to urine, as both have excellent negative predictive values (>99%) at similar specificities

TABLE 11.2 Clinical score for the likelihood of pheochromocytoma (PCC) and paraganglioma (PGL) (range −1 to +7 points)[a]: A score of 3 or more is associated with a 5.8 higher probability of PCC or PGL.

Clinical score for the likelihood of PCC[b,c]	Point score
Pallor	+1 point
Palpitations	+1 point
Heart rate ≥85 bpm	+1 point
Tremor	+1 point
Nausea	+1 point
Body mass index (BMI) > 30 kg/m^2	−1 point
BMI < 25 kg/m^2	+1 point

BMI, body mass index.
[a]Adapted from From Geroula A, Deutschbein T, Langton K, Masjkur J, Pamporaki C, Peitzsch M, Fliedner S, Timmers HJLM, Bornstein SR, Beuschlein F, Stell A, Januszewicz A, Prejbisz A, Fassnacht M, Lenders JWM, Eisenhofer G. Pheochromocytoma and paraganglioma: clinical feature-based disease probability in relation to catecholamine biochemistry and reason for disease suspicion. Eur J Endocrinol. 2019;181(4):409−20. https://doi.org/10.1530/EJE-19-0159.
[b]Cluster 1 tumors usually are associated with lower scores but sustained hypertension.
[c]Cluster 2 tumors usually are associated with higher scores and episodic "flares".

($\sim$94%) [38,39]. Thus, a negative plasma free metanephrine or urinary fractionated metanephrine test virtually rules out a PCC/PGL except in those with very small tumors or in those with nonsecretory head and neck PGLs [10].

The plasma free metanephrines have an equivalent diagnostic accuracy to urinary fractionated metanephrines in those with low risk for PCC/PGL as in those with symptoms suggestive of PCC/PGL. However, plasma free metanephrines have a superior diagnostic accuracy in those with high risk for PCC/PGL as in those with adrenal incidentaloma or in those on surveillance [10]. The analytic method of choice is liquid chromatography-tandem mass spectrometry (LC-MS/MS), as it provides greater diagnostic performance when compared to alternative detection methods in the form of superior accuracy, cost-effectiveness and minimal analytical interferences with the drugs [40].

Detection of dopamine-producing tumors or biochemically silent PCC/PGL remains a challenge, as these tumors rarely produce excessive amounts of adrenaline and noradrenaline. Therefore, a personalized approach for biochemical screening must consider phenotype-genotype-biochemical correlations. Upon suspicion of this type of tumor (specially *SDHx*-related tumors), the inclusion of plasma 3-methoxytyramine (3MT; the dopamine metabolite) measurement has been proposed and endorsed by the European Society of Endocrinology clinical practice guideline [41], as well as by the European Society of Hypertension working group on endocrine hypertension position statements [10], as a tool to increase the diagnostic sensitivity [42,43].

In a recent research study that evaluated adrenal incidentalomas, an approach that targeted plasma metabolomics (including 19 steroids, normetanephrine, and metanephrine) combined with adrenal lesion size provides 95% sensitivity and 99% specificity for PCC diagnosis. Nevertheless, discrimination of PCC from other adrenal secreting tumors is utterly dependent on plasma free metanephrines [44]. Chromogranin A (CgA) can be a valuable plasma biomarker for patients with *SDHB*-related PCCs and sympathetic paragangliomas with normal plasma/urine metanephrines [45].

The personalized interpretation of the test report is essential since conditions associated with blood sampling (e.g., supine, at rest), as well as chronic kidney disease, might alter the test results [46]. Higher upper cut-off values are needed in patients with chronic kidney disease [10]. Several drugs may cause falsely elevated results for the plasma or urinary metanephrines, both due to pharmacodynamic interference (e.g., antidepressants, sympathomimetics, MAO-inhibitors, levodopa, phenoxybenzamine) or analytical interference (e.g., acetaminophen, sotalol) (minimal for LC-MS/MS). A list of the most common interfering drugs can be found in the European and Endocrine Society guidelines [10,37].

Conditions with chronic sympathetic overactivity, including heart failure and obstructive sleep apnea, inappropriate sampling, drug interferences, and incorrect cut-off values can cause false-positive metanephrines test tests [10]. Food items interfere with the 3MT estimation, hence overnight fasting and avoidance of certain foods are relevant for 3MT analysis [37]. Solitary elevation of metanephrines/normetanephrines by 2-fold or simultaneous elevation of two or more metabolites (metanephrines, normetanephrines, and/or 3MT) are less likely to be false-positive [10]. These situations need further diagnostic imaging, regardless of the pretest probability. On the other hand, in those with less than 2-fold elevation of a single metabolite with no other possible explanation for a false-positive test result, especially in those with a high pretest probability for PCC/PGL based on the clinical score given in Table 11.2, a clonidine suppression test can be done to differentiate the false-positive test from the true-positive. However, those with a low pretest probability for PCC/PGL do not need further tests [10,47].

Diagnostic imaging

Anatomical imaging

Ideally, imaging studies should be carried out only after biochemical confirmation of the disease. Exceptions for this rule might be patients critically ill and/or in the intensive care setting [48], as well in those where nonsecretory tumors are suspected. Appearance of PCC in the anatomical imaging is highly variable, as tumors can contain necrosis, hemorrhage, cystic changes, and calcifications. Upon suspicion of PCC, a contrast-enhanced computed tomography (CT) is the first-choice imaging modality because of its adequate spatial resolution and high sensitivity [37,49]. The demonstration of an adrenal tumor with an unenhanced CT attenuation value ≤ 10 Hounsfield Units (HU) has a high diagnostic predictive value to exclude the presence of PCC (sensitivity of >99%) [50,51]. Magnetic resonance imaging (MRI) also has good sensitivity and specificity for the diagnosis of PCC. It is the method of choice in patients allergic to iodinated contrast agents, and in those for whom radiation exposure should be limited (i.e., children, and pregnant women). A high intensity (bright) T2-weighted signal on MRI is highly specific for PCC, but it lacks sensitivity, as it occurs in less than half of the tumors [52].

Functional imaging

The choice of the most appropriate method depends on each patient's genotypical and/or phenotypical findings. Molecular imaging tracers for the diagnosis of PPGL can be classified according to their target ligand (Table 11.3). Functional imaging modalities can benefit patients at high risk for metastatic disease, including those with large tumors, extra-adrenal tumors, and multifocal disease.

[123]I-metaiodobenzylguanidine (MIBG) scintigraphy is the most classical functional imaging for PCC evaluation. Nevertheless, ^{123}I-MIBG scintigraphy may provide false-positive results in approximately 10% of the cases, mainly because the normal adrenal glands can demonstrate a physiological tracer uptake [53]. Moreover, it has poor sensitivity for small PCCs and those that secrete dopamine. Drugs such as tricyclic antidepressants, calcium channel blockers, and some combined α- and β-adrenoceptor blockers such as labetalol can interfere with ^{123}I-MIBG accumulation. They should be withheld 2 weeks before the test [54]. In a multicentric retrospective study with 340 patients, ^{123}I-MIBG scintigraphy did not significantly add to CT/MRI imaging modalities for PCC/PGL diagnosis. Therefore, this test should be considered especially for patients with suspicion of metastatic PPGL who might benefit from ^{131}I-MIBG radiotherapy [55].

[18]Fluorine-Fluorodeoxyglucose positron emission tomography/CT (^{18}F-FDG PET/CT) can be used in patients with metastatic disease, as it outperforms ^{123}I-MIBG scintigraphy as a functional imaging modality [56]. This test's sensitivity is high (80%−100%), while the specificity is low, as observed for any type of malignancy. In one study, ^{18}F-FDG uptake was higher in *SDHx* and *VHL*-related tumors than in MEN2 related tumors [57].

Functional imaging with somatostatin receptor analogues (SSAs), especially the use of ^{68}Ga-DOTA-SSA, has shown excellent results in localizing PCCs. In a recent systematic review and meta-analysis, the PPGL detection rate for ^{68}Ga-DOTA-SSA PET/CT was 93%, which was significantly higher compared to ^{18}F-labeled fluorodihydroxyphenylalanine (^{18}F-FDOPA)-PET/CT (80%), ^{18}F-FDG PET/CT (74%) and [123/131]I-MIBG scintigraphy (38%) [58], suggesting that ^{68}Ga-DOTA-SSA is the most sensitive tool for detecting PPGLs in the context of unknown genetic status. In another study, ^{68}Ga-DOTATATE PET/CT was evaluated for initial staging (*n* = 28) and restaging (*n* = 18, including 8 metastatic cases) for PCCs. Overall, ^{68}Ga-DOTATATE PET/CT had a sensitivity of 84% for PCC (21/24). Further, ^{68}Ga-DOTATATE PET/CT resulted in management change in 50% PCC (23/46) cases [59]. ^{68}Ga-DOTA-SSA PET/CT should also be performed when planning peptide receptor radionuclide therapy (PRRT).

^{18}F-FDOPA PET/CT demonstrates high tumor uptake in PPGLs with *VHL, RET, NF1, MAX, HIF2A,* and *FH* mutations [60]. Considering only PCCs, ^{18}F-FDOPA PET/CT showed better patient-based and lesion-based detection rates than did ^{68}Ga-DOTA-SSA PET/CT in 10 cases (100% vs. 90% and 94% vs. 81%, respectively) in one study [61]. Still, a preliminary study from the National Institute of Health (NIH) demonstrated that ^{68}Ga-DOTA-SSA performs similar to ^{18}F-FDOPA PET/CT for sporadic PCCs [62]. ^{18}F-Fluorodopamine (^{18}F-FDA) is a tracer specific for chromaffin tumors and should be restricted to primary PCCs or sympathetic PGLs. In cases of sporadic primary PCCs, a study comparing six different imaging modalities in 14 patients found that ^{18}F-FDOPA performed better in the evaluation of sporadic tumors. ^{18}F-FDOPA was the only imaging modality that received a conspicuity score of 5 for all patients for both interpreters and had the highest SUVmax (maximum standardized uptake values) ratios between the adrenal lesion and either the contralateral normal adrenal gland or normal liver [63].

A practical approach for functional imaging in PCC evaluation is the following: when the genetic status is unknown, and in the absence of tumor multifocality, ^{18}F-FDOPA or ^{123}I-MIBG is proposed as first-line imaging in sporadic PCC and metastatic cases, but ^{68}Ga-DOTATE is also an adequate choice. For those associated with *NF1/RET/VHL/MAX*, ^{18}F-FDOPA PET/CT is recommended as the first option but could be replaced by ^{68}Ga-DOTATE or ^{123}I-MIBG if the former is not available [60]. For tumors associated with *SDHx* mutations, ^{68}Ga-DOTATATE is the first-line choice, with ^{18}F-FDG or ^{18}F-DOPA as alternatives (Fig. 11.1, Table 11.3).

MEN2 and VHL PCCs

Specifically, MEN2-related PCCs exhibit an adrenergic biochemical phenotype; Consequently, positive biochemistry and CT or MRI images showing adrenal glands tumors can confirm the presence of PCCs. In this context, functional imaging is not needed. MEN2 and VHL-related PCCs are rarely metastatic (<5%) [64]. Thus, whole-body imaging is indicated only if a lesion cannot be found in the adrenal glands. Exceptions may be extra-adrenal tumors or PCCs measuring >5 cm, which are likely to become metastatic. However, such cases are rare.

For further reading on imaging of PCCs, please refer to Chapter 20.

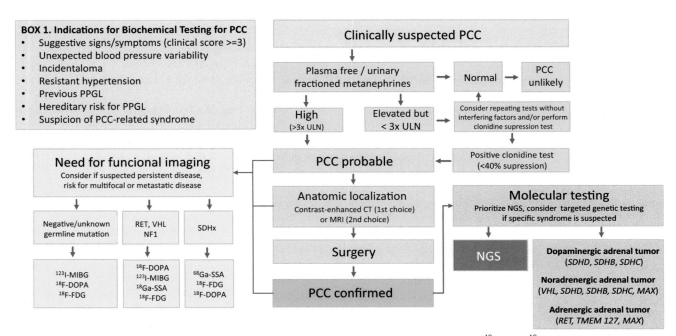

FIGURE 11.1 Suggested approach for PCC diagnosis and initial management. *CT*, computed tomography; *18F-FDG*, 18Fluorine-Fluorodeoxyglucose; *F-FDOPA*, 18F-fluoro-dihydroxyphenylalanine; *68Ga-SSA*, 68Ga-somatostatin analog; *123I-MIBG*, 123I-metaiodobenzylguanidine; *MAX,* myc-associated factor X; *MRI*, magnetic resonance imaging; *NGS*, next-generation sequencing; *PCC*, pheochromocytoma; *PPGL*, pheochromocytoma/paraganglioma; *18SDHD*, succinate dehydrogenase complex subunit D; *SDHB*, succinate dehydrogenase complex subunit B; *SDHC*, succinate dehydrogenase complex subunit C; *TMEM127*, transmembrane protein 127; *ULN*, the upper limit of normal; *VHL*, Von Hippel-Lindau.

TABLE 11.3 Functional imaging and its specific characteristics.

Target ligand	Tracer	Indication	Comments
Catecholamine storage and synthesis	123I-MIBG	Metastatic PCC when radiotherapy with 131I-MIBG is planned	Uptake by the normal adrenal gland. Lower accuracy for *SDHx*-related PPGLs
	18F-FDA	Primary PCCs	Unavailable in most centers
	18F-FDOPA	Cluster 1B and 2	Reduced sensitivity for *SDHx*-related PPGLs. Lack of uptake by healthy adrenal tissue
Glucose metabolism	18F-FDG	Scanning patients with metastatic disease	Better than 123I-MIBG for scanning patients with metastatic disease. Complementary with other functional imaging studies.
Somatostatin receptor	111Indium-pentetreotide (OctreoscanTM)	Complementary investigation	Provides complementary information to 123I-MIBG for detection of metastatic PCCs
	68Ga-DOTATATE	Diagnosis staging; considered for evaluation of metastases and multifocality; planning PRRT	High sensitivity for PCC with unknown genetic status

FDA, fluorodopamine; *FDOPA*, fluorodihydroxyphenylalanine; *FDG*, fluorodeoxyglucose; *68Ga-DOTATATE,* 68Gallium DOTA-conjugated peptide; *MIBG*, metaiodobenzylguanidine; *PCC*, pheochromocytoma; *PPGL*, pheochromocytoma/paraganglioma; *PRRT*, peptide receptor radionuclide treatment; *SDHx*, succinate dehydrogenase complex.

Molecular diagnosis

All patients with PCC should be offered molecular testing due to the high prevalence of germline genetic alterations. As discussed previously, several driver genes are involved in the development of PCC. Although clinical and biochemical characteristics can suggest a specific causal gene, they do not always predict the underlying genotype [65]. If available, targeted Next Generation Sequencing (NGS), is the recommended approach by enabling testing of several genes in one panel. Nevertheless, if a specific syndrome is suspected (e.g., MEN2, VHL), targeted gene analysis is appropriate for the genetic diagnosis [10] (Fig. 11.1).

Management

Presurgical and surgical management of PCC

Surgical resection is the only curative treatment option for a PCC. Nevertheless, tumor manipulation during the surgical procedure can induce a massive release of catecholamines from the tumor, resulting in hypertensive crises, cardiac arrhythmias, myocardial infarction, and acute pulmonary edema. On the other hand, the sudden withdrawal of catecholamines from the circulation after tumor resection can result in severe and refractory hypotension. Therefore, adequate presurgical medical preparation is indicated to avoid intraoperative cardiovascular complications and promote optimal hemodynamic stability during the procedure. This approach also applies to normotensive patients with normal levels of catecholamines or metanephrines before surgery [37].

Administration of alpha-adrenoceptor blockers is the first choice and should be initiated at least 7–14 days before the surgery. Doses should be increased gradually until the blood pressure targets are achieved. Generally, patients are advised liberal oral intake of salt and fluids during this period to replenish the catecholamine-induced volume contraction [7,66]. This approach can reduce the risk of undesirable hypotension and postural hypotension while sufficient α-blockade is achieved. Choices of α-blockers usually include phenoxybenzamine, a nonselective and noncompetitive α_1-and α_2-adrenergic receptor blocker, or doxazosin, a selective and competitive α_1-adrenergic receptor blocker. Most studies do not demonstrate the superiority of one versus another. Phenoxybenzamine was associated with more hemodynamic stability during surgery, but not with better clinical outcomes [67].

After adequate α-adrenergic blockade has been achieved, the β-adrenergic blockade can be initiated. Apart from improving hypertension control, this also helps to reduce the undesirable tachycardia from the alpha-blockade. The β-adrenergic blocker is never used as monotherapy or started first because β-adrenergic blockade with unopposed α-adrenoceptor stimulation can cause a further elevation in blood pressure and even a pheochromocytoma crisis.

Calcium channel blockers may be added for further optimization of blood pressure control. A high-sodium diet and increased fluid intake presurgically also help to minimize the effects of vascular volume expansion that occur after the tumor removal [37]. Additionally, intravenous administration of 1–2 L of saline 24-hour before surgery is usually performed, except in situations of volume overload in at-risk patients (e.g., heart or renal failure). Preoperative blood pressure targets have not been well defined. An upright systolic blood pressure of less than 90 mmHg is associated with more hemodynamic instability [67]. Therefore, a seated blood pressure target of less than 130/80 mmHg, and an upright systolic blood pressure target of more than 90 mmHg are commonly accepted as adequate, as are heart rates of 60–70 beats per minute (bpm) in seated, and 70–80 bpm in an upright position, respectively.

Regarding the operative approach, minimally invasive surgery is the procedure of choice, as it is associated with a shorter operative time, shorter length of hospital stay, and a decreased need for intensive care support [68]. Due to the high risk of recurrence and metastatic spread, adrenalectomy is preferred for Cluster 1 tumors. Cortical-sparing adrenal surgery may be considered for the removal of less aggressive PCCs associated with *RET* or *VHL* mutations, but the risk of recurrent disease is still significant ($\sim$13%) [69]. A recent study comparing robotic versus laparoscopic minimally invasive adrenalectomy for adrenal malignancies found that a laparoscopic approach was associated with a greater conversion (to open surgery) rate (18.3%, vs. 7.8% $P = .005$) and poorer outcomes [70]. Nevertheless, only 30% of these cases were PCCs and half of the tumors were larger than 5 cm. Although controversial, surgical removal of the primary tumor or debulking surgery in the context of metastatic disease can also be considered to reduce the tumor burden and the biochemical consequences. Recent studies suggest that this approach might be associated with improved overall survival [71]. Moreover, removing the primary lesion may enhance the uptake of radiopharmaceuticals by the target metastatic lesions [72].

Locoregional approaches

External beam radiotherapy

External beam radiation therapy (EBRT) is frequently used to treat patients with PCC and bone metastasis. Studies have shown an 81%–94% rate of symptom improvement when both PCCs and PGLs are evaluated together. Despite favorable disease response/control of the treated lesion, most patients later develop disease progression at distant sites outside the irradiated field [73]. EBRT should be considered, especially for symptomatic relief, in patients with localized diseases that are unsuitable for other options such as surgical resection or percutaneous ablation.

Other approaches

Locoregional therapy approaches besides EBRT include stereotactic radiosurgery to alleviate symptoms related to tumor growth and mass effects. Radiofrequency ablation or cryoablation are the alternatives, especially for single-site metastasis [12].

Systemic therapy

Systemic therapy must be considered for metastatic PCCs once locoregional approaches have been exhausted.

Chemotherapy

For a rapidly progressive disease with a significant tumor burden, treatment with a combination of cyclophosphamide, vincristine, and dacarbazine (CVD) is preferred. Disease control with this approach ranges from 48% to 83%, and progression-free survival of 40 months has been described [74,75]. Temozolomide (TMZ) is an oral chemotherapeutic alternative to intravenous dacarbazine. The efficacy of TMZ therapy is related to the expression of O-6-methylguanine-DNA methyltransferase (MGMT) and/or its promoter methylation. Therefore, TMZ has higher efficacy in MGMT deficient tumors. In a recent study with TMZ, where half of the patients (8/15) had metastatic PCCs, there was partial response in 5 patients, stable disease in 7, and progressive disease in 3 patients. Partial responses were only observed in patients with *SDHB* mutation [76]. TMZ can be used as monotherapy after CVD cycles or as the first alternative in less aggressive cases depending on the individual contexts.

Radionuclide therapy

For PCCs with a slow to moderate progression, radionuclide therapy is an appropriate choice in most cases. Classically, ^{131}I-MIBG targeting norepinephrine transporter system is recommended for ^{123}I-MIBG positive patients. In a study that evaluated long-term outcomes of patients with metastatic PCC and PGL treated with ^{131}I-MIBG, 1% of patients experienced complete response, 33% partial response, 53% stability, and 13% progression. However, 51% showed subsequent progression with a median progression-free survival of 2.0 years. Having PCC was not related to response (as opposed to having PGL) in a multivariate analysis [77]. Moreover, Cluster 1 *SDHx*-related disease might be less frequently positive on a ^{123}I-MIBG scan, and therefore less sensitive to ^{131}I-MIBG radionuclide therapy.

More recently, ^{68}Ga/^{90}Y/^{177}Lu-DOTA-SSA analogs targeting peptide (somatostatin) receptors (SSTR) have been introduced as potential new theragnostic agents for PCCs. As PCCs (especially *SDHx*-associated tumors) show high SSTR2 expression [78], SSTR-based radionuclide therapy is promising. However, most studies to date include both PGL and PCC cases. Therefore, the response rate exclusively for PCCs is limited. One study that evaluated SSTR-based therapy and ^{131}I-MIBG therapy in 22 patients (7 PCCs and 14 PGL) reported a clear difference in overall survival, progression-free survival (PFS), event-free survival (EFS), and response to treatment in favor of peptide receptor radionuclide treatment when comparing only patients with metastatic PGLs, as opposed to incorporating PCCs in the comparison, suggesting that efficacy of treatment is different between PCCs and PGLs, and that these pathologies should be treated differently [79].

Tyrosine kinase inhibitors (TKIs)

TKIs have been investigated as an alternative treatment option in the context of disease progression despite radionuclide therapy or chemotherapy, or when these are not acceptable options [8]. These include sunitinib, cabozantinib, axitinib, and pazopanib, all with antiangiogenic effects. Nevertheless, for PCC, the results are not very promising. In a study that evaluated sunitinib for patients with metastatic PCC/PGL, 9/11 patients with PCC demonstrated disease progression with treatment [80]. There are ongoing trials with TKIs that will probably shed more light on the efficacy of these agents in PCC in near future.

Other agents

For an extensive review of ongoing trials and systemic therapy for PCCs, including mTORC1 inhibitor everolimus, immunotherapy, and "cold" SSTR2 analogs, an interesting article has been published recently [12]. Though the response rates with these agents were in the range of ∼70% based on small-scale clinical trial data, long-term follow-up results are yet to emerge to make firm recommendations for clinical practice. With the recent advances in the knowledge about the molecular and genetic alterations of PCCs, personalized treatment strategies are being incorporated into clinical practice. Genomic profiling to enhance the tumor-oriented personalized treatment algorithms is being tested for clinically advanced PCCs [36].

Follow-up

Adjustments in the antihypertensive agents and their dosages are usually necessary after successful tumor resection with the improvement of hypertension. Patients who undergo bilateral adrenalectomy will need lifelong steroid replacement if the adrenal cortex is not spared. Metanephrine levels should be evaluated 2—6 weeks after the surgery, as the plasma pool may remain elevated in the immediate postoperative period. Normalization of the previously altered hormones usually implies successful tumor removal.

For asymptomatic *RET*-mutation carriers, the initial biochemical screening depends on the type of *RET* mutation, but usually starts between 11 and 16 years of age, then yearly, while imaging should be considered every 3—5 years [81]. For *NF1* asymptomatic mutation carriers, the biochemical screening should begin around the age of 10—14 years, then every 3 years, while a CT/MRI is recommended only if biochemical testing is positive [82]. In patients with VHL syndrome, abdominal imaging should be performed every 2 years to look for kidney, pancreas, and other potential tumors.

Generally, for patients with previous PCC and cluster 2 mutations, yearly screening with plasma free metanephrines or urinary fractionated metanephrines is recommended. Imaging studies are optional for patients with low-risk mutations but are recommended every 3—5 years in those with moderate to high-risk mutations [12]. For follow-up of cluster 1 patients, please refer to Chapter 12 (Paraganglioma and Hypertension).

Areas of uncertainty/emerging concepts

Several therapies have emerged as potential treatment options for advanced PCC, such as systemic drugs and peptide receptor radionuclide therapy (see above). Nevertheless, questions remain regarding the adequate timing and the sequence of these therapeutic agents to be used for the optimal care of patients with PCC [8].

Besides the metastatic risk associated with specific germline mutations, we still lack adequate biomarkers that can accurately determine the malignant potential of PCCs. Recent studies demonstrate that mechanisms occurring in other types of carcinomas, such as immortalization through telomere deregulation, also play a role in PCC progression. Indeed, activation of telomerase (*TERT*), NOP10 overexpression, and loss of function of the ATRX chromatin remodeler gene (*ATRX*) relate to poor prognosis in PCC [83—85]. Hopefully, emerging research will shed light on the mechanisms that facilitate the metastatic potential of PCCs.

The development of mouse and cell lines as the disease models for PCC research has proved to be much more challenging than expected. The lack of an *SDH*-specific PPGL model limits the study of the downstream causal tumor-igenic mechanisms in these neoplasms. Moreover, the lack of numerous different human cell lines and animal models that mimic each mutation-driven oncogenic process still hinders the progress in the basic science for new therapeutics in PCC [86].

Finally, defining the penetrance of each PCC-causing pathogenic mutation is still a challenge. Adequate evaluation of the degree of penetrance requires large observational cohorts. Most pathogenic variants involved in PCC are rare. Penetrance estimates vary considerably for each gene, ranging from ∼3% for *NF1* mutations to 90% for *SDHD* mutations [87]. Future studies could more accurately determine the gene-based risk for PCC in germline mutation carriers and, therefore, could help define rational protocols for biochemical and imaging surveillance [88].

Summary and conclusions

The knowledge of the diagnosis and management of PCC has evolved dramatically in recent years. Diagnostic algorithms have expanded from symptom-based investigations to the detection of asymptomatic patients with PCCs based on familial genetic testing. Moreover, advances in functional imaging have made precise tumor localization possible. Treatment decisions and surveillance protocols are now individualized based on the identification of pathogenic germline mutations that cause PCC. If curative surgery is performed, the prognosis of PCC is considered excellent. However, large, metastatic extraadrenal tumors are associated with progressive disease and poor outcomes despite systemic treatment.

Learning points

- PCCs are uncommon causes of hypertension, for the diagnosis of which high-level clinical suspicion is needed. More than 90% of cases present with persistent or paroxysmal hypertension. Biochemical testing with plasma free metanephrines or urinary fractionated metanephrines should be performed as the initial screening of patients.
- PCCs are classified into three specific clusters based on their underlying mutations, reflecting the different biochemical and molecular characteristics. Personalized management must consider these biochemical, molecular, and genetic profiles as well as the aggressiveness of each mutation-dependent tumor.
- All patients with PCC and all asymptomatic mutation carriers will need lifelong follow-up individualized according to the patient's mutation status.
- Laparoscopic/open resection of the tumor is the only curative treatment option and should be conducted with adequate presurgical preparation, whenever possible. Systemic therapy, including chemotherapy, radionuclide therapy, and tyrosine kinase inhibitors are alternatives for inoperable/metastatic disease.

References

[1] Noilhan C, Barigou M, Bieler L, Amar J, Chamontin B, Bouhanick B. Causes of secondary hypertension in the young population: a monocentric study. Ann Cardiol Angeiol 2016;65(3):159−64. https://doi.org/10.1016/j.ancard.2016.04.016.

[2] Omura M, Saito J, Yamaguchi K, Kakuta Y, Nishikawa T. Prospective study on the prevalence of secondary hypertension among hypertensive patients visiting a general outpatient clinic in Japan. Hypertens Res 2004;27(3):193−202. https://doi.org/10.1291/hypres.27.193.

[3] Zhang L, Li J, Li N, Sun N, Xie L, Han Q, Li Y, Lu XZ, Sun P, Li Y, Shi Y, Wang H, Zhang Y, Chen H, Huo Y. Trends in cause-related comorbidities in hospitalized patients with secondary hypertension in China from 2013 to 2016: a retrospective analysis of hospital quality monitoring system data. J Hypertens 2021;39(10):2015−21. https://doi.org/10.1097/HJH.0000000000002891.

[4] Stenström G, Svårdsudd K. Pheochromocytoma in Sweden 1958−1981: an analysis of the national cancer registry data. Acta Med Scand 1986;220(3):225−32. https://doi.org/10.1111/j.0954-6820.1986.tb02755.x.

[5] Young WF. Management approaches to adrenal incidentalomas: a view from Rochester, Minnesota. Endocrinol Metab Clin North Am 2000;29(1):159−85. https://doi.org/10.1016/s0889-8529(05)70122-5.

[6] Zelinka T, Eisenhofer G, Pacak K. Pheochromocytoma as a catecholamine producing tumor: implications for clinical practice. Stress 2007;10(2):195−203. https://doi.org/10.1080/10253890701395896.

[7] Desai AS, Chutkow WA, Edelman E, Economy KE, Dec GW. A crisis in late pregnancy. N Engl J Med 2009;361(23):2271−7. https://doi.org/10.1056/NEJMcps0708258.

[8] Winzeler B, Challis BG, Casey RT. Precision medicine in phaeochromocytoma and paraganglioma. J Personalized Med 2021;11(11):1239. https://doi.org/10.3390/jpm11111239.

[9] Castro-Vega LJ, Lepoutre-Lussey C, Gimenez-Roqueplo AP, Favier J. Rethinking pheochromocytomas and paragangliomas from a genomic perspective. Oncogene 2016;35(9):1080−9. https://doi.org/10.1038/onc.2015.172.

[10] Lenders JWM, Kerstens MN, Amar L, Prejbisz A, Robledo M, Taieb D, Pacak K, Crona J, Zelinka T, Mannelli M, Deutschbein T, Timmers HJLM, Castinetti F, Dralle H, Widimský J, Gimenez-Roqueplo AP, Eisenhofer G. Genetics, diagnosis, management and future directions of research of phaeochromocytoma and paraganglioma: a position statement and consensus of the Working Group on Endocrine Hypertension of the European Society of Hypertension. J Hypertens 2020;38(8):1443−56. https://doi.org/10.1097/HJH.0000000000002438.

[11] Fishbein L, Leshchiner I, Walter V, Danilova L, Robertson AG, Johnson AR, et al. Comprehensive molecular characterization of pheochromocytoma and paraganglioma. Cancer Cell 2017 Feb 13;31(2):181−93. https://doi.org/10.1016/j.ccell.2017.01.001.

[12] Nölting S, Bechmann N, Taieb D, Beuschlein F, Fassnacht M, Kroiss M, Eisenhofer G, Grossman A, Pacak K. Personalized management of pheochromocytoma and paraganglioma. Endocr Rev 2022 Mar 9;43(2):199−239. https://doi.org/10.1210/endrev/bnab019. Erratum in: Endocr Rev. 2021 Dec 14;: Erratum in: Endocr Rev. 2021 Dec 14.

[13] Favier J, Gimenez-Roqueplo AP. Pheochromocytomas: the (pseudo)-hypoxia hypothesis. Best Pract Res Clin Endocrinol Metabol 2010;24(6):957−68. https://doi.org/10.1016/j.beem.2010.10.004.

[14] Eisenhofer G, Goldstein DS, Sullivan P, Csako G, Brouwers FM, Lai EW, Adams KT, Pacak K. Biochemical and clinical manifestations of dopamine-producing paragangliomas: utility of plasma methoxytyramine. J Clin Endocrinol Metab 2005;90(4):2068−75. https://doi.org/10.1210/jc.2004-2025.

[15] Eisenhofer G, Huynh TT, Pacak K, Brouwers FM, Walther MM, Linehan WM, Munson PJ, Mannelli M, Goldstein DS, Elkahloun AG. Distinct gene expression profiles in norepinephrine- and epinephrine-producing hereditary and sporadic pheochromocytomas: activation of hypoxia-driven angiogenic pathways in von Hippel-Lindau syndrome. Endocr Relat Cancer 2004;11(4):897−911. https://doi.org/10.1677/erc.1.00838.

[16] Eisenhofer G, Klink B, Richter S, Lenders JWM, Robledo M. Metabologenomics of phaeochromocytoma and paraganglioma: an integrated approach for personalised biochemical and genetic testing. Clin Biochem Rev 2017;38(2):69−100. https://www.aacb.asn.au/documents/item/4777.

[17] Eisenhofer G, Lenders JWM, Timmers H, Mannelli M, Grebe SK, Hofbauer LC, Bornstein SR, Tiebel O, Adams K, Bratslavsky G, Linehan WM, Pacak K. Measurements of plasma methoxytyramine, normetanephrine, and metanephrine as discriminators of different hereditary forms of pheochromocytoma. Clin Chem 2011;57(3):411−20. https://doi.org/10.1373/clinchem.2010.153320.

[18] Eisenhofer G, Walther MM, Huynh TT, Li ST, Bornstein SR, Vortmeyer A, Mannelli M, Goldstein DS, Linehan WM, Lenders JWM, Pacak K. Pheochromocytomas in von Hippel-Lindau syndrome and multiple endocrine neoplasia type 2 display distinct biochemical and clinical phenotypes. J Clin Endocrinol Metab 2001;86(5):1999−2008. https://doi.org/10.1210/jcem.86.5.7496.

[19] Proye C, Fossati P, Fontaine P, Lefebvre J, Decoulx M, Wemeau JL, Dewailly D, Rwamasirabo E, Cecat P. Dopamine-secreting pheochromocytoma: an unrecognized entity? Classification of pheochromocytomas according to their type of secretion. Surgery 1986;100(6):1154−62.

[20] Lips CJ, Höppener JW, Van Nesselrooij BP, Van der Luijt RB. Counselling in multiple endocrine neoplasia syndromes: from individual experience to general guidelines. J Intern Med 2005;257(1):69−77.

[21] Schovanek J, Martucci V, Wesley R, Fojo T, del Rivero J, Huynh T, et al. The size of the primary tumor and age at initial diagnosis are independent predictors of the metastatic behavior and survival of patients with SDHB-related pheochromocytoma and paraganglioma: a retrospective cohort study. BMC Cancer 2014;14(1):523. https://doi.org/10.1186/1471-2407-14-523.

[22] Crona J, Lamarca A, Ghosal S, Welin S, Skogseid B, Pacak K. Genotype-phenotype correlations in pheochromocytoma and paraganglioma: a systematic review and individual patient meta-analysis. Endocr Relat Cancer 2019;26(5):539−50. https://doi.org/10.1530/ERC-19-0024.

[23] Kumar A, Pappachan JM, Fernandez CJ. Catecholamine-induced cardiomyopathy: an endocrinologist's perspective. Rev Cardiovasc Med 2021;22(4):1215−28. https://doi.org/10.31083/j.rcm2204130.

[24] Zuber SM, Kantorovich V, Pacak K. Hypertension in pheochromocytoma: characteristics and treatment. Endocrinol Metab Clin North Am 2011;40(2):295−311. https://doi.org/10.1016/j.ecl.2011.02.002.

[25] Jones C, Hamilton C, Whyte K, Elliott H, Reid JL. Acute and chronic regulation of alpha 2-adrenoceptor number and function in man. Clin Sci (Lond) 1985;68(Suppl 10):129s−32s.

[26] Lam AKy. Update on adrenal tumours in 2017 World Health Organization (WHO) of endocrine tumours. Endocr Pathol 2017;28(3):213−27. https://doi.org/10.1007/s12022-017-9484-5.

[27] Koh JM, Ahn SH, Kim H, Kim BJ, Sung TY, Kim YH, et al. Validation of pathological grading systems for predicting metastatic potential in pheochromocytoma and paraganglioma. PLoS One 2017;12(11):e0187398. https://doi.org/10.1371/journal.pone.0187398.

[28] Pierre C, Agopiantz M, Brunaud L, Battaglia-Hsu S-F, Max A, Pouget C, Nomine C, Lomazzi S, Vignaud J-M, Weryha G, Oussalah A, Gauchotte G, Busby-Venner H. COPPS, a composite score integrating pathological features, PS100 and SDHB losses, predicts the risk of metastasis and progression-free survival in pheochromocytomas/paragangliomas. Virchows Arch 2019;474(6):721−34. https://doi.org/10.1007/s00428-019-02553-5.

[29] Thompson LDR. Pheochromocytoma of the adrenal gland scaled score (PASS) to separate benign from malignant neoplasms: a clinicopathologic and immunophenotypic study of 100 cases. Am J Surg Pathol 2002;26(5):551−66. https://doi.org/10.1097/00000478-200205000-00002.

[30] Kimura N, Takekoshi K, Naruse M. Risk stratification on pheochromocytoma and paraganglioma from laboratory and clinical medicine. J Clin Med 2018;7(9):242. https://doi.org/10.3390/jcm7090242.

[31] Geroula A, Deutschbein T, Langton K, Masjkur J, Pamporaki C, Peitzsch M, Fliedner S, Timmers HJLM, Bornstein SR, Beuschlein F, Stell A, Januszewicz A, Prejbisz A, Fassnacht M, Lenders JWM, Eisenhofer G. Pheochromocytoma and paraganglioma: clinical feature-based disease probability in relation to catecholamine biochemistry and reason for disease suspicion. Eur J Endocrinol 2019;181(4):409−20. https://doi.org/10.1530/EJE-19-0159.

[32] Soltani A, Pourian M, Davani BM. Does this patient have pheochromocytoma? A systematic review of clinical signs and symptoms. J Diabetes Metab Disord 2016;15(1):6. https://doi.org/10.1186/S40200-016-0226-x.

[33] Falhammar H, Kjellman M, Calissendorff J. Initial clinical presentation and spectrum of pheochromocytoma: a study of 94 cases from a single center. Endocr Connect 2018;7(1):186−92. https://doi.org/10.1530/EC-17-0321.

[34] Thomas RM. Endocrine hypertension: an overview on the current etiopathogenesis and management options. World J Hypertens 2015;5(2):14. https://doi.org/10.5494/wjh.v5.i2.14.

[35] Baguet JP, Hammer L, Mazzuco TL, Chabre O, Mallion JM, Sturm N, Chaffanjon P. Circumstances of discovery of phaeochromocytoma: a retrospective study of 41 consecutive patients. Eur J Endocrinol 2004;150(5):681−6. https://doi.org/10.1530/eje.0.1500681.

[36] Bratslavsky G, Sokol ES, Daneshvar M, Necchi A, Shapiro O, Jacob J, Liu N, Sanford TS, Pinkhasov R, Goldberg H, Killian JK, Ramkissoon S, Severson EA, Huang RSP, Danziger N, Mollapour M, Ross JS, Pacak K. Clinically advanced pheochromocytomas and paragangliomas: a comprehensive genomic profiling study. Cancers 2021;13(13):3312. https://doi.org/10.3390/cancers13133312.

[37] Lenders JWM, Duh QY, Eisenhofer G, Gimenez-Roqueplo AP, Grebe SKG, Murad MH, Naruse M, Pacak K, Young WF. Pheochromocytoma and paraganglioma: an endocrine society clinical practice guideline. J Clin Endocrinol Metab 2014;99(6):1915–42. https://doi.org/10.1210/jc.2014-1498.

[38] Chen Y, Xiao H, Zhou X, Huang X, Li Y, Xiao H, Cao X. Accuracy of plasma free metanephrines in the diagnosis of pheochromocytoma and paraganglioma: a systematic review and meta-analysis. Endocr Pract 2017;23(10):1169–77. https://doi.org/10.4158/EP171877.OR.

[39] Eisenhofer G, Prejbisz A, Peitzsch M, Pamporaki C, Masjkur J, Rogowski-Lehmann N, Langton K, Tsourdi E, Peczkowska M, Fliedner S, Deutschbein T, Megerle F, Timmers HJLM, Sinnott R, Beuschlein F, Fassnacht M, Januszewicz A, Lenders JWM. Biochemical diagnosis of chromaffin cell tumors in patients at high and low risk of disease: plasma versus urinary free or deconjugated o-methylated catecholamine metabolites. Clin Chem 2018;64(11):1646–56. https://doi.org/10.1373/clinchem.2018.291369.

[40] Mullins F, O'Shea P, FitzGerald R, Tormey W. Enzyme-linked immunoassay for plasma-free metanephrines in the biochemical diagnosis of phaeochromocytoma in adults is not ideal. Clin Chem Lab Med 2012;50(1):105–10. https://doi.org/10.1515/CCLM.2011.742.

[41] Plouin PF, Amar L, Dekkers OM, Fassnacht M, Gimenez-Roqueplo AP, Lenders JWM, Lussey-Lepoutre C, Steichen O. European Society of Endocrinology Clinical Practice Guideline for long-term follow-up of patients operated on for a phaeochromocytoma or a paraganglioma. Eur J Endocrinol 2016;174(5):G1–10. https://doi.org/10.1530/EJE-16-0033.

[42] Liu L, Xie W, Song Z, Wang T, Li X, Gao Y, Li Y, Zhang J, Guo X. Addition of 3-methoxytyramine or chromogranin A to plasma free metanephrines as the initial test for pheochromocytoma and paraganglioma: which is the best diagnostic strategy. Clin Endocrinol 2022;96(2):132–8. https://doi.org/10.1111/cen.14585.

[43] Rao D, Peitzsch M, Prejbisz A, Hanus K, Fassnacht M, Beuschlein F, Brugger C, Fliedner S, Langton K, Pamporaki C, Gudziol V, Stell A, Januszewicz A, Timmers HJLM, Lenders JWM, Eisenhofer G. Plasma methoxytyramine: clinical utility with metanephrines for diagnosis of pheochromocytoma and paraganglioma. Eur J Endocrinol 2017;177(2):103–13. https://doi.org/10.1530/EJE-17-0077.

[44] März J, Kurlbaum M, Roche-Lancaster O, Deutschbein T, Peitzsch M, Prehn C, et al. Plasma metabolome profiling for the diagnosis of catecholamine producing tumors. Front Endocrinol 2021;12:722656. https://doi.org/10.3389/fendo.2021.722656.

[45] Timmers HJLM, Pacak K, Huynh TT, Abu-Asab M, Tsokos M, Merino MJ, Baysal BE, Adams KT, Eisenhofer G. Biochemically silent abdominal paragangliomas in patients with mutations in the succinate dehydrogenase subunit B gene. J Clin Endocrinol Metab 2008;93(12):4826–32. https://doi.org/10.1210/jc.2008-1093.

[46] Pamporaki C, Prejbisz A, Małecki R, Pistrosch F, Peitzsch M, Bishoff S, Mueller P, Meyer I, Reimann D, Hanus K, Januszewicz A, Bornstein SR, Parmentier S, Kunath C, Lenders JWM, Eisenhofer G, Passauer J. Optimized reference intervals for plasma free metanephrines in patients with CKD. Am J Kidney Dis 2018;72(6):907–9. https://doi.org/10.1053/j.ajkd.2018.06.018.

[47] Lenders JWM, Pacak K, Walther MM, Linehan WM, Mannelli M, Friberg P, Keiser HR, Goldstein DS, Eisenhofer G. Biochemical diagnosis of pheochromocytoma: which test is best? JAMA 2002;287(11):1427–34.

[48] Amar L, Eisenhofer G. Diagnosing phaeochromocytoma/paraganglioma in a patient presenting with critical illness: biochemistry versus imaging. Clin Endocrinol 2015;83(3):298–302. https://doi.org/10.1111/cen.12745.

[49] Ku EJ, Kim KJ, Kim JH, Kim MK, Ahn CH, Lee KA, et al. Diagnosis for pheochromocytoma and paraganglioma: A joint position statement of the Korean pheochromocytoma and paraganglioma task force. Endocrinol Metab (Seoul) 2021 Apr;36(2):322–38. https://doi.org/10.3803/EnM.2020.908.

[50] Buitenwerf E, Korteweg T, Visser A, Haag CMSC, Feelders RA, Timmers HJLM, Canu L, Haak HR, Bisschop PHLT, Eekhoff EMW, Corssmit EPM, Krak NC, Rasenberg E, Van Den Bergh J, Stoker J, Greuter MJW, Dullaart RPF, Links TP, Kerstens MN. Unenhanced CT imaging is highly sensitive to exclude pheochromocytoma: a multicenter study. Eur J Endocrinol 2018;178(5):431–7. https://doi.org/10.1530/EJE-18-0006.

[51] Canu L, Van Hemert JAW, Kerstens MN, Hartman RP, Khanna A, Kraljevic I, et al. CT Characteristics of Pheochromocytoma: Relevance for the Evaluation of Adrenal Incidentaloma. J Clin Endocrinol Metab 2019 Feb 1;104(2):312–8. https://doi.org/10.1210/jc.2018-01532.

[52] Raja A, Leung K, Stamm M, Girgis S, Low G. Multimodality imaging findings of pheochromocytoma with associated clinical and biochemical features in 53 patients with histologically confirmed tumors. Am J Roentgenol 2013;201(4):825–33. https://doi.org/10.2214/AJR.12.9576.

[53] Mozley PD, Kim CK, Mohsin J, Jatlow A, Gosfield E, Alavi A. The efficacy of iodine-123-MIBG as a screening test for pheochromocytoma. J Nucl Med 1994;35(7):1138–44.

[54] Solanki KK, Bomanji J, Moyes J, Mather SJ, Trainer PJ, Britton KE. A pharmacological guide to medicines which interfere with the biodistribution of radiolabelled meta-iodobenzylguanidine (MIBG). Nucl Med Commun 1992;13(7):513–21. https://doi.org/10.1097/00006231-199207000-00006.

[55] Rao D, Berkel A, Piscaer I, Young W, Gruber L, Deutschbein T, et al. Impact of 123 I-MIBG scintigraphy on clinical decision making in pheochromocytoma and paraganglioma. J Clin Endocrinol Metab 2019;104:3812–20. https://doi.org/10.1210/jc.2018-02355.

[56] Shulkin BL, Thompson NW, Shapiro B, Francis IR, Sisson JC. Pheochromocytomas: imaging with 2-[fluorine-18]fluoro-2-deoxy-D-glucose PET. Radiology 1999;212(1):35–41. https://doi.org/10.1148/radiology.212.1.r99jl3035.

[57] Timmers HJLM, Chen CC, Carrasquillo JA, Whatley M, Ling A, Eisenhofer G, King KS, Rao JU, Wesley RA, Adams KT, Pacak K. Staging and functional characterization of pheochromocytoma and paraganglioma by 18F-fluorodeoxyglucose (18F-FDG) positron emission tomography. J Natl Cancer Inst 2012;104(9):700–8. https://doi.org/10.1093/jnci/djs188.

[58] Han S, Suh CH, Woo S, Kim YJ, Lee JJ. Performance of 68 Ga-DOTA–conjugated somatostatin receptor–targeting peptide PET in detection of pheochromocytoma and paraganglioma: a systematic review and metaanalysis. J Nucl Med 2019;60(3):369–76. https://doi.org/10.2967/jnumed.118.211706.

[59] Gild ML, Naik N, Hoang J, Hsiao E, McGrath RT, Sywak M, Sidhu S, Delbridge LW, Robinson BG, Schembri G, Clifton-Bligh RJ. Role of DOTATATE-PET/CT in preoperative assessment of phaeochromocytoma and paragangliomas. Clin Endocrinol 2018;89(2):139−47. https://doi.org/10.1111/cen.13737.

[60] Taïeb D, Pacak K. Molecular imaging and theranostic approaches in pheochromocytoma and paraganglioma. Cell Tissue Res 2018;372(2):393−401. https://doi.org/10.1007/s00441-018-2791-4.

[61] Archier A, Varoquaux A, Garrigue P, Montava M, Guerin C, Gabriel S, Beschmout E, Morange I, Fakhry N, Castinetti F, Sebag F, Barlier A, Loundou A, Guillet B, Pacak K, Taïeb D. Prospective comparison of 68Ga-DOTATATE and 18F-FDOPA PET/CT in patients with various pheochromocytomas and paragangliomas with emphasis on sporadic cases. Eur J Nucl Med Mol Imag 2016;43(7):1248−57. https://doi.org/10.1007/s00259-015-3268-2.

[62] Jha A, Ling A, Millo C, Chen C, Gonzales M, Patel M, et al. Diagnostic performance of PET/CT utilizing 68Ga-DOTATATE, 18F-FDG, 18F-DOPA, and 18F-FDA, and anatomic imaging in the detection of sporadic primary pheochromocytoma - a comparative prospective study. J Nucl Med 2019;60(Suppl 1):439.

[63] Jha A, Patel M, Carrasquillo JA, Ling A, Millo C, Saboury B, Chen CC, Wakim P, Gonzales MK, Meuter L, Knue M, Talvacchio S, Herscovitch P, Rivero JD, Chen AP, Nilubol N, Taïeb D, Lin FI, Civelek AC, Pacak K. F-FDA. AJR Am J Roentgenol 2022;218(2):342−50. https://doi.org/10.2214/AJR.21.26071.

[64] Kumar S, Lila AR, Memon SS, Sarathi V, Patil VA, Menon S, Mittal N, Prakash G, Malhotra G, Shah NS, Bandgar TR. Metastatic cluster 2-related pheochromocytoma/paraganglioma: a single-center experience and systematic review. Endocr Connect 2021;10(11):1463−76. https://doi.org/10.1530/ec-21-0455.

[65] Ben Aim L, Pigny P, Castro-Vega LJ, Buffet A, Amar L, Bertherat J, Drui D, Guilhem I, Baudin E, Lussey-Lepoutre C, Corsini C, Chabrier G, Briet C, Faivre L, Cardot-Bauters C, Favier J, Gimenez-Roqueplo A-P, Burnichon N. Targeted next-generation sequencing detects rare genetic events in pheochromocytoma and paraganglioma. J Med Genet 2019;56(8):513−20. https://doi.org/10.1136/jmedgenet-2018-105714.

[66] Ross JJ, Desai AS, Chutkow WA, Economy KE, Dec GW. Interactive medical case. A crisis in late pregnancy. N Engl J Med 2009;361(20):e45. https://doi.org/10.1056/NEJMimc0806409.

[67] Buitenwerf E, Osinga TE, Timmers HJLM, Lenders JWM, Feelders RA, Eekhoff EMW, Haak HR, Corssmit EPM, Bisschop PHLT, Valk GD, Veldman RG, Dullaart RPF, Links TP, Voogd MF, Wietasch GJKG, Kerstens MN. Efficacy of α-blockers on hemodynamic control during pheochromocytoma resection: a randomized controlled trial. J Clin Endocrinol Metab 2020;105(7):2381−91. https://doi.org/10.1210/clinem/dgz188.

[68] Galati SJ, Said M, Gospin R, Babic N, Brown K, Geer EB, Kostakoglu L, Krakoff LR, Leibowitz AB, Mehta L, Muller S, Owen RP, Pertsemlidis DS, Wilck E, Xiao GQ, Levine AC, Inabnet WB. The Mount Sinai clinical pathway for the management of pheochromocytoma. Endocr Pract Off J Am Coll Endocrinol Am Assoc Clin Endocrinol 2015;21(4):368−82. https://doi.org/10.4158/EP14036.RA.

[69] Castinetti F, Qi XP, Walz MK, Maia AL, Sansó G, Peczkowska M, et al. Outcomes of adrenal-sparing surgery or total adrenalectomy in phaeochromocytoma associated with multiple endocrine neoplasia type 2: an international retrospective population-based study. Lancet Oncol 2014;15(6):648−55. https://doi.org/10.1016/S1470-2045(14)70154-8.

[70] Hue JJ, Ahorukomeye P, Bingmer K, Drapalik L, Ammori JB, Wilhelm SM, et al. A comparison of robotic and laparoscopic minimally invasive adrenalectomy for adrenal malignancies. Surg Endosc 2022 Jul;36(7):5374-5381. 2022;36(7):5374−81. https://doi.org/10.1007/s00464-021-08827-x.

[71] Roman-Gonzalez A, Zhou S, Ayala-Ramirez M, Shen C, Waguespack SG, Habra MA, Karam JA, Perrier N, Wood CG, Jimenez C. Impact of surgical resection of the primary tumor on overall survival in patients with metastatic pheochromocytoma or sympathetic paraganglioma. Ann Surg 2018;268(1):172−8. https://doi.org/10.1097/SLA.0000000000002195.

[72] Arnas-Leon C, Sánchez V, Santana Suárez AD, Quintana Arroyo S, Acosta C, Martinez Martin FJ. Complete remission in metastatic pheochromocytoma treated with extensive surgery. Cureus 2016;8(1):e447. https://doi.org/10.7759/cureus.447.

[73] Breen W, Bancos I, Young WF, Bible KC, Laack NN, Foote RL, Hallemeier CL. External beam radiation therapy for advanced/unresectable malignant paraganglioma and pheochromocytoma. Adv Radiat Oncol 2018;3(1):25−9. https://doi.org/10.1016/j.adro.2017.11.002.

[74] Averbuch SD, Steakley CS, Young RC, Gelmann EP, Goldstein DS, Stull R, Keiser HR. Malignant pheochromocytoma: effective treatment with a combination of cyclophosphamide, vincristine, and dacarbazine. Ann Intern Med 1988;109(4):267−73. https://doi.org/10.7326/0003-4819-109-4-267.

[75] Tanabe A, Naruse M, Nomura K, Tsuiki M, Tsumagari A, Ichihara A. Combination chemotherapy with cyclophosphamide, vincristine, and dacarbazine in patients with malignant pheochromocytoma and paraganglioma. Horm Cancer 2013;4(2):103−10. https://doi.org/10.1007/s12672-013-0133-2.

[76] Hadoux J, Favier J, Scoazec JY, Leboulleux S, Ghuzlan AA, Caramella C, Deandreis D, Borget I, Loriot C, Chougnet C, Letouze E, Young J, Amar L, Bertherat J, Libe R, Dumont F, Deschamps F, Schlumberger M, Gimenez-Roqueplo AP, Baudin E. SDHB mutations are associated with response to temozolomide in patients with metastatic pheochromocytoma or paraganglioma. Int J Cancer 2014;135(11):2711−20. https://doi.org/10.1002/ijc.28913.

[77] Thorpe MP, Kane A, Zhu J, Morse MA, Wong T, Borges-Neto S. Long-term outcomes of 125 patients with metastatic pheochromocytoma or paraganglioma treated with 131-I MIBG. J Clin Endocrinol Metab 2020;105(3):dgz074. https://doi.org/10.1210/clinem/dgz074.

[78] Ziegler CG, Brown JW, Schally AV, Erler A, Gebauer L, Treszl A, Young L, Fishman LM, Engel JB, Willenberg HS, Petersenn S, Eisenhofer G, Ehrhart-Bornstein M, Bornstein SR. Expression of neuropeptide hormone receptors in human adrenal tumors and cell lines: antiproliferative effects of peptide analogues. Proc Natl Acad Sci U S A 2009;106(37):15879−84. https://doi.org/10.1073/pnas.0907843106.

[79] Nastos K, Cheung VTF, Toumpanakis C, Navalkissoor S, Quigley AM, Caplin M, Khoo B. Peptide Receptor Radionuclide Treatment and (131)I-MIBG in the management of patients with metastatic/progressive phaeochromocytomas and paragangliomas. J Surg Oncol 2017;115(4):425−34. https://doi.org/10.1002/jso.24553.

[80] Ayala-Ramirez M, Chougnet CN, Habra MA, Palmer JL, Leboulleux S, Cabanillas ME, Caramella C, Anderson P, Al Ghuzlan A, Waguespack SG, Deandreis D, Baudin E, Jimenez C. Treatment with sunitinib for patients with progressive metastatic pheochromocytomas and sympathetic paragangliomas. J Clin Endocrinol Metab 2012;97(11):4040−50. https://doi.org/10.1210/jc.2012-2356.

[81] Wells SA, Asa SL, Dralle H, Elisei R, Evans DB, Gagel RF, Lee N, MacHens A, Moley JF, Pacini F, Raue F, Frank-Raue K, Robinson B, Rosenthal MS, Santoro M, Schlumberger M, Shah M, Waguespack SG. Revised American thyroid association guidelines for the management of medullary thyroid carcinoma. Thyroid 2015;25(6):567−610. https://doi.org/10.1089/thy.2014.0335.

[82] Geurts JL, Strong EA, Wang TS, Evans DB, Clarke CN. Screening guidelines and recommendations for patients at high risk of developing endocrine cancers. J Surg Oncol 2020;121(6):975−83. https://doi.org/10.1002/jso.25869.

[83] Dwight T, Flynn A, Amarasinghe K, Benn DE, Lupat R, Li J, Cameron DL, Hogg A, Balachander S, Candiloro ILM, Wong SQ, Robinson BG, Papenfuss AT, Gill AJ, Dobrovic A, Hicks RJ, Clifton-Bligh RJ, Tothill RW. TERT structural rearrangements in metastatic pheochromocytomas. Endocr Relat Cancer 2018;25(1):1−9. https://doi.org/10.1530/ERC-17-0306.

[84] Job S, Draskovic I, Burnichon N, Buffet A, Cros J, Lépine C, Venisse A, Robidel E, Verkarre V, Meatchi T, Sibony M, Amar L, Bertherat J, de Reyniès A, Londoño-Vallejo A, Favier J, Castro-Vega LJ, Gimenez-Roqueplo A-P. Telomerase activation and ATRX mutations are independent risk factors for metastatic pheochromocytoma and paraganglioma. Clin Cancer Res 2019;25(2):760−70. https://doi.org/10.1158/1078-0432.ccr-18-0139.

[85] Monteagudo M, Martínez P, Leandro-García LJ, Martínez-Montes Á M, Calsina B, Pulgarín-Alfaro M, et al. Analysis of telomere maintenance related genes reveals NOP10 as a new metastatic-risk marker in pheochromocytoma/paraganglioma. Cancers (Basel) 2021;13(19):4758. https://doi.org/10.3390/cancers13194758.

[86] Bayley JP, Devilee P. Advances in paraganglioma-pheochromocytoma cell lines and xenografts. Endocr Relat Cancer 2020;27(12):R433−50. https://doi.org/10.1530/ERC-19-0434.

[87] Benn DE, Zhu Y, Andrews KA, Wilding M, Duncan EL, Dwight T, et al. Bayesian approach to determining penetrance of pathogenic SDH variants. J Med Genet 2018;55(11):729−34. https://doi.org/10.1136/jmedgenet-2018-105427.

[88] White G, Velusamy A, Anandappa S, Masucci M, Breen LA, Joshi M, et al. Tumour detection and outcomes of surveillance screening in SDHB and SDHD pathogenic variant carriers. Endocr Connect 11(2):e210602 2022;11(2):e210602. https://doi.org/10.1530/ec-21-0602.

Chapter 12

Paragangliomas and hypertension

Tomáš Zelinka and Ondřej Petrák

Department of Medicine — Department of Endocrinology and Metabolism, General Faculty Hospital and First Faculty of Medicine, Charles University in Prague, Prague, Czech Republic

Visit the *Endocrine Hypertension: From Basic Science to Clinical Practice, First Edition* companion web site at: https://www.elsevier.com/books-and-journals/book-companion/9780323961202.

Graphical Abstract

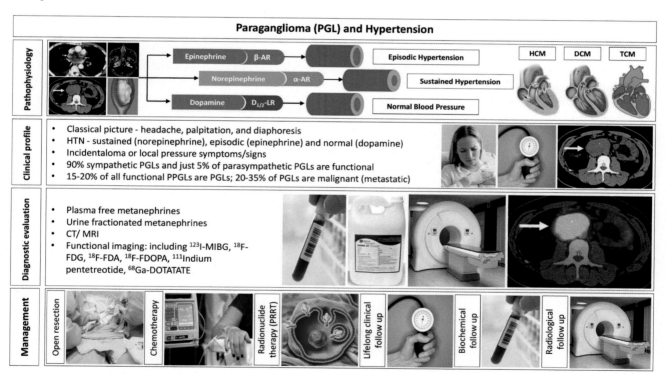

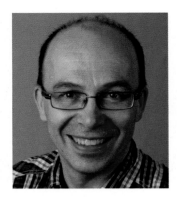

Tomáš Zelinka

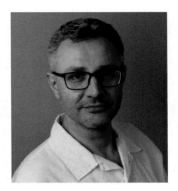

Ondřej Petrák

Introduction

Paragangliomas (PGLs) are rare neuroendocrine tumors that arise from the extra-adrenal autonomic paraganglia, a diffuse neuroendocrine system dispersed from the skull base to the pelvic floor, derived from the embryonic neural crest cells [1–3]. Paragangliomas arising from the sympathetic ganglia of the thorax, abdomen and pelvis may be catecholamine secreting, and form 15%–20% of the PPGLs (pheochromocytomas and paragangliomas), whereas paragangliomas originating from the parasympathetic ganglia of the head and neck region (HNPGLs) are often nonsecretary. While hypertension is present in the vast majority (95%) of patients with adrenal pheochromocytomas, the extraadrenal sympathetic PGLs of the thorax, abdomen and pelvis may not always present with hypertension. For example, dopamine secreting PPGLs usually present without hypertension [4]. There are distinct differences between the adrenal pheochromocytomas and the extraadrenal PGLs in the clinical presentation, genetic characteristics, malignant potentials, management algorithms, and prognostic factors [1,5]. We outline an evidence-based review of the epidemiology, pathophysiology, genetics, clinical characteristics, diagnostic algorithms, and therapeutic aspects of PGLs in this chapter.

Epidemiology of paragangliomas and hypertension

Parasympathetic paragangliomas of the head and neck (HNPGLs) arise from the autonomic ganglia located along the glossopharyngeal and vagal nerves in the neck and at the base of the skull, and rarely within the anterior mediastinum [1]. Generally, there are four distinct areas for the HNPGLs — carotid body, vagal, middle ear, and the larynx [6]. The commonest among the HNPGLs are the carotid body tumors (CBTs) and are followed by jugulotympanic PGLs (JTPGLs) and vagal PGLs (VPGLs). This is followed by PGLs of larynx, trachea, thyroid, orbit, and nasal cavity [7]. These tumor cells are chromaffin-negative (meaning that they do not stain brown when exposed to potassium dichromate), and usually do not secrete catecholamines. Only up to 4% of HNPGLs are functional, and produce clinically significant levels of catecholamines [8].

An estimated annual clinical incidence of HNPGL is 1/100,000 persons and is most frequently diagnosed in middle-aged adults (mean age 40–50 years), with equal frequency in men and women in hereditary forms, but the sporadic form is more common in women (Table 12.1) [9]. The association of chronic hypoxia in the development of carotid body PGL (the older term chemodectoma or CBT) is well known, with a higher incidence in people living at high altitudes, and in the setting of chronic obstructive pulmonary disease [10]. Genetic cases are more than a decade younger, and often multifocal [11]. A positive family history increases the risk of multifocality: up to 78% of the cases with a positive family history and 17%–37% of the unselected cases are multicentric [12]. In a large series, evidence of malignancy has been found in 3%–5% of HNPGL cases, with a lower risk for carotid body and middle ear HNPGLs (2%–6%) and a higher risk for vagal paragangliomas (16%) [6].

Sympathetic PGLs are chromaffin-positive tumors located in the sympathetic paravertebral ganglia of the thorax, abdomen, and pelvis that generally synthesize, store, and secrete catecholamines. They are also known as functional PGLs. Because the clinical patterns of PGLs are commonly described together with those of pheochromocytomas, the specific incidence of functional PGLs is largely unknown. The incidence of PGLs is estimated at 1/300,000 and is diagnosed in the third to fifth decades, with no gender differences. A nationwide study of PPGLs in the Netherlands revealed age-

TABLE 12.1 Clinical and pathologic features of head and neck paragangliomas (HNPGLs) divided by anatomic site.

	Carotid body PGL	Vagal PGL	Middle ear PGL	Laryngeal PGL
Localization	Carotid body	Along the nerve and nodose ganglion	Adventitia of jugular bulb or along the middle ear medial promontory wall	Superior/supraglottic (80%) and inferior paired paraganglion
Percentage	60	10	30	Very rare
Mean age	50–60	50	60	40–60
Female: Male	2:1 (8:1 at high altitudes)	2:1–8:1	3:1–9:1	3:1
Clinical symptoms	Asymptomatic	70% asymptomatic, <4% clinically functional	Pulsatile tinnitus, hearing loss, aural fullness	Dyspnea, hoarseness, stridor
Bilateral/ multifocal	10–25%	16%	2%	2%
Hereditary	~33%	~33%	~33%	Unknown

From Williams MD. Paragangliomas of the head and neck: an overview from diagnosis to genetics. Head Neck Pathol. 2017;11(3):278–87. https://doi.org/10.1007/s12105-017-0803-4.

standardized incidence rates for PGLs at 0.11 (95% CI: 0.09–0.13) per 100,000 person-years [13]. Similar to HNPGLs, hereditary paragangliomas tend to develop disease about a decade earlier than in the sporadic form [11]. However, the incidence of these tumors is much higher at autopsy (~0.05%), probably due to the often-asymptomatic clinical course [14]. Of these neuroendocrine tumors (PPGLs), 80%–85% are pheochromocytomas, and 15%–20% are PGLs [15]. The vast majority of functional PGLs (70%–80%) arises from the infradiaphragmatic sympathetic ganglia in the abdomen, most often at the junction of the vena cava and the left renal vein, or at the organ of Zuckerkandl located near the origin of the inferior mesenteric artery at the aortic bifurcation. It is less frequently found in the retroperitoneal area around the kidney and adrenal, and in the bladder. Approximately 10% of PGLs are in the mediastinal and pericardial locations within the thorax. Sympathetic PGLs can very rarely also arise in the thyroid gland, adjacent to the thoracic spine, and at the level of the cauda equina [8].

About 26% of PGLs are multiple, and one-third to one-half are associated with a hereditary syndrome. Multiplicity is far more common in hereditary cases [16]. The incidence of malignancy depends on the genetic background and anatomical location [17]. Approximately 20% of the secretory PGLs (abdominal and mediastinal) are malignant. The highest malignancy rates are seen in PGLs associated with *SDHB* mutation, which are usually abdominal and secretory [17].

Pathophysiology of paraganglioma and hypertension

There exists distinct secretory pathways in PPGLs. Eisenhofer *et al.* showed that the norepinephrine-producing tumor is associated with less maturity of chromaffin cells with a constitutive form of secretion, and a reduced response to secretagogue stimuli, whereas the epinephrine-producing tumor is related to a regulated secretory pathway and higher sensitivity to various stimuli [18]. Chromaffin cells of the secreting PGLs do not have the ability to produce epinephrine, compared to the adrenal medulla, due to a lack of the relevant enzyme machinery.

Norepinephrine acts primarily on alpha-adrenoceptors and induces vasoconstriction of vessels, volume contraction with an increased peripheral vascular resistance, and leads to sustained arterial hypertension [4]. Dopamine targets D_1 and D_2 dopaminergic receptors. Activation of D_1 receptors results in vasodilation of the renal arteries, while D2 activation will inhibit norepinephrine secretion from sympathetic nerve terminals and have a mild negative inotropic effect on the heart [19]. The signaling net result would explain the clinical phenomenon of lack of hypertension and palpitations in patients with dopamine secreting PGLs.

While normal levels of dopamine do not affect the adrenergic receptors, it can stimulate both α and β adrenoceptors when dopamine increases in the circulation, as in the case of tumors that exclusively secrete dopamine. Dopamine overproduction may be due to further tumor dedifferentiation and may indicate a malignant potential for PGLs [17].

Desensitization of adrenergic receptors has always been a hot topic in both research and clinical care. There have been numerous studies that reported significant desensitization of both α and β adrenergic receptors in either healthy humans or patients with PPGLs as well as in animal models [19].

Genetics of paragangliomas

PGLs are tumors which present with a high degree of heritability, perhaps the highest among other cancers. More than 40% of cases may carry a germline mutation—its prevalence depends mostly on the population studied: for example, it is very high in the Netherlands, due to the presence of a founder mutation of the *SDHD* gene. During the last 2 decades, more than 20 susceptibility genes associated with the development of PGLs or pheochromocytoma have been identified. According to the Cancer Genome Atlas, these genes were divided into three distinct molecular groups: Pseudohypoxia-related (Cluster 1), and Kinase signaling-related (Cluster 2), and Wnt-related (Cluster 3) [20,21]. Unlike pheochromocytoma, which is associated with gene mutations of all three groups, the vast majority of PGLs is caused by mutations of the Cluster 1-related genes. Only a few PGL cases have been published in the kinase signaling group and none in the Cluster 3 [22].

The pseudohypoxic group is characterized by activation of pathways which mimic hypoxia signaling. It is divided into two subgroups—according to the position of the gene mutation, either in the Krebs cycle (Cluster 1A) or the hypoxia-signaling pathway (Cluster 1B). Cluster 1A-related genes include succinate dehydrogenase subunits (*SDHx*), succinate dehydrogenase complex assembly factor 2 (*SDHAF2*), fumarate hydrogenase (*FH*), malate dehydrogenase 2 (*MDH2*), mitochondrial glutamic-oxaloacetic transaminase (*GOT2*), 2-oxoglutarate-malate carrier (*SLC25A11*), dihydrolipoamide S-succinyl transferase (*DLST*), and isocitrate dehydrogenase1 (*IDH1*). The Cluster 1B-related group consists of mutations of Egl-9 prolyl hydroxylase-1 and -2 (*EGLN1/2* encoding PHD1/2), von Hippel−Lindau (*VHL*) tumor suppressor, hypoxia-inducible factor 2α (*HIF2A/EPAS1*) and iron regulatory protein 1 (*IRP1*) genes [20]. Moreover, mutations in other genes associated with PGLs (alone or in combination with pheochromocytoma), such as genes involved in DNA hypermethylation: histone subunit gene (*H3F3A*) [23], and DNA methyltransferase (*DNMT3A*), have been described [24].

In Cluster 2, PGLs were described in a few subjects with multiple endocrine neoplasia type 2 [mutation in the rearranged-during-transfection (*RET*) proto-oncogene], or with mutation in the *MERTK* gene [24]. Interestingly, somatic mutations of the *HRAS* and *FGFR1* genes were described predominantly in Chinese patients with epinephrine producing PGLs, but not in the European population [25].

In contrast to pheochromocytoma (Cluster 2-related genes), in which mutations of involved genes may occur as germline or somatic, most PGLs-related mutations are reported only as germline (except for Cluster 1B-related, which are more frequently somatic). Underlining mutations predispose its carrier to specific tumor development (HNPGLs or sympathetic PGLs), metastatic or multifocal involvement, disease penetration, and other syndrome-related tumors (Table 12.2).

All subjects with PGLs should be involved in the discussion about genetic testing, irrespective of age or tumor location. This is performed using next-generation sequencing, either on DNA acquired from peripheral blood or buccal swab or, more recently, from tumor tissue. The latter approach enables not only the germline mutations (mutation found in tumorous and peripheral DNA) to be identified, but also somatic mutations (mutation found only in tumorous DNA) [2,26]. Another way of screening for *SDHx* mutations is *SDHA/SDHB* immunohistochemistry [27]. Genetic testing allows earlier detection of primary tumors or metastases, and has a positive impact on the prognosis of subjects with *SDHx* or *VHL* mutation [28]. Screening for tumors should be started between 6 and 10 years of age in asymptomatic *SDHB* mutation carriers (first PGLs reported at the age of 6), and between 10 and 15 years in *SDHA, SDHC* and *SDHD* mutation carriers [29].

Compared to *SDHD* mutation carriers, which have a normal standardized mortality ratio (SMR) even in affected subjects, *SDHB* mutation carriers have an increased mortality rate (SMR of 1.89 increasing to 2.88 in subjects with PGLs), due to susceptibility for metastatic disease [30].

Clinical presentation

Paragangliomas are clinically heterogenous in their presentation [31]. Initial symptoms vary widely and can be caused by local growth. HNPGLs typically present as slow-growing, painless lateral neck masses [6,32]. In advanced disease, there can be hoarseness, dysphonia, dysphagia, hearing loss, shoulder weakness/pain, and dysarthria. Horner's syndrome and facial paralysis may be present due to the involvement of the cranial (VII and IX−XII) or cervical nerves. Pulsatile tinnitus

TABLE 12.2 Paraganglioma-associated clusters, genes, and syndromes and its clinical characteristics.

Gene	Type	Germline/Somatic	Inheritance	Syndrome	Presentation					Lifetime penetrance	Biochemical phenotype	PET	Other presentation
					HNPGL	TPGL	APPGL	PHEO	Metastases				
Pseudohypoxic—Tricarboxylic acid cycle—related													
SDHA (succinate dehydrogenase complex flavoprotein subunit A)	TS	Germline	AD	FPGL5	+	+	+	+	++	1.7%	NA/D	68Ga-DOTATATE PET/CT	GIST, pituitary adenomas, pulmonary chordomas, RCC[a]
SDHB (succinate dehydrogenase complex iron sulfur subunit B)	TS	Germline	AD	FPGL4	++	++	+++	+	+++	22%	NA/D	68Ga-DOTATATE PET/CT	
SDHC (succinate dehydrogenase complex subunit C)	TS	Germline	AD	FPGL3	++	+/-	+	+/-	+	8.3%	NA/D	68Ga-DOTATATE PET/CT	
SDHD (succinate dehydrogenase complex subunit D)	TS	Germline	AD, paternal	FPGL1	+++ (multifocal)	+	+	+	+	43,2%[b]	NA/D	68Ga-DOTATATE PET/CT	
SDHAF2 (succinate dehydrogenase complex assembly factor 2)	TS	Germline	AD, paternal	FPGL2	+++ (multifocal)	+/-	+/-	+/-	-		NA/D	68Ga-DOTATATE PET/CT	
FH (fumarate hydratase)	TS	Germline	AD		+/-		+	+	+		NA/D	18F-DOPA PET/CT	Leiomyomatosis, RCC
Pseudohypoxic group—VHL/EPAS													
VHL (von Hippel–Lindau tumor suppressor)	TS	Germline/Somatic	AD	Von Hippel-Lindau	+/-	+/-	+/-	+++ (bilateral)	+/-	15%–20%	NA	18F-DOPA PET/CT	Hemangioblastoma, RCC, epididymal cystadenoma, pancreatic Neuroendocrine tumors, retinal Abnormalities
EPAS 1 (Endothelial PAS domain protein 1)	OG	Postzygotic/ somatic		Pacák-Zhuang	+/-	+	+++	+++	+		NA	18F-DOPA PET/CT	Polycythemia, somatostatinoma, retinal abnormalities, organ cysts

AD, autosomal dominant; APPGL, abdominopelvic paraganglioma, D, dopamine or methoxytyramine; FPGL, familial paraganglioma syndrome; GIST, gastrointestinal stromal tumor; HNPGL, head and neck paraganglioma; NA, norepinephrine or normetanephrine; OC, oncogen; PHEO, pheochromocytoma; RCC, renal cell carcinoma; TPGL, thoracic paraganglioma; TS, tumor suppressor.

[a]Patients with FPGL due to mutations of SDHA-SDHD genes may present with Carney Stratakis syndrome (PGL and GIST) or Carney syndrome (PGL, GIST and pulmonary chondroma).

[b]Penetrance by the age of 60.

Modified from Lenders JWM, Kerstens MN, Amar L, Prejbisz A, Robledo M, Taïeb D, Pacak K, Crona J, Zelinka T, Mannelli M, Deutschbein T, Timmers HJLM, Castinetti F, Dralle H, Widimský J, Gimenez-Roqueplo A-P, Eisenhofer G. Genetics, diagnosis, management and future directions of research of phaeochromocytoma and paraganglioma: a position statement and consensus of the Working Group on Endocrine Hypertension of the European Society of Hypertension. J Hypertens. 2020;38(8):1443–56. https://doi.org/10.1097/HJH.0000000000002438.

may also be appreciated on the side of the tumor, caused by the high-flow state due to hypervascularization. Physical examination often demonstrates a pulsatile lateral neck mass that is characteristically less mobile in the cephalocaudal direction, due to adherence to the carotid artery (Table 12.1) [33].

Another clinical attribute comes from catecholamine synthesis and release, which are inherently linked to cell differentiation. Functional PGLs secrete the catecholamines, norepinephrine and/or dopamine. In the case of norepinephrine overproduction, arterial hypertension is typical, either sustained or paroxysmal with characteristic, but nonspecific symptoms such as episodic headache, sweating, and palpitations [31]. Patients with pure norepinephrine phenotype usually present with sustained and more severe hypertension as compared to adrenergic subtypes [34]. Hypertension is very often characterized by an enhanced blood pressure (BP) variability, and impaired circadian BP rhythm [34,35]. Most patients with concomitant dopamine overproduction may be normotensive due to the vasodilatory actions of dopamine that might counteract the vasoconstrictor actions of norepinephrine. In patients with dopamine-secreting PGLs, tumors are usually discovered either as an incidental finding on imaging studies for an unrelated condition, or because of space-occupying complications of the lesions [36]. Primary tumors are generally larger, and often metastatic. Presumably, the attainment of a large size in such tumors, compared with those more usually encountered, reflects the relatively mild signs and symptoms associated with predominantly dopamine-secreting tumors [36]. Nausea, sometimes accompanied by vomiting, may be related to the emetic effects of dopamine [36]. Table 12.3 shows the variety of clinical symptoms and signs of PGLs [31].

Episodes of symptoms caused by PGLs can occur at any time. They can also be triggered by various stimuli as shown in Table 12.4.

TABLE 12.3 Clinical symptoms and signs of paragangliomas.

Organ system	Clinical signs and symptoms
Cardiovascular	Paroxysmal or sustained arterial hypertension Hypotension including postural hypotension Tachycardia Shortness of breath Chest pain Episodic syncope
Gastrointestinal	Obstipation Dry mouth Dysphagia Nausea and vomiting Abdominal pain
Neurologic	Tremors or shakiness Cephalgia Tingling of fingers
Psychiatric	Panic symptoms Fidgetiness
Musculoskeletal	Generalized fatigue
Urologic	Micturition symptoms
Skin	Diaphoresis (sweating) Extreme paleness in the face Clammy skin
Endocrine and metabolic	Hyperglycemia Weight loss Polyuria and polydipsia Fever

Lenders JW, Pacak K, Walther MM et al. Biochemical diagnosis of pheochromocytoma: which test is best? Jama 2002;287:1427−34.

TABLE 12.4 Conditions and factors that can trigger a catecholamine storm.

Physical activity

Physical injury and pain

Stress or anxiety

Drinking coffee

Medical procedures, such as anesthesia or surgery

Drugs
Dopamine (D2) receptor antagonists (including metoclopramide, tiapride), beta-blockers, sympathomimetics, opioid analgesics, antidepressants, corticosteroids, peptides (ACTH, glucagon) neuromuscular blocking agents

Eating food items high in tyramine, such as red wine, dried meats, chocolate, bananas, pineapples, peppers, and cheese

The act of micturition, in people with a PGLs in the bladder

Childbirth

Modified from Lenders JWM, Duh Q-Y, Eisenhofer G, Gimenez-Roqueplo A-P, Grebe SKG, Murad MH, Naruse M, Pacak K, Young WF. Pheochromocytoma and paraganglioma: an endocrine society clinical practice guideline. J Clin Endocrinol Metab. 2014;99(6):1915—42. https://doi.org/10.1210/jc.2014-1498.

Biochemical investigations

For diagnosis, it is necessary first to validate the overproduction of catecholamines and then only to proceed with tumor imaging. The gold standard is the measurement of plasma-free metanephrines (metanephrine, normetanephrine, 3-methoxytyramine), the inactive metabolites of catecholamines, which have a high sensitivity of 99% and an acceptable specificity of 89% [37].

The reason for testing plasma-free metanephrines is that these are produced continuously by the metabolism of catecholamines within tumor cells. This contrasts with episodic secretion of catecholamines by the normal adrenal gland [38]. Furthermore, sympathoadrenal excitation causes large increases in catecholamine release, whereas plasma-free metanephrines remain relatively unaffected [38]. Checking urinary vanillylmandelic acid (VMA) is obsolete; it reflects production in different parts of the body by metabolic processes not directly related to the tumor itself, and finally VMA is produced mainly in the liver.

In addition, urinary metanephrines can be determined. However, this test is more difficult and cumbersome for the patient, as a 24-hour urine collection is required, which must be acidified with hydrochloric acid [38].

There can be false elevation of plasma/urinary metanephrines in several situations. A list of drugs, substances, and conditions that affect metanephrine and catecholamine levels, leading to a false positive biochemical result is provided in Table 12.5.

Specific blood collection conditions must be ensured during blood sampling to avoid false-positives [39]. Collection is performed after insertion of a venous cannula and the patient should be lying down for a minimum of 20 min before collection, and during collection.

The determination of chromogranin A (CGA), located in the secretory vesicles of neurons and endocrine cells including chromaffin tissue, can also serve as an auxiliary marker [40]. Falsely elevated CGA levels are observed in patients treated with proton pump inhibitors (PPIs) or other acid-blocking medications. This effect of PPIs is fully eliminated after discontinuation of the PPI for 2 weeks [40].

Anatomical and functional imaging studies

Most sympathetic PGLs are diagnosed incidentally during examinations for other reasons. Unlike pheochromocytoma, PGLs are frequently not included in the differential diagnosis of incidentally discovered abdominal masses (mostly lymph nodes or other neurogenic tumors such as sarcomas are often taken into consideration) and may be only diagnosed either during operation or even during histopathology. In certain cases, biopsies are performed, which can be catastrophic in catecholamine-producing tumors. In the case of suspected sympathetic (elevated urine or plasma normetanephrine values) or HNPGLs, magnetic resonance imaging (MRI) may be advantageous because of better soft tissue contrast compared to computed tomography (CT). CT provides better spatial resolution, fewer motion artifacts, and better determination of

TABLE 12.5 Medications that may cause falsely elevated test results for plasma and urinary metanephrines.

Antidepressants	Selective serotonin reuptake inhibitors
	Serotonin-norepinephrine reuptake inhibitors
	Norepinephrine and specific serotonergic antidepressants
	Tricyclic antidepressants
	Serotonin antagonists and reuptake inhibitors
	Monoamine oxidase inhibitors
Antipsychotics	Lithium
Antiparkinsonics	Levodopa
Antihypertensives	Clonidine
	Methyldopa
	Reserpine
NSA	Acetaminophen
Steroids	Dexamethasone
Asthma medications	Aminophylline
	Theophylline
Antibiotics	Tetracycline
Drugs	Amphetamines
	Cocaine
Food and drink	Caffeine, alcohol, nicotine, bananas, pineapples, and peppers
Stressful condition	Various acute illnesses

From Lenders JWM, Duh Q-Y, Eisenhofer G, Gimenez-Roqueplo A-P, Grebe SKG, Murad MH, Naruse M, Pacak K, Young WF. Pheochromocytoma and paraganglioma: an endocrine society clinical practice guideline. J Clin Endocrinol Metab. 2014;99(6):1915—42. https://doi.org/10.1210/jc.2014-1498.

tumor extension into the temporal bone. Moreover, CT has better availability and lower costs, compared to MRI. MRI enables the detection of succinate using ^{1}H-nuclear magnetic resonance (NMR) spectrometry to confirm SDH-deficiency [41]. To protect from radiation exposure, MRI should be preferred in children and young females. Rapid-sequence noncontrast MRI from the skull base to the pelvis is very useful for lifelong tumor surveillance [42].

To confirm the diagnosis of suspected PGLs, functional imaging should be performed. It plays an irreplaceable role in evaluating the extent of PGLs (multifocal or metastatic involvement), and in monitoring the treatment effect (and for indication of radionuclide therapy—theranostic application) [2]. Functional imaging is also a part of initial screening in adult carriers of the mutation of the *SDHx* gene [29]. Positron emission tomography (PET)-based techniques are preferred to single photon emission computed tomography (SPECT), due to better spatial resolution.

^{68}Ga-DOTA-SSA (somatostatin analog) should be considered as tracer of choice for functional imaging of PGLs using PET/CT [43]. ^{68}Ga-DOTA-SSAs include DOTATOC [somatostatin receptors (SSTR) 2 and 5], DOTANOC (SSTRs 2, 3, and 5), and DOTATATE (SSTR 2), but only the latter is approved for use in the USA and in the European Union [44]. If not available, it can be substituted either with 99mTc-HYNIC-octreotide or ^{111}In-pentetreotide SPECT, especially if SSTR-based radionuclide therapy (PRRT) comes into consideration for management of the tumor. In vitro, PGLs express predominantly SSTR2 and SSTR3 [45]. Compared to other radiopharmaceuticals, ^{68}Ga-DOTA-SSA provides the best detection rate of lesions in sympathetic or parasympathetic PGLs, in particular *SDHx*-related (Table 12.2 and Fig. 12.1) [43]. Another diagnostic option is ^{18}F-FDOPA (not available in the USA), which is transported into PGL cells via large neutral amino acid transporter 1 and further sequestered into secretory vesicles via vesicular monoamine transporters [44]. It provides very good results in HNPGLs (Fig. 12.2), but shows low sensitivity in less differentiated PGLs, such as those with *SDHB* mutation. The exceptions to the rule are very rare PGLs in Pacák-Zhuang or in VHL syndromes which are ^{18}F-FDOPA avid (Table 12.2). Another alternative is ^{18}F-FDG, which is a surrogate marker of glucose metabolism. It provides best results in less differentiated PGLs—*SDHB*-related (Fig. 12.1). The last imaging modality is MIBG (either labeled with ^{123}I for SPECT or with ^{124}I for PET) which binds to norepinephrine transporters. For PGLs, it has only a complementary role—due its low sensitivity in lesion detection—in the decision whether the patient may be suitable for therapeutic MIBG (Fig. 12.1) [43].

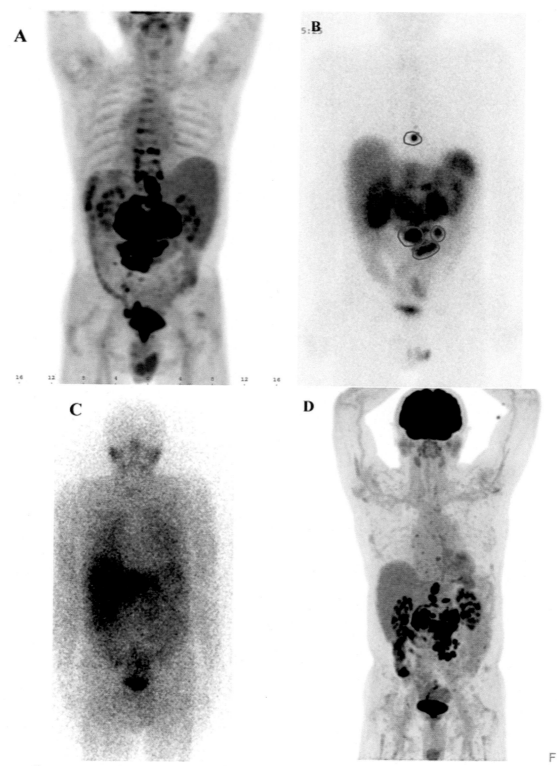

FIGURE 12.1 ^{18}F-FDG PET/CT before and after peptide receptor radionuclide therapy and octreoscan and ^{123}I-MIBG before peptide receptor radionuclide therapy in subjects with mutation of the *SDHB* gene. A 65-year-old patient was investigated because of pain in his left hip for 2 years. Previously, a retroperitoneal mass was found, and open biopsy was performed in the local hospital. Histopathology report concluded a diagnosis of "Benign paraganglioma" and the patient was subsequently followed by a hematologist. Due to progression of pain and tumoral mass, the patient was sent for further evaluation. While ^{18}F-FDG (A) and octreoscan (B) showed large masses in the retroperitoneal region and metastatic involvement of the spine and sternum, ^{123}I-MIBG (C) did not show any uptake in the affected regions. Laboratory examination showed significantly elevated serum chromogranin values and mild elevation of plasma normetanephrine and methoxytyramine. Genetic examinations confirmed the clinical suspicion of *SDHB*-mutation. The patient underwent two cycles of PRRT which led to significant decrease of tumoral lesion (^{18}F-FDG, D) but treatment was later terminated due to bone marrow toxicity (secondary myelodysplastic syndrome). His tumoral involvement has progressed despite the hyertment with somatostatin analogues and metronomic capecitabine.

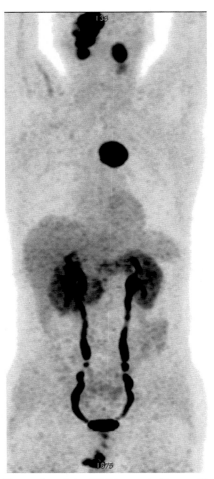

FIGURE 12.2 ^{18}F-FDOPA PET/CT in subject with mutation of the *SDHD* gene. A 47-year-old male patient noticed peripheral palsy of right facial nerve. A large right jugular paraganglioma was found 3 years earlier, and embolization was performed. On the left side, a smaller carotid paraganglioma was found. Ten years after initial diagnosis, the patient was sent to our ward for further investigation. ^{18}F-DOPA PET/CT revealed large mass of one of the two paraganglioma(s) extending from carotid bifurcation to skull base with the brainstem involvement on the right side and a larger carotid paraganglioma on the left side. An additional paraganglioma was found in the anterior mediastinum which was previously not diagnosed (no whole-body examination performed). Genetic testing revealed a mutation in the *SDHD* gene. Laboratory examination showed elevated serum chromogranin and normal values of plasma metanephrines.

Perioperative medical management of paragangliomas

Hypertension in functional PGLs should be treated with α-adrenoceptor antagonists, which leads not only to BP reduction but also to the amelioration of paroxysmal symptoms. Treatment with α-adrenoceptor antagonists should be initiated with small doses, due to a significant first dose effect (with possible significant BP drop), and then increased to the maximally tolerated dose (=very mild orthostatic hypotension). Treatment with α-adrenoceptor antagonists may be hindered by various reasons. The first reason may be the combination of hypertension and orthostatic hypotension, which could rarely occur in functional PGLs; others are leg swelling or urine incontinence in females. Doses of α-adrenoceptor antagonists frequently exceed those doses recommended as maximal in summaries of product characteristics (e.g., 8 mg for doxazosin). α-adrenoceptor antagonists are divided into two classes—nonselective and noncompetitive antagonist phenoxybenzamine and $α_1$-selective and competitive antagonist doxazosin (others, such as terazosin are used less frequently). The blockade of $α_2$-adrenoceptors with phenoxybenzamine is associated with significant sinus tachycardia, which requires treatment with β-blockers. Treatment with β-blockers should be started only after reaching the effective blockade of vasoconstrictive $α_1$-adrenoceptors—usually after 3–5 days. As functional PGLs usually do not secret epinephrine, the addition of β-blockers is not often needed in subjects treated with doxazosin. Calcium channel blockers may be used either as add-on medication to α-adrenoceptor antagonists, or as substitution for α-adrenoceptor antagonists, if they are not tolerated [46]. In some cases, metyrosine, a tyrosine hydroxylase inhibitor may be used as an add-on to conventional treatment in the case of difficult PPGL resection, or in the anticipated large release of catecholamines (e.g., chemotherapy) [47]. Unfortunately, treatment with metyrosine is unavailable in many countries and, if available, it is expensive.

According to available recommendations, all subjects with functional PGLs (not only hypertensive, but also normotensive) should be medically prepared at least 7−14 days before surgery [2]. To date, no data have shown the superiority of one α-adrenoceptor antagonist over the other. Phenoxybenzamine may prevent hemodynamic instability during tumor resection, compared to doxazosin. However, this was not associated with a better clinical outcome [48] All subjects with functional PGLs should also adhere to a high-sodium diet to reduce hypotensive episodes in the early postoperative period.

Perhaps the most important preparation for surgery is the information about tumor secretory activity and the subsequent risk of hemodynamic instability. Due to progress in perioperative management (hemodynamic monitoring and the availability of short-acting vasoactive drugs), some authors do not recommend routine preoperative preparation with α-adrenoceptor antagonists [15]. Hemodynamic instability may be expected in subjects with high preoperative BP or high levels of norepinephrine [49].

Treatment with α-adrenoceptor antagonists is not indicated in pure dopamine-secreting PGLs because of the risk of severe hypotension [36].

Surgery for management of paragangliomas

Curative surgery

The only curative treatment of PGLs is tumor removal. Unlike pheochromocytomas, even a small sympathetic PGL may represent a surgical challenge, due to its close relation to adjacent blood vessels or other organs such as pancreas. In some cases, suspicion of a functional PGL may arise only during operation of an incidentally found retroperitoneal mass, because of unanticipated peroperative hemodynamic instability.

Due to their rarity, patients with PGLs should be operated only in centers with adequate experience in treating these tumors. Close collaboration between different surgical specializations, such as vascular and cardiac surgeons (heart or pericardial PGLs), thoracic, and abdominal surgeons, or urologists (PGLs of the urinary bladder) is required in the case of sympathetic PGLs. The location of sympathetic PGLs in most cases determines the need for open surgery, which differs from pheochromocytoma, where minimally invasive surgery is the preferred approach. Not only improvement in surgical techniques but also the hemodynamic management has led to a dramatic improvement in the perioperative outcomes [48].

Surgery of parasympathetic PGLs is also challenging and requires surgeons experienced in skull base surgery, microsurgery, vascular surgery, and aural surgery. Due to the close relationship to cranial nerves VII, IX, X, XI, XII, and their branches (e.g., laryngeal nerve), the decision for surgery should be made on an individual basis to keep the surgical complication rate as low as possible, which is dependent not only on local tumor characteristics (Shamblin-status, Fitch-status, or Netterville-status for the carotid body, jugulotympanic or vagal PGLs), but also on the functional status of the patient (age, life expectancy, and comorbidities). A large meta-analysis of surgery results of Shamblin III carotid body PGLs (complete involvement of carotid vessels) revealed a high complication rate, including stroke in 4%, and cranial nerve injury in 17% [50]. In some centers, preoperative embolization is performed, but this is not associated with an improvement in postoperative outcomes [50].

Due to the low growth rate of head and neck PGLs, the watch-and-wait policy may be a reasonable strategy in older patients. To preserve cranial nerve function, incomplete resection may be performed, with subsequent stereotactic radiosurgery such as Gamma Knife, Cyber Knife or, less frequently, linear accelerator. Stereotactic radiosurgery may achieve local tumor growth control in about 94% of patients with a very low complication rate [51].

Metastatic paragangliomas

Depending on the population studied, the incidence of metastatic disease may occur in up to 35%—the highest is among carriers of the mutation of the *SDHB* gene. Only metastases are diagnostic for malignancy in PGLs, which may be found either in lymph nodes or in the bones, lungs, and liver. In about 35%−50% of patients, metastases are found at the time of diagnosis. In the remaining 50%−65% of patients, metastases develop even decades after the first PGL presentation. Compared to pheochromocytoma, PGLs metastasize more frequently to bones and less frequently to the liver and are diagnosed at a younger age. The natural course of metastatic PGLs varies from a very indolent one (stable disease for more than 10 years) on one side, to a very progressive course (survival less than 1 year, despite different treatment modalities) on the other hand [32]. Overall survival depends on the age at initial diagnosis, functional phenotype, and size of the primary tumor [52]. Survival may also be limited due to catecholamine-induced reduction of gastrointestinal motility, which is usually associated with constipation and but may lead to severe difficulty in treating complications such as toxic mega-colon or paralytic ileus [53].

Palliative surgery

Patients with metastatic PGLs often benefit from surgical resection of the primary tumor and/or locoregional/distant metastases [32]. Resection of a large primary tumor decreases catecholamine secretion, with subsequent improvement of catecholamine-related symptoms. The preferred surgical approach is an open one, which not only provides better visualization of the surgical field and facilitates tumor removal, but also lowers the risk of tumor rupture. In the case of pathological fracture from skeletal metastatic involvement, surgical stabilization of the pathological fracture/resection is required. Subjects with bone involvement benefit from antiresorptive therapy (bisphosphonates or deno-sumab) [54].

Systemic therapy

Systemic therapy is indicated in patients with either rapidly progressive disease (evaluated over a 3-month interval), or with high tumor burden (large liver metastases, larger pulmonary nodules, or higher number of bone metastases). According to disease progression, either chemotherapy or radionuclide therapy (alone or in combination) are indicated. However, due to the rarity of these tumors and different clinical courses, most of the treatment recommendations are based mainly on retrospective studies, but not on randomized controlled trials. In some cases, local ablative therapy, or radiotherapy may be helpful.

Chemotherapy

Chemotherapy is the mainstay of management for rapidly progressive disease. The mostly used combination is the Averbuch's (CVD) scheme with cyclophosphamide, vincristine and dacarbazine on day 1−2 at 21-day intervals. Initial response may be expected after six to nine cycles, which can be prolonged up to 20 cycles. CVD chemotherapy is more effective in patients with *SDHB* mutations [55]. In these patients, temozolomide (oral equivalent of dacarbazine) is effective, either as maintenance therapy after CVD chemotherapy, or as an alternative to CVD in less aggressive disease, or in patients with comorbidities [20]. Temozolimide alone or in combination with capecitabine may also be tried. In Cluster 1 tumors, poly (ADP-ribose) polymerase (PARP) inhibitors, in combination with temozolomide may be an alternative [20]. Another systemic therapeutic option is treatment with antiangiogenic therapy, such as tyrosin-kinase inhibitors (TKI)—sunitinib or cabozantinib. As this treatment regime may be more effective in kinase signaling-related Cluster 2 tumors, it would be of great importance to compare the efficacy of this targeted therapy with temozolomide in Cluster 1-related tumors. Small studies were also reported on mTORC1 inhibitor everolimus (a signaling pathway inhibitor), and with immunotherapy (checkpoint inhibitors) in subjects without any alternative treatment option [20]. As in other neuroendocrine tumors, long-acting somatostatin analogs (lanreotide or octreotide LAR) could be efficacious in *SDHx*-related PGLs which show the highest expression of SSTR2 [56], although a small previous study with metastatic pheochromocytoma did not report promising results [57].

Radionuclide therapy

Slowly or moderately progressive metastatic PGLs are best treated with radionuclide therapy, either with ^{131}I-MIBG or peptide receptor radionuclide therapy (PRRT). Both therapies are relatively well tolerated with acceptable bone narrow toxicity (both) and nephrotoxicity (more pronounced in PRRT). Infusion of ^{131}I-MIBG (more frequently with low specific activity) may be associated with sudden BP rise. As most metastatic PGLs are *SDHx*-related, the preferred therapy would be PRRT, due to the high expression of SSTR2 on one side, and the low expression of norepinephrine transporter system on the other side [58,59].

^{177}Lu-DOTATATE has already been approved by the FDA and European Medicines Agency for therapeutic use, and is also recommended for first-line use by a recent Guideline of the National Comprehensive Cancer Network [60]. A meta-analysis of studies with PRRT found an objective response in 25% of patients, and disease control rate in 84% of patients. Clinical and biochemical responses were noted in 61% and 64% of patients, respectively. No difference was found between [177]Lu- and ^{90}Y-based agents (available only in academic centers) [61].

Local ablative therapy

Bone metastases in metastatic PGL may be treated by interventional radiological techniques, such as cementoplasty, osteosynthesis, or thermal-ablation to prolong the time to first skeletal-related event [62]. Radiological local control of metastases may be achieved with radiofrequency ablation, cryoablation or percutaneous ethanol injection in 86% of lesions [63]. External beam radiation therapy may help to control pain and local growth of bone or soft tissue metastases [64].

Follow-up care of patients with paragangliomas

People treated for PGLs need lifelong follow-up care. This is important because PGLs can recur years after initial treatment. Generally, people treated for catecholamine producing PGLs should have their blood tested annually for increased levels of metanephrines suggestive of recurrence.

Special emphasis needs to be placed on all mutation carriers, who should be considered for annual biochemical surveillance for PGLs. The nature of this surveillance should, however, consider the gene affected according to the genotype-phenotype relationships described above, as well as considerations of the penetrance and potential severity of the disease.

In the case of *SDHx* gene mutations, regular annual review by laboratory tests, including metanephrines, is strongly recommended, as well as MRI imaging of the head and neck, abdomen and pelvis, every 2—3 years. Screening tests should be delayed to every 5 years after 70 years of age, and follow-up may be stopped at 80 years of age [29].

Management in special populations
Children

Compared to adults, PPGLs in children are more likely to be familial, multicentric, or malignant. Children showed a higher prevalence than adults of extraadrenal (66.3% vs. 35.1%), multifocal (32.6% vs. 13.5%), metastatic (49.5% vs. 29.1%), and recurrent (29.5% vs. 14.2%) disease. In addition, children were more likely than adults to have pathogenic variants in Cluster 1 genes (76.1% vs. 39.3%), especially *VHL* and *SDHB* [65]. Therefore, long-term monitoring is necessary in all patients, even in those who are apparently cured. All patients should be evaluated annually by biochemical testing. Surveillance with MRI every 2—3 years is indicated in patients who had a nonfunctioning PGL and with any *SDHx* pathogenic variant [29].

Apart from the typical symptoms (arterial hypertension, sweating, tachycardia, and headache—although a typical triad is not common in children) described above, a common manifestation in children is the symptomatology of attention deficit hyperactivity disorder (ADHD). In pediatric patients with hypertension and ADHD, an evaluation to rule out pheochromocytoma and PGL is warranted prior to treatment with stimulant medications, which may exacerbate a hypertension crisis [66].

Pregnancy

Pregnancies complicated by a pheochromocytoma or functional PGL are very rare, and estimated to occur in one in 15,000 pregnancies [67]. PGLs are less common than pheochromocytomas (81% vs. 19%) [68]. Due to the rarity, management in pregnancy is based on the experience of the individual case studies and the opinion of experts. Early diagnosis of the disease improves mortality in pregnancy. If PGL is detected antenatally, it leads to 12% fetal mortality and almost zero maternal mortality. However, if the diagnosis is made late, during or soon after delivery, it is associated with up to 29% fetal and maternal mortality [68]. For imaging, MRI is recommended for PGL, due to the associated risk of fetal exposure to ionizing radiation with CT imaging.

The management of blood pressure in pregnant woman is a careful balance between providing the adequate catecholamine blockade to reduce the risk of catecholamine excess, while not compromising placental blood flow by lowering the BP excessively. The available literature shows that the use of nonselective α-adrenoceptor antagonist (phenoxybenzamine), or selective α_1-adrenoceptor antagonist (doxazosin) during pregnancy is considered safe, and expectant mothers should be provided with this treatment [67,69]. Caution should be exercised with phenoxybenzamine, because it does cross the placenta and may cause neonatal hypotension and respiratory depression [69]. It is therefore necessary to monitor the newborn's blood pressure and respiratory function in the first days of life. The use of a low-dose alpha-blockade in combination with a high-salt diet and fluid loading is also recommended in normotensive PGL, to prevent marked blood pressure fluctuation and life-threating arrhythmias, especially during delivery [69].

If PGL is diagnosed in the first trimester of pregnancy, laparoscopic tumor extirpation in the second trimester is recommended. On the other hand, if PGL is discovered during the third trimester, surgery should be postponed until the fetus is viable and able to be delivered, with the tumor being removed either immediately after delivery or later [70]. Delivery should be by caesarean section, as vaginal delivery is associated with higher mortality. The delivery can be performed under a spinal anesthetic. If the blockage is high enough (Th5—Th12), it can reduce nerve stimulation of the sympathetic chain. In any case, this is a multidisciplinary approach in a tertiary hospital, and the decision on the method of delivery depends on the circumstances—pharmacological pretreatment, secretory activity of the PGL, and catecholamine phenotype. Some papers mention a completely uncomplicated vaginal delivery, especially in purely dopaminergic tumors [70]. Finally, drugs potentially inducing a hypertensive crisis, such as metoclopramide, should also be avoided [70].

Elderly

In the case of HNPGL in elderly patients, or those with significant comorbidities, a wait-and-watch approach with serial scans, or radiation therapy may be entertained [71]. More controversy arises in the management of jugulotympanic tumors. Small jugulotympanic tumors generally are resected easily with little morbidity. Larger tumors generally require lateral skull base or infratemporal fossa approaches that are associated with significant risks such as cerebrospinal fluid leak, meningitis, death, stroke, hearing loss, and multiple lower cranial nerve palsies. Thus, for these tumors, serial scanning, and regular clinical examination only may be considered as follow-up options [33]. If the patient experiences significant clinical symptoms, surgery can then be performed. Another option for these tumors is radiation therapy. Radiation therapy has also been advocated for patients with multiple PGLs, to minimize the risks of multiple surgeries. There has been ongoing development of newer surgical techniques to minimize intraoperative and postoperative complications.

In the case of functional PGL, a curative procedure is recommended regardless of age, except in patients with poor performance status.

Areas of uncertainty/emerging research

(1) How to prepare the asymptomatic patient with sympathetic PGL for surgery?
  Although available guidelines recommend the presurgical preparation with α-adrenoceptor antagonists for all patients, some patients tolerate only very small doses of α-adrenoceptor antagonists. Some reports state no difference between hemodynamic parameters in subjects pretreated with or without α-adrenoceptor antagonists. Therefore, it is interesting to compare these strategies in a prospective way.
(2) There are no prediction markers, apart from genetic background (mutation of *SDHB* gene) to predict potential metastatic spread. This would necessitate targeting close follow-up in the high-risk group on one side and performing more liberal follow-up in the low-risk group on the other side.
(3) Due to the rarity of metastatic PGL and its very different clinical behavior, the optimal therapy and follow up strategies are still unclear. There is hope in the new targeted therapies (radionuclide therapy, immunotherapy, demethylating agents, HIF-2α or tyrosine kinase inhibitors) based on genetic background (germline or somatic mutations).

Summary and conclusions

PGLs are rare tumors with different clinical profiles and pathobiological behavior. The most important part of PGL diagnosis is the timely consideration of its probability. Catecholamine secretion may lead to variable degrees of arterial hypertension, paroxysmal symptoms, and metabolic abnormalities, such as disturbances of the glucose metabolism. The only curative treatment is surgery. In some cases, the watch-and-wait approach may be acceptable especially for subjects with HNPGLs, and those with higher operative risk. All subjects with PGL should be offered genetic testing to search for mutations in PGL-related culprit genes. The management of PGL patients requires a multidisciplinary approach and should be concentrated in large-volume centers with sufficient experience.

Learning points

- Paragangliomas (PGLs) are rare neural crest-derived neuroendocrine tumors with a high degree of inheritance.
- Paragangliomas frequently present as incidentally discovered masses, but the diagnosis of paraganglioma is often not considered in its differential diagnosis of such masses. Therefore, PGLs frequently undergo biopsies or surgery without ruling out the secretory activity.

- The only curative treatment is surgery. Due to the peculiar localizations close to larger blood vessels or other organs, PGL surgery should be performed only in experienced centers.
- Lifelong follow-up is necessary, due to the high risk of tumor recurrence and metastatic disease.

References

[1] Lenders JWM, Duh Q-Y, Eisenhofer G, Gimenez-Roqueplo A-P, Grebe SKG, Murad MH, Naruse M, Pacak K, Young WF. Pheochromocytoma and paraganglioma: an endocrine society clinical practice guideline. J Clin Endocrinol Metab 2014;99(6):1915–42. https://doi.org/10.1210/jc.2014-1498.

[2] Lenders JWM, Kerstens MN, Amar L, Prejbisz A, Robledo M, Taieb D, Pacak K, Crona J, Zelinka T, Mannelli M, Deutschbein T, Timmers HJLM, Castinetti F, Dralle H, Widimský J, Gimenez-Roqueplo A-P, Eisenhofer G. Genetics, diagnosis, management and future directions of research of phaeochromocytoma and paraganglioma: a position statement and consensus of the Working Group on Endocrine Hypertension of the European Society of Hypertension. J Hypertens 2020;38(8):1443–56. https://doi.org/10.1097/HJH.0000000000002438.

[3] Lumb R, Schwarz Q. Sympathoadrenal neural crest cells: the known, unknown and forgotten? Dev Growth Differ 2015;57(2):146–57. https://doi.org/10.1111/dgd.12189.

[4] Soltani A, Pourian M, Davani BM. Does this patient have pheochromocytoma? a systematic review of clinical signs and symptoms. J Diabetes Metab Disord 2015;15:6. https://doi.org/10.1186/s40200-016-0226-x.

[5] Pappachan JM, Tun NN, Arunagirinathan G, Sodi R, Hanna FWF. Pheochromocytomas and hypertension. Curr Hypertens Rep 2018;20(1):3. https://doi.org/10.1007/s11906-018-0804-z.

[6] Williams MD. Paragangliomas of the head and neck: an overview from diagnosis to genetics. Head Neck Pathol 2017;11(3):278–87. https://doi.org/10.1007/s12105-017-0803-4.

[7] Cleere EF, Martin-Grace J, Gendre A, Sherlock M, O'Neill JP. Contemporary management of paragangliomas of the head and neck. Laryngoscope Investig Otolaryngol 2021;7(1):93–107. https://doi.org/10.1002/lio2.706. Published 2021 Nov 26.

[8] Martins R, Bugalho MJ. Paragangliomas/pheochromocytomas: clinically oriented genetic testing. Int J Endocrinol 2014;2014:794187. https://doi.org/10.1155/2014/794187.

[9] Boedeker CC, Neumann HPH, Maier W, Bausch B, Schipper J, Ridder GJ. Malignant head and neck paragangliomas in SDHB mutation carriers. Otolaryngol Head Neck Surg 2007;137(1):126–9. https://doi.org/10.1016/j.otohns.2007.01.015.

[10] Cerecer-Gil NY, Figuera LE, Llamas FJ, Lara M, Escamilla JG, Ramos R, Estrada G, Hussain AK, Gaal J, Korpershoek E, de Krijger RR, Dinjens WNM, Devilee P, Bayley JP. Mutation of SDHB is a cause of hypoxia-related high-altitude paraganglioma. Clin Cancer Res 2010;16(16):4148. https://doi.org/10.1158/1078-0432.CCR-10-0637.

[11] Neumann HPH, Young WF, Eng C. Pheochromocytoma and paraganglioma. N Engl J Med 2019;381(6):552–65. https://doi.org/10.1056/NEJMra1806651.

[12] Capatina C, Ntali G, Karavitaki N, Grossman AB. The management of head-and-neck paragangliomas. Endocr Relat Cancer 2013;20(5):R291–305. https://doi.org/10.1530/ERC-13-0223.

[13] Berends AMA, Buitenwerf E, de Krijger RR, Veeger NJGM, van der Horst-Schrivers ANA, Links TP, Kerstens MN. Incidence of pheochromocytoma and sympathetic paraganglioma in The Netherlands: a nationwide study and systematic review. Eur J Intern Med 2018;51:68–73. https://doi.org/10.1016/j.ejim.2018.01.015.

[14] Platts JK, Drew PJ, Harvey JN. Death from phaeochromocytoma: lessons from a post-mortem survey. J R Coll Physicians Lond 1995;29(4):299–306.

[15] Groeben H, Nottebaum BJ, Alesina PF, Traut A, Neumann HP, Walz MK. Perioperative alpha-receptor blockade in phaeochromocytoma surgery: an observational case series. Br J Anaesth 2017;118(2):182–9. https://doi.org/10.1093/bja/aew392.

[16] Mannelli M, Castellano M, Schiavi F, Filetti S, Giacche M, Mori L, Pignataro V, Bernini G, Giache V, Bacca A, Biondi B, Corona G, Di Trapani G, Grossrubatscher E, Reimondo G, Arnaldi G, Giacchetti G, Veglio F, Loli P, Opocher G. Clinically guided genetic screening in a large cohort of Italian patients with pheochromocytomas and/or functional or nonfunctional paragangliomas. J Clin Endocrinol Metab 2009;94(5):1541–7. https://doi.org/10.1210/jc.2008-2419.

[17] Garcia-Carbonero R, Matute Teresa F, Mercader-Cidoncha E, Mitjavila-Casanovas M, Robledo M, Tena I, Alvarez-Escola C, Arístegui M, Bella-Cueto MR, Ferrer-Albiach C, Hanzu FA. Multidisciplinary practice guidelines for the diagnosis, genetic counseling and treatment of pheochromocytomas and paragangliomas. Clin Transl Oncol 2021;23(10):1995–2019. https://doi.org/10.1007/s12094-021-02622-9.

[18] Eisenhofer G, Huynh T-T, Elkahloun A, Morris JC, Bratslavsky G, Linehan WM, Zhuang Z, Balgley BM, Lee CS, Mannelli M, Lenders JWM, Bornstein SR, Pacak K. Differential expression of the regulated catecholamine secretory pathway in different hereditary forms of pheochromocytoma. Am J Physiol Endocrinol Metab 2008;295(5):E1223–33. https://doi.org/10.1152/ajpendo.90591.2008.

[19] Zuber SM, Kantorovich V, Pacak K. Hypertension in pheochromocytoma: characteristics and treatment. Endocrinol Metabol Clin 2011;40(2):295–311. https://doi.org/10.1016/j.ecl.2011.02.002.

[20] Nölting S, Bechmann N, Taieb D, Beuschlein F, Fassnacht M, Kroiss M, et al. Personalized management of pheochromocytoma and paraganglioma. Endocr Rev 2022;43(2):199–239. https://doi.org/10.1210/endrev/bnab019.

[21] Fishbein L, Leshchiner I, Walter V, Danilova L, Robertson AG, Johnson AR, Lichtenberg TM, Murray BA, Ghayee HK, Else T, Ling S, Jefferys SR, de Cubas AA, Wenz B, Korpershoek E, Amelio AL, Makowski L, Rathmell WK, Gimenez-Roqueplo A-P, Wilkerson MD.

Comprehensive molecular characterization of pheochromocytoma and paraganglioma. Cancer Cell 2017;31(2):181–93. https://doi.org/10.1016/j.ccell.2017.01.001.

[22] Boedeker CC, Erlic Z, Richard S, Kontny U, Gimenez-Roqueplo A-P, Cascon A, Robledo M, de Campos JM, van Nederveen FH, de Krijger RR, Burnichon N, Gaal J, Walter MA, Reschke K, Wiech T, Weber J, Ruckauer K, Plouin PF, Darrouzet V, Neumann HPH. Head and neck paragangliomas in von Hippel-Lindau disease and multiple endocrine neoplasia type 2. J Clin Endocrinol Metab 2009;94(6):1938–44. https://doi.org/10.1210/jc.2009-0354.

[23] Remacha L, Currás-Freixes M, Torres-Ruiz R, Schiavi F, Torres-Pérez R, Calsina B, Letón R, Comino-Méndez I, Roldán-Romero JM, Montero-Conde C, Santos M, Pérez LI, Pita G, Alonso MR, Honrado E, Pedrinaci S, Crespo-Facorro B, Percesepe A, Falcioni M, Cascón A. Gain-of-function mutations in DNMT3A in patients with paraganglioma. Genet Med 2018;20(12):1644–51. https://doi.org/10.1038/s41436-018-0003-y.

[24] Toledo RA, Qin Y, Cheng Z-M, Gao Q, Iwata S, Silva GM, Prasad ML, Ocal IT, Rao S, Aronin N, Barontini M, Bruder J, Reddick RL, Chen Y, Aguiar RCT, Dahia PLM. Recurrent mutations of chromatin-remodeling genes and kinase receptors in pheochromocytomas and paragangliomas. Clin Cancer Res 2016;22(9):2301. https://doi.org/10.1158/1078-0432.CCR-15-1841.

[25] Jiang J, Zhang J, Pang Y, Bechmann N, Li M, Monteagudo M, Calsina B, Gimenez-Roqueplo A-P, Nölting S, Beuschlein F, Fassnacht M, Deutschbein T, Timmers HJLM, Åkerström T, Crona J, Quinkler M, Fliedner SMJ, Liu Y, Guo J, Eisenhofer G. Sino-European differences in the genetic landscape and clinical presentation of pheochromocytoma and paraganglioma. J Clin Endocrinol Metab 2020;105(10):3295–307. https://doi.org/10.1210/clinem/dgaa502.

[26] Toledo RA, Burnichon N, Cascon A, Benn DE, Bayley J-P, Welander J, Tops CM, Firth H, Dwight T, Ercolino T, Mannelli M, Opocher G, Clifton-Bligh R, Gimm O, Maher ER, Robledo M, Gimenez-Roqueplo A-P, Dahia PLM, The NGS in PPGL (NGSnPPGL) Study Group. Consensus Statement on next-generation-sequencing-based diagnostic testing of hereditary phaeochromocytomas and paragangliomas. Nat Rev Endocrinol 2017;13(4):233–47. https://doi.org/10.1038/nrendo.2016.185.

[27] Papathomas TG, Oudijk L, Persu A, Gill AJ, van Nederveen F, Tischler AS, Tissier F, Volante M, Matias-Guiu X, Smid M, Favier J, Rapizzi E, Libe R, Currás-Freixes M, Aydin S, Huynh T, Lichtenauer U, van Berkel A, Canu L, de Krijger RR. SDHB/SDHA immunohistochemistry in pheochromocytomas and paragangliomas: a multicenter interobserver variation analysis using virtual microscopy: a multinational study of the European Network for the Study of Adrenal Tumors (ENS@T). Mod Pathol 2015;28(6):807–21. https://doi.org/10.1038/modpathol.2015.41.

[28] Buffet A, Ben Aim L, Leboulleux S, Drui D, Vezzosi D, Libé R, Ajzenberg C, Bernardeschi D, Cariou B, Chabolle F, Chabre O, Darrouzet V, Delemer B, Desailloud R, Goichot B, Esvant A, Offredo L, Herman P, Laboureau S, Gimenez-Roqueplo A-P. Positive impact of genetic test on the management and outcome of patients with paraganglioma and/or pheochromocytoma. J Clin Endocrinol Metab 2019;104(4):1109–18. https://doi.org/10.1210/jc.2018-02411.

[29] Amar L, Pacak K, Steichen O, Akker SA, Aylwin SJB, Baudin E, Buffet A, Burnichon N, Clifton-Bligh RJ, Dahia PLM, Fassnacht M, Grossman AB, Herman P, Hicks RJ, Januszewicz A, Jimenez C, Kunst HPM, Lewis D, Mannelli M, Lussey-Lepoutre C. International consensus on initial screening and follow-up of asymptomatic SDHx mutation carriers. Nat Rev Endocrinol 2021;17(7):435–44. https://doi.org/10.1038/s41574-021-00492-3.

[30] Rijken JA, van Hulsteijn LT, Dekkers OM, Niemeijer ND, Leemans CR, Eijkelenkamp K, et al. Increased mortality in SDHB but not in SDHD pathogenic variant carriers. Cancers 2019;11(1):103. https://doi.org/10.3390/cancers11010103.

[31] Lenders JW, Eisenhofer G, Mannelli M, Pacak K. Phaeochromocytoma. Lancet 2005;366(9486):665–75. https://doi.org/10.1016/S0140-6736(05)67139-5.

[32] Hamidi O, Young Jr WF, Gruber L, Smestad J, Yan Q, Ponce OJ, Prokop L, Murad MH, Bancos I. Outcomes of patients with metastatic phaeochromocytoma and paraganglioma: a systematic review and meta-analysis. Clin Endocrinol 2017;87(5):440–50. https://doi.org/10.1111/cen.13434.

[33] Moore MG, Netterville JL, Mendenhall WM, Isaacson B, Nussenbaum B. Head and neck paragangliomas: an update on evaluation and management. Otolaryngol Head Neck Surg 2016;154(4):597–605. https://doi.org/10.1177/0194599815627667.

[34] Petrák O, Rosa J, Holaj R, Štrauch B, Krátká Z, Kvasnička J, Klímová J, Waldauf P, Hamplová B, Markvartová A, Novák K, Michalský D, Widimský Jr J, Zelinka T. Blood pressure profile, catecholamine phenotype, and target organ damage in pheochromocytoma/paraganglioma. J Clin Endocrinol Metab 2019;104(11):5170–80. https://doi.org/10.1210/jc.2018-02644.

[35] Zelinka T, Štrauch B, Petrák O, Holaj R, Vranková A, Weisserová H, et al. Increased blood pressure variability in pheochromocytoma compared to essential hypertension patients. J Hypertens 2005;23(11):2033–9. https://doi.org/10.1097/01.hjh.0000185714.60788.52.

[36] Poirier É, Thauvette D, Hogue J-C. Management of exclusively dopamine–secreting abdominal pheochromocytomas. J Am Coll Surg 2013;216(2):340–6. https://doi.org/10.1016/j.jamcollsurg.2012.10.002.

[37] Lenders JWM, Pacak K, Walther MM, Linehan WM, Mannelli M, Friberg P, Keiser HR, Goldstein DS, Eisenhofer G. Biochemical diagnosis of pheochromocytoma: which test is best? JAMA 2002;287(11):1427–34. https://doi.org/10.1001/jama.287.11.1427.

[38] Eisenhofer G, Rundquist B, Aneman A, Friberg P, Dakak N, Kopin IJ, Jacobs MC, Lenders JW. Regional release and removal of catecholamines and extraneuronal metabolism to metanephrines. J Clin Endocrinol Metab 1995;80(10):3009–17. https://doi.org/10.1210/jcem.80.10.7559889.

[39] Lenders JW, Willemsen JJ, Eisenhofer G, Ross HA, Pacak K, Timmers HJ, Sweep C, Fred). Is supine rest necessary before blood sampling for plasma metanephrines? Clin Chem 2007;53(2):352–4. https://doi.org/10.1373/clinchem.2006.076489.

[40] Bílek R, Vlček P, Šafařík L, Michalský D, Novák K, Dušková J, et al. Chromogranin A in the laboratory diagnosis of pheochromocytoma and paraganglioma. Cancers 2019;11(4):586. https://doi.org/10.3390/cancers11040586.

[41] Lussey-Lepoutre C, Bellucci A, Burnichon N, Amar L, Buffet A, Drossart T, Fontaine S, Clement O, Benit P, Rustin P, Groussin L, Meatchi T, Gimenez-Roqueplo A-P, Tavitian B, Favier J. Succinate detection using in vivo 1H-MR spectroscopy identifies germline and somatic SDHx mutations in paragangliomas. Eur J Nucl Med Mol Imag 2020;47(6):1510–7. https://doi.org/10.1007/s00259-019-04633-9.

[42] Daniel E, Jones R, Bull M, Newell-Price J. Rapid-sequence MRI for long-term surveillance for paraganglioma and phaeochromocytoma in patients with succinate dehydrogenase mutations. Eur J Endocrinol 2016;175(6):561–70. https://doi.org/10.1530/EJE-16-0595.

[43] Taïeb D, Hicks RJ, Hindié E, Guillet BA, Avram A, Ghedini P, Timmers HJ, Scott AT, Elojeimy S, Rubello D, Virgolini IJ, Fanti S, Balogova S, Pandit-Taskar N, Pacak K. European association of nuclear medicine practice guideline/society of nuclear medicine and molecular imaging procedure standard 2019 for radionuclide imaging of phaeochromocytoma and paraganglioma. Eur J Nucl Med Mol Imag 2019;46(10):2112–37. https://doi.org/10.1007/s00259-019-04398-1.

[44] Carrasquillo JA, Chen CC, Jha A, Ling A, Lin FI, Pryma DA, Pacak K. Imaging of pheochromocytoma and paraganglioma. J Nucl Med 2021;62(8):1033. https://doi.org/10.2967/jnumed.120.259689.

[45] Leijon H, Remes S, Hagström J, Louhimo J, Mäenpää H, Schalin-Jäntti C, Miettinen M, Haglund C, Arola J. Variable somatostatin receptor subtype expression in 151 primary pheochromocytomas and paragangliomas. Hum Pathol 2019;86:66–75. https://doi.org/10.1016/j.humpath.2018.11.020.

[46] Brunaud L, Boutami M, Nguyen-Thi P-L, Finnerty B, Germain A, Weryha G, Fahey TJ, Mirallie E, Bresler L, Zarnegar R. Both preoperative alpha and calcium channel blockade impact intraoperative hemodynamic stability similarly in the management of pheochromocytoma. Surgery 2014;156(6):1410–8. https://doi.org/10.1016/j.surg.2014.08.022.

[47] Gruber LM, Hartman RP, Thompson GB, McKenzie TJ, Lyden ML, Dy BM, Young Jr WF, Bancos I. Pheochromocytoma characteristics and behavior differ depending on method of discovery. J Clin Endocrinol Metab 2019;104(5):1386–93. https://doi.org/10.1210/jc.2018-01707.

[48] Buitenwerf E, Osinga TE, Timmers HJLM, Lenders JWM, Feelders RA, Eekhoff EMW, Haak HR, Corssmit EPM, Bisschop PHLT, Valk GD, Veldman RG, Dullaart RPF, Links TP, Voogd MF, Wietasch GJKG, Kerstens MN, for the PRESCRIPT Investigators. Efficacy of α-blockers on hemodynamic control during pheochromocytoma resection: a randomized controlled trial. J Clin Endocrinol Metab 2020;105(7):2381–91. https://doi.org/10.1210/clinem/dgz188.

[49] Gaujoux S, Bonnet S, Lentschener C, Thillois J-M, Duboc D, Bertherat J, Samama CM, Dousset B. Preoperative risk factors of hemodynamic instability during laparoscopic adrenalectomy for pheochromocytoma. Surg Endosc 2016;30(7):2984–93. https://doi.org/10.1007/s00464-015-4587-x.

[50] Robertson V, Poli F, Hobson B, Saratzis A, Ross Naylor A. A systematic review and meta-analysis of the presentation and surgical management of patients with carotid body tumours. Eur J Vasc Endovasc Surg 2019;57(4):477–86. https://doi.org/10.1016/j.ejvs.2018.10.038.

[51] Fatima N, Pollom E, Soltys S, Chang SD, Meola A. Stereotactic radiosurgery for head and neck paragangliomas: a systematic review and meta-analysis. Neurosurg Rev 2021;44(2):741–52. https://doi.org/10.1007/s10143-020-01292-5.

[52] Hescot S, Curras-Freixes M, Deutschbein T, van Berkel A, Vezzosi D, Amar L, de la Fouchardière C, Valdes N, Riccardi F, Do Cao C, Bertherat J, Goichot B, Beuschlein F, Drui D, Canu L, Niccoli P, Laboureau S, Tabarin A, Leboulleux S, Prognosis of Malignant Pheochromocytoma and Paraganglioma (MAPP-Prono Study). A European Network for the Study of Adrenal Tumors Retrospective Study. J Clin Endocrinol Metab 2019;104(6):2367–74. https://doi.org/10.1210/jc.2018-01968.

[53] Thosani S, Ayala-Ramirez M, Román-González A, Zhou S, Thosani N, Bisanz A, Jimenez C. Constipation: an overlooked, unmanaged symptom of patients with pheochromocytoma and sympathetic paraganglioma. Eur J Endocrinol 2015;173(3):377–87. https://doi.org/10.1530/EJE-15-0456.

[54] Ayala-Ramirez M, Palmer JL, Hofmann M-C, de la Cruz M, Moon BS, Waguespack SG, Habra MA, Jimenez C. Bone metastases and skeletal-related events in patients with malignant pheochromocytoma and sympathetic paraganglioma. J Clin Endocrinol Metab 2013;98(4):1492–7. https://doi.org/10.1210/jc.2012-4231.

[55] Fishbein L, Ben-Maimon S, Keefe S, Cengel K, Pryma DA, Loaiza-Bonilla A, Fraker DL, Nathanson KL, Cohen DL. SDHB mutation carriers with malignant pheochromocytoma respond better to CVD. Endocr Relat Cancer 2017;24(8):L51–5. https://doi.org/10.1530/ERC-17-0086.

[56] Patel M, Tena I, Jha A, Taieb D, Pacak K. Somatostatin Receptors and Analogs in Pheochromocytoma and Paraganglioma. Old Players in a New Precision Medicine World. Front Endocrinol (Lausanne) 2021;12:625312. https://doi.org/10.3389/fendo.2021.625312.

[57] Lamarre-Cliche M, Gimenez-Roqueplo A-P, Billaud E, Baudin E, Luton J-P, Plouin P-F. Effects of slow-release octreotide on urinary metanephrine excretion and plasma chromogranin A and catecholamine levels in patients with malignant or recurrent phaeochromocytoma. Clin Endocrinol 2002;57(5):629–34. https://doi.org/10.1046/j.1365-2265.2002.01658.x.

[58] Fonte JS, Robles JF, Chen CC, Reynolds J, Whatley M, Ling A, Mercado-Asis LB, Adams KT, Martucci V, Fojo T, Pacak K. False-negative 123I-MIBG SPECT is most commonly found in SDHB-related pheochromocytoma or paraganglioma with high frequency to develop metastatic disease. Endocr Relat Cancer 2012;19(1):83–93. https://doi.org/10.1530/ERC-11-0243.

[59] Janssen I, Chen CC, Millo CM, Ling A, Taïeb D, Lin FI, Adams KT, Wolf KI, Herscovitch P, Fojo AT, Buchmann I, Kebebew E, Pacak K. PET/CT comparing 68Ga-DOTATATE and other radiopharmaceuticals and in comparison with CT/MRI for the localization of sporadic metastatic pheochromocytoma and paraganglioma. Eur J Nucl Med Mol Imag 2016;43(10):1784–91. https://doi.org/10.1007/s00259-016-3357-x.

[60] Shah MH, Goldner WS, Benson AB, Bergsland E, Blaszkowsky LS, Brock P, Chan J, Das S, Dickson PV, Fanta P, Giordano T, Halfdanarson TR, Halperin D, He J, Heaney A, Heslin MJ, Kandeel F, Kardan A, Khan SA, Hochstetler C. Neuroendocrine and Adrenal Tumors, Version 2.2021, NCCN Clinical Practice Guidelines in Oncology. J Natl Compr Cancer Netw 2021;19(7):839–68. https://doi.org/10.6004/jnccn.2021.0032.

[61] Satapathy S, Mittal BR, Bhansali A. Peptide receptor radionuclide therapy in the management of advanced pheochromocytoma and paraganglioma: a systematic review and meta-analysis. Clin Endocrinol 2019;91(6):718–27. https://doi.org/10.1111/cen.14106.

[62] Gravel G, Leboulleux S, Tselikas L, Fassio F, Berraf M, Berdelou A, Ba B, Hescot S, Hadoux J, Schlumberger M, Al Ghuzlan A, Nguyen F, Faron M, de Baere T, Baudin E, Deschamps F. Prevention of serious skeletal-related events by interventional radiology techniques in patients with malignant paraganglioma and pheochromocytoma. Endocrine 2018;59(3):547–54. https://doi.org/10.1007/s12020-017-1515-y.

[63] Kohlenberg J, Welch B, Hamidi O, Callstrom M, Morris J, Sprung J, et al. Efficacy and safety of ablative therapy in the treatment of patients with metastatic pheochromocytoma and paraganglioma. Cancers 2019;11(2):195. https://doi.org/10.3390/cancers11020195.

[64] Breen W, Bancos I, Young Jr WF, Bible KC, Laack NN, Foote RL, Hallemeier CL. External beam radiation therapy for advanced/unresectable malignant paraganglioma and pheochromocytoma. Adv Radiat Oncol 2018;3(1):25−9. https://doi.org/10.1016/j.adro.2017.11.002.

[65] Pamporaki C, Hamplova B, Peitzsch M, Prejbisz A, Beuschlein F, Timmers HJLM, Fassnacht M, Klink B, Lodish M, Stratakis CA, Huebner A, Fliedner S, Robledo M, Sinnott RO, Januszewicz A, Pacak K, Eisenhofer G. Characteristics of pediatric vs adult pheochromocytomas and paragangliomas. J Clin Endocrinol Metab 2017;102(4):1122−32. https://doi.org/10.1210/jc.2016-3829.

[66] Batsis M, Dagalakis U, Stratakis CA, Prodanov T, Papadakis GZ, Adams K, Lodish M, Pacak K. Attention deficit hyperactivity disorder in pediatric patients with pheochromocytoma and paraganglioma. Horm Metab Res 2016;48(08):509−13.

[67] Wing LA, Conaglen JV, Meyer-Rochow GY, Elston MS. Paraganglioma in pregnancy: a case series and review of the literature. J Clin Endocrinol Metab 2015;100(8):3202−9. https://doi.org/10.1210/jc.2015-2122.

[68] Biggar MA, Lennard TWJ. Systematic review of phaeochromocytoma in pregnancy. Br J Surg 2013;100(2):182−90. https://doi.org/10.1002/bjs.8976.

[69] Aplin SC, Yee KF, Cole MJ. Neonatal effects of long-term maternal phenoxybenzamine therapy. Anesthesiology 2004;100(6):1608−10. https://doi.org/10.1097/00000542-200406000-00039.

[70] Lenders JWM, Langton K, Langenhuijsen JF, Eisenhofer G. Pheochromocytoma and pregnancy. Endocrinol Metabol Clin 2019;48(3):605−17. https://doi.org/10.1016/j.ecl.2019.05.006.

[71] Gujrathi CS, Donald PJ. Current trends in the diagnosis and management of head and neck paragangliomas. Curr Opin Otolaryngol Head Neck Surg 2005;13(6):339−42. https://doi.org/10.1097/01.moo.0000188707.35494.6b.

Chapter 13

ACTH-dependent Cushing's syndrome

Stuti Fernandes[1], Elena V. Varlamov[2] and Maria Fleseriu[3]

[1]*Department of Medicine, Division of Endocrinology, Diabetes and Clinical Nutrition, Oregon Health & Science University and Veterans Affairs Medical Center Hospital, Portland, OR, United States;* [2]*Departments of Medicine (Division of Endocrinology, Diabetes and Clinical Nutrition) and Neurological Surgery, and Pituitary Center, Oregon Health & Science University, Portland, OR, United States;* [3]*Departments of Medicine (Division of Endocrinology, Diabetes and Clinical Nutrition) and Neurological Surgery, and Pituitary Center, Oregon Health & Science University, Portland, OR, United States*

Visit the *Endocrine Hypertension: From Basic Science to Clinical Practice, First Edition* companion web site at: https://www.elsevier.com/books-and-journals/book-companion/9780323961202.

Graphical Abstract

Adrenocorticotropin (ACTH)-Dependent Cushing's Syndrome and Hypertension

Pathophysiology

Pituitary adenoma

Ectopic ACTH

- Activation of MC receptor
- Overwhelming of 11-β-HSD2
- Initial ↓ urine Na⁺ excretion

- Insulin resistance
- Upregulation of sympathetic nervous system
- Sleep apnea

- ↓ production of vasodilators (ANP, NO, PGI2, PGE2, and Kallikrein)
- ↑ plasma VGEF
- ↓ Na⁺-Ca²⁺ exchanger
- ↑ angiotensinogen

Diagnosis

Clinical Picture
- Weight gain, central obesity, hypertension, fatigue, decreased libido, menstrual abnormalities, hirsutism, dorsocervical fat pad, supraclavicular fullness, mood disturbances, and peripheral edema
- Facial plethora, easy bruising, purple striae, osteoporosis & proximal myopathy

- Biochemical Tests
- Screening: DST, LNSC, and 24-Hr UFC
- Confirmation: Dex-CRH/desmopressin test
- Localization: ACTH (high or normal) + imaging

Imaging
- MRI pituitary
- IPSS
- Dotatate scan+ whole body CT

Complications
- Cardiovascular disease, hyperglycemia, hyperlipidemia
- Hypokalemia
- Hypercoagulability
- Infections (PJP)
- Osteoporosis
- Infertility
- Neuropsychiatric disorders

Management
- Transsphenoidal surgery (TSS) for CD or Resection of ectopic ACTH source
- Pharmacotherapy for hypercortisolemia
- Pharmacotherapy for hypertension
- Pituitary radiotherapy (after failed TSS if not controlled medically)
- Bilateral adrenalectomy

Endocrine Hypertension. https://doi.org/10.1016/B978-0-323-96120-2.00011-X

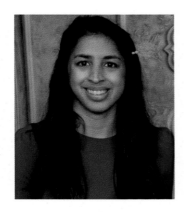

Stuti Fernandes

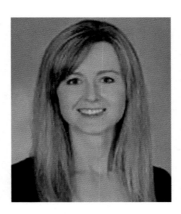

Elena V. Varlamov

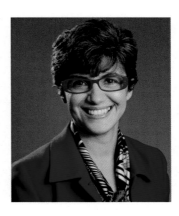

Maria Fleseriu

Introduction

Cushing's syndrome (CS) is an important cause of secondary hypertension. Hypertension is the most prevalent comorbidity and present in 75%—85% of adults and 47%—51% of children and adolescents with endogenous Cushing's. In patients with ectopic CS, the prevalence of hypertension is 95% [1—5]. Complex pathophysiological mechanisms are involved in the etiology of hypertension in patients with CS. Signs and symptoms of CS overlap with other conditions such as obesity, metabolic syndrome, and depression and thus it can take years to diagnose CS. Once there is clinical suspicion for CS, a complex testing algorithm including obtaining serum cortisol, salivary cortisol, urinary cortisol, and imaging studies are required to confirm the presence and to localize the disease source [6—8], leading to further delay in the diagnosis and treatment. In fact, the mean time to diagnosis for patients with CS is 34 months (14 months for ectopic CS, 30 months for adrenal CS, and 38 months for pituitary CS) [9]. Timely diagnosis is important to minimize morbidity and mortality, especially since there is evidence that duration of CS can impact outcome of surgery [9]. Even after curative surgery, many of the sequelae of CS persist; hypertension is still present in more than 75% of such patients, perhaps due to irreversible vascular remodeling that might develop after prolonged glucocorticoid excess states [5].

Moreover, hypertension can complicate the management of CS and the perioperative care of patients contemplating potentially curative surgical treatment. Therefore, it is imperative for clinicians to have a thorough understanding of the epidemiology, pathophysiology, clinical characteristics, management algorithms, and follow-up care of patients with CS-related hypertension. This chapter is an attempt to compile up-to-date evidence for this purpose.

Clinical presentation, screening, and diagnosis of Cushing's syndrome

Cushing's syndrome is a severe medical condition caused by chronic exposure to elevated cortisol levels. Patients often present with weight gain, central obesity, hypertension, fatigue, decreased libido, menstrual abnormalities, hirsutism, dorsocervical fat pad, supraclavicular fullness, mood disturbances, and peripheral edema. However, these signs and symptoms are common in the general population, especially with the rise in global prevalence of obesity. Signs and symptoms with a higher specificity for CS include facial plethora, easy bruising, reddish purple striae >1 cm, osteoporosis, and proximal myopathy or muscle weakness [7]. On laboratory work up, these patients may have hypokalemia (from excess cortisol acting on the mineralocorticoid (MC) receptor [10]), hyperglycemia [11], leukocytosis [12], elevated liver enzymes [13], secondary hyperparathyroidism [14], and hyperandrogenism [15].

Endogenous CS is caused by an adrenocorticotropin (ACTH)-secreting pituitary adenoma, cortisol secreting adrenal tumor, or an ectopic ACTH- or corticotrophin-releasing hormone (CRH)-producing tumor. Endogenous CS is rare and occurs in approximately 3/100,000 people [16]. On the other hand, CS due to exogenous administration of glucocorticoids is much more common. Therefore, if there is suspicion of CS, the first step is to rule out exogenous glucocorticoid exposure (oral, injectable, inhaled, or topical preparations). Then cortisol excess should be confirmed with one or more of the following tests: 24-hour urinary free cortisol (UFC), late night salivary cortisol (LNSC), and/or dexamethasone suppression testing (DST) [6—8]. UFC measures cortisol not bound to cortisol binding globulin (CBG). Urine collection should be done at least twice and collected along with urine creatinine and volume to ensure adequate collection. This test may not be accurate in those patients with chronic renal insufficiency [7].

Patients with CS lose their normal circadian rhythm of cortisol production and overnight drop in cortisol levels and thus patients with CS have high late night salivary cortisol (LNSC) values. LSNC should be checked multiple times at bedtime or midnight [6]. LSNC may not be accurate in smokers, shift workers or those with oral bleeding and infection [7].

In healthy patients, 1 mg of dexamethasone should inhibit ACTH production and cortisol concentrations. A normal response to dexamethasone given at 11 p.m.−12 a.m. is cortisol suppression to <1.8 ug/dL. Dexamethasone levels should be checked as well to ensure that the patient does not have malabsorption, increased dexamethasone metabolism (caused by medications such as carbamazepine and phenytoin), decreased dexamethasone clearance (renal or liver insufficiency), or performed the test incorrectly. DST is recommended as the first-line screening test for CS in those with an adrenal incidentaloma. This test may not be accurate in patients with alterations in cortisol binding globulin and albumin, such as those on estrogen [6−8]. Though these tests have high sensitivity, they do not have high specificity.

Physicians should use the results of several screening tests and clinical judgment to confirm the diagnosis of CS [7]. Patients with severe obesity, psychiatric disorders, alcohol overuse, polycystic ovary syndrome, and some other metabolic disorders may have clinical features simulating CS and abnormal screening tests, known as non-neoplastic hypercortisolism or pseudo-Cushing's. Special testing with dexamethasone-CRH test and/or desmopressin test are pursued to rule out pseudo-Cushing's [6].

Localization testing: distinguishing between ACTH-dependent and ACTH-independent Cushing's syndrome

Once the diagnosis is confirmed, healthcare providers should determine if the CS is ACTH dependent (∼80%) or ACTH independent (∼20%) [6−8,16]. In patients with ACTH independent CS, ACTH is usually suppressed (<10 pg/mL), and adrenal imaging should be pursued to look for an adrenal adenoma or bilateral adrenal hyperplasia [8]. However, an ACTH level of 10−20 pg/mL can also occur in those with adrenal CS. Raised dehydroepiandrosterone sulfate (DHEA-S) levels in the setting of low ACTH increase suspicion of adrenal carcinoma [8]. For further reading on adrenal CS, please refer Chapter 14.

In cases of ACTH dependence, ACTH level is high or normal (>20 pg/mL); differential diagnosis includes an ACTH producing pituitary adenoma (∼80%; Cushing's Disease, CD) or ectopic ACTH secretion by a tumor (EAS; ∼20%) [7,8]. There is no single test that can easily distinguish between CD and ectopic CS. It is recommended to use a combination of imaging and diagnostic testing within the clinical context to determine the source of ACTH [6]. Pituitary MRI should be obtained looking for a pituitary adenoma as it is the most common cause of ACTH-dependent CS. A finding of an adenoma >10 mm lends support to the diagnosis of CD [6−8]. However, ∼12% of patients with EAS can also have abnormal pituitary imaging [14]. On the other hand, normal pituitary MRI does not rule out pituitary source of CS because up to 40% of corticotroph adenomas are not visible on MRI [17]. Inferior petrosal sinus sampling (IPSS) is recommended to localize the source of ACTH in cases of pituitary adenomas < 6−9 mm or in uncertain cases [6,7]. IPSS measures ACTH in the pituitary drainage versus peripheral venous sample; a central to peripheral ACTH gradient >2 before or >3 after stimulation (with CRH or desmopressin) is consistent with a pituitary source [6,8]. IPSS is highly sensitive and specific (∼95%) for differentiating pituitary from ectopic ACTH secretion, but is invasive and only available at specialized centers [8]. Peripheral CRH and desmopressin tests are potential alternative noninvasive tests. They rely on robust ACTH and cortisol responses in CD versus a poor response in EAS. However, overlap in responses exists and the diagnostic accuracy of these tests is lower than IPSS [18]. High dose dexamethasone suppression testing with 8 mg of dexamethasone has been used to differentiate between CD and EAS. In theory, patients with CD retain the ability to inhibit ACTH secretion in response to high dose dexamethasone, whereas ACTH production is not affected by dexamethasone in those with EAS [6]. However, some patients with EAS (especially benign carcinoid tumors) do have ACTH suppression in response to high dose dexamethasone not making this test sufficiently accurate [6,8]. A combination of CRH and desmopressin testing, pituitary MRI, and whole-body CT has been proposed as an alternative to IPSS in specialized centers for selected patients [6−8].

If the pituitary is confirmed to be the source of ACTH overproduction, then pituitary surgery is the first line treatment in most patients [6,7].

If an ectopic source is suspected, then localization imaging should be pursued. EAS is commonly caused by carcinoid tumors of the lung, islet cell tumors of the pancreas, medullary carcinoma of the thyroid, small cell tumors of the lung, and tumors of the thymus [19]. CT scan of cervical, thoracic, abdominal, and pelvic regions is the initial imaging modality for localization of the tumor. In the cases of negative anatomic imaging and a strong suspicion for EAS, nuclear imaging ([65]Ga DOTATATE- and/or FDG-PET) is recommended [6].

A diagnostic algorithm for CS from the Pituitary Society Guidelines is depicted in Fig. 13.1 [6].

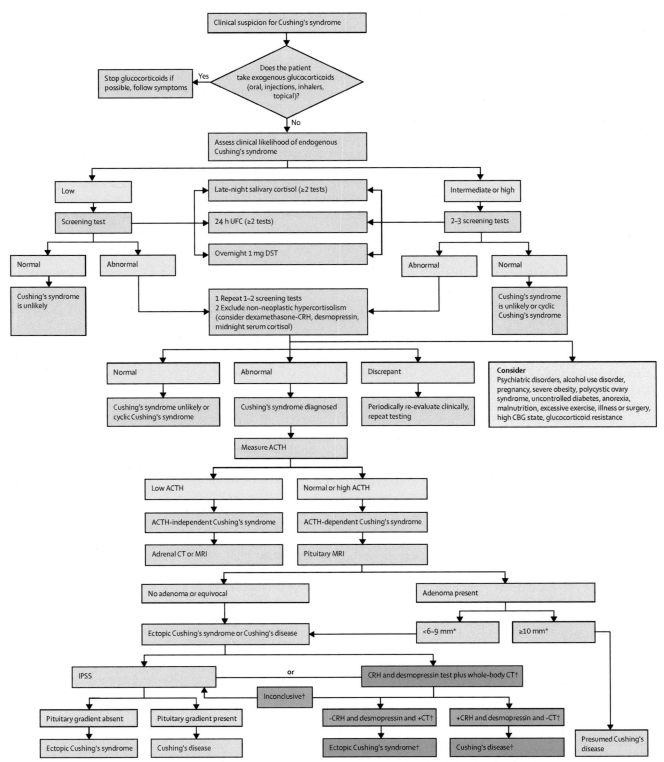

FIGURE 13.1   Algorithm for diagnosis of Cushing's syndrome ACTH, adrenocorticotropic hormone; CBG, corticosteroid-binding globulin; CRH, corticotropin-releasing hormone; DST, dexamethasone suppression test; IPSS, inferior petrosal sinus sampling; UFC, urinary free cortisol. *There is consensus that all patients with lesions smaller than 6 mm in diameter should have IPSS and those with lesions of ≥10 mm do not need IPSS, but expert opinions differed for lesions 6–9 mm in diameter. †This alternative option does not have clear consensus and needs further research, and this is indicated by darker boxes. Blue boxes indiate points to consider; darker colours indicate less validated testing pathways. *Adapted with permission from Fleseriu, M., Auchus, R., Bancos, I., Ben-Shlomo, A., Bertherat, J., Biermasz, N. R., Boguszewski, C. L., Bronstein, M. D., Buchfelder, M., Carmichael, J. D., Casanueva, F. F., Castinetti, F., Chanson, P., Findling, J., Gadelha, M., Geer, E. B., Giustina, A., Grossman, A., Gurnell, M., ... Biller, B. M. K. (2021). Consensus on diagnosis and management of Cushing's disease: a guideline update. The Lancet. Diabetes & Endocrinology, 9(12), 847–875. https:// doi.org/10.1016/S2213-8587(21)00235-7.*

Epidemiology of hypertension in Cushing's syndrome

Elevated blood pressure is more prevalent in EAS, and one study reported it was more common in adrenal CS versus Cushing's disease (CD) [20]. The incidence is much lower in those with iatrogenic CS (20%), and in these patients, hypertension is usually dose dependent [21,22]. There is debate over or as to whether the severity of blood pressure elevation in CS is related to the magnitude of cortisol elevation [5,20]. Hypertension appears to be associated with older age and longer exposure to excess glucocorticoids [5]. There appears to be no sex differences in hypertension prevalence among patients with CD [23]. Most patients present with mild to moderate hypertension, but some patients (17%) have severe blood pressure elevations [24]. On the other hand, the prevalence of CS is 0.5% in hypertensive patients and <1% in those with resistant hypertension [25]. Thus, not all patients with hypertension should be screened for CS. Screening should occur in those with other clinical findings suggestive of a diagnosis of CS. Additionally many patients with CS may also have essential hypertension that predates the CS [26].

The risk of cardiovascular disease is 4–5 fold higher in CS patients than in the general population, and risk factors include hypertension, hypercoagulability, obesity, dyslipidemia, and diabetes mellitus [22]. Thus, proper evaluation and management of all other comborbidities is promptly needed after diagnosis.

Pathophysiology of hypertension in Cushing's syndrome

Early in the disease process, there is an altered blood pressure circadian rhythm in patients with CS [20], while circadian rhythm is preserved in those with essential hypertension or primary aldosteronism. The abnormal circadian rhythm in blood pressure elevation is seen in both untreated and treated patients, and often there is no nocturnal fall; some patients even have a rise in blood pressure at night. Interestingly, patients on exogenous glucocorticoids (GCs) also lose the diurnal variation [27–29]. The absence of nocturnal blood pressure fall is associated with a higher rate of cardiovascular events, increased left ventricular hypertrophy, faster progression of microalbuminuria and renal damage, increased vascular stiffness, and an overall increased cardiovascular mortality [28].

The pathogenesis of hypertension in CS is complex and not fully understood [30]. There are several mechanisms for hypertension in those with CS including: MC receptor activation, activation of the renin-angiotensin system, increased sensitivity to vasoconstrictors, increased beta-adrenergic receptor sensitivity to catecholamines, suppression of vasodilators, sleep apnea, and insulin resistance [20,22,24]. These mechanisms are summarized in Table 13.1.

Cortisol binds to the glucocorticoid receptor (GR) and MC receptor. **Activation of the MC receptor** causes reabsorption of sodium in the kidneys, and intravascular volume expansion due to overactivity of the epithelial sodium channel (ENaC) [20,26]. Sodium reabsorption in the distal nephron is coupled with tubular secretion of potassium and protons,

TABLE 13.1 Mechanisms of hypertension in Cushing's syndrome.

Mineralocorticoid receptor activation	11 β HSD2 saturation and decreased activity [24,29,31–33] ↑ Plasma volume [22]
Renin angiotensin system (RAS) activation	↑ Angiotensinogen [34,35] ↑ Angiotensin II 1A receptors I in blood cell [36] ↑ Pressor response to angiotensin II [22,31,34]
Sympathetic nervous system	↑ Sensitivity of β adrenergic receptors [20,22]
Vasoregulatory system	↑ Endothelin 1 [1,20,28,37] (some studies indicate no role of ET1 [26,37–39]) ↓ Sodium calcium exchanger in vascular smooth muscle = ↑ cytosolic calcium = vasoconstriction [22,40] ↑ Erythropoietin [22] ↓ Response to atrial natriuretic peptide [22] ↓ Nitric oxide and L arginine [22,31] ↓ Prostacyclin [22] ↓ Prostaglandin E2 [22] ↓ Kallikrein [22] ↑ VGEF [22]
Other	Sleep apnea [20,26] Insulin resistance [22]

leading to hypokalemia and metabolic alkalosis [24]. Hypokalemia leads to activation of the sodium chloride cotransporter (NCC) leading to further volume expansion [20]. Volume expansion leads to lower levels of renin [1]. The MC receptor has a similar binding affinity for both aldosterone and cortisol in vitro. However, in vivo **11-β-hydroxysteroid dehydrogenase-2 (11-βHSD2)** converts cortisol to cortisone, which does not activate the MC receptor. This enzyme is overwhelmed in CS leading to impaired cortisol-to-cortisone metabolism. Of note, there is significant variability in the activity of 11-βHSD2, and there is evidence of a positive association between 11-βHSD2 activity and BMI [20]. Additionally, in cultured human cells, ACTH decreased the activity of 11-βHSD2 in a dose-dependent manner [24,29]. Excess MC activity contributes directly to endothelial dysfunction, left ventricular hypertrophy, and cardiomyopathy [26]. MC excess is most prevalent in patients with EAS and these patients often have hypokalemic alkalosis, which is only present in <10% of those with other etiologies of CS [31]. Patients with EAS also have increased production of other adrenal metabolites such as deoxycorticosterone (DOC) and corticosterone, which cause sodium retention [22]. Thus MC excess may not be a significant mechanism of hypertension in other forms of CS besides EAS [31]. Supporting this is the fact that MC receptor antagonism does not fully normalize blood pressure in CS patients, suggesting that there are other mechanisms of hypertension [20]. Long-term use of mifepristone, a GR blocker that does not bind the MC receptor, can normalize blood pressure in CS in some patients, while worsening it in others. Thus, it appears that activation of MC receptor and sodium retention can amplify hypertension but is not required for its development [31].

Patients with CS have **increased angiotensinogen levels**, the renin substrate. However, plasma concentrations of angiotensin II, aldosterone, and renin are often normal and thus there is speculation of increased throughput in the renin-angiotensin-aldosterone (RAAS) system [34,35]. There are conflicting data on renin levels in CS patients with some studies showing normal and other studies showing low levels, while a few studies even show elevated levels. One study focused on patients with CD found low renin and aldosterone levels, thus suggesting, in these patients, hypertension is not renin-mediated [41]. CS patients have an increased pressor response to angiotensin II; in rats, steroid exposure results in increased angiotensin II receptor type 1 expression in brain and peripheral tissues, and increases angiotensin II converting enzyme (ACE) [34]. In humans with CS, there are greater number of angiotensin II 1A receptors in blood cells [36]. Glucocorticoids also enhance the central actions of angiotensin II to increase blood pressure [24,31], and intravenous angiotensin II antagonist administration attenuates glucocorticoid induced hypertension [34].

Glucocorticoids cause increased secretion of **endothelin-1** (ET-1), a vasoconstrictor produced by smooth muscle cells and vascular endothelial cells [28]. Levels are significantly elevated in patients with untreated CS [1] and there is a decline in ET-1 in Cushing's patients following remission [20]. Studies of the role of ET-1 in rats with glucocorticoid induced hypertension have been conflicting. In animal studies, 11-βHSD2 inhibitor impairs cortisol-to-cortisone metabolism and increases vascular ET-1 levels. Chronic use of an endothelin type-A receptor antagonist normalizes vascular ET-1 concentration and reduces blood pressure, supporting a role of ET-1 in glucocorticoid mediated hypertension [37]. However, bosentan (a nonselective endothelin antagonist) has no effect on blood pressure in rats with ACTH-induced hypertension, indicating there is no major role of ET-1 in Cushing's syndrome-mediated hypertension [26,37−39].

Additionally, glucocorticoids downregulate the expression of the **sodium-calcium exchanger** in vascular smooth muscle [40]. This results in higher cytosolic calcium levels causing vasoconstriction. High cortisol levels cause increased concentrations of **erythropoietin (EPO)** leading to polycythemia. EPO has a direct vasoconstrictor effect and may also contribute to elevated blood pressure [22].

Cortisol results in the upregulation of the **sympathetic nervous system** by potentiating the action of catecholamines [22]. Chromaffin cells convert norepinephrine to epinephrine using the enzyme phenylethanolamine N-methyltransferase (transcription is glucocorticoid dependent) [20]. The sensitivity of β-adrenergic receptors is increased in states of cortisol excess, though catecholamine levels are normal. This results in increased vascular tone. Increased pressor response to angiotensin II and noradrenaline, and greater negative chronotropism to phenylephrine has been shown in patients with CS. Additionally, there is an increase in the number of α_{1B}-adrenergic receptors in vascular smooth muscle which further increases vascular tone [22].

Glucocorticoids impair the action or production of **vasodilators** such as **atrial natriuretic peptide (ANP), nitric oxide (NO), prostacyclin, prostaglandin E2, and kallikrein** [22]. Circulating levels of ANP are normal or increased in CS; however, patients have a decreased response to ANP as compared with healthy subjects. Glucocorticoids inhibit the enzyme NO synthase leading to lower NO levels [31]. Decreased NO activity is associated with increased production of vascular superoxide, which is important in the development of hypertension and atherosclerosis. There is also decreased transmembrane transport of L-arginine, the substrate for NO production. L-arginine has been shown to have beneficial endothelial effects [22]. Glucocorticoids also inhibit production of prostacyclin [31].

Plasma levels of **vascular endothelial growth factor (VGEF)**, an important angiogenic factor, are increased in patients with CS. This leads to increased angiotensin converting enzyme activity in endothelial cells, and likely increased local angiotensin II production [22].

With weight gain there is an initial **reduction in urine sodium excretion**. Additionally plasma volume, extracellular fluid volume, and exchangeable sodium are increased significantly and contribute to elevated blood pressure [22].

Sleep apnea is also common in patients with CS. These patients have disproportionate weight gain from adiposity in the head, neck, and waist areas. There are also myopathic changes in genioglossal and geniohyoid muscles responsible for the patency of the airway which contributes to development of sleep apnea [26]. Sympathetic tone is increased during hypoxemic episodes leading to hypertension. Regular use of continuous positive airway pressure (CPAP) has been found to markedly improve blood pressure in these patients [20]. Central hypothyroidism is also common in patients with CS and can contribute to development of sleep apnea [26].

Insulin resistance is also thought to play a role in the development of hypertension in CS patients [22].

Other complications of Cushing's syndrome

Other complications of CS include cardiovascular disease, hyperglycemia, hyperlipidemia, hypokalemia, hypercoagulability, infection, osteoporosis, infertility, and neuropsychiatric disorders [19,35].

Cardiovascular risk is markedly elevated in patients with CS. Dyslipidemia is present in 16%−64% and type 2 diabetes mellitus in 30%. The increased mortality in CS patients is driven primarily by myocardial infarction, stroke, and other vascular events [6]. Predictors for mortality are older age at diagnosis, duration of active disease, and presence of diabetes and hypertension [42]. This cardiovascular risk is reduced, but not normalized with treatment of CS [6]. It is important to treat cardiovascular and metabolic complications simultaneously with treatment of CS itself in order to improve outcomes.

Patients with CS are at high risk for venous thromboembolic (VTE) and arterial thrombotic events which occur in about 18% [43]. The incidence of venous thromboembolism is more than 10-fold increased as compared with the normal population [44,45]. The pathogenesis of hypercoagulability in CS is not completely understood; patients have increased production of procoagulant factors (factor VII and Von Willebrand factor ristocetin cofactor), and activation of the coagulation cascade [46]. In patients who have had curative surgery for CD, the increased thromboembolic risk continues to persist in the first months after surgery. Thus, prophylactic anticoagulation has been recommended by many experts, particularly for patients with risk factors (history of VTE or thrombophilia, severe CS, estrogen/testosterone use, poor mobility, or prolonged hospitalization) [6,35,47,48]. The choice of regimen and duration is individualized; longer prophylaxis (up to 2 months post-operatively or longer) has been proposed for the highest risk patients and after bilateral adrenalectomy [6,43].

Patients with CS are also at risk of various bacterial, viral, and fungal infections due to suppression of the immune system. *Pneumocystis jirovecii* pneumonia (PJP) is a high-mortality opportunistic fungal infection that sometimes develops in patients with severe CS. Elevated cortisol levels result in deprivation of T lymphocytes and macrophages [49]. Additionally, treatment of CS leads to recovery of the T cells which can result in an inflammatory reaction to PJP, similar to immune reconstitution syndrome (IRIS) in HIV patients [49]. The risk of PJP has been found to be associated with the degree of cortisol elevation. Prophylaxis with trimethoprim-sulfamethoxazole (TMP-SMX) should be considered in patients with severe CS [49].

Patients with cortisol excess are at risk for osteoporosis and bone fractures. Osteopenia is present in 60%−80% and osteoporosis in 30%−65% of patients with CS [50]. Fractures may be the first clinical manifestation of CS and occur most commonly at the thoracic and lumbar vertebrae [6,50]. Glucocorticoids inhibit osteoblast function, thereby suppressing bone formation [50]. Glucocorticoids also inhibit calcium reabsorption in the kidney and reduce calcium absorption in the intestine, thus leading to secondary hyperparathyroidism, increased bone resorption and risk of kidney stones [51,52]. CS patients have suppressed sex and growth hormones, further contributing to decreased osteoblast function [6]. Bone mineral density improves with treatment of CS, and may be completely reversed in some [50]. Conventional osteoporosis treatment with calcium, vitamin D, and bisphosphonate may result in more rapid improvement in bone mineral density than treatment of hypercortisolism alone [6].

Glucocorticoids can inhibit growth hormone secretion, thus many patients with CS have growth hormone deficiency (GHD) and low hepatic production of insulin-like growth factor 1 (IGF-1). In patients with CD, GHD is more prevalent in children, younger patients and/or women; notably, diabetes mellitus and hypertension are more prevalent in patients with both CS and GHD [6−8]. A recent study found that low IGF-1 at 6 months was also predictive of more severe muscle weakness postremission of CS [53]. GHD has been shown in a meta-analysis to increase mortality in patients with hypopituitarism of various causes [54]. However, though GH replacement ameliorates several complications associated with metabolic syndrome, prospective trials failed to show reversal of metabolic syndrome or cardiovascular complications [55].

Treatment of Cushing's syndrome and associated hypertension

Once the source of cortisol or ACTH excess is identified, initial resection of the primary lesion is recommended. In the case of an adrenal adenoma causing CS, patients may undergo unilateral adrenalectomy. Virtually all patients are cured by adrenalectomy and mortality is low, especially with a laparoscopic approach [56,57]. Bilateral macronodular adrenal hyperplasia (BMAH) and primary pigmented adrenal nodular adrenocortical disease are treated with bilateral adrenalectomy (or unilateral adrenalectomy for BMAH in selected cases) [6–8]. Patients with CD should undergo transsphenoidal surgery (TSS), unless they are not candidates due to high surgical risk, they decline surgery, or surgery is not possible. Remission rate varies in the literature, up to 80% for microadenomas, while remission for macroadenomas in specialized centers is up to 60% [6–8]. Remission is more likely in patients who have a noninvasive microadenoma visible on preoperative imaging and histopathological analysis, a postoperative serum cortisol nadir <55 nmol/L (<2 µg/dL) and an experienced surgeon [6–8,58]. In EAS, the source of ACTH production should be actively sought and surgically resected if feasible [6,14]. For curative purposes, EAS tumors should be well localized on imaging and in an accessible area without distant metastases [19]. It is hard to determine outcomes of surgery in patients with EAS given the rarity of EAS, different underlying etiology and varying degree of metastases. From one study, surgical cure is achieved in 83% of those with bronchial carcinoid [59]; patients with squamous cell and thymic carcinoid causing EAS tend to have poor prognosis [60].

The role of preoperative management of hypercortisolism in CS is unclear. A retrospective database study found no differences at 6-month follow-up in morbidity or remission rates between those treated with medical therapy prior to and those proceeded directly to surgery. However, patients with more severe clinical features were more likely to receive medical therapy, which confounds the analysis. Also, medical treatment is recommended in patients with occult EAS to treat acute and possibly potentially life-threatening morbidities caused be severe hypercortisolism [61]. There is no specific guidance on preoperative blood pressure management for CS patients; noncardiac surgery guidelines recommend a preoperative blood pressure <180–200/100–110 mmHg [62–65]. In the long-term, blood pressure goal is <130/80 mmHg for patients with increased cardiovascular risk (atherosclerotic cardiovascular disease, ASCVD >10%–15%) and diabetes, and <140/90 mmHg for patients without increased cardiovascular risk [66,67]. Additionally, management of hyperglycemia, hyperlipidemia, as well as antiplatelet therapy for secondary and, in some patients, for primary prevention of CVD is recommended to reduce potential cardiovascular events perioperatively and long term [35]. Patients with multiple comorbidities due to CS are likely to benefit from multidisciplinary management in conjunction with endocrinology, primary care provider, surgery, and cardiology consultations in case of suspected CVD.

Medical therapy for CS is implemented when the surgery is not possible or is delayed, in patients with severe hypercortisolism while awaiting surgery, and in case of persistent CS after an unsuccessful surgery. Options for medical treatment include adrenal steroidogenesis inhibitors (Osilodrostat, Metyrapone, Levoketoconazole, Ketoconazole, Etomidate, Mitotane), pituitary directed drugs for CD (Pasireotide, Cabergoline) and GR blockers (Mifepristone). These medications and their effects on blood pressure are summarized in Table 13.2. Radiotherapy is used for incompletely resected or significantly enlarging pituitary adenomas causing persistent CD [6,14]. Finally, bilateral adrenalectomy and subsequent replacement of adrenal steroids can be considered in cases where rapid eucortisolism is necessary, or when other therapies have failed, or are not appropriate [6,8].

A management algorithm from the Pituitary Society guidelines for patients with CD is depicted in Fig. 13.2 [6].

Achievement of eucortisolism or hypocortisolemia by surgery, generally results in significant improvement of hypertension, though often does not eradicate it. While the patient is awaiting surgery, treatment of hypertension should be implemented to reduce the risk of cardiovascular events. If the patient is already receiving antihypertensive treatment, this should be further optimized in the preoperative period. Postoperatively, antihypertensive agents may need to be reduced, or even discontinued to prevent hypotension and hyperkalemia especially in patients who achieve biochemical remission [35].

Medical treatment of hypercortisolemia also helps to control hypertension, particularly in severe cases. However, it is not typically used routinely for mild and moderate disease in centers where surgery can be undertaken without delay [6–8]. Patients with persistent CS treated medically may also require ongoing antihypertensive treatment [35].

Antihypertensive therapy in Cushing's syndrome

Patients with active and uncontrolled CS will often require more than one agent to control their blood pressure [22]. However, no controlled studies on combination therapies are available in patients with CS to guide treatment [73]. Thus,

TABLE 13.2 Summary of medications for treatment of HTN or CS, their effects on blood pressure and common adverse effects.

Medication	Mechanism of action	Doses	Effect on blood pressure	Possible side effects
Antihypertensives				
Captopril [68,69] Trandolapril	Angiotensin converting enzyme inhibition	Captopril 3.75 mg TID Trandolapril 2 mg/day	Trandolapril ↓ in 50% Captopril and ramipril ↓	Dry cough, hyperkalemia, angioedema
Losartan [70,71] Saralasin[a]	Angiotensin receptor blockers	Losartan 50 mg	Losartan ↓ in 50% Saralasin ↓	Hyperkalemia, angioedema
Spironolactone [21,26,72—74]	Mineralocorticoid receptor antagonist Androgen receptor blocker	25—100 mg/day	May not affect blood pressure significantly	Hyperkalemia Irregular or absent menses Gynecomastia, reduced libido, erectile dysfunction
Eplerenone [26,75]	Mineralocorticoid receptor antagonist	50—200 mg/day	No studies in CS	Hypokalemia Fewer androgen side effects than spironolactone
Triamterene [76]	Potassium sparing diuretic Blocks epithelial sodium channel	50—100 mg/day	No studies in CS	Dizziness, fatigue, hypokalemia, diarrhea
Chlorthalidone Hydrochlorothiazide (HCTZ) [20,73,77]	Diuretic Impairs sodium transport in distal convoluted tubule	HCTZ 6.25—50 mg/day	No studies in CS	Hypokalemia, hyperuricemia, diabetes May reduce kidney stones in CS patients
Isosorbide Mononitrate [21]	Donor of nitric oxide	60 mg	↓ in patients given GC	Headache, tachycardia, flushing, nausea
Atenolol [20,73,78—80] Carvedilol Labetalol Nebivolol	Selective beta blockers [20]	Carvedilol 25 mg BID Nebivolol 2.5—10 mg/day	No change in patients given GC Consider in patients with hx of MI, active angina, HF	Bradycardia, fatigue Avoid in patients with pheochromocytoma
Doxazosin [20,81]	Alpha 1 receptor antagonist causing vasodilation	1—16 mg/day (usual dose 7 mg)	No specific studies in CS 3rd line therapy in resistant HTN	Dizziness, fatigue, headache, vertigo, edema
Medications used for Cushing syndrome treatment [6—8]				
Pituitary directed drugs				
Cabergoline [82—84]	D2 receptor agonist	0.5—7 mg/week	Relaxes vascular smooth muscle ↓ cortisol in some patients ↓BP in some patients	Dizziness, nausea, mood changes, valvular heart disease (high dose)
Bromocriptine [85—88] Not used for CS anymore, rarely used for Nelson's syndrome	D2 receptor agonist	2.5—40 mg/day	Variable reports on change in cortisol ↓ BP in non-CS patients	Nasal congestion, nausea, and postural hypotension

Continued

TABLE 13.2 Summary of medications for treatment of HTN or CS, their effects on blood pressure and common adverse effects.—cont'd

Medication	Mechanism of action	Doses	Effect on blood pressure	Possible side effects
Pasireotide [82,89,90]	Somatostatin receptor ligand (SSTR5 especially)	600–900 μg BID 10–30 mg monthly (long acting)	↓ BP even with partial UFC control	Nausea, gall stones, diarrhea, prolonged QTc, hyperglycemia (frequent)
Retinoic Acid [20,73,91,92]	↓ ACTH production through inhibition of AP-I and Nur77/Nurrl transcriptional activities	10–80 mg/day	↓ cortisol ↓ BP in some patients	Conjunctival irritation, cheilitis, mucositis, nausea, headache, arthralgias, elevated triglyceride, transaminitis
Steroidogenesis inhibitors				
Osilodrostat [16,93 –95]	Inhibits CYP11B1 and aldosterone synthase	1–30 mg BID (doses required for most patients are 2 –14 mg/day)	↓ cortisol and aldosterone but ↑ DOC BP ↓ [93,94] but no change in one study [95]	Hypokalemia, edema, HTN, hirsutism, nausea, diarrhea, adrenal insufficiency, QT prolongation
Metyrapone [26,82,96–100]	Inhibitor of 11 hydroxylase and aldosterone synthase Inhibits CYP11B1 mainly), CYP17, CYP11B2, CYP19	0.5–4.5 g (3–4 x/day)	↓ cortisol ↑ DOC BP: ↓ [96–98], ↑ [99] or no change [100]	Hypokalemia, HTN, edema, hirsutism, alopecia, acne, clitoromegaly, voice deepening, adrenal insufficiency, gastrointestinal distress
Ketoconazole [82,101–105]	Inhibits StAR[b], CYP11A1, CYP11B1, CYP17	400–1600 mg (BID or TID administration)	BP control appears to be related to cortisol control BP ↓ in 40% of patients or more	Adrenal insufficiency, transaminitis, gastrointestinal distress, hypogonadism, drug –drug interactions
Levoketoconazole [106]	Inhibits CYP17A1, CYP11A1, CYP11B1, and CYP21A2	150–600 mg BID	No change in BP overall, though BP would improve in some patients with UFC decreased	Nausea, headache, adrenal insufficiency, transaminitis, gastrointestinal distress, drug–drug interactions, QT prolongation
Etomidate [82,107,108]	Inhibits StAR[b], CYP11A1, CYP11B1, CYP17	Bolus 5 mg (1 x) followed by IV 0.02 –0.3 mg/kg/hr	↓ BP	Sedation, adrenal insufficiency, propylene glycol toxicity
Mitotane [82,104,109]	Inhibits StAR[b], CYP11A1, CYP11B1, CYP11B2, 3β-HSD Adrenolytic	2–5 g/day	↓ cortisol ↓ aldosterone No change in BP in one study	Adrenal insufficiency, dizziness, altered cognition, gastrointestinal distress, teratogenic, cytopenia, hyperglycemia low T4 m, drug–drug interactions
Glucocorticoid receptor antagonist				
Mifepristone [82,110,111]	Glucocorticoid receptor antagonist	300–1200 mg/day	↓ action of cortisol on GR	Hypokalemia, HTN, adrenal insufficiency,

Continued

TABLE 13.2 Summary of medications for treatment of HTN or CS, their effects on blood pressure and common adverse effects.—cont'd

Medication	Mechanism of action	Doses	Effect on blood pressure	Possible side effects
			↑ action of cortisol on MR ↓BP in some, ↑ in some and treat with MR blocker	vaginal bleeding, endometrial hyperplasia, nausea, fatigue, edema, arthralgias, edema, QTc prolongation

[a]no longer used to treat patients.
[b]steroidogenic acute regulatory protein.

treatment recommendations are extrapolated from the general hypertension guidelines while keeping in mind CS-specific issues. The goal of treatment is to achieve a blood pressure of <140/80 mmHg in those with atherosclerotic cardiovascular disease (ASCVD) risk <10%−15% or <130/80 mmHg in those with diabetes mellitus and ASCVD >10%−15% [35,66].

Since glucocorticoid-mediated hypertension may be augmented by alterations in the renin-angiotensin-aldosterone (RASS) system, ACE inhibitors and angiotensin receptor II blockers (ARBs) are preferred. Angiotensin II blockers (losartan) and ACE inhibitors (trandolapril, captopril) have been found to normalize the blood pressure in 50% of CS patients [22]. These agents have also been shown to have cardiovascular benefit in patients with diabetes mellitus, and heart failure [66]. These classes of antihypertensives are recommended by some as the first line agents for treatment of hypertension in CS [73].

Agents that block MC receptors and spare potassium (spironolactone or eplerenone) can be used as they also reduce the edema and hypokalemia associated with hypercortisolism. Spironolactone also blocks the androgen receptors, and may be useful in treatment of hirsutism, acne, and alopecia in women, but the progesterone agonism results in irregular or absent menses. However, spironolactone can cause gynecomastia, reduced libido, and erectile dysfunction in men [22,26]. Eplerenone is a more selective MC receptor antagonist that can be used if the antiandrogen side effects of sprinolactone are not tolerable [26]. As monotherapy, this class of antihypertensives may not affect the blood pressure significantly [21,73,74]. However, they are effective at reducing MC effects of cortisol excess and its precursors that may be present in high amounts in patients treated with mifepristone, metyrapone, or osilodrostat. Triamterene is a nonreceptor blocking potassium sparing diuretic that can be used, though there are no studies of its use in CS [26]. Importantly, MC receptor blockers also have benefits in patients with heart failure [66].

Atenolol, a beta blocker, was shown to decrease cardiac output and blood pressure, but did not prevent increase in blood pressure in study patients given glucocorticoids to induce hypertension [31]. Beta blockers are generally not the first-line treatment in uncomplicated hypertension in CS, but may be beneficial in patients with myocardial infarction, active angina, heart failure, and for rate control [79].

Felodipine, a calcium channel blocker, has not been shown to be useful in managing glucocorticoid-induced hypertension [31,66]. However, this class of medications may be useful in combination [31] and there is evidence of synergism when used with an ACE inhibitor in non-CS hypertension management [81].

Isosorbide mononitrate, a nitrate that results in release of NO, may have a role in management of hypertension in CS. One study showed a decrease in blood pressure in patients with iatrogenic glucocorticoid-induced HTN [21].

Doxazosin, an alpha blocker, has effectively been used as third-line therapy in resistant hypertension and does not have any specific contraindications related to CS [81].

Due to frequent hypokalemia in patients with CS, medications such as thiazides, indapamide, furosemide, and ethacrynic acid should be used sparingly. Additionally, furosemide causes renal losses of calcium, and this may further increase the risk of osteoporotic fractures and kidney stones [22,26]. If used, furosemide should be paired with calcium supplementation, and an antiresorptive agent (bisphosphonate) [22]. Hydrochlorothiazide may be preferred over furosemide to avoid osteoporosis and kidney stones risk [73].

Peroxisome proliferator-activated receptor gamma (PPARγ) receptor antagonists, such as pioglitazone and rosiglitazone, showed antiproliferative and proapoptotic effects on corticotroph cells in vitro, and have antiinflammatory,

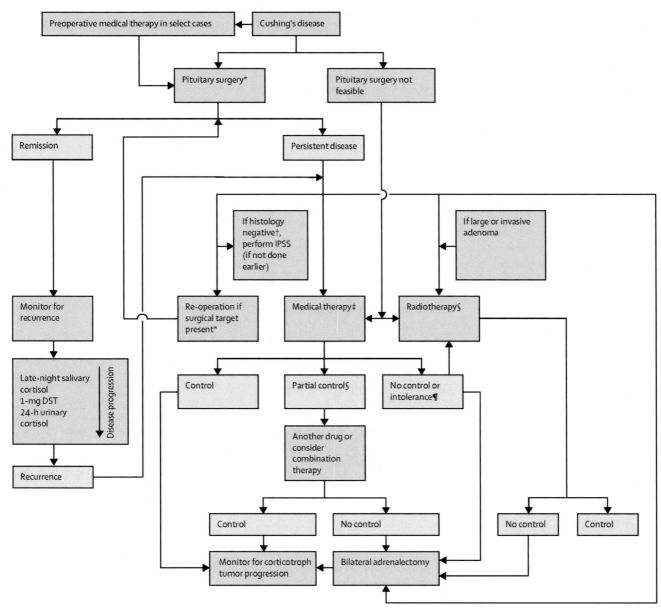

FIGURE 13.2 Algorithm for management of Cushing's disease. ACTH adrenocorticotropic hormone; DST, dexamethasone suppression test; IPSS, inferior petrosal sinus sampling. *Pituitary surgery should be performed by an experienced surgeon. †Absence of ACTH-staining adenoma. §Lifelong monitoring for hypopituitarism and secondary neoplasia in the radiation field required. ¶On maximum tolerated dose of the drug. ‡See Table 2 and panel 3 for considerations regarding selection of medical therapy of the article Fleseriu, M., Auchus, R., Bancos, I., Ben-Shlomo, A., Bertherat, J., Biermasz, N. R., Boguszewski, C. L., Bronstein, M. D., Buchfelder, M., Carmichael, J. D., Casanueva, F. F., Castinetti, F., Chanson, P., Findling, J., Gadelha, M., Geer, E. B., Giustina, A., Grossman, A., Gurnell, M., … Biller, B. M. K. (2021). Consensus on diagnosis and management of Cushing's disease: a guideline update. The Lancet. Diabetes & Endocrinology, 9(12), 847–875. https://doi.org/10.1016/S2213-8587(21)00235-7 (from which the figure is adapted with permission).

antioxidative, and antiproliferative effects on the cells of the vessel walls [20]. This class of medications has been shown to reduce blood pressure in patients with type 2 diabetes mellitus and cause downregulation of 11β-HSD1, thus decreasing availability of biologically active glucocorticoids. Thus, it was hypothesized PPARγ antagonists could be used in the treatment of CS [112]. Though PPARγ antagonists were shown in some studies to reduce UFC, significant blood pressure reductions have not been demonstrated [113].

Role of medical therapy for CS in the treatment of hypertension

Treatment of CS and normalization of UFC has shown to be the most efficacious treatment for glucocorticoid induced hypertension [73].

Adrenal steroidogenesis inhibitors

Medications that suppress adrenal steroid production such as osilodrostat, metyrapone, ketoconazole, levoketoconazole, and mitotane are most frequently used in CS and have been shown to improve hypertension in CS (Table 13.2). However, some of these treatments can also worsen hypertension.

Metyrapone and osilodrostat inhibit 11-β-hydroxylase and aldosterone synthase, which results in decreased cortisol and aldosterone levels but causes increases in deoxycorticosterone (DOC) levels, a potent MC [22,104]. Both are approved in Europe, while in the US Metyrapone is used off-label. Patients may develop hypertension, hypokalemia, and edema, but these can be treated and prevented by using MC receptor blockers. In addition to changes in blood pressure, steroidogenesis inhibitors can help to improve blood glucose, lipids (except mitotane), weight, and muscle strength [114]. However, side effects and drug-drug interactions should be considered.

Ketoconazole blocks several enzymes involved in steroidogenesis, and reductions in blood pressure appear to be related to reductions in UFC. Ketoconazole is approved in Europe, but is used off-label in the US [102,103,110]; use requires frequent monitoring of liver enzymes and it has an FDA warning for hepatoxicity. It also decreases adrenal androgen synthesis and can contribute to hypogonadism and gynecomastia in men. Ketoconazole prolongs the QT interval and should be used with caution if other QT prolonging drugs are prescribed [104,105]. Lastly, ketoconazole is a potent inhibitor of CYP3A4 and other hepatic cytochromes, and can elevate concentrations of many medications commonly used in CS, such as eplerenone, amlodipine, nifedipine, losartan, statins (contraindicated with simvastatin and lovastatin), sulfonylureas, and pioglitazone [104,105].

Levoketoconazole, a more potent enantiomer of ketoconazole with a neutral effect on blood pressure based on a phase III clinical trial, has been recently FDA approved [106]. In addition to providing sustained reductions in UFC, it has shown to lower total and LDL cholesterol, glycemic parameters, and weight [106]. It has potential for liver toxicity (FDA warning for hepatoxicity); however, this was mild and reversible in clinical trials. Levoketoconazole also has the risk of drug-drug interactions and QT prolongation.

Etomidate is the only parenteral option for treating CS. It inhibits several enzymes involved in the steroidogenesis pathway. Studies show improvement in hypertension [107,108].

Mitotane is a steroidogenesis inhibitor and adrenolytic agent used most often in the management of adrenocortical carcinoma. Use results in reduced cortisol and aldosterone levels which, in theory, should result in reductions in blood pressure [6–8,82]. There are not many studies on its use and one study showed no change in blood pressure [109].

Aminoglutethimide inhibits steroid production early and blocks conversion of cholesterol to pregnenolone [115], and was used in the past as an adjunct to metyrapone therapy and has been found to decrease blood pressure in patients with low renin hypertension [116], but it is not available anymore.

Pituitary targeted agents

Pasireotide, a somatostatin receptor ligand approved for treatment of CD, has been found to improve hypertension in clinical trials in both biochemically controlled and partially controlled patients [42]. Favorable lipid and weight effects were also noted in clinical trials. However, development of hyperglycemia is common and often leads to discontinuation of its use [89]. Octreotide and lanreotide are used in treatment of neuroendocrine tumors; however, their effectiveness in treatment of EAS is low [19]. In rats, treatment with somatostatin and octreotide has been shown to decrease the volume of the adrenal zona glomerulosa and serum concentrations of aldosterone. Human arterial endothelial cells express somatostatin receptor subtypes 1, 2, and 4, and thus medications targeting these receptors may affect vasoconstriction. In fact, octreotide and pasireotide have been found to reduce vasoconstriction of the iliac arteries in rats [41], but despite this potential blood-pressure lowering effect, hypertension has persisted in some patients treated with pasireotide in both clinical trials and post trial studies [42,89,90,117].

In a study of patients with CD taking cabergoline, 8/20 had long-term normalization of UFC and resolution of hypertension. Blood pressure decreased after short-term treatment, and nearly normalized in the majority of patients during long-term treatment. Hypertension improved even in patients without improvement in UFC [83], though the mechanism is not clear. Dopamine receptors in the vascular system could mediate a relaxing effect resulting in decreased peripheral resistance [83,84]. Additionally, in vitro studies showed that cabergoline inhibited aldosterone secretion in primary cultures of human adrenal glands [41,118]. Bromocriptine, another dopamine agonist, has been shown to inhibit ACTH secretion in rats, but outcomes in humans with CS have been variable. It is rarely used to treat patients with CD but has been used in Nelson's syndrome [85,86]. Bromocriptine has been found to reduce blood pressure in patients with essential hypertension [87].

Retinoic acid has antiproliferative action on corticotroph cells and can rarely used for CD, though it is off label. Studies have shown a significant decrease in UFC as well as systolic and diastolic blood pressure [20,91,92].

Glucocorticoid receptor blockers

Mifepristone, a GR and progesterone receptor antagonist could mildly improve blood pressure in some patients, mostly diastolic pressure [111]. It also has a positive effect on blood glucose, lipids, and weight and is approved just in the US for hyperglycemia associated with CS. However, it leads to further elevation of cortisol levels, leading to oversaturation of the 11-βHSD2 enzyme that normally inactivates cortisol. These excessive cortisol levels cause inappropriate MC activation and can worsen hypertension [22,35,119]; hypertension was noted in 24%, peripheral edema in 26%, and hypokalemia in 34% of patients in a clinical trial [111]. As with osilodrostat and metyrapone, MC receptor blockers often need to be used concurrently to reduce these effects [22]. Additionally, mifepristone also has significant drug—drug interactions and is contraindicated with simvastatin and lovastatin and should be used with caution with QT prolonging drugs [104].

Follow up of Cushing syndrome and hypertension

After surgical treatment for CS, patients should be closely followed. Patients who achieve surgical remission may have adrenal insufficiency and require glucocorticoid replacement. They usually experience a gradual resolution of symptoms and slow recovery of the hypothalamic-pituitary-adrenal axis [8]. Patients with CD should be monitored lifelong for recurrence of cortisol excess clinically and biochemically, as recurrence occurs in approximately one third of patients [6—8]. Patients with persistent CD or recurrence require further treatment for hypercortisolemia (reoperation, medical therapy, radiation, or bilateral adrenalectomy), and ongoing management for cortisol-dependent morbidities.

In patients with surgical remission of CD, there is a significant decrease in systolic and diastolic blood pressure [28]. Therefore, proactive reductions or withdrawal of blood pressure medications is often necessary [35]. However, a third of patients have persistent systolic hypertension and 75% have diastolic hypertension [20,22]. Patients with CS often have essential hypertension, which is not expected to be cured after surgery [22]. Many still have a lack of diurnal variation (nondippers) even after cure, which may account for the persistently increased cardiovascular risk (50% were nondippers preoperatively, and 28% were nondippers at 3 years) [28]. However, those with adrenal adenomas appear to have restoration of circadian rhythm [120]. There does not appear to be a correlation between severity of hypertension before cure and persistence after. Longer duration of hypertension is associated with persistence of hypertension after surgical cure, likely reflecting irreversible remodeling of vasculature [22]. One study showed that lower baseline UFC predicted the persistence of hypertension several years after remission of CS, and may be reflective of longer time of exposure to excess cortisol in patients with milder CS [5].

Bilateral adrenalectomy can be considered rarely after failed pituitary surgery for CD, for example, in women desiring pregnancy, but is mostly employed for unlocalized EAS or severe CS requiring rapid control of hypercortisolemia. In one study, hypertension was present in 85% and resolved in 40% after removal of the adrenal glands. Patients also had improvement in weight, diabetes mellitus, hirsutism, and proximal muscle weakness. Risks of this procedure include adrenal crisis, and corticotroph tumor progression (Nelson syndrome). This procedure is not as risky as it once was (13.6% mortality), but risk factors for mortality include male sex, EAS, and prolonged postoperative ventilator dependence [121].

Children and adolescents are more likely to have resolution of hypertension after surgical cure. As in adults, duration of hypertension is correlated with persistence of hypertension. Younger patients may be more protected from permanent remodeling, potentially through the antigrowth and anticytokine effects of glucocorticoids [22]. However some pediatric patients will continue to have persistent hypertension, which might be from vascular remodeling or excess cortisol replacement dosing [20].

A summary of medications for treatment of HTN and CS, their effects on blood pressure, and the common adverse effects are shown in Table 13.2.

Summary

Cushing's syndrome should be suspected in patients with hypertension and other clinical features of CS (central obesity, striae, myopathy, or osteoporosis). It is important to have high clinical suspicion for CS since these patients are at increased risk for morbidity and mortality. After suspecting CS, several laboratory tests should be performed to confirm the diagnosis, followed by localization for ACTH dependent or independent CS. For most patients, where tumor is seen on imaging, surgical resection is the mainstay of treatment. Most patients have improvement in hypertension after surgery, but many require continued blood pressure management. If surgery is not possible or noncurative, medical therapy should be pursued. Medications for CS might improve or worsen blood pressure, thus specific medications for blood pressure are often needed.

Learning points

- Cushing's syndrome is a condition of cortisol excess that has devastating health consequences and increased mortality if not appropriately treated.
- Cushing's syndrome work-up is complex. Once cortisol excess is confirmed, it should be determined if cortisol production is ACTH dependent or independent.
- Surgical cure is ideal when the source of cortisol excess is removed and is the best treatment for cortisol induced hypertension.
- Medications used to treat CS usually improve, but sometimes can worsen hypertension; understanding the mechanisms of these drugs and using antihypertensives concurrently can help mitigate rise in blood pressure.

References

[1] Ross EJ, Linch DC. Cushing's syndrome—killing disease: discriminatory value of signs and symptoms aiding early diagnosis. Lancet 1982;320(8299):646—9.

[2] Terzolo M, et al. Adrenal incidentaloma: a new cause of the metabolic syndrome? J Clin Endocrinol Metab 2002;87(3):998—1003.

[3] Magiakou MA, et al. Blood pressure in children and adolescents with Cushing's syndrome before and after surgical cure. J Clin Endocrinol Metab 1997;82(6):1734—8.

[4] Plotz CM, Knowlton AI, Ragan C. The natural history of Cushing's syndrome. Am J Med 1952;13(5):597—614.

[5] Schernthaner-Reiter MH, et al. Factors predicting long-term comorbidities in patients with Cushing's syndrome in remission. Endocrine 2019;64(1):157—68.

[6] Fleseriu M, et al. Consensus on diagnosis and management of Cushing's disease: a guideline update. Lancet Diabetes Endocrinol 2021;9(12):847—75.

[7] Nieman LK, et al. The diagnosis of Cushing's syndrome: an endocrine society clinical practice guideline. J Clin Endocrinol Metab 2008;93(5):1526—40.

[8] Lacroix A, et al. Cushing's syndrome. Lancet 2015;386(9996):913—27.

[9] Rubinstein G, et al. Time to diagnosis in Cushing's syndrome: a meta-analysis based on 5367 patients. J Clin Endocrinol Metab 2020;105(3):dgz136.

[10] Fan L, et al. Association of hypokalemia with cortisol and ACTH levels in Cushing's disease. Ann N Y Acad Sci 2020;1463(1):60—6.

[11] Mazziotti G, Gazzaruso C, Giustina A. Diabetes in Cushing syndrome: basic and clinical aspects. Trends Endocrinol Metabol 2011;22(12):499—506.

[12] Masri-Iraqi H, et al. Elevated white blood cell counts in Cushing's disease: association with hypercortisolism. Pituitary 2014;17(5):436—40.

[13] Hazlehurst JM, Tomlinson JW. Non-alcoholic fatty liver disease in common endocrine disorders. Eur J Endocrinol 2013;169(2):R27—37.

[14] Nieman LK, et al. Treatment of Cushing's syndrome: an endocrine society clinical practice guideline. J Clin Endocrinol Metab 2015;100(8):2807—31.

[15] Arnaldi G, Martino M. Androgens in Cushing's syndrome. Front Horm Res 2019;53:77—91.

[16] Barbot M, Zilio M, Scaroni C. Cushing's syndrome: overview of clinical presentation, diagnostic tools and complications. Best Pract Res Clin Endocrinol Metab 2020;34(2):101380.

[17] Patronas N, et al. Spoiled gradient recalled acquisition in the steady state technique is superior to conventional postcontrast spin echo technique for magnetic resonance imaging detection of adrenocorticotropin-secreting pituitary tumors. J Clin Endocrinol Metab 2003;88(4):1565—9.

[18] Vassiliadi DA, Tsagarakis S. Diagnosis of endocrine disease: the role of the desmopressin test in the diagnosis and follow-up of Cushing's syndrome. Eur J Endocrinol 2018;178(5):R201—r214.

[19] Young J, et al. Management of endocrine disease: Cushing's syndrome due to ectopic ACTH secretion: an expert operational opinion. Eur J Endocrinol 2020;182(4):R29—58.

[20] Barbot M, Ceccato F, Scaroni C. The pathophysiology and treatment of hypertension in patients with Cushing's syndrome. Front Endocrinol 2019;10. pp. 321—321.

[21] Williamson PM, Kelly JJ, Whitworth JA. Dose-response relationships and mineralocorticoid activity in cortisol-induced hypertension in humans. J Hypertens Suppl 1996;14(5):S37–41.

[22] Magiakou MA, Smyrnaki P, Chrousos GP. Hypertension in Cushing's syndrome. Best Pract Res Clin Endocrinol Metab 2006;20(3):467–82.

[23] Giraldi FP, Moro M, Cavagnini F. Gender-related differences in the presentation and course of Cushing's disease. J Clin Endocrinol Metab 2003;88(4):1554–8.

[24] Cicala MV, Mantero F. Hypertension in Cushing's syndrome: from pathogenesis to treatment. Neuroendocrinology 2010;92(1):44–9.

[25] Rimoldi SF, Scherrer U, Messerli FH. Secondary arterial hypertension: when, who, and how to screen? Eur Heart J 2013;35(19):1245–54.

[26] Sacerdote A, et al. Hypertension in patients with Cushing's disease: pathophysiology, diagnosis, and management. Curr Hypertens Rep 2005;7(3):212–8.

[27] Imai Y, et al. Altered circadian blood pressure rhythm in patients with Cushing's syndrome. Hypertension 1988;12(1):11–9.

[28] Pecori Giraldi F, et al. Circadian blood pressure profile in patients with active Cushing's disease and after long-term cure. Horm Metab Res 2007;39(12):908–14.

[29] Imai Y, et al. Exogenous glucocorticoid eliminates or reverses circadian blood pressure variations. J Hypertens 1989;7(2):113–20.

[30] Pappachan JM, Buch HN. Endocrine hypertension: a practical approach. Adv Exp Med Biol 2017;956:215–37.

[31] Baid S, Nieman LK. Glucocorticoid excess and hypertension. Curr Hypertens Rep 2004;6(6):493–9.

[32] Ulick S, et al. Cortisol inactivation overload: a mechanism of mineralocorticoid hypertension in the ectopic adrenocorticotropin syndrome. J Clin Endocrinol Metab 1992;74(5):963–7.

[33] Stewart PM, et al. 11 beta-hydroxysteroid dehydrogenase activity in Cushing's syndrome: explaining the mineralocorticoid excess state of the ectopic adrenocorticotropin syndrome. J Clin Endocrinol Metab 1995;80(12):3617–20.

[34] Scheuer DA, Bechtold AG. Glucocorticoids potentiate central actions of angiotensin to increase arterial pressure. Am J Physiol Regul Integr Comp Physiol 2001;280(6):R1719–26.

[35] Varlamov EV, et al. Management of endocrine disease: cardiovascular risk assessment, thromboembolism, and infection prevention in Cushing's syndrome: a practical approach. Eur J Endocrinol 2021;184(5):R207–24.

[36] Shibata H, et al. Gene expression of angiotensin II receptor in blood cells of Cushing's syndrome. Hypertension 1995;26(6 Pt 1):1003–10.

[37] Ruschitzka F, et al. Endothelin 1 type a receptor antagonism prevents vascular dysfunction and hypertension induced by 11beta-hydroxysteroid dehydrogenase inhibition: role of nitric oxide. Circulation 2001;103(25):3129–35.

[38] Bailey MA. 11β-hydroxysteroid dehydrogenases and hypertension in the metabolic syndrome. Curr Hypertens Rep 2017;19(12):100.

[39] Sharma ST, Nieman LK. Cushing's syndrome: all variants, detection, and treatment. Endocrinol Metab Clin North Am 2011;40(2). 379–91-viii-ix.

[40] Smith L, Smith JB. Regulation of sodium-calcium exchanger by glucocorticoids and growth factors in vascular smooth muscle. J Biol Chem 1994;269(44):27527–31.

[41] van der Pas R, et al. Cushing's disease and hypertension: in vivo and in vitro study of the role of the renin-angiotensin-aldosterone system and effects of medical therapy. Eur J Endocrinol 2014;170(2):181–91.

[42] Pivonello R, et al. Complications of Cushing's syndrome: state of the art. Lancet Diabetes Endocrinol 2016;4(7):611–29.

[43] Suarez MG, et al. Hypercoagulability in Cushing syndrome, prevalence of thrombotic events: a large, single-center, retrospective study. J Endocr Soc 2019;4(2):bvz033.

[44] Stuijver DJ, et al. Incidence of venous thromboembolism in patients with Cushing's syndrome: a multicenter cohort study. J Clin Endocrinol Metab 2011;96(11):3525–32.

[45] Van Zaane B, et al. Hypercoagulable state in Cushing's syndrome: a systematic review. J Clin Endocrinol Metab 2009;94(8):2743–50.

[46] van der Pas R, et al. Hypercoagulability in Cushing's syndrome: prevalence, pathogenesis and treatment. Clin Endocrinol (Oxf) 2013;78(4):481–8.

[47] McCormick JP, et al. Venous thromboembolic (VTE) prophylaxis in Cushing disease patients undergoing transsphenoidal surgery. Interdiscip Neurosurg 2022;27:101371.

[48] Boscaro M, et al. Anticoagulant prophylaxis markedly reduces thromboembolic complications in Cushing's syndrome. J Clin Endocrinol Metab 2002;87(8):3662–6.

[49] van Halem K, et al. Characteristics and mortality of pneumocystis pneumonia in patients with Cushing's syndrome: a plea for timely initiation of chemoprophylaxis. Open Forum Infect Dis 2017;4(1):ofx002.

[50] Tóth M, Grossman A. Glucocorticoid-induced osteoporosis: lessons from Cushing's syndrome. Clin Endocrinol (Oxf) 2013;79(1):1–11.

[51] Mirza F, Canalis E. Management of endocrine disease: secondary osteoporosis: pathophysiology and management. Eur J Endocrinol 2015;173(3):R131–51.

[52] Canalis E, et al. Glucocorticoid-induced osteoporosis: pathophysiology and therapy. Osteoporos Int 2007;18(10):1319–28.

[53] Vogel F, et al. Patients with low IGF-I after curative surgery for Cushing's syndrome have an adverse long-term outcome of hypercortisolism-induced myopathy. Eur J Endocrinol 2021;184(6):813–21.

[54] Pappachan JM, et al. Excess mortality associated with hypopituitarism in adults: a meta-analysis of observational studies. J Clin Endocrinol Metab 2015;100(4):1405–11.

[55] Verhelst J, et al. The prevalence of the metabolic syndrome and associated cardiovascular complications in adult-onset GHD during GH replacement: a KIMS analysis. Endocr Connect 2018;7(5):653–62.

[56] Conzo G, et al. Long-term outcomes of laparoscopic adrenalectomy for Cushing disease. Int J Surg 2014;12:S107–11.

[57] Mishra AK, et al. Outcome of adrenalectomy for Cushing's syndrome: experience from a tertiary care center. World J Surg 2007;31(7):1425–32.

[58] Stroud A, et al. Outcomes of pituitary surgery for Cushing's disease: a systematic review and meta-analysis. Pituitary 2020;23(5):595–609.

[59] Isidori AM, et al. The ectopic adrenocorticotropin syndrome: clinical features, diagnosis, management, and long-term follow-up. J Clin Endocrinol Metab 2006;91(2):371−7.

[60] Salgado LR, et al. Cushing's disease arising from a clinically nonfunctioning pituitary adenoma. Endocr Pathol 2006;17(2):191−9.

[61] Webb SM, Valassi E. Morbidity of Cushing's syndrome and impact of treatment. Endocrinol Metab Clin North Am 2018;47(2):299−311.

[62] Howell SJ. Preoperative hypertension. Curr Anesthesiol Rep 2018;8(1):25−31.

[63] Goldman L, Caldera DL. Risks of general anesthesia and elective operation in the hypertensive patient. Anesthesiology 1979;50(4):285−92.

[64] Fleisher LA, et al. 2014 ACC/AHA guideline on perioperative cardiovascular evaluation and management of patients undergoing noncardiac surgery: executive summary: a report of the American College of Cardiology/American Heart Association Task Force on Practice Guidelines. Circulation 2014;130(24):2215−45.

[65] Gill R, Goldstein S. Evaluation and management of perioperative hypertension. In: StatPearls. Treasure Island (FL): StatPearls Publishing Copyright © 2022, StatPearls Publishing LLC; 2022.

[66] 10. Cardiovascular disease and risk management: standards of medical care in diabetes-2021. Diabetes Care 2021;44(1):S125−50.

[67] Arnett DK, et al. 2019 ACC/AHA guideline on the primary prevention of cardiovascular disease: a report of the American College of Cardiology/American Heart Association task force on clinical practice guidelines. Circulation 2019;140(11):e596−646.

[68] Saruta T, et al. Multiple factors contribute to the pathogenesis of hypertension in Cushing's syndrome. J Clin Endocrinol Metab 1986;62(2):275−9.

[69] Zacharieva S, et al. Trandolapril in Cushing's disease: short-term trandolapril treatment in patients with Cushing's disease and essential hypertension. Methods Find Exp Clin Pharmacol 1998;20(5):433−8.

[70] Zacharieva S, et al. Losartan in Cushing's syndrome. Methods Find Exp Clin Pharmacol 1998;20(2):163−8.

[71] Dalakos TG, et al. Evidence for an angiotensinogenic mechanism of the hypertension of Cushing's syndrome. J Clin Endocrinol Metab 1978;46(1):114−8.

[72] Batterink J, et al. Spironolactone for hypertension. Cochrane Database Syst Rev 2010;(8):Cd008169.

[73] Isidori AM, et al. The hypertension of Cushing's syndrome: controversies in the pathophysiology and focus on cardiovascular complications. J Hypertens 2015;33(1):44−60.

[74] Whitworth JA, Mangos GJ, Kelly JJ. Cushing, cortisol, and cardiovascular disease. Hypertension 2000;36(5):912−6.

[75] Tam TS, et al. Eplerenone for hypertension. Cochrane Database Syst Rev 2017;2(2):Cd008996.

[76] Gong H, et al. Modulatory effects of hydrochlorothiazide and triamterene on resistant hypertension patients. Exp Ther Med 2017;13(6):3217−22.

[77] Musini VM, et al. Blood pressure-lowering efficacy of monotherapy with thiazide diuretics for primary hypertension. Cochrane Database Syst Rev 2014;(5):Cd003824.

[78] Pirpiris M, et al. Hydrocortisone-induced hypertension in men. The role of cardiac output. Am J Hypertens 1993;6(4):287−94.

[79] Unger T, et al. 2020 International Society of Hypertension global hypertension practice guidelines. Hypertension 2020;75(6):1334−57.

[80] Choi DJ, et al. Assessment of clinical effect and treatment quality of immediate-release carvedilol-IR versus SLOW release carvedilol-SR in Heart Failure patients (SLOW-HF): study protocol for a randomized controlled trial. Trials 2018;19(1):103.

[81] Chapman N, et al. Effect of doxazosin gastrointestinal therapeutic system as third-line antihypertensive therapy on blood pressure and lipids in the Anglo-Scandinavian Cardiac Outcomes Trial. Circulation 2008;118(1):42−8.

[82] Fernandes S, Varlamov EV, Fleseriu M. Abrupt weight gain, hypertension, and severe hypokalemia in a young male. In: Davies TF, editor. A case-based guide to clinical endocrinology. Cham: Springer International Publishing; 2022. p. 27−41.

[83] Pivonello R, et al. The medical treatment of Cushing's disease: effectiveness of chronic treatment with the dopamine agonist cabergoline in patients unsuccessfully treated by surgery. J Clin Endocrinol Metab 2009;94(1):223−30.

[84] Murphy MB. Dopamine: a role in the pathogenesis and treatment of hypertension. J Hum Hypertens 2000;14(1):S47−50.

[85] Lamberts SW, et al. The mechanism of the suppressive action of bromocriptine on adrenocorticotropin secretion in patients with Cushing's disease and Nelson's syndrome. J Clin Endocrinol Metab 1980;51(2):307−11.

[86] Burman P, et al. Limited value of cabergoline in Cushing's disease: a prospective study of a 6-week treatment in 20 patients. Eur J Endocrinol 2016;174(1):17−24.

[87] Schobel HP, et al. Effects of bromocriptine on cardiovascular regulation in healthy humans. Hypertension 1995;25(5):1075−82.

[88] Morris D, Grossman A. The medical management of Cushing's syndrome. Ann N Y Acad Sci 2002;970:119−33.

[89] Pivonello R, et al. Pasireotide treatment significantly improves clinical signs and symptoms in patients with Cushing's disease: results from a Phase III study. Clin Endocrinol (Oxf) 2014;81(3):408−17.

[90] Colao A, et al. A 12-month phase 3 study of pasireotide in Cushing's disease. N Engl J Med 2012;366(10):914−24.

[91] Pecori Giraldi F, et al. Potential role for retinoic acid in patients with Cushing's disease. J Clin Endocrinol Metab 2012;97(10):3577−83.

[92] Vilar L, et al. The role of isotretinoin therapy for Cushing's disease: results of a prospective study. Int J Endocrinol 2016;2016:8173182.

[93] Bertagna X, et al. LCI699, a potent 11β-hydroxylase inhibitor, normalizes urinary cortisol in patients with Cushing's disease: results from a multicenter, proof-of-concept study. J Clin Endocrinol Metab 2014;99(4):1375−83.

[94] Pivonello R, et al. Efficacy and safety of osilodrostat in patients with Cushing's disease (LINC 3): a multicentre phase III study with a double-blind, randomised withdrawal phase. Lancet Diabetes Endocrinol 2020;8(9):748−61.

[95] Fleseriu M, et al. Osilodrostat, a potent oral 11β-hydroxylase inhibitor: 22-week, prospective, Phase II study in Cushing's disease. Pituitary 2016;19(2):138−48.

[96] Puglisi S, et al. Preoperative treatment with metyrapone in patients with Cushing's syndrome due to adrenal adenoma. Endocr Connect 2018;7(11):1227−35.

[97] Jeffcoate WJ, et al. Metyrapone in long-term management of Cushing's disease. Br Med J 1977;2(6081):215−7.

[98] Verhelst JA, et al. Short and long-term responses to metyrapone in the medical management of 91 patients with Cushing's syndrome. Clin Endocrinol (Oxf) 1991;35(2):169−78.

[99] Valassi E, et al. A reappraisal of the medical therapy with steroidogenesis inhibitors in Cushing's syndrome. Clin Endocrinol (Oxf) 2012;77(5):735−42.

[100] Ceccato F, et al. Metyrapone treatment in Cushing's syndrome: a real-life study. Endocrine 2018;62(3):701−11.

[101] Castinetti F, et al. Ketoconazole revisited: a preoperative or postoperative treatment in Cushing's disease. Eur J Endocrinol 2008;158(1):91−9.

[102] Winquist EW, et al. Ketoconazole in the management of paraneoplastic Cushing's syndrome secondary to ectopic adrenocorticotropin production. J Clin Oncol 1995;13(1):157−64.

[103] Sonino N, et al. Ketoconazole treatment in Cushing's syndrome: experience in 34 patients. Clin Endocrinol (Oxf) 1991;35(4):347−52.

[104] Varlamov EV, Han AJ, Fleseriu M. Updates in adrenal steroidogenesis inhibitors for Cushing's syndrome − a practical guide. Best Pract Res Clin Endocrinol Metab 2021;35(1):101490.

[105] Castinetti F, et al. Ketoconazole in Cushing's disease: is it worth a try? J Clin Endocrinol Metab 2014;99(5):1623−30.

[106] Fleseriu M, et al. Efficacy and safety of levoketoconazole in the treatment of endogenous Cushing's syndrome (SONICS): a phase 3, multicentre, open-label, single-arm trial. Lancet Diabetes Endocrinol 2019;7(11):855−65.

[107] Carroll TB, et al. Continuous etomidate infusion for the management of severe Cushing syndrome: validation of a standard protocol. J Endocr Soc 2018;3(1):1−12.

[108] Preda VA, et al. Etomidate in the management of hypercortisolaemia in Cushing's syndrome: a review. Eur J Endocrinol 2012;167(2):137−43.

[109] Baudry C, et al. Efficiency and tolerance of mitotane in Cushing's disease in 76 patients from a single center. Eur J Endocrinol 2012;167(4):473−81.

[110] Castinetti F, Conte-Devolx B, Brue T. Medical treatment of Cushing's syndrome: glucocorticoid receptor antagonists and mifepristone. Neuroendocrinology 2010;92(1):125−30.

[111] Fleseriu M, et al. Mifepristone, a glucocorticoid receptor antagonist, produces clinical and metabolic benefits in patients with Cushing's syndrome. J Clin Endocrinol Metab 2012;97(6):2039−49.

[112] Whitworth JA, et al. Cardiovascular consequences of cortisol excess. Vasc Health Risk Manag 2005;1(4):291−9.

[113] Pecori Giraldi F, et al. Effect of protracted treatment with rosiglitazone, a PPARgamma agonist, in patients with Cushing's disease. Clin Endocrinol (Oxf) 2006;64(2):219−24.

[114] Pivonello R, et al. The treatment of Cushing's disease. Endocr Rev 2015;36(4):385−486.

[115] Gross BA, et al. Medical management of Cushing disease. Neurosurg Focus 2007;23(3):E10.

[116] Woods JW, et al. Effect of an adrenal inhibitor in hypertensive patients with suppressed renin. Arch Intern Med 1969;123(4):366−70.

[117] Manetti L, et al. Long-term safety and efficacy of subcutaneous pasireotide in patients with Cushing's disease: interim results from a long-term real-world evidence study. Pituitary 2019;22(5):542−51.

[118] Pivonello R, et al. Dopamine receptor expression and function in human normal adrenal gland and adrenal tumors. J Clin Endocrinol Metab 2004;89(9):4493−502.

[119] Fleseriu M, et al. A new therapeutic approach in the medical treatment of Cushing's syndrome: glucocorticoid receptor blockade with mifepristone. Endocr Pract 2013;19(2):313−26.

[120] Zacharieva S, et al. Circadian blood pressure profile in patients with Cushing's syndrome before and after treatment. J Endocrinol Invest 2004;27(10):924−30.

[121] Prajapati OP, et al. Bilateral adrenalectomy for Cushing's syndrome: pros and cons. Ind J Endocrinol Metab 2015;19(6):834−40.

Chapter 14

Adrenal Cushing's syndrome

Oskar Ragnarsson[1,2]

[1]Department of Internal Medicine and Clinical Nutrition, Institute of Medicine at Sahlgrenska Academy, University of Gothenburg, Gothenburg, Sweden; [2]Department of Endocrinology, Sahlgrenska University Hospital, Gothenburg, Sweden

Visit the *Endocrine Hypertension: From Basic Science to Clinical Practice, First Edition* companion web site at: https://www.elsevier.com/books-and-journals/book-companion/9780323961202.

Graphical Abstract

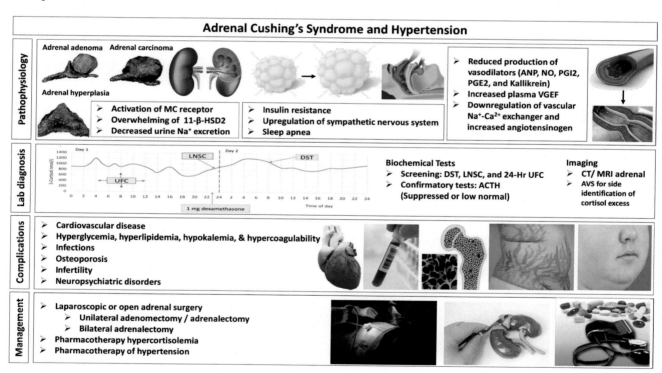

Adrenal Cushing's Syndrome and Hypertension

Pathophysiology

Adrenal adenoma   Adrenal carcinoma

Adrenal hyperplasia

➢ Activation of MC receptor
➢ Overwhelming of 11-β-HSD2
➢ Decreased urine Na⁺ excretion

➢ Insulin resistance
➢ Upregulation of sympathetic nervous system
➢ Sleep apnea

➢ Reduced production of vasodilators (ANP, NO, PGI2, PGE2, and Kallikrein)
➢ Increased plasma VGEF
➢ Downregulation of vascular Na⁺-Ca²⁺ exchanger and increased angiotensinogen

Lab diagnosis

Biochemical Tests
➢ Screening: DST, LNSC, and 24-Hr UFC
➢ Confirmatory tests: ACTH (Suppressed or low normal)

Imaging
➢ CT/ MRI adrenal
➢ AVS for side identification of cortisol excess

Complications
➢ Cardiovascular disease
➢ Hyperglycemia, hyperlipidemia, hypokalemia, & hypercoagulability
➢ Infections
➢ Osteoporosis
➢ Infertility
➢ Neuropsychiatric disorders

Management
➢ Laparoscopic or open adrenal surgery
  ➢ Unilateral adenomectomy / adrenalectomy
  ➢ Bilateral adrenalectomy
➢ Pharmacotherapy hypercortisolemia
➢ Pharmacotherapy of hypertension

Endocrine Hypertension. https://doi.org/10.1016/B978-0-323-96120-2.00006-6

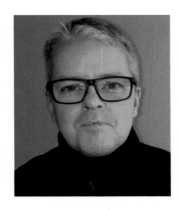

Oskar Ragnarsson

Introduction

Endogenous Cushing's syndrome (CS) is a rare disorder caused by chronic overproduction of cortisol. The most common causes of endogenous CS are adrenocorticotropin (ACTH)-producing pituitary adenoma (Cushing's disease), ectopic ACTH-producing tumors (ectopic CS) and cortisol-producing adrenal adenoma (commonest cause of adrenal CS) [1]. Less common causes of adrenal CS are cortisol-producing adrenocortical carcinoma and bilateral micro- and macronodular adrenal hyperplasia. Far more common than endogenous CS is exogenous CS, that is, patients who develop cushingoid features due to prolonged glucocorticoid treatment in supraphysiological doses.

CS, irrespective of the etiology, may have serious consequences on health. The risk for cerebro- and cardiovascular diseases, psychiatric illnesses, skeletal fractures, and severe infections are greatly increased in patients with CS [2]. Consequently, mortality is increased, not only in patients with untreated hypercortisolism, but also in patients who have achieved biochemical remission following treatment. Thus, CS is a serious disorder that needs to be diagnosed and treated properly without delay.

This chapter summarizes the epidemiology, genetics, clinical characteristics, management, follow-up, and outcome in patients with adrenal CS. A special emphasis is put on the pathophysiology and treatment of hypertension, a complication seen in most of the patients, as well as cardiovascular morbidity.

Causes and epidemiology of adrenal Cushing syndrome

Approximately 20%–30% of patients with endogenous CS have adrenal CS [3,4]. Since the cortisol production in all forms of adrenal CS is autonomous, and not dependent on stimuli from the pituitary gland, these together are also referred to as ACTH-independent CS (Table 14.1). The most common cause of adrenal CS is a cortisol-producing adrenocortical

TABLE 14.1

Etiologies of endogenous CS	Proportion of patients with CS
ACTH-dependent CS	
ACTH-producing pituitary adenoma	60%–70%
ACTH-producing pituitary carcinoma	Very rare
Ectopic ACTH-producing tumors	5%–10%
ACTH-independent (Adrenal CS)	
Cortisol producing adrenal adenoma	10%–20%
Cortisol producing adrenal carcinoma	5%
Bilateral macronodular adrenal hyperplasia	<2%
Bilateral micronodular adrenal hyperplasia	<2%

adenoma. Less common are cortisol-producing adrenocortical carcinoma and bilateral adrenal hyperplasia [1]. Several forms of adrenal hyperplasia exist; bilateral micronodular adrenal hyperplasia, characterized by either pigmented or nonpigmented micronodules (<10 mm), and bilateral macronodular adrenal hyperplasia that present either as macronodules (>10 mm) with internodular atrophy (primary bilateral macronodular adrenocortical hyperplasia; or PBMAH) or with internodular hyperplasia (massive macronodular adrenocortical disease; or MMAD) [5,6].

The etiologies of endogenous Cushing's syndrome are shown in Table 14.1.

Epidemiological studies that have estimated the incidence of adrenal CS are few. In two nationwide studies, one from New Zealand [7], and one from Denmark [3], the annual incidence of cortisol-producing adrenal adenoma was 0.3 and 0.6 cases per million per year, respectively. Similarly, in a recent study from Sweden, the incidence of adrenal CS was 0.5 cases per million per year [8]. In that study, 22 out of 82 (27%) patients with endogenous CS had adrenal CS; 14 had cortisol-producing adrenocortical adenoma, 5 had cortisol-producing adrenocortical carcinoma, two had bilateral micronodular adrenal hyperplasia, and one had bilateral macronodular adrenal hyperplasia. Finally, in a nationwide study from Korea, the incidence of adrenal CS was 1.3 per million per and year between 2002 and 2017 [9]. The vast majority (94%) of 1199 patients included in the study had benign adrenal CS.

The majority (80%–90%) of patients with cortisol-producing adrenal adenoma are women [4,9]. In patients with bilateral adrenal hyperplasia, the gender distribution is more or less equal [5,10]. Cortisol-producing adrenal adenoma and bilateral macronodular adrenal hyperplasia are most often diagnosed at an age between 40 and 60 years [4,5], while the median age at diagnosis of bilateral micronodular adrenal hyperplasia is 20 years [10].

In children, although rare, ACTH-producing pituitary adenomas are the most common cause of endogenous CS (as in adults) [11]. However, in neonates and infants, adrenal CS is more common [11,12], mainly due to rare genetic syndromes associated with adrenal CS as discussed below.

Genetic syndromes associated with adrenal Cushing syndrome

Several genetic syndromes are associated with adrenal CS [6].

Multiple endocrine neoplasia type 1 (MEN-1) is an autosomal dominant disorder, typically considered to be a syndrome characterized by development of hyperparathyroidism, pituitary adenoma, and pancreatic neuroendocrine tumors. However, patients with MEN-1 are also at increased risk for developing several other tumors, including adrenal tumors that affect at least 10% of individuals with this syndrome [13]. In fact, 5% of patients with MEN-1 develop CS, that may either be ACTH-dependent due to ACTH-producing pituitary adenoma or ectopic ACTH-production, or ACTH-independent due to benign or malignant adrenocortical tumors as well as bilateral adrenal hyperplasia [6,13].

McCune-Albright syndrome is a rare genetic disorder characterized by fibrous dysplasia of the bone, café-au-lait skin pigmentation, and various endocrinopathies, including precocious puberty, hyperthyroidism, and overproduction of growth hormone [14]. Adrenal CS is a rare but serious component of McCune-Albright syndrome, seen in 7% of the patients [15]. CS in these patients presents in the neonatal period and may be fatal if not adequately treated [12].

Carney complex is an autosomal dominant disorder that can present with a wide variety of features, including lentiginosis, cutaneous-, cardiac-, and breast-myxomas, thyroid and testicular tumors, psammomatous melanotic schwannomas, and acromegaly [16]. Adrenal CS is one of the most common manifestations of Carney complex, affecting approximately 70% of the women and 20% of the men [16]. CS in patients with Carney complex is caused by bilateral micronodular adrenal hyperplasia, also called primary pigmented nodular adrenocortical disease (PPNAD).

Other syndromes that rarely cause adrenal CS are Beckwith-Wiedemann syndrome and Li-Fraumeni syndrome [6].

Genetics of ACTH -independent Cushing syndrome

Significant progress has been made in the understanding of the genetic basis of adrenal CS [17]. Specifically, genetic alterations resulting in abnormal function of the cAMP-dependent protein kinase A (PKA) system, a major cell-signaling pathway in humans and other species, is of great importance. This was first discovered in patients with McCune-Albright syndrome who have an activating mutation in *GNAS,* a gene that encodes the alpha subunit of the G-protein complex, an important regulator of the cAMP-dependent PKA system [18]. Similarly, the majority (70%) of patients with Carney complex have a mutation in *PRKAR1A*, encoding another regulatory protein of PKA (Protein Kinase CAMP-Dependent Type I Regulatory Subunit Alpha) [19]. Furthermore, mutations in *PRKACA*, a gene encoding the Cα subunit of PKA, have been found in 35%–65% of patients with cortisol-producing adrenal adenoma and overt CS [20–23]. Thus, genetic variants responsible for activation of the cAMP-dependent PKA system, resulting in increased cell proliferation and cortisol-production, appear to be an important player in the pathogenesis of adrenal CS.

Another recent and important discovery was that one-fourth of the patients with primary bilateral macronodular adrenal hyperplasia (PBMAH) have a damaging mutation of the gene encoding armadillo repeat-containing protein 5 (ARMC5), a protein that inhibits the cell cycle and stimulates cell apoptosis in the adrenal gland [5,24]. Interestingly, patients with cortisol-producing adrenal adenoma secondary to *PRKACA* mutation, as well as patients with PBMAH secondary to *ARMC5* mutation, both have a more severe phenotype with higher cortisol concentrations than patients with same disorders but without these mutations [5,20].

Clinical features

Patients with CS may present with various symptoms and signs. The degree of cortisol secretion varies greatly in patients with CS, from a marginally elevated concentration causing mild symptoms, to greatly increased plasma levels causing a severe phenotype. The most common symptoms are fatigue and weight gain [1,4,25], where a central fat accumulation with an increased waist circumference, supraclavicular and dorsocervical fat pads, and round face are characteristic (Table 14.2). Due to the presence of muscle atrophy, the extremities are often disproportionally thin compared to the rest of the body, and muscle weakness is common. Cutaneous symptoms are also common, including skin atrophy, striae, easy bruising, plethora, and acne. Most patients with CS have hypertension, which can be therapy-resistant, and one-third have diabetes mellitus. Other common symptoms are depression, anxiety, cognitive impairment, insomnia, menstrual disorders, and osteoporosis with an increased fracture risk. Some symptoms such as bluish-purple striae, facial plethora, proximal muscle weakness, easy bruising, and unexpected osteoporotic fractures are more specific for CS [26]. These are, however, often absent in patients with mild CS.

None of the symptoms of endogenous CS can be used to determine the etiology of the hypercortisolism, i.e., whether it is caused by adrenal, pituitary, or ectopic source. However, patients with ectopic CS often have a shorter disease course, and more severe hypercortisolism, characterized by severe muscle weakness, hyperglycemia, therapy-resistant hypertension, hypokalemia, and sometimes disorientation and/or psychosis. Also, due to pronounced catabolism, weight gain and the otherwise characteristic central fat accumulation may not be present in these patients with severe hypercortisolism.

Many of the symptoms and clinical signs of CS are nonspecific and are common in the general population. A long diagnostic delay is, therefore, unfortunately common, especially in patients with mild hypercortisolism. In a study from Germany, the mean time from the first contact with a physician due to symptoms caused by CS until a correct diagnosis was made was 3 years [27]. On an average, the patients met with five different specialists before being diagnosed; most

TABLE 14.2 Clinical characteristics of Cushing's syndrome.

Clinical characteristics of CS	Proportion
Fatigue	90%
Weight gain with central fat accumulation, increased waist circumference, supraclavicular and dorsocervical fat pads and round face	80%—90%
Hypertension	75%—85%
Skin changes including skin atrophy, **blue-violet striae, easy bruising, facial plethora,** hirsutism, and acne	70%—80%
Proximal muscle atrophy and muscle weakness	60%—70%
Cognitive dysfunction including memory and concentration defects and impaired attention	60%—80%
Oligomenorrhoea or amenorrhoea	50%—60%
Sleeping difficulties	50%
Decreased libido and erectile dysfunction	50%
Depression	40%—60%
Diabetes mellitus	30%
Osteoporotic fractures	20%

Symptoms that are more specific for CS are in bold italic style.

common specialists were general practitioners, gynecologists, dermatologists, internists, and/or orthopedists [27]. In a meta-analysis, including data from more than 5000 patients with CS, the mean diagnostic delay was 38 months in patients with ACTH-producing pituitary adenoma, 30 months in patients with adrenal CS, and 14 months in patients with ectopic CS [28]. This delay is unfortunate. The quality of life is greatly reduced in patients with CS and does not improve until successful treatment has been provided [29]. Also, severe comorbidities such as cardiovascular disease, fractures, thromboembolic disease, and psychiatric illness are common before diagnosis [2]. Furthermore, a long diagnostic delay is associated with increased mortality, emphasizing the importance of early diagnosis and treatment [30].

Pathophysiology of hypertension in adrenal Cushing syndrome

Hypertension is one of the most commonly occurring features of CS, being present in 80%—85% of the patients [4,31—33], and seem to be equally common in patients with adrenal CS as in patients with pituitary CS [4,33]. When evaluated with 24-hour ambulatory blood pressure monitoring, most patients with CS lack the nocturnal blood pressure dip that is normally seen in healthy individuals and in patients with essential hypertension [34—36]. The blood pressure in patients with untreated CS can be greatly increased. In fact, a recent study from Austria showed that 9% of patients with CS had required in-patient management for hypertensive crisis on some occasions before they were diagnosed with the syndrome [33].

The pathogenesis of hypertension in patients with CS is not fully understood [37]. However, one of the major pathophysiological mechanisms for the development of hypertension in patients with CS is the direct stimulatory effects of cortisol on the mineralocorticoid receptor in the kidneys (Fig. 14.1). In healthy individuals the mineralocorticoid receptor is protected from the actions of cortisol by the 11β-hydroxysteroid-dehydrogenase type 2 (11β-HSD2), an enzyme that converts cortisol to its inactive form, cortisone. In patients with CS, especially in patients with very high cortisol production, the enzyme becomes saturated, allowing the excessive amounts of cortisol to activate the mineralocorticoid receptor. This, in turn, leads to sodium retention, expansion of plasma volume, and hypertension [38,39].

The activation of the mineralocorticoid receptor is not the only explanation for the development of hypertension in patients with CS, and several other factors have been suggested (Fig. 14.1). However, most of the available literature on this topic dates back to the 1980s and 1990s, the studies often include a small number of subjects, and the findings are frequently based on administration of glucocorticoids to healthy subjects, rodents or in vitro cells, and not on patients with endogenous CS. Nevertheless, among suggested mechanisms are increased concentrations of angiotensinogen [40], increased expression of the angiotensin II type 1 gene in smooth muscle cells [41], increased vascular sensitivity to angiotensin II and/or catecholamines [42—45], and increased cardiac sensitivity to catecholamines [46]. Decreased

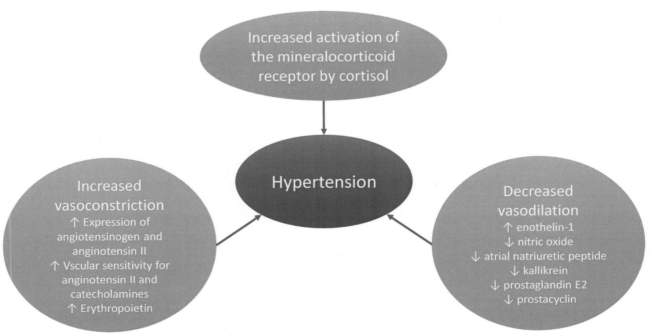

FIGURE 14.1 Pathophysiological mechanisms of hypertension in Cushing's syndrome.

production of vasodilating mediators have also been suggested including kallikrein, prostacyclin (prostaglandin I_2), prostaglandin E_2 [44,47], and nitric oxide [48,49]. Similarly, increased production of vasoconstricting mediator like enothelin-1 [50] is also suggested. Furthermore, erythropoietin-mediated reduction of vasodilating mediators and increased vasoconstriction has also been proposed [51].

Investigations for adrenal CS

Upon clinical suspicion of CS, a screening for the disorder should be initiated without a delay. Three tests are useful for this purpose: 24-h urinary free cortisol (UFC), overnight 1 mg dexamethasone suppression test (DST), and late-night salivary cortisol (LNSC) [26,52]. With these tests, three cardinal features of endogenous CS are utilized to diagnose the syndrome, that is, the increased cortisol production (UFC), the nonsuppressible autonomous cortisol production by the administration of exogenous glucocorticoids (DST), and the lack of normal circadian cortisol rhythm (LNSC) (Fig. 14.2).

Which test is chosen depends on the local availability of these tests with a validated analytical method and well-defined diagnostic cut-offs, as well as certain patient characteristics such as renal function, severity of the hypercortisolism, and the use of medications that either increase the concentrations of corticosteroid-binding globulin (e.g., oral estrogen) or induce a more rapid degradation of dexamethasone (e.g., carbamazepine) (Table 14.3). All the tests have a high sensitivity for identifying patients with CS. DST has slightly higher sensitivity than the other two tests while the specificity is lower [53]. More details on the initial diagnostic evaluation of CS are discussed in Chapter 13: ACTH-dependent Cushing's syndrome (Fernandes et al. 2022).

The next step in the investigation of patients with biochemically confirmed CS is to measure plasma ACTH level. Patients with adrenal CS have low ACTH levels, while those with ACTH-dependent CS have normal or high plasma ACTH. For patients with adrenal CS, computed tomography (CT) of the adrenal glands is primarily recommended, although magnetic resonance imaging (MRI) can also be used [54]. The most common cause of adrenal CS, an adrenal adenoma, is almost always larger than 1 cm in diameter, and therefore easy to detect. The most important differential diagnoses in patients with adrenal CS and unilateral adrenal lesion are cortisol-producing adrenal adenoma and adrenocortical carcinoma. Some of the radiological characteristics are useful to differentiate between these two disorders. Adrenal adenomas, compared to adrenocortical carcinoma, are smaller (mean 3.5 cm, [range 2−7 cm], vs. mean 14.5, [range 7.5−21] cm), have lower unenhanced attenuation [mean 11, range −16 to +41 Hounsfield units (HU), versus mean 28, range +20 to +31 HU] and have homogenous texture [55]. Differential diagnoses in patients with CS and bilateral adrenal

FIGURE 14.2 Screening tests for Cushing's syndrome based on cortisol circadian rhythm in health and disease. *DST*, Dexamethasone suppression test; *LNSC*, Late night salivary cortisol; *UFC*, Urinary free cortisol.

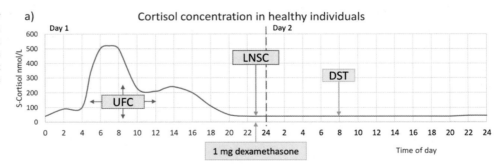

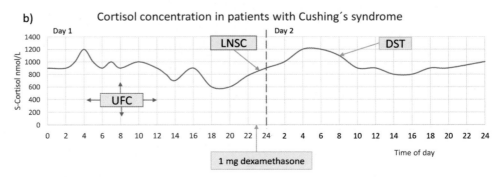

TABLE 14.3 Summary of the principles, strengths, and limitations with the three tests recommended for screening of CS.

Screening tests	Principles	Strengths	Limitations
Urinary free cortisol (UFC)	Reflects total cortisol production for 24 h	• Measures unbound (free) cortisol • Independent of concentrations of corticosteroid-binding globulin (CBG)	• Cumbersome for the patient • Dependent on complete urinary collection for 24 h • Low sensitivity in patients with mild hypercortisolism and impaired renal function
Dexamethasone suppression test (DST)	Reflects the autonomous cortisol production in CS that cannot be suppressed by administration of exogenous glucocorticoids	High sensitivity	• Low specificity • Total cortisol is measured • False-positive results are common in patients with increased CBG levels (e.g., use of oral estrogen and pregnancy) • False-positive results are common in patients on medications that induce the metabolism of dexamethasone (e.g., carbamazepine)
Late-night salivary cortisol (LNSC)	Reflects the lack of normal circadian cortisol rhythm in CS patients with high concentrations in the evening (e.g., 10–11 p.m.)	• Measures unbound (free) cortisol • Independent of concentrations of CBG • Easy to perform and can be done at home	• Reference values are not established at all laboratories • Falsely elevated if contaminated with blood or hydrocortisone

lesions are bilateral adenomas, bilateral micro- and macronodular hyperplasia, and ACTH-dependent CS [54]. Of note is that patients with bilateral micronodular hyperplasia may have morphologically normal adrenal glands on imaging.

Adrenal venous sampling in patients with ACTH-independent hypercortisolism, and either bilateral adrenal lesions or normally appearing adrenals on imaging, has been found to be useful for differentiating between unilateral and bilateral overproduction of cortisol, both in patients with overt adrenal CS and autonomous cortisol secretion (see below) [56–59]. Although the studies are based on a limited number of patients, adrenal venous sampling should be considered in patients who are considered to be candidates for surgical treatment.

Treatment of adrenal CS

First-line treatment for patients with CS due to cortisol-producing adrenal adenoma is unilateral adrenalectomy, performed by either retroperitoneal or transabdominal laparoscopic technique [60]. Adrenalectomy in these cases is always curative when performed by an experienced surgeon. Unilateral adrenalectomy is also the primary treatment for patients with cortisol-producing adrenocortical cancer. However, many patients with adrenocortical cancer have metastatic disease at the time of diagnosis, which makes curative treatment only rarely possible.

Bilateral adrenalectomy is the treatment of choice in patients with overt CS due to micro- and macronodular adrenal hyperplasia [60,61]. Recently, however, unilateral adrenalectomy where the larger gland is removed has been suggested for patients with PBMAH in a French study [62]. In this study, all patients were considered to be in biochemical remission following surgery, and CS recurred in only two out of 15 patients during the 5 years of follow-up. In contrast, two other studies have shown a significantly higher recurrence rate; and not more than one-third of the patients were still biochemically controlled after few years of follow-up [63,64]. Similarly, recurrence is common in patients with PPNAD treated with unilateral adrenalectomy [65,66].

Cortisol-lowering medical treatment is rarely used as a long-term treatment option for patients with adrenal CS, e.g., patients with mild hypercortisolism and the elderly with multiple comorbidities [67]. However, they are mainly used preoperatively to reduce the risk of perioperative complications (see below).

Preoperative treatment of adrenal CS

Hypertension and diabetes mellitus should be adequately controlled preoperatively in patients with CS in order to reduce the risk of complications during and after surgery. Pharmacotherapy with adrenal steroidogenesis inhibitors is effective in lowering the cortisol concentrations, and subsequently reducing the blood pressure and the plasma glucose concentrations. Preoperative cortisol-lowering treatment is also important for patients with severe hypercortisolism, especially when they present with serious comorbidities such as pronounced muscle weakness and neuropsychiatric symptoms including psychosis [67,68].

Cortisol-lowering medical therapy alone is not always sufficient in reducing the high blood pressure in patients with CS. In these cases, treatment with either of the mineralocorticoid receptor antagonists, spironolactone or eplerenone, is often useful, especially in patients with moderate to severe hypercortisolemia and/or hypokalemia. Based on studies on the pathophysiology of hypertension in patients with CS, angiotensin-converting enzyme inhibitors or angiotensin II receptor blockers are also considered to be a good choices [37,69,70], either as monotherapy or in combination with calcium channel blockers [37]. Detailed discussion of the management of hypertension in patients with CS can be found in chapter 13: ACTH-dependent Cushing's syndrome.

Patients with CS have a greatly increased risk of developing deep vein thrombosis and pulmonary embolism [33,71−73]. In fact, in a meta-analysis of 48 studies including data from more than 7000 patients with CS, a 17-fold higher risk of perioperative venous thromboembolic events was demonstrated [74]. Thus, administration of perioperative thromboprophylaxis with low molecular weight heparin should be considered in all patients with CS, especially in patients with moderate to severe hypercortisolism [70].

Another serious complication in patients with CS is severe infections, caused by both commonly acquired bacteria, and by opportunistic microorganisms [70]. In a recent study from Sweden, a 14-fold increased risk for sepsis was observed from diagnosis until one year after treatment [72]. Also, in a large study from the European Registry on CS (ERCUSYN), the most common causes of perioperative death were infections [75]. Prophylactic broad-spectrum antibiotics as well as prophylactic treatment against *Pneumocystis jirovecii* should be considered, especially in patients with severe hypercortisolism [70].

Postoperative treatment of adrenal CS

All patients with adrenal CS who are successfully treated with unilateral adrenalectomy develop adrenal insufficiency and, therefore, need glucocorticoid replacement therapy postoperatively for several months [76]. In a study from Germany, the median time to recovery of normal hypothalamic−pituitary−adrenal (HPA) axis function in patients treated for unilateral adrenal CS was 2.5 years [77]. Other studies have shown that adrenal CS patients regain their normal cortisol production on an average within 6−18 months postoperatively [78,79]. In all these studies, however, 10%−20% fail to restore normal HPA axis function [77−80]. Interestingly, preoperative cortisol-lowering medical treatment seems to reduce duration of postoperative adrenal insufficiency [67]. Since adrenal insufficiency can be a life-threatening condition, it is of great importance to thoroughly counsel the patients about this possibility [76,81]. Specifically, the patients should be informed about which actions are needed in situations associated with increased physical or psychological stress, that is, the need of increased dose of oral glucocorticoids during intercurrent illness with fever as well as before minor procedures, such as tooth extractions, and the need of parenterally administered glucocorticoids in the case of severe illness, major surgery, or adrenal crisis [76].

Long-term outcome of adrenal CS

The cardiometabolic risk profile in patients with CS significantly improves following the treatment and resolution of the hypercortisolism as shown in (Fig. 14.3). In a study from Italy including 14 patients with ACTH-producing pituitary adenoma, and 15 patients with cortisol producing adrenal adenoma, the prevalence of hypertension, diabetes mellitus, impaired glucose tolerance, and dyslipidemia before treatment was 72%, 24%, 27%, and 59%, respectively, compared to 10%, 0%, 10%, and 21% in controls matched for age, sex, and BMI [82]. One year following adrenalectomy, the prevalence of hypertension in patients with adrenal CS due to cortisol producing adrenal adenoma fell from 80% to 40%, the prevalence of impaired glucose tolerance/diabetes mellitus from 53% to 7%, and dyslipidemia from 53% to 27%. In another study, including 18 patients with adrenal CS, 83% had hypertension at diagnosis, but only 17% following surgery [36]. Interestingly, the outcome, in both studies, was better in patients with adrenal CS compared to patients with ACTH-producing pituitary adenoma [36,82]. In a

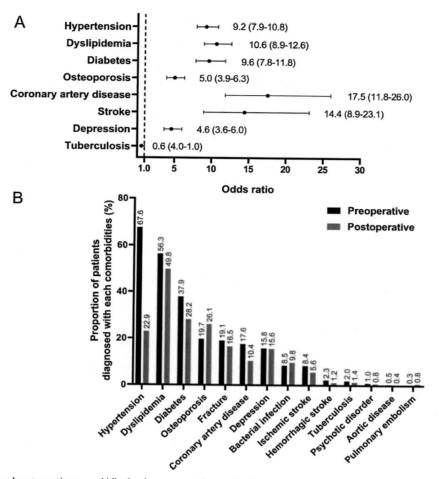

FIGURE 14.3 The pre- and postoperative comorbidity burden among patients with CS.
Figure adapted from Ahn C.H., Kim J.H., Park M.Y., Kim S.W. Epidemiology and comorbidity of adrenal Cushing syndrome: a nationwide cohort study. J Clin Endocrinol Metab 2021;106(3):E1362—E1372. https://doi.org/10.1210/clinem/dgaa752.

recent study from the Mayo clinic, including patients with CS of various etiologies and hyperglycemia, a significant improvement in glycemic control following treatment was observed [83].

Before treatment, patients with CS more often have left ventricular hypertrophy, diastolic dysfunction [84], increased carotid intima-media thickness, and more commonly atherosclerotic plaques in the common carotid artery [85], as compared to controls. In fact, at diagnosis, 32% of patients with CS have atherosclerotic plaques in the common carotid artery as compared to 6% of BMI-matched controls [85]. Following treatment for CS, the intima-media thickness decreases [85], and left ventricular structure and function improves [84]. Nevertheless, the adverse cardiovascular risk profile is still prevalent following successful treatment for CS [82,85]. Furthermore, during long-term follow-up, both coronary artery calcifications and noncalcified plaques are more prevalent in patients with CS compared to controls [86]. Large register-based epidemiological studies have also demonstrated significant burdens of cardiovascular morbidity in patients with CS. In Denmark, a sixfold increased risk of heart failure and a four- to fivefold increased risk of stroke was observed before the CS was diagnosed, and a threefold increased risk of acute myocardial infarction was observed during long-term follow-up [71]. The increased risk was similar between patients with ACTH-producing pituitary adenoma and adrenal CS. Similarly, in a nationwide study from Sweden, a fourfold increased risk of myocardial infarction was observed before treatment and a threefold increased risk for stroke was observed during long-term follow-up [72]. In the same cohort, out of 133 deaths, 63 were due to cardiovascular diseases, where the expected number in the background population was only 19, giving a hazard ratio of more than three [87] (Fig. 14.4).

Most studies on mortality rate in patients with CS have focused on patients with ACTH-producing pituitary adenoma and demonstrated a significantly increased standardized mortality ratio (SMR) [87—89]. Until recently only a limited

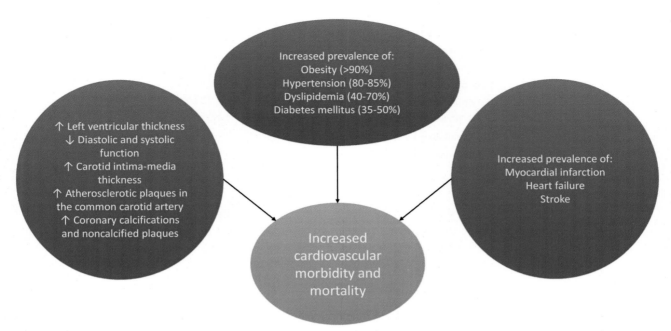

FIGURE 14.4 The risk factors and pathophysiological aspects of increased cardiovascular morbidity and mortality in patients with CS.

number of studies with a limited number of patients ($n = 16-84$) had provided mortality data from patients with adrenal CS, indicating that mortality was not increased in this subgroup of patients with CS [3,7,90,91]. However, in a nationwide Danish study, including data from 211 patients with pituitary CS and 132 patients with adrenal CS, a more than twofold higher mortality risk was observed, with no difference between the two groups [71]. Also, last year, results from an exceptionally large nationwide cohort of 1199 patients with adrenal CS, diagnosed from 2002 to 2017 in Korea, were published [9] (Fig. 14.3). In this study, the SMR for patients with benign adrenal CS ($n = 1127$) was 3.0 (95% CI 2.4−3.7) and that for patients with malignant adrenal CS ($n = 72$) was 13 (95% CI 7.6−19).

Quality of life is severely affected in patients with CS [29]. Quality of life improve, but does not normalize following treatment [29,92]. According to the data from the ERCUSYN, the improvement in quality of life at long-term follow-up seems to be greater in patients with adrenal CS compared to patients with pituitary CS [92]. However, when only patients in biochemical remission were included, no difference was seen between the groups. Various factors contribute to the impaired quality of life at long-term follow-up after treatment for CS, including a high burden of various comorbidities [9,71,72], a high prevalence of psychiatric symptoms [25,93,94], impaired neurocognitive function [25,94], as well as long-standing muscle atrophy and weakness [95].

Lifelong follow-up is necessary for all patients who have been treated for CS. Apart from general support, special emphasis should be put on evaluation of cardiovascular risk and mental health [96].

Autonomous cortisol secretion in adrenal incidentaloma

Adrenal lesions, detected on imaging that is performed for investigation of symptoms unrelated to diseases of the adrenal glands, are called adrenal incidentalomas [97]. Approximately 2% of the general population (at any age), and more than 7% of individuals who are 70 years or older have an adrenal incidentaloma. Autonomous cortisol secretion in patients with adrenal incidentaloma (formerly called subclinical CS), defined as ACTH-independent cortisol excess without clinical signs and symptoms characteristic of overt CS, is seen in up to 20% of these patients [97]. Furthermore, 15%−20% of patients with adrenal incidentaloma have bilateral lesions where mild autonomous hypercortisolism is even more common. Autonomous cortisol secretion is associated with increased prevalence of obesity, hypertension, insulin resistance, type 2 diabetes, dyslipidemia, and osteoporosis [97].

Even the mortality seems to be increased in these patients with autonomous cortisol secretion compared to patients with nonsecreting adrenal incidentaloma. In a single-center study from Italy on 198 consecutive patients diagnosed with adrenal incidentaloma between 1995 and 2010, the overall survival rate for cardiovascular mortality was 97% in patients with nonsecreting adrenal incidentaloma, 78% for patients with stable autonomous cortisol secretion, and 60% in patients with worsening autonomous cortisol secretion [98]. Also, in a study from the UK, including 206 patients (95 with nonsecreting adrenal incidentaloma and 111 autonomous cortisol secretion) with a mean follow-up time 4.2 years, 17 of the 18 patients who died during the follow-up had autonomous cortisol secretion [99].

Outcome following surgical treatment for autonomous cortical secretion has been studied in a meta-analysis including 26 studies, with a total of 584 patients with autonomous cortical secretion [100]. The prevalence of obesity, hypertension, diabetes mellitus, and dyslipidemia decreased significantly following surgery. All but one of the studies in the analysis was nonrandomized cohort studies. In the only randomized study, however, improvement in cardiovascular risk factors was seen in comparison with conservatively treated patients with autonomous cortical secretion [101]. Nevertheless, there is still a lack of well-designed randomized controlled trials where cardiovascular morbidity and mortality in patients with autonomous cortical secretion is studied, and preferably compared to both conservatively treated patients as well as patients with nonsecreting adrenal incidentaloma.

Unfortunately, no international consensus exists on a diagnostic criterion for autonomous cortisol secretion in patients with adrenal incidentaloma [26,102,103]. In fact, numerous different criteria have been used in studies published to date [reviewed by Ref. [97]]. Thus, until a consensus has been reached, and the results are available from studies that convincingly demonstrated a beneficial effect on outcome variables that are clinically important, the benefits of the surgical treatment for patients with autonomous cortisol secretion will remain controversial.

Areas of uncertainty/emerging concepts

Many topics concerning optimal management of patients with CS are inadequately studied and randomized controlled trials are lacking. Most of the recommendations in clinical guidelines and consensus documents are, therefore, based on retrospective observational studies, case series, or clinical experience. Among the issues that would benefit from well-designed prospective trials include (a) the influence of strict control and treatment of cardiovascular risk factors on long-term outcome, (b) the effects of preoperative cortisol-lowering treatment on perioperative complications and recovery of normal cortisol production, (c) the benefits of perioperative thromboprophylaxis, inclusive the optimal dosing and length of treatment, weighted against the risk of serious adverse events such as major hemorrhage, (d) the effect of chronic medical treatment as a therapeutic alternative instead of adrenalectomy for patients with adrenal CS on the long-term outcome including mortality.

For patients with adrenal incidentaloma(s), an international consensus on a well-defined diagnostic criterion for autonomous cortisol secretion is needed. Also, randomized controlled trials where the effect of surgical treatment for autonomous cortisol secretion on the cardiovascular outcome, skeletal health, and quality of life are urgently needed, considering the high prevalence and increased detection rates in the recent years.

Summary and conclusions

CS is a serious disorder associated with a greatly increased risk for various severe comorbidities, including cardiovascular diseases, psychiatric illnesses, skeletal fractures, and severe infections. Consequently, the mortality is increased, not only in patients with untreated hypercortisolism, but also in those who have achieved biochemical remission following treatment. To improve the clinical outcome, as well as quality of life, patients with CS should be diagnosed and treated appropriately without a delay.

Learning points

- Endogenous Cushing's syndrome (CS) is a rare disorder caused by chronic overproduction of cortisol.
- Approximately 20%−30% of patients with endogenous CS have adrenal CS, also called ACTH-independent CS, that is, overproduction of cortisol due to an adrenal disorder.
- CS is a serious disorder that needs to be diagnosed and treated promptly without any delay.
- The risk for cardiovascular diseases, psychiatric illnesses, skeletal fractures, and severe infections is greatly increased in patients with CS.
- The overall and cardiovascular prognosis improves significantly following treatment. Nevertheless, patients treated for CS still have increased cardiovascular risk during long-term follow-up, necessitating life-long surveillance.

References

[1] Lacroix A, Feelders RA, Stratakis CA, Nieman LK. Cushing's syndrome. Lancet 2015;386(9996):913−27. https://doi.org/10.1016/S0140-6736(14)61375-1.

[2] Pivonello R, Isidori AM, De Martino MC, Newell-Price J, Biller BMK, Colao A. Complications of Cushing's syndrome: state of the art. Lancet Diabetes Endocrinol 2016;4(7):611−29. https://doi.org/10.1016/S2213-8587(16)00086-3.

[3] Lindholm J, Juul S, Jørgensen JOL, Astrup J, Bjerre P, Feldt-Rasmussen U, Hagen C, Jørgensen J, Kosteljanetz M, Kristensen LØ, Laurberg P, Schmidt K, Weeke J. Incidence and late prognosis of Cushing's syndrome: a population-based study 1. J Clin Endocrinol Metab 2001;86(1):117−23. https://doi.org/10.1210/jcem.86.1.7093.

[4] Valassi E, Santos A, Yaneva M, Tóth M, Strasburger CJ, Chanson P, Wass JAH, Chabre O, Pfeifer M, Feelders RA, Tsagarakis S, Trainer PJ, Franz H, Zopf K, Zacharieva S, Lamberts SW, Tabarin A, Webb SM. The European Registry on Cushing's syndrome: 2-Year experience. Baseline demographic and clinical characteristics. Eur J Endocrinol 2011;165(3):383−92. https://doi.org/10.1530/EJE-11-0272.

[5] Espiard S, Drougat L, Libé R, Assié G, Perlemoine K, Guignat L, Barrande G, Brucker-Davis F, Doullay F, Lopez S, Sonnet E, Torremocha F, Pinsard D, Chabbert-Buffet N, Raffin-Sanson M-L, Groussin L, Borson-Chazot F, Coste J, Bertagna X, Bertherat J. ARMC5 mutations in a large cohort of primary macronodular adrenal hyperplasia: clinical and functional consequences. J Clin Endocrinol Metab 2015;100(6):E926−35. https://doi.org/10.1210/jc.2014-4204.

[6] Tatsi C, Flippo C, Stratakis CA. Cushing syndrome: old and new genes. Best Pract Res Clin Endocrinol Metab 2020;34(2):101418. https://doi.org/10.1016/j.beem.2020.101418.

[7] Bolland MJ, Holdaway IM, Berkeley JE, Lim S, Dransfield WJ, Conaglen JV, Croxson MS, Gamble GD, Hunt PJ, Toomath RJ. Mortality and morbidity in Cushing's syndrome in New Zealand. Clin Endocrinol 2011;75(4):436−42. https://doi.org/10.1111/j.1365-2265.2011.04124.x.

[8] Wengander S, Trimpou P, Papakokkinou E, Ragnarsson O. The incidence of endogenous Cushing's syndrome in the modern era. Clin Endocrinol 2019;91(2):263−70. https://doi.org/10.1111/cen.14014.

[9] Ahn CH, Kim JH, Park MY, Kim SW. Epidemiology and comorbidity of adrenal Cushing syndrome: a nationwide cohort study. J Clin Endocrinol Metab 2021;106(3):E1362−72. https://doi.org/10.1210/clinem/dgaa752.

[10] Stratakis CA, Kirschner LS, Carney JA. Clinical and molecular features of the carney complex: diagnostic criteria and recommendations for patient evaluation. J Clin Endocrinol Metab 2001;86(9):4041−6. https://doi.org/10.1210/jcem.86.9.7903.

[11] Stratakis CA. Cushing syndrome in pediatrics. Endocrinol Metab Clin North Am 2012;41(4):793−803. https://doi.org/10.1016/j.ecl.2012.08.002.

[12] Tatsi C, Stratakis CA. Neonatal Cushing syndrome: a rare but potentially devastating disease. Clin Perinatol 2018;45(1):103−18. https://doi.org/10.1016/j.clp.2017.10.002.

[13] Gatta-Cherifi B, Chabre O, Murat A, Niccoli P, Cardot-Bauters C, Rohmer V, Young J, Delemer B, Du Boullay H, Verger MF, Kuhn JM, Sadoul JL, Ruszniewski P, Beckers A, Monsaingeon M, Baudin E, Goudet P, Tabarin A. Adrenal involvement in MEN1. Analysis of 715 cases from the Groupe d'étude des Tumeurs Endocrines database. Eur J Endocrinol 2012;166(2):269−79. https://doi.org/10.1530/EJE-11-0679.

[14] Spencer T, Pan KS, Collins MT, Boyce AM. The clinical spectrum of McCune-Albright syndrome and its management. Horm Research Paediatr 2019;92(6):347−56. https://doi.org/10.1159/000504802.

[15] Brown RJ, Kelly MH, Collins MT. Cushing syndrome in the McCune-Albright syndrome. J Clin Endocrinol Metab 2010;95(4):1508−15. https://doi.org/10.1210/jc.2009-2321.

[16] Correa R, Salpea P, Stratakis CA. Carney complex: an update. Eur J Endocrinol 2015;173(4):M85−97. https://doi.org/10.1530/EJE-15-0209.

[17] Kamilaris CDC, Stratakis CA, Hannah-Shmouni F. Molecular genetic and genomic alterations in Cushing's syndrome and primary aldosteronism. Front Endocrinol 2021;12. https://doi.org/10.3389/fendo.2021.632543.

[18] Weinstein LS, Shenker A, Friedman E, Spiegel AM, Gejman PV, Merino MJ. Activating mutations of the stimulatory G protein in the McCune−Albright syndrome. N Engl J Med 1991;325(24):1688−95. https://doi.org/10.1056/NEJM199112123252403.

[19] Kirschner LS, Carney JA, Pack SD, Taymans SE, Giatzakis C, Cho YS, Cho-Chung YS, Stratakis CA. Mutations of the gene encoding the protein kinase A type I-α regulatory subunit in patients with the Carney complex. Nat Genet 2000;26(1):89−92. https://doi.org/10.1038/79238.

[20] Beuschlein F, Fassnacht M, Assié G, Calebiro D, Stratakis CA, Osswald A, Ronchi CL, Wieland T, Sbiera S, Faucz FR, Schaak K, Schmittfull A, Schwarzmayr T, Barreau O, Vezzosi D, Rizk-Rabin M, Zabel U, Szarek E, Salpea P, Allolio B. Constitutive activation of PKA catalytic subunit in adrenal Cushing's syndrome. N Engl J Med 2014;370(11):1019−28. https://doi.org/10.1056/NEJMoa1310359.

[21] Cao Y, He M, Gao Z, Peng Y, Li Y, Li L, Zhou W, Li X, Zhong X, Lei Y, Su T, Wang H, Jiang Y, Yang L, Wei W, Yang X, Jiang X, Liu L, He J, Ning G. Activating hotspot L205R mutation in PRKACA and adrenal Cushing's syndrome. Science 2014;344(6186):913−7. https://doi.org/10.1126/science.1249480.

[22] Sato Y, Maekawa S, Ishii R, Sanada M, Morikawa T, Shiraishi Y, Yoshida K, Nagata Y, Sato-Otsubo A, Yoshizato T, Suzuki H, Shiozawa Y, Kataoka K, Kon A, Aoki K, Chiba K, Tanaka H, Kume H, Miyano S, Ogawa S. Recurrent somatic mutations underlie corticotropin-independent Cushing's syndrome. Science 2014;344(6186):917−20. https://doi.org/10.1126/science.1252328.

[23] Thiel A, Reis AC, Haase M, Goh G, Schott M, Willenberg HS, Scholl UI. PRKACA mutations in cortisol-producing adenomas and adrenal hyperplasia: a single-center study of 60 cases. Eur J Endocrinol 2015;172(6):677−85. https://doi.org/10.1530/EJE-14-1113.

[24] Chevalier B, Vantyghem MC, Espiard S. Bilateral adrenal hyperplasia: pathogenesis and treatment. Biomedicines 2021;9(10). https://doi.org/10.3390/biomedicines9101397.

[25] Piasecka M, Papakokkinou E, Valassi E, Santos A, Webb SM, de Vries F, Pereira AM, Ragnarsson O. Psychiatric and neurocognitive consequences of endogenous hypercortisolism. J Intern Med 2020;288(2):168−82. https://doi.org/10.1111/joim.13056.

[26] Nieman LK, Biller BMK, Findling JW, Newell-Price J, Savage MO, Stewart PM, Montori VM, Edwards H. The diagnosis of Cushing's syndrome: an endocrine society clinical practice guideline. J Clin Endocrinol Metab 2008;93(5):1526–40. https://doi.org/10.1210/jc.2008-0125.

[27] Kreitschmann-Andermahr I, Psaras T, Tsiogka M, Starz D, Kleist B, Siegel S, Milian M, Kohlmann J, Menzel C, Führer-Sakel D, Honegger J, Sure U, Müller O, Buchfelder M. From first symptoms to final diagnosis of Cushing's disease: experiences of 176 patients. Eur J Endocrinol 2015;172(3):285–9. https://doi.org/10.1530/EJE-14-0766.

[28] Rubinstein G, Osswald A, Hoster E, Losa M, Elenkova A, Zacharieva S, Machado MC, Hanzu FA, Zopp S, Ritzel K, Riester A, Braun LT, Kreitschmann-Andermahr I, Storr HL, Bansal P, Barahona MJ, Cosaro E, Dogansen SC, Johnston PC, Reincke M. Time to diagnosis in Cushing's syndrome: a meta-analysis based on 5367 patients. J Clin Endocrinol Metab 2020;105(3). https://doi.org/10.1210/clinem/dgz136.

[29] Broersen LHA, Andela CD, Dekkers OM, Pereira AM, Biermasz NR. Improvement but no normalization of quality of life and cognitive functioning after treatment of Cushing syndrome. J Clin Endocrinol Metab 2019;104(11):5325–37. https://doi.org/10.1210/jc.2019-01054.

[30] Lambert JK, Goldberg L, Fayngold S, Kostadinov J, Post KD, Geer EB. Predictors of mortality and long-term outcomes in treated Cushing's disease: a study of 346 patients. J Clin Endocrinol Metab 2013;98(3):1022–30. https://doi.org/10.1210/jc.2012-2893.

[31] Giraldi FP, Moro M, Cavagnini F. Gender-related differences in the presentation and course of Cushing's disease. J Clin Endocrinol Metab 2003;88(4):1554–8. https://doi.org/10.1210/jc.2002-021518.

[32] Mancini T, Kola B, Mantero F, Boscaro M, Arnaldi G. High cardiovascular risk in patients with Cushing's syndrome according to 1999 WHO/ISH guidelines. Clin Endocrinol 2004;61(6):768–77. https://doi.org/10.1111/j.1365-2265.2004.02168.x.

[33] Schernthaner-Reiter MH, Siess C, Micko A, Zauner C, Wolfsberger S, Scheuba C, Riss P, Knosp E, Kautzky-Willer A, Luger A, Vila G. Acute and life-threatening complications in Cushing syndrome: prevalence, predictors, and mortality. J Clin Endocrinol Metab 2021;106(5):E2035–46. https://doi.org/10.1210/clinem/dgab058.

[34] Avenatti E, Rebellato A, Iannaccone A, Battocchio M, Dassie F, Veglio F, Milan A, Fallo F. Left ventricular geometry and 24-h blood pressure profile in Cushing's syndrome. Endocrine 2017;55(2):547–54. https://doi.org/10.1007/s12020-016-0986-6.

[35] Pecori Giraldi F, Toja PM, De Martin M, Maronati A, Scacchi M, Omboni S, Cavagnini F, Parati C. Circadian blood pressure profile in patients with active Cushing's disease and after long-term cure. Horm Metab Res 2007;39(12):908–14. https://doi.org/10.1055/s-2007-992813.

[36] Zacharieva S, Orbetzova M, Stoynev A, Shigarminova R, Yaneva M, Kalinov K, Nachev E, Elenkova A. Circadian blood pressure profile in patients with Cushing's syndrome before and after treatment. J Endocrinol Invest 2004;27(10):924–30. https://doi.org/10.1007/BF03347534.

[37] Isidori AM, Graziadio C, Paragliola RM, Cozzolino A, Ambrogio AG, Colao A, Corsello SM, Pivonello R. The hypertension of Cushing's syndrome: controversies in the pathophysiology and focus on cardiovascular complications. J Hypertens 2015;33(1):44–60. https://doi.org/10.1097/HJH.0000000000000415.

[38] Stewart PM, Walker BR, Holder G, O'Halloran D, Shackleton CH. 11 beta-hydroxysteroid dehydrogenase activity in Cushing's syndrome: explaining the mineralocorticoid excess state of the ectopic adrenocorticotropin syndrome. J Clin Endocrinol Metab 1995;80(12):3617–20. https://doi.org/10.1210/jcem.80.12.8530609.

[39] Ulick S, Wang JZ, Blumenfeld JD, Pickering TG. Cortisol inactivation overload: a mechanism of mineralocorticoid hypertension in the ectopic adrenocorticotropin syndrome. J Clin Endocrinol Metab 1992;74(5):963–7. https://doi.org/10.1210/jcem.74.5.1569172.

[40] Van Der Pas R, Van Esch JHM, De Bruin C, Danser AHJ, Pereira AM, Zelissen PM, Netea-Maier R, Sprij-Mooij DM, Van Den Berg-Garrelds IM, Van Schaik RHN, Lamberts SWJ, Van Den Meiracker AH, Hofland LJ, Feelders RA. Cushing's disease and hypertension: in vivo and in vitro study of the role of the renin-Angiotensin-Aldosterone system and effects of medical therapy. Eur J Endocrinol 2014;170(2):181–91. https://doi.org/10.1530/EJE-13-0477.

[41] Sato A, Suzuki H, Murakami M, Nakazato Y, Iwaita Y, Saruta T. Glucocorticoid increases angiotensin II type 1 receptor and its gene expression. Hypertension 1994;23(1):25–30. https://doi.org/10.1161/01.HYP.23.1.25.

[42] McKnight JA, Rooney DP, Whitehead H, Atkinson AB. Blood pressure responses to phenylephrine infusions in subjects with Cushing's syndrome. J Hum Hypertens 1995;9(10):855–8.

[43] Pirpiris M, Sudhir K, Yeung S, Jennings G, Whitworth JA. Pressor responsiveness in corticosteroid-induced hypertension in humans. Hypertension 1992;19(6):567–74. https://doi.org/10.1161/01.HYP.19.6.567.

[44] Saruta T, Suzuki H, Handa M, Igarashi Y, Kondo K, Senba S. Multiple factors contribute to the pathogenesis of hypertension in Cushing's syndrome. J Clin Endocrinol Metab 1986;62(2):275–9. https://doi.org/10.1210/jcem-62-2-275.

[45] Yasuda G, Shionoiri H, Umemura S, Takasaki I, Ishii M. Exaggerated blood pressure response to angiotensin II in patients with Cushing's syndrome due to adrenocortical adenoma. Eur J Endocrinol 1994;131(6):582–8. https://doi.org/10.1530/eje.0.1310582.

[46] Ritchie CM, Sheridan B, Fraser R, Hadden DR, Kennedy AL, Riddell J, Atkinson AB. Studies on the pathogenesis of hypertension in Cushing's disease and acromegaly. QJM 1990;76(2):855–67. https://doi.org/10.1093/oxfordjournals.qjmed.a068490.

[47] Axelrod L. Inhibition of prostacyclin production mediates permissive effect of glucocorticoids on vascular tone. Perturbations of this mechanism contribute to pathogenesis of Cushing's syndrome and Addison's disease. Lancet 1983;321(8330):904–6. https://doi.org/10.1016/S0140-6736(83)91330-2.

[48] Kelly JJ, Tam SH, Williamson PM, Lawson J, Whitworth JA. The nitric oxide system and cortisol-induced hypertension in humans. Clin Exp Pharmacol Physiol 1998;25(11):945–6. https://doi.org/10.1111/j.1440-1681.1998.tb02349.x.

[49] Wallerath T, Witte K, Schafer SC, Schwarz PM, Prellwitz W, Wohlfart P, Kleinert H, Lehr HA, Lemmer B, Forstermann U. Down-regulation of the expression of endothelial NO synthase is likely to contribute to glucocorticoid-mediated hypertension. Proc Natl Acad Sci U S A 1999;96(23):13357–62. https://doi.org/10.1073/pnas.96.23.13357.

[50] Kirilov G, Tomova A, Dakovska L, Kumanov P, Shinkov A, Alexandrov AS. Elevated plasma endothelin as an additional cardiovascular risk factor in patients with Cushing's syndrome. Eur J Endocrinol 2003;149(6):549−53. https://doi.org/10.1530/eje.0.1490549.

[51] Kelly J, Martin A, Whitworth J. Role of erythropoietin in cortisol-induced hypertension. J Hum Hypertens 2000;14(3):195−8. https://doi.org/10.1038/sj.jhh.1000959.

[52] Fleseriu M, Auchus R, Bancos I, Ben-Shlomo A, Bertherat J, Biermasz NR, Boguszewski CL, Bronstein MD, Buchfelder M, Carmichael JD, Casanueva FF, Castinetti F, Chanson P, Findling J, Gadelha M, Geer EB, Giustina A, Grossman A, Gurnell M, Biller BMK. Consensus on diagnosis and management of Cushing's disease: a guideline update. Lancet Diabetes Endocrinol 2021;9(12):847−75. https://doi.org/10.1016/S2213-8587(21)00235-7.

[53] Galm BP, Qiao N, Klibanski A, Biller BMK, Tritos NA. Accuracy of laboratory tests for the diagnosis of Cushing syndrome. J Clin Endocrinol Metab 2020;105(6). https://doi.org/10.1210/clinem/dgaa105.

[54] Yalniz C, Morani AC, Waguespack SG, Elsayes KM. Imaging of adrenal-related endocrine disorders. Radiol Clin 2020;58(6):1099−113. https://doi.org/10.1016/j.rcl.2020.07.010.

[55] Rockall AG, Babar SA, Aslam Sohaib SA, Isidori AM, Diaz-Cano S, Monson JP, Grossman AB, Reznek RH. CT and MR imaging of the adrenal glands in ACTH-independent Cushing syndrome. Radiographics 2004;24(2):435−52. https://doi.org/10.1148/rg.242035092.

[56] Acharya R, Dhir M, Bandi R, Yip L, Challinor S. Outcomes of adrenal venous sampling in patients with bilateral adrenal masses and ACTH-independent Cushing's syndrome. World J Surg 2019;43(2):527−33. https://doi.org/10.1007/s00268-018-4788-2.

[57] Papakokkinou E, Jakobsson H, Sakinis A, Muth A, Wängberg B, Ehn O, Johannsson G, Ragnarsson O. Adrenal venous sampling in patients with ACTH-independent hypercortisolism. Endocrine 2019;66(2):338−48. https://doi.org/10.1007/s12020-019-02038-0.

[58] Ueland G, Methlie P, Eirik Jøssang D, Sagen JV, Viste K, Thordarson HB, Heie A, Grytaas M, Løvås K, Biermann M, Husebye ES. Adrenal venous sampling for assessment of autonomous cortisol secretion. J Clin Endocrinol Metab 2018;103(12):4553−60. https://doi.org/10.1210/jc.2018-01198.

[59] Young WF, Du Plessis H, Thompson GB, Grant CS, Farley DR, Richards ML, Erickson D, Vella A, Stanson AW, Carney JA, Abboud CF, Carpenter PC. The clinical conundrum of corticotropin-independent autonomous cortisol secretion in patients with bilateral adrenal masses. World J Surg 2008;32(5):856−62. https://doi.org/10.1007/s00268-007-9332-8.

[60] Nieman LK, Biller BMK, Findling JW, Murad MH, Newell-Price J, Savage MO, Tabarin A. Treatment of Cushing's syndrome: an endocrine society clinical practice guideline. J Clin Endocrinol Metab 2015;100(8):2807−31. https://doi.org/10.1210/jc.2015-1818.

[61] Albiger NM, Regazzo D, Iacobone M, Scaroni C. Different therapeutic options in patients with Cushing's syndrome due to bilateral macronodular adrenal hyperplasia. Minerva Endocrinol 2019;44(2):205−20. https://doi.org/10.23736/S0391-1977.17.02771-7.

[62] Debillon E, Velayoudom-Cephise FL, Salenave S, Caron P, Chaffanjon P, Wagner T, Massoutier M, Lambert B, Benoit M, Young J, Tabarin A, Chabre O. Unilateral adrenalectomy as a first-line treatment of Cushing's syndrome in patients with primary bilateral macronodular adrenal hyperplasia. J Clin Endocrinol Metab 2015;100(12):4417−24. https://doi.org/10.1210/jc.2015-2662.

[63] Albiger NM, Ceccato F, Zilio M, Barbot M, Occhi G, Rizzati S, Fassina A, Mantero F, Boscaro M, Iacobone M, Scaroni C. An analysis of different therapeutic options in patients with Cushing's syndrome due to bilateral macronodular adrenal hyperplasia: a single-centre experience. Clin Endocrinol 2015;82(6):808−15. https://doi.org/10.1111/cen.12763.

[64] Osswald A, Quinkler M, Di Dalmazi G, Deutschbein T, Rubinstein G, Ritzel K, Zopp S, Bertherat J, Beuschlein F, Reincke M. Long-term outcome of primary bilateral macronodular adrenocortical hyperplasia after unilateral adrenalectomy. J Clin Endocrinol Metab 2019;104(7):2985−93. https://doi.org/10.1210/jc.2018-02204.

[65] Kyrilli A, Lytrivi M, Bouquegneau MS, Demetter P, Lucidi V, Garcia C, Moreno-Reyes R, Tabarin A, Corvilain B, Driessens N. Unilateral adrenalectomy could be a valid option for primary nodular adrenal disease: evidence from twins. J Endocr Soc 2019;3(1):129−34. https://doi.org/10.1210/js.2018-00261.

[66] Powell AC, Stratakis CA, Patronas NJ, Steinberg SM, Batista D, Alexander HR, Pingpank JF, Keil M, Bartlett DL, Libutti SK. Operative management of Cushing Syndrome secondary to micronodular adrenal hyperplasia. Surgery 2008;143(6):750−8. https://doi.org/10.1016/j.surg.2008.03.022.

[67] Valassi E, Franz H, Brue T, Feelders RA, Netea-Maier R, Tsagarakis S, Webb SM, Yaneva M, Reincke M, Droste M, Komerdus I, Maiter D, Kastelan D, Chanson P, Pfeifer M, Strasburger CJ, Tóth M, Chabre O, Krsek M, Zosin I. Preoperative medical treatment in Cushing's syndrome: frequency of use and its impact on postoperative assessment: data from ERCUSYN. Eur J Endocrinol 2018;178(4):399−409. https://doi.org/10.1530/EJE-17-0997.

[68] Marques JVO, Boguszewski CL. Medical therapy in severe hypercortisolism. Best Pract Res Clin Endocrinol Metab 2021;35(2):101487. https://doi.org/10.1016/j.beem.2021.101487.

[69] Nieman LK. Hypertension and cardiovascular mortality in patients with Cushing syndrome. Endocrinol Metab Clin North Am 2019;48(4):717−25. https://doi.org/10.1016/j.ecl.2019.08.005.

[70] Varlamov EV, Langlois F, Vila G, Fleseriu M. Cardiovascular risk assessment, thromboembolism, and infection prevention in Cushing's syndrome: a practical approach. Eur J Endocrinol 2021;184(5):R207−24. https://doi.org/10.1530/EJE-20-1309.

[71] Dekkers OM, Horvath-Puho; E, Jørgensen JOL, Cannegieter SC, Ehrenstein V, Vandenbroucke JP, Pereira AM, Srøensen HT. Multisystem morbidity and mortality in Cushing's syndrome: a cohort study. J Clin Endocrinol Metab 2013;98(6):2277−84. https://doi.org/10.1210/jc.2012-3582.

[72] Papakokkinou E, Olsson DS, Chantzichristos D, Dahlqvist P, Segerstedt E, Olsson T, Petersson M, Berinder K, Bensing S, Höybye C, Edén-Engström B, Burman P, Bonelli L, Follin C, Petranek D, Erfurth EM, Wahlberg J, Ekman B, Åkerman AK, Ragnarsson O. Excess morbidity persists in patients with

Cushing's disease during long-term remission: a Swedish nationwide study. J Clin Endocrinol Metab 2020;105(8):2616−24. https://doi.org/10.1210/clinem/dgaa291.

[73] Suarez MG, Stack M, Hinojosa-Amaya JM, Mitchell MD, Varlamov EV, Yedinak CG, Cetas JS, Sheppard B, Fleseriu M. Hypercoagulability in Cushing syndrome, prevalence of thrombotic events: a large, single-center, retrospective study. J Endocr Soc 2020;4(2). https://doi.org/10.1210/jendso/bvz033.

[74] Wagner J, Langlois F, Lim DST, McCartney S, Fleseriu M. Hypercoagulability and risk of venous thromboembolic events in endogenous Cushing's syndrome: a systematic meta-analysis. Front Endocrinol 2019;9. https://doi.org/10.3389/fendo.2018.00805.

[75] Valassi E, Tabarin A, Brue T, Feelders RA, Reincke M, Netea-Maier R, Tóth M, Zacharieva S, Webb SM, Tsagarakis S, Chanson P, Pfeifer M, Droste M, Komerdus I, Kastelan D, Maiter D, Chabre O, Franz H, Santos A, Zosin I. High mortality within 90 days of diagnosis in patients with Cushing's syndrome: results from the ERCUSYN Registry. Eur J Endocrinol 2019;181(5):461−72. https://doi.org/10.1530/EJE-19-0464.

[76] Broersen LHA, Van Haalen FM, Kienitz T, Dekkers OM, Strasburger CJ, Pereira AM, Biermasz NR. The incidence of adrenal crisis in the postoperative period of HPA axis insufficiency after surgical treatment for Cushing's syndrome. Eur J Endocrinol 2019;181(2):201−10. https://doi.org/10.1530/EJE-19-0202.

[77] Berr CM, Di Dalmazi G, Osswald A, Ritzel K, Bidlingmaier M, Geyer LL, Treitl M, Hallfeldt K, Rachinger W, Reisch N, Blaser R, Schopohl J, Beuschlein F, Reincke M. Time to recovery of adrenal function after curative surgery for Cushing's syndrome depends on etiology. J Clin Endocrinol Metab 2015;100(4):1300−8. https://doi.org/10.1210/jc.2014-3632.

[78] Hurtado MD, Cortes T, Natt N, Young WF, Bancos I. Extensive clinical experience: hypothalamic-pituitary-adrenal axis recovery after adrenalectomy for corticotropin-independent cortisol excess. Clin Endocrinol 2018;89(6):721−33. https://doi.org/10.1111/cen.13803.

[79] Kim HK, Yoon JH, Jeong YA, Kang HC. The recovery of hypothalamic-pituitary-adrenal axis is rapid in subclinical Cushing syndrome. Endocrino Metab 2016;31(4):592−7. https://doi.org/10.3803/EnM.2016.31.4.592.

[80] Klose M, Jorgensen K, Kristensen LO. Characteristics of recovery of adrenocortical function after treatment for Cushing's syndrome due to pituitary or adrenal adenomas. Clin Endocrinol 2004;61(3):394−9. https://doi.org/10.1111/j.1365-2265.2004.02111.x.

[81] Acree R, Miller CM, Abel BS, Neary NM, Campbell K, Nieman LK. Patient and provider perspectives on postsurgical recovery of Cushing syndrome. J Endocr Soc 2021;5(8). https://doi.org/10.1210/jendso/bvab109.

[82] Giordano R, Picu A, Marinazzo E, D'Angelo V, Berardelli R, Karamouzis I, Forno D, Zinnà D, MacCario M, Ghigo E, Arvat E. Metabolic and cardiovascular outcomes in patients with Cushing's syndrome of different aetiologies during active disease and 1 year after remission. Clin Endocrinol 2011;75(3):354−60. https://doi.org/10.1111/j.1365-2265.2011.04055.x.

[83] Herndon J, Kaur RJ, Romportl M, Smith E, Koenigs A, Partlow B, Arteaga L, Bancos I. The effect of curative treatment on hyperglycemia in patients with Cushing syndrome. J Endocr Soc 2022;6(1). https://doi.org/10.1210/jendso/bvab169.

[84] Pereira AM, Delgado V, Romijn JA, Smit JWA, Bax JJ, Feelders RA. Cardiac dysfunction is reversed upon successful treatment of Cushing's syndrome. Eur J Endocrinol 2010;162(2):331−40. https://doi.org/10.1530/EJE-09-0621.

[85] Faggiano A, Pivonello R, Spiezia S, De Martino MC, Filippella M, Di Somma C, Lombardi G, Colao A. Cardiovascular risk factors and common carotid artery caliber and stiffness in patients with Cushing's disease during active disease and 1 year after disease remission. J Clin Endocrinol Metab 2003;88(6):2527−33. https://doi.org/10.1210/jc.2002-021558.

[86] Barahona MJ, Resmini E, Viladés D, Pons-Lladó G, Leta R, Puig T, Webb SM. Coronary artery disease detected by multislice computed tomography in patients after long-term cure of Cushing's syndrome. J Clin Endocrinol Metab 2013;98(3):1093−9. https://doi.org/10.1210/jc.2012-3547.

[87] Ragnarsson O, Olsson DS, Papakokkinou E, Chantzichristos D, Dahlqvist P, Segerstedt E, Olsson T, Petersson M, Berinder K, Bensing S, Hoybye C, Eden-Engstrom B, Burman P, Bonelli L, Follin C, Petranek D, Erfurth EM, Wahlberg J, Ekman B, Johannsson G. Overall and disease-specific mortality in patients with Cushing disease: a Swedish nationwide study. J Clin Endocrinol Metab 2019;104(6):2375−84. https://doi.org/10.1210/jc.2018-02524.

[88] Clayton RN, Jones PW, Reulen RC, Stewart PM, Hassan-Smith ZK, Ntali G, Karavitaki N, Dekkers OM, Pereira AM, Bolland M, Holdaway I, Lindholm J. Mortality in patients with Cushing's disease more than 10 years after remission: a multicentre, multinational, retrospective cohort study. Lancet Diabetes Endocrinol 2016;4(7):569−76. https://doi.org/10.1016/S2213-8587(16)30005-5.

[89] Van Haalen FM, Broersen LHA, Jorgensen JO, Pereira AM, Dekkers OM. Management of endocrine disease: mortality remains increased in Cushing's disease despite biochemical remission: a systematic review and meta-analysis. Eur J Endocrinol 2015;172(4):R143−9. https://doi.org/10.1530/EJE-14-0556.

[90] Ntali G, Asimakopoulou A, Siamatras T, Komninos J, Vassiliadi D, Tzanela M, Tsagarakis S, Grossman AB, Wass JAH, Karavitaki N. Mortality in Cushing's syndrome: systematic analysis of a large series with prolonged follow-up. Eur J Endocrinol 2013;169(5):715−23. https://doi.org/10.1530/EJE-13-0569.

[91] Yaneva M, Kalinov K, Zacharieva S. Mortality in Cushing's syndrome: data from 386 patients from a single tertiary referral center. Eur J Endocrinol 2013;169(5):621−7. https://doi.org/10.1530/EJE-13-0320.

[92] Valassi E, Feelders R, Maiter D, Chanson P, Yaneva M, Reincke M, Krsek M, Tóth M, Webb SM, Santos A, Paiva I, Komerdus I, Droste M, Tabarin A, Strasburger CJ, Franz H, Trainer PJ, Newell-Price J, Wass JAH, Zosin I. Worse Health-Related Quality of Life at long-term follow-up in patients with Cushing's disease than patients with cortisol producing adenoma. Data from the ERCUSYN. Clin Endocrinol 2018;88(6):787−98. https://doi.org/10.1111/cen.13600.

[93] Bengtsson D, Ragnarsson O, Berinder K, Dahlqvist P, Edén Engström B, Ekman B, Höybye C, Burman P, Wahlberg J. Psychotropic drugs in patients with Cushing's disease before diagnosis and at long-term follow-up: a nationwide study. J Clin Endocrinol Metab 2021;106(6):1750−60. https://doi.org/10.1210/clinem/dgab079.

[94] Lin TY, Hanna J, Ishak WW. Psychiatric symptoms in Cushing's syndrome: a systematic review. Innov Clin Neurosci 2020;17(1−3):30−5. https://www.ncbi.nlm.nih.gov/pmc/articles/PMC7239565/pdf/icns_17_1-3_30.pdf.

[95] Martel-Duguech L, Alonso-Jimenez A, Bascuñana H, Díaz-Manera J, Llauger J, Nuñez-Peralta C, Montesinos P, Webb SM, Valassi E. Prevalence of sarcopenia after remission of hypercortisolism and its impact on HRQoL. Clin Endocrinol 2021;95(5):735−43. https://doi.org/10.1111/cen.14568.

[96] Ragnarsson O, Johannsson G. Cushing's syndrome: a structured short- and long-term management plan for patients in remission. Eur J Endocrinol 2013;169(5):R139−52. https://doi.org/10.1530/EJE-13-0534.

[97] Sherlock M, Scarsbrook A, Abbas A, Fraser S, Limumpornpetch P, Dineen R, Stewart PM. Adrenal incidentaloma. Endocr Rev 2020;41(6):775−820. https://doi.org/10.1210/endrev/bnaa008.

[98] Di Dalmazi G, Vicennati V, Garelli S, Casadio E, Rinaldi E, Giampalma E, Mosconi C, Golfieri R, Paccapelo A, Pagotto U, Pasquali R. Cardiovascular events and mortality in patients with adrenal incidentalomas that are either non-secreting or associated with intermediate phenotype or subclinical Cushing's syndrome: a 15-year retrospective study. Lancet Diabetes Endocrinol 2014;2(5):396−405. https://doi.org/10.1016/S2213-8587(13)70211-0.

[99] Debono M, Bradburn M, Bull M, Harrison B, Ross RJ, Newell-Price J. Cortisol as a marker for increased mortality in patients with incidental adrenocortical adenomas. J Clin Endocrinol Metab 2014;99(12):4462−70. https://doi.org/10.1210/jc.2014-3007.

[100] Bancos I, Alahdab F, Crowley RK, Chortis V, Delivanis DA, Erickson D, Natt N, Terzolo M, Arlt W, Young WF, Murad MH. Therapy of endocrine disease: improvement of cardiovascular risk factors after adrenalectomy in patients with adrenal tumors and subclinical Cushing's syndrome: a systematic review and meta-analysis. Eur J Endocrinol 2016;175(6):R283−95. https://doi.org/10.1530/eje-16-0465.

[101] Toniato A, Merante-Boschin I, Opocher G, Pelizzo MR, Schiavi F, Ballotta E. Surgical versus conservative management for subclinical Cushing syndrome in adrenal incidentalomas: a prospective randomized study. Ann Surg 2009;249(3):388−91. https://doi.org/10.1097/SLA.0b013e31819a47d2.

[102] Fassnacht M, Arlt W, Bancos I, Dralle H, Newell-Price J, Sahdev A, Tabarin A, Terzolo M, Tsagarakis S, Dekkers OM. Management of adrenal incidentalomas: European society of endocrinology clinical practice guideline in collaboration with the European network for the study of adrenal tumors. Eur J Endocrinol 2016;175(2):G1−34. https://doi.org/10.1530/EJE-16-0467.

[103] Yanase T, Oki Y, Katabami T, Otsuki M, Kageyama K, Tanaka T, Kawate H, Tanabe M, Doi M, Akehi Y, Ichijo T. New diagnostic criteria of adrenal subclinical Cushing's syndrome: opinion from the Japan Endocrine Society. Endocr J 2018;65(4):383−93. https://doi.org/10.1507/endocrj.EJ17-0456.

Chapter 15

Hypertension in growth hormone excess and deficiency

Gabriela Mihai and Márta Korbonits

Centre for Endocrinology, William Harvey Research Institute, Barts and The London School of Medicine and Dentistry, Queen Mary University of London, London, United Kingdom

Visit the *Endocrine Hypertension: From Basic Science to Clinical Practice, First Edition* companion web site at: https://www.elsevier.com/books-and-journals/book-companion/9780323961202.

Graphical Abstract

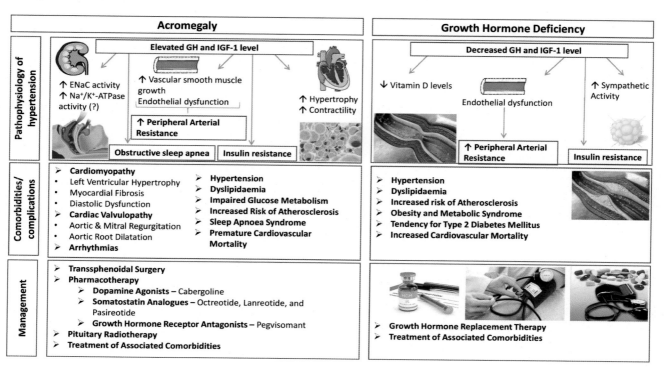

Endocrine Hypertension. https://doi.org/10.1016/B978-0-323-96120-2.00017-0

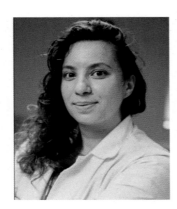

Gabriela Mihai

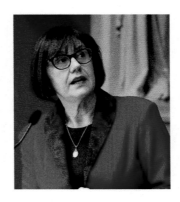

Márta Korbonits

GH and IGF-1 physiological effects

Growth hormone (GH) plays an important role in the postnatal body growth and composition. Several actions of GH are mediated through insulin-like growth factor 1 (IGF-1). The original hypothesis postulated that GH acts on its receptor in the liver to stimulate IGF-1 synthesis which in turn promotes growth by acting on the peripheral tissues [1]. This concept, however, was later challenged by the data from liver-specific GH receptor of IGF-1 knockout mice, as in these animals the concentration of circulating IGF-1 in the serum was drastically reduced, but body growth was close to normal suggesting that locally produced IGF-1 rather than circulating (mostly liver-derived) IGF-1 determines body growth [2,3]. In this review, we summarize the effects of GH on blood pressure (BP), with more concentration on states with GH excess or deficiency.

GH and IGF-1 in the blood vessels

The vascular endothelium covers the internal surface of blood vessels and has the ability to control vascular tone by releasing vasoconstrictors or vasodilatory agents such as nitric oxide (NO) and prostacyclin [4]. GH infusion in the brachial artery has been shown to acutely increase the blood flow in the forearm and to lower the peripheral vascular resistance in healthy subjects [5]. This vasodilatory effect was paralleled by an augmented forearm NO release. As circulating IGF-1 did not change, the vasodilatory effect could be due to GH per se, or due to local IGF-1 production. Similarly, intravascular IGF-1 infusion led to an increased response in forearm blood flow [6] through a NO-dependent mechanism [7]. Indirect evidence from animal studies points that both GH and IGF-1 can stimulate NO synthesis by regulating the expression of endothelial nitric oxide synthase (eNOS), the enzyme required for NO production in the endothelium [8].

Decreased bioavailability of NO and subsequent increased vascular resistance can be encountered both in GH excess and GH deficiency (GHD). GH/IGF-1 may exert endothelium-independent vasodilatory effects by upregulating gene expression of the vascular smooth muscle ATP-sensitive potassium channel (KATP) [9], or by enhancing vascular smooth muscle sodium-pump (Na^+/K^+-ATPase) activity [10]. The main effects of GH and IGF-1 on blood vessels are summarized in Fig. 15.1.

In addition to the vasodilatory effect, GH and IGF-1 have mitogenic activity in the vascular cells since they can induce proliferation of the endothelial cells [11−13] and vascular smooth muscle cells [14]. This aspect may play a role in acromegaly-related hypertension.

The role of GH and IGF-1 in the myocardium

In vitro studies showed that IGF-1 exerts a physiological hypertrophic effect on cardiomyocytes via enhancing the gene transcription and protein synthesis for cardiac and skeletal muscle-specific proteins [15]. IGF-1 also has calcium-dependent positive inotropic effect on cardiomyocytes, resulting in increased contractility. The proposed mechanisms underlying the increased contractility include modulation of membrane channel activity [16], enhancement of myofilament sensitivity to calcium [17], or by upregulating the sarcoplasmic reticulum calcium-ATPase [18]. The main effects of GH and IGF-1 in the myocardium are summarized in Fig. 15.1.

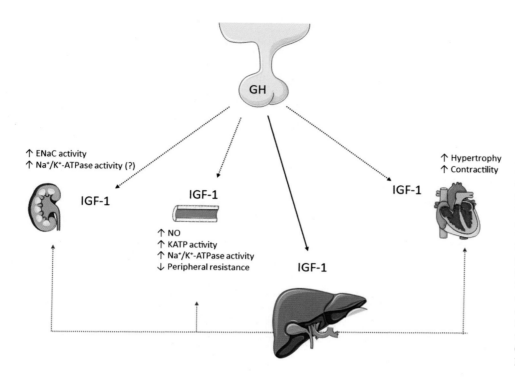

FIGURE 15.1 Schematic representation of physiological GH and IGF-1 stimulatory effects on target tissues *Black filled arrow*, indicates GH direct effects on the liver; *dotted arrow*, indicates GH indirect effects, through locally produced IGF-1 (*black dotted arrow*) or liver-derived IGF-1 (*blue dotted arrow*); *GH*, growth hormone; *IGF-1*, insulin-like growth factor 1; ENaC-amilorid-sensitive epithelial sodium channel; Na$^+$/K$^+$-ATPase, sodium potassium pump in the collecting duct cells; *NO*, nitric oxide; *KATP*, ATP-sensitive K channels in the vascular smooth muscle cells of blood vessels; Na$^+$/K$^+$-ATPase activity, sodium potassium pump in the vascular smooth muscle cells of blood vessels; ↑, increased; ↓, decreased; (?), possible effects; Parts of the figure were drawn using Servier Medical Art in compliance with the terms of the Creative Commons Attribution 3.0 Unported License (https://smart.servier.com/).

The role of GH and IGF-1 in the kidney

The kidney plays a significant role in the regulation of body fluid homeostasis and BP by adjusting the sodium and water excretion depending on the dietary intake [19]. The main effects of GH and IGF-1 in the kidneys are summarized in Fig. 15.1. Short-term treatment with GH in human subjects provided the direct evidence for its effects on the kidney: (1) an increased glomerular filtration rate (GFR) and renal plasma flow; (2) sodium retention, (3) phosphate retention, and (4) hypercalciuria [20]. A decrease in the arteriolar resistance is followed by an increased glomerular perfusion and consequently an increased GFR. The effect on the vascular resistance requires IGF-1-related NO and prostaglandin release [21]. Data suggest that the sodium retention effect of GH/IGF-1 in the kidney is achieved by stimulating the amiloride-sensitive epithelial sodium channel (ENaC) [19] in the aldosterone-sensitive distal nephron (the distal convoluted tubule, connecting tubule, and collecting duct) [22]. Renal effects of both IGF-1 [23,24] and GH [25,26] suggest a co-operative model between GH and IGF-1 to explain the sodium-retaining effect in the distal nephron [25]. In addition to the increased ENaC activity, enhanced Na$^+$/K$^+$-ATPase activity in the collecting duct cells may represent another mechanism responsible for the increased sodium reabsorption in the distal nephron [25]; however, the role of GH/IGF-1 on the Na$^+$/K$^+$-ATPase pump in the sodium-retaining effect remains yet to be fully elucidated [19,21]. GH/IGF-1 also modulates the phosphate and calcium metabolism in the kidney. IGF-1 stimulates the phosphate reabsorption via increased expression and activity of the sodium-dependent phosphate transport protein 2A (NaPi-2a) in the proximal tubule [21]. Studies on animal models and human subjects suggest that GH (either directly or indirectly through IGF-1) increases the circulating levels of calcitriol (bioactive vitamin D) by stimulating 1-alpha hydroxylase, the enzyme responsible for calcitriol production in the kidney [27]. The hypercalciuric effect observed after GH treatment is rather transient [28]; however, in acromegaly, enhanced intestinal calcium absorption secondary to increased calcitriol synthesis is linked to absorptive hypercalciuria [29].

Acromegaly and hypertension

Epidemiology

The global prevalence of hypertension in adults aged 30–79 years is 32% in women and 34% in men [30]. Acromegaly, on the other hand, has a prevalence between 2.8 and 13.7 cases per 100,000 people with an annual incidence between 0.2 and

TABLE 15.1 The prevalence of hypertension in patients with acromegaly from analysis of previous studies.

Number of studies analyzed	Publication period for the included studies	Hypertension prevalence	Publication year for the study analysis	Reference
18	1962–2001	18.0%–57.0%	2001	[14]
19	1987–2002	17.5%–57.0%	2004	[33]
14	2004–2017	11.0%–54.7%	2019	[34]

1.1 cases/100,000 people [31]. While hypertension is a cardinal feature in acromegaly, it only represents a negligible percent of the global hypertension burden.

Hypertension is the most frequent cardiovascular comorbidity accompanying acromegaly [32]. The prevalence of hypertension in patients with acromegaly is ranging between 11% and 57% (Table 15.1) [14,33,34]. Results from a recent large international study (ACROSTUDY, a global noninterventional surveillance study of long-term treatment with pegvisomant) showed that 56% of patients with acromegaly had hypertension at study entry and the percentage increased up to 64% during the follow-up period [35]. However, the prevalence in this cohort is not representative of the true disease burden because it includes cases of uncontrolled acromegaly with a longer disease duration, as pegvisomant is generally used in patients who failed to achieve disease control after surgery and somatostatin analogue treatment [36].

This wide range in the prevalence might be the result of different criteria used to define hypertension over different periods of recruitment, or because of different clinical characteristics of the selected patients [33]. In addition, the majority of the aforementioned studies did not use ambulatory blood pressure monitoring (ABPM) for the assessment of hypertension, as this was reported only in three studies out of 19 in a meta-analysis [33]. This is relevant as clinic-based BP measurements can overestimate the actual frequency of hypertension in patients with acromegaly compared with ABPM: 42.5% with office BP assessment versus 17.5% with ABPM in a study from 40 patients or 32.4% with office BP measurement versus 23.9% ABPM among 37 patients [37,38]. In a 10-year long retrospective observational study of 205 newly diagnosed patients with acromegaly and 410 age- and sex-matched controls, patients with acromegaly had 1.67-fold and 1.58-fold higher risk to develop mild and severe hypertension, respectively compared to the general population. Moreover, the risk was extremely high for patients with a diagnostic delay of more than 10 years from the onset of the disease [39]. In acromegaly, hypertension occurs a decade earlier compared to the general population [33]. The prevalence of hypertension increases with age, as nearly 50% of the patients with acromegaly older than 55 years were hypertensive, according to the data from an Italian registry ($n = 1512$) [40].

Pathophysiology of hypertension in acromegaly

Hypertension in acromegaly is considered to be multifactorial, but exact mechanisms are unclear. Proposed mechanisms (Fig. 15.2) include increased plasma volume due to the fluid retention [19], and increased vascular resistance due to vascular remodeling, and endothelial dysfunction [34]. In addition, sleep apnea, insulin resistance, and increased cardiac output may contribute to the pathophysiology of hypertension [32]. The way each factor contributes to hypertension is detailed below.

Plasma volume expansion
Sodium-retaining effect and the role of ENaC in acromegaly

In a set of elegant studies, Kamenický's group established that enhanced action of ENaC is responsible for the sodium and water retention seen in acromegaly. Because it was suggested previously that the Na^+-K^+-$2Cl^-$ (NKCC2) cotransporter located in the thick ascending limb of Henle's loop is indirectly activated by GH [41], they evaluated the natriuretic and kaliuretic responses to furosemide (the drug that blocks NKCC2) or to amiloride (the drug that blocks ENaC) before and after treatment of acromegaly in 16 patients on a high-sodium diet. They observed that the urinary Na/K ratio was higher after amiloride and lower after furosemide in patients before treatment of acromegaly. By blocking NKCC2 with furosemide there is a higher amount of sodium delivered to the distal nephron, where an enhanced ENaC retains sodium (and water in response to the osmotic gradient created by sodium) and secretes potassium. Therefore, the urinary Na/K is lower after furosemide. In contrast, by blocking an active ENaC with amiloride, a potassium-sparing diuretic, potassium is

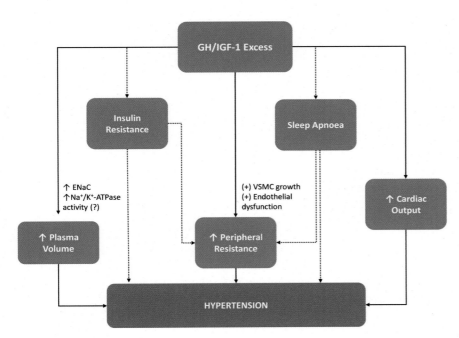

FIGURE 15.2 Possible mechanisms involved in acromegaly-related hypertension *Black filled arrow*, indicates GH/IGF-1 direct mechanisms; *black dotted arrow*, indicates GH/IGF-1 indirect mechanisms; *GH*, growth hormone; *IGF-1*, insulin-like growth factor 1; ENaC-amilorid-sensitive epithelial sodium channel; Na^+/K^+-ATPase, sodium potassium pump in the collecting duct cells; VSMC, vascular smooth muscle growth; (+), stimulatory effects; GH/IGF-1-promoting effects; ↑, increased; ↓, decreased; (?), possible effects.

preserved while sodium is lost in the urine, meaning a higher urinary Na/K ratio. Successful treatment of acromegaly reduced the effect of amiloride and enhanced the effect of furosemide on the urinary Na/K ratio. The stable natriuretic response after furosemide in acromegaly before and after treatment suggests that NKCC2 does not mediate sodium reabsorption with GH excess. In contrast, it appears that enhanced ENaC is responsible for the sodium and water retention effect seen in acromegaly [26].

Overview of other possible mechanisms for enhanced fluid retention in acromegaly

Insulin can stimulate the sodium reabsorption through ENaC, but to be able to obtain the same effect as that of IGF-1 on the sodium transport in murine collecting duct-derived cells, insulin concentration had to be 50 times higher than IGF-1. This effect was achieved through the IGF-1 receptor (IGF-1R), as insulin can bind IGF-1R but with a lower affinity [24].

The amiloride-sensitive ENaC is also positively modulated by aldosterone [42]; therefore, an indirect antinatriuretic effect for GH excess through activation of renin—angiotensin—aldosterone system (RAAS) has been suggested [14,34]. This hypothesis remains controversial. Early results from GH treatment in adrenalectomized rats showed that the sodium-retaining effect after GH treatment was preserved, suggesting an aldosterone independent effect [43]. On the other hand, by blocking RAAS, the fluid retention effect was prevented after GH treatment in human subjects [44]. In patients with acromegaly, plasma aldosterone was increased which significantly dropped after successful treatment, while plasma renin was unaffected [45]. In contrast, in another study, RAAS was partially supressed in patients with acromegaly on a high sodium diet and did not change after acromegaly treatment. Therefore, RAAS was not responsible for the antinatriuretic effect observed in GH/IGF-1 excess.

An inadequate response of natriuretic peptides to sodium retention and hypervolemia was suggested to be one of the factors responsible for hypertension in acromegaly [46]; however, plasma atrial natriuretic peptide was normal in patients with acromegaly compared to controls [47], and plasma brain natriuretic peptide did not change before and after acromegaly treatment [26].

Sympathetic nervous system activity is commonly increased in hypertension and involves sodium and water retention as well. But there is controversy over the role of adrenergic system in acromegaly [34,48]. Plasma catecholamine concentrations [49] and the mean 24-h plasma catecholamine levels did not differ between patients with acromegaly and controls [50]. Normally, BP has a circadian variability, and there is a nocturnal dip. Subjects who have a blunted nocturnal dip are called nondippers and this pattern reflects deficient mechanisms to regulate BP [51]. Patients with acromegaly manifest a nondipper behavior [38,52]. In spite of the fact that plasma catecholamine levels did not differ between patients and controls, a normal circadian rhythm of catecholamine levels and BP was observed only in cured patients, which might suggest an impaired sympathetic activity in GH excess. In addition, one of the mechanisms responsible for hypertension is sleep apnea, which is common in acromegaly, associated with an increased adrenergic tone [53]; however, further studies are needed for a firm conclusion regarding the sympathetic overactivity among patients with acromegaly.

Finally, another possible player in the sodium-retaining effect of chronic GH excess might be the sodium pump Na^+/K^+-ATPase in the distal nephron. Enhanced Na^+/K^+-ATPase activity was found in leukocytes and skeletal muscles of patients with acromegaly, but its activity in the kidney remains unclear [19]. The main mechanisms related to hypertension in acromegaly are summarized in Fig. 15.2.

Increased peripheral vascular resistance

Small arteries and arterioles are the main determinants of peripheral resistance and play an important role in the pathophysiology of hypertension. Hypertension is associated with increased wall-to-lumen ratio in these arterial segments resulting from vascular (eutrophic or hypertrophic) remodeling [54]. The increased wall-to-lumen ratio is a marker of vascular remodeling.

Vascular remodeling of the resistance arteries

Smooth muscle cells play an important role in the remodeling process of vascular structures, and GH may have mitogenic activity on these cells either directly or through IGF-1 [55]. Vascular remodeling in the small arteries and arterioles narrow the lumen of the vessels and even minor changes in the lumen of these arteries significantly increase the peripheral resistance. In essential hypertension, there are two types of vascular remodeling: eutrophic and hypertrophic. In eutrophic remodeling, vascular smooth muscle cells rearrange around a smaller lumen without an actual hypertrophy or hyperplasia, while in hypertrophic remodeling vascular smooth muscle cells show hypertrophy [56]. Using pressure myography, the vascular structure of subcutaneous small arteries was studied in patients with essential hypertension ($n = 12$) and acromegaly ($n = 9$). Hypertrophic remodeling and greater wall thickening were seen in patients with acromegaly compared to those with essential hypertension, who had eutrophic remodeling. IGF-1 levels in acromegaly were correlated to the wall-to-lumen ratio suggesting that the hypertrophic remodeling is probably due to the growth-promoting properties of GH or IGF-I [55]. Similar structural changes were described in 41 patients (18 with active acromegaly and 23 in remission) and additional impaired endothelial-dependent relaxation was also reported. Successful treatment of acromegaly significantly improved the vascular structure and function, although without fully returning to normal [57].

More recently, retinal imaging in 60 patients (19 with active disease vs. 41 with controlled disease) and 60 controls found that the wall-to-lumen ratio was increased in active acromegaly, while in controlled disease the ratio did not differ from controls. The vascular pattern described was eutrophic remodeling. Possible explanations for this discrepancy in vascular pattern include different vascular territories and techniques used for exploration. The lack of hypertrophy in their cohorts may be attributable to a reversible process in the treatment-stabilized patients [58]. Although the precise pattern involved in the vascular remodeling is not clear, there is a positive relationship between the wall-to-lumen ratio and plasma IGF-1 level, suggesting that an active disease influences vascular structure, but acromegaly induced remodeling may be (partially or totally) reversible if IGF-1 is normalized [55,57,58].

Endothelial dysfunction

The NO pathway regulates the peripheral resistance, and it has been shown that patients with essential hypertension have an altered endothelium-dependent vasodilation and reduced NO [59]. The same hypothesis was suggested to be applicable in acromegaly [14,34]. This is an interesting hypothesis because GH and IGF-1 at physiological levels stimulate endothelial NO production, as we explained before (Fig. 15.1). However, comparing cutaneous vasoreactivity responses in patients with active acromegaly ($n = 10$) and normotensive subjects ($n = 10$), it was confirmed that endothelium-dependent vasodilatation mediated through NO was impaired in acromegaly [60], while in another study NO concentrations inversely correlated with GH and IGF-1 levels and disease duration, probably due to reduced expression of eNOS protein [61]. Possible mechanism to explain a reduced NO includes increased levels of oxidative stress or the presence of asymmetric dimethylarginine (ADMA), an endogenous eNOS inhibitor. Overproduction of reactive oxygen species by mitochondria diminishes NO by transforming it into peroxynitrite which is a toxic compound for endothelial cells [62]. In fact, acromegaly has been associated with increased levels of oxidative stress and endothelial dysfunction [63]. Endogenous ADMA, on the other hand, inhibits eNOS and, therefore, reduces NO formation. Patients with acromegaly ($n = 13$) compared to matched controls ($n = 12$) had impaired endothelial function assessed by flow-mediated dilatation of the brachial artery [64], a method used to reflect NO production. ADMA levels did not differ between patients with acromegaly and matched controls, but there was a positive correlation between ADMA and arterial stiffness and negative correlation with small vessel compliance, suggesting a harmful effect on the small arterial elasticity [64].

Impaired glucose metabolism

GH has the ability to antagonize the hepatic and peripheral effects of insulin on glucose metabolism, likely due to concomitant increase in lipid metabolites and uptake [65]. Insulin resistance, glucose intolerance, and diabetes mellitus are common features of acromegaly [66]. A relationship between insulin and indices of subcutaneous small resistance artery structure, hypertrophic remodeling, and endothelial dysfunction along with reduced NO bioavailability have been described in patients with noninsulin-dependent diabetes mellitus [67], which is similar to the evidence obtained in patients with acromegaly when IGF-1 was analyzed. In clinical terms, impaired glucose tolerance and diabetes mellitus significantly contribute to increased BP values seen in acromegaly [68,69]. Suggested mechanisms include an impaired NO-mediated vasodilatation, activation of RAAS, or increased sympathetic activity [66]. Indirect evidence supports that insulin stimulates angiotensinogen and vascular smooth muscle cell growth, thus promoting vascular hypertrophy through RAAS activation [70]. Hyperinsulinemia increases peripheral resistance through an adrenergic-mediated vasoconstriction effect [71]. However, the role of RAAS and sympathetic activity in the acromegaly related hypertension remains inconclusive [34,48].

Sleep apnea syndrome

Obstructive sleep apnea is a frequent complication of GH excess and is characterized by five or more episodes of apnea (air flow cessation ≥ 10 s) and hypopnoea (diminished airflow of $\geq 30\%$ for ≥ 10 s) on a sleep study (respiratory polygraphy or polysomnography) [72]. GH excess is linked to sleep apnea because of tissue infiltration of the upper respiratory system (tongue, soft palate, pharyngeal and laryngeal swelling as well as vocal cord thickening due to enhanced fluid retention), or anatomical changes in the cranio-facial region (maxilla and mandibular overgrowth) [19,73]. Up to a third of patients have a central component of the sleep apnea without the obstruction of airflow, and this may be related to high GH or IGF-1 [32]. The reported prevalence for sleep apnea varies between 44% and 87.5% in active acromegaly [74].

Sleep apnea is independently associated with hypertension and one of the mechanisms involved is an increased adrenergic tone (due to brief awakening and hypoxia during breathing cessation). Additionally, hypoxia promotes the formation of reactive oxygen species, potentially resulting in oxidative stress, inflammation, endothelial dysfunction, and ultimately increased BP [53]. Similar to acromegaly [38,52], sleep apnea is associated with a nondipper BP behavior [75]. In a cohort of 37 patients with acromegaly (including patients with active disease, controlled disease, or those in remission), the risk assessment for sleep apnea was done using a screening tool (STOP-bang questionnaire). Although a respiratory polygraphy or polysomnography were not used to confirm sleep apnea in patients at high risk, a trend toward an inverse correlation was described between a high risk for sleep apnea and a nondipper behavior in acromegaly, the small sample size accounting possibly for the borderline association. Furthermore, all hypertensive patients ($n = 22$) had a high risk for sleep apnea compared to normotensive patients ($n = 15$) where only 18% had this high risk [38]. Sleep apnea improves with acromegaly treatment [76], but it still persists in controlled acromegaly among 35%−58% of the cases [74]. These aspects suggest that active disease is not the only determinant of sleep apnea in acromegaly. Even so, treatment with continuous positive airway pressure or mandibular advancement devices is associated with reductions in BP in unselected sleep apnea population [77].

Hypertension phenotype and cardiovascular comorbidities

Characteristics of acromegaly related hypertension

Baseline characteristics for patients enrolled in the ACROSTUDY before pegvisomant treatment showed that patients with acromegaly-related hypertension had higher body mass index (BMI), higher prevalence of diabetes mellitus, hyperlipidemia, and cardiovascular disease (CVD) and were older compared to normotensive patients with acromegaly. Because pegvisomant is a second- or third-line treatment, patients in this cohort were older and had a longer duration of active disease which might explain the higher cardiovascular risk profile in hypertensive patients. Other findings include more frequent pituitary deficiencies in hypertensive patients. In addition, patients with hypertension had less likelihood of undergoing pituitary surgery and this might be related to the older age and multiple comorbidities compared to the normotensive patients [35]. Although this study does not describe baseline characteristics at acromegaly diagnosis, it has the advantage to include a large number of patients with inadequate control of acromegaly.

Predictive factors (Fig. 15.3) identified for acromegaly-related hypertension are the following: IGF-1 levels, age at diagnosis [40], glucose levels, estimated disease duration [33], and BMI [78]. IGF-1 levels are not universally seen as a predictive factor since hypertension was poorly related to IGF-1 levels at diagnosis in other studies [33,79]. Hypertension

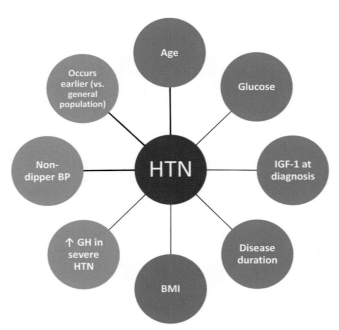

FIGURE 15.3 **Hypertension (HTN) characteristics and predictive factors for acromegaly-related hypertension** Darker blue indicates predictive factors for acromegaly-related hypertension; lighter blue indicates characteristics of hypertension; (clockwise): *IGF-1*, insulin-like growth factor 1; *BMI*, body mass index; *GH*, growth hormone; *BP*, blood pressure; ↑, increased.

is usually not very severe [40]; however, in patients with severe hypertension, GH was found to be higher at baseline compared to those with controlled or mild hypertension [80]. The predictive factors for hypertension and characteristics of acromegaly related factors are summarized in Fig. 15.3. Results from a case—control study of 200 patients with '*acromegaly and hypertension*' matched with 200 hypertensive controls for age, sex, BMI, and smoking habits showed a preferential increase in diastolic BP (DBP) in acromegaly. This could be attributed to the increased peripheral resistance through the vascular remodeling induced by GH/IGF-1 excess [33]. However, this was not confirmed in a similar although smaller cohort [81]. A sex-dependent difference has been observed in some studies: a Mexican registry found hypertension being more common among female patients [79], and the German Pegvisomant Observational Study showed that acromegalic men had increased DBP only, whereas women had both increased SBP and DBP [82]. However, these differences were not seen in other studies [33,35,39,40,79,80,83].

Acromegaly and comorbidities

Cardiomyopathy

Acromegaly related cardiomyopathy is a cardinal feature and develops in three stages [84,85]: (i) in the first stage, patients display a hyperkinetic cardiac syndrome which denotes increased cardiac contractility and output due to myocardial hypertrophy; (ii) the second stage is characterized by progressive hypertrophy, myocardial fibrosis, and damaged heart function which is mainly diastolic dysfunction and impaired systolic performance on effort; (iii) in the last stage, if acromegaly is untreated or uncontrolled, systolic dysfunction and heart failure occur. Left ventricular hypertrophy in acromegaly was observed in 11%—78% when analyzed by cardiac ultrasound and this wide variation in prevalence estimate may be the consequence of different methodologies used to define left ventricular hypertrophy, different study designs, or the characteristics of study population [73]. A significantly lower frequency for left ventricular hypertrophy was detected using cardiac magnetic resonance imaging (cardiac MRI) when compared to cardiac ultrasound in patients with acromegaly ($n = 30$) before treatment (5% vs. 31%) suggesting that cardiac ultrasound might overestimate the prevalence. Cardiac MRI has higher accuracy and reproducibility, and lower variability in comparison with echocardiography and this may explain the dissimilar results between the two methods of imaging [86]. SBP, followed by GH levels [68], and disease duration were found to be the most important predictors of left ventricular hypertrophy [39]. Diastolic dysfunction assessed by ultrasound was observed in 11%—58% of patients, but it is usually mild with no clinical consequence and the progression to systolic dysfunction is infrequent in more recent studies [73].

Valvulopathy

Aortic valve regurgitation has been described in a third of patients with acromegaly (30%−31% vs. controls 7%) [87,88]. Mild aortic root dilatation observed in some patients does not have any clinically relevant complications [89]; however, gross aortic root dilation with heart failure was described in young women with acromegaly, necessitating aortic root replacement with a composite aortic graft prosthesis [90]. A wider range of prevalence of mitral regurgitation has also been described (5%−26% vs. controls 0%−7%) [87,88].

Arrhythmias

Arrhythmias have been reported in 7%−40% of patients with acromegaly, more frequent during exercise [32]. The prevalence of arrhythmia may vary depending on the presence of left ventricular hypertrophy because ventricular arrhythmias occurred more often in those with left ventricular hypertrophy [91], whereas a low frequency of ventricular and supraventricular arrhythmias were reported in patients with lack of cardiac structural changes [92]. Several types of arrhythmias have been linked to acromegaly such as paroxysmal atrial fibrillation and supraventricular tachycardia, sick sinus syndrome, isolated and paired ventricular ectopic beats, ventricular tachycardia as well as abnormally long or dispersed QT interval and a higher frequency of late potentials [73,84]. Malignant ventricular tachyarrhythmia may be the cause of repeated syncope and sudden cardiac death in patients with acromegaly [85].

Diabetes mellitus

The prevalence of diabetes mellitus at the time of acromegaly diagnosis varies between 20% and 35% [66]. Data from the Mexican registry ($n = 2057$) showed that nearly two thirds of patients have abnormal glucose metabolism at diagnosis, since 30% of patients had diabetes mellitus, whereas 33% of patients displayed glucose intolerance or impaired fasting glucose [79]. These data could be influenced by ethnic differences, as the prevalence of diabetes mellitus is higher in Mexicans than the average prevalence in the world (9.4% vs. 8.5%) [93]. Furthermore, IGF-1 levels at diagnosis and the concomitant presence of hypertension were significantly associated with the presence of diabetes mellitus [79]. In the ACROSTUDY ($n = 2090$), diabetes mellitus was significantly more frequent in the hypertensive group compared with normotensive patients (20.2% vs. 11.4%) [35].

Hyperlipidemia

GH stimulates free fatty acid release into the circulation from the adipose tissue [65], and, therefore, dyslipidemia is expected at presentation. The prevalence of hyperlipidemia varies from 13% to 51%, typically with higher levels of triglycerides or reduced HDL levels compared to controls [73]. Other lipid parameters such as total cholesterol, very low-density lipoprotein (VLDL), and low-density lipoprotein (LDL) levels were found to be significantly higher in 62 patients with acromegaly (50 with active disease) compared to controls [94]. In the ACROSTUDY ($n = 2090$), dyslipidemia was significantly more frequent in the hypertensive group compared with normotensive patients (17.0% vs. 5.6%) [35].

Atherosclerosis and mortality

Patients with acromegaly present with risk factors for coronary artery disease such as hypertension, dyslipidaemia, and diabetes mellitus [73]. Early markers of the peripheral vascular damage and predictors of cardiovascular events such as intima-media thickness (IMT) of common carotid arteries, flow- mediated dilatation (FMD), and arterial pulse wave velocity (PWV) were assessed in a meta-analysis. Results showed that patients with acromegaly had higher IMT, impaired FMD, and higher PWV compared to controls, yet controlled disease showed a significant improvement in IMT and FMD. This suggests that patients with acromegaly may be at increased risk of atherosclerosis, especially if the disease is active [95]. The Framingham risk score is an algorithm used to calculate the likelihood of coronary artery disease over a period of 10 years, and this score was shown to be significantly higher in patients with acromegaly compared with controls [82]. However, the incidence of myocardial infarction and stroke in acromegaly was found to be similar compared to controls in two national registries [96,97]. Hypertension rather than active acromegaly was linked to a higher rate of cardiovascular events since myocardial infarction or stroke were more common in patients with hypertension compared to those without (94% vs. 43.4%), whereas the proportion of patients with active disease was similar between the groups [97]. An association between pituitary radiotherapy and cerebrovascular mortality has been described [98] and similarly, in patients with acromegaly, treatment with radiotherapy was associated with increased mortality and cerebrovascular-related deaths. Compared to those without radiotherapy, the increased mortality risk persisted even after adjusting for GH and IGF-1 levels [99].

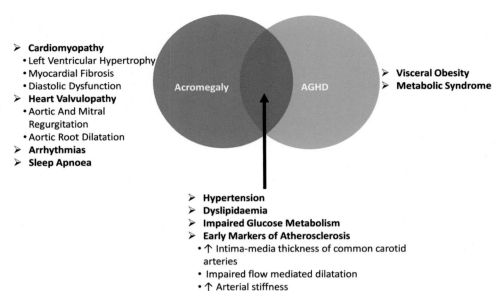

FIGURE 15.4 Clinical consequences of acromegaly and adult growth hormone deficiency (AGHD) Comorbidities of acromegaly and AGHD overlap for several clinical aspects (black filled arrow), whereas particular clinical features are represented on the left of the diagram for acromegaly or on the right for AGHD. *Adapted from Mazziotti G, Marzullo P, Doga M, Aimaretti G, Giustina A. Growth hormone deficiency in treated acromegaly. Trends Endocrinol Metab. 2015;26:11—21*

➤ **Cardiomyopathy**
  • Left Ventricular Hypertrophy
  • Myocardial Fibrosis
  • Diastolic Dysfunction
➤ **Heart Valvulopathy**
  • Aortic And Mitral Regurgitation
  • Aortic Root Dilatation
➤ **Arrhythmias**
➤ **Sleep Apnoea**

Acromegaly   AGHD

➤ **Visceral Obesity**
➤ **Metabolic Syndrome**

➤ **Hypertension**
➤ **Dyslipidaemia**
➤ **Impaired Glucose Metabolism**
➤ **Early Markers of Atherosclerosis**
  • ↑ Intima-media thickness of common carotid arteries
  • Impaired flow mediated dilatation
  • ↑ Arterial stiffness

Cardiovascular and cerebrovascular complications are among the leading causes of death in acromegaly [100], but it seems that other factors such as hypertension [97] or radiotherapy [99] are linked to coronary artery disease rather than acromegaly itself. The limited use of radiotherapy [96] due to improvement in the surgical and medical treatment of acromegaly or optimal hypertension management (82% of the patients without myocardial infarction and stroke were on antihypertensive drugs) [97] could explain the lower risk for cardiovascular events described in the two national registries of acromegaly.

In the ACROSTUDY, a total of 68 deaths (5.1%) were observed in hypertensive patients with acromegaly compared to 10 deaths (1.3%) in patients with acromegaly and normal BP. The mortality rate was 13.2 per 1000 patient years in the hypertension group and 4 per 1000 patient years in the normotensive group. The main causes of death in these patients were cardiovascular disease (31%), cerebrovascular disease (18%), cancer (18%), and respiratory problems/sepsis (13%). The most frequent cause of death due to cardiovascular disease was heart failure, which accounted for nine cases. Two deaths were caused by ventricular fibrillation, and aortic aneurysm rupture was the cause of death in one patient. Cardiovascular disease and pituitary deficiencies at study entry predicted mortality independently. In hypertensive patients, pituitary deficiency was present in 72% of hypertensive patients who died, and in 51% of survivors. However, in patients with acromegaly and hypertension the survival was reduced in the presence of concomitant cardiovascular disease rather than pituitary deficiency [35]. Hypopituitarism is linked to increased cardiovascular mortality, and GHD is suggested to be the culprit [101], but this was not the case for the acromegaly cohort. Over-replacement of glucocorticoids increases the risks of metabolic and cardiovascular disease [102], and given the fact that study is lacking information on how adequately pituitary deficiencies were treated, mortality related to overreplacement of glucocorticoids cannot be excluded [35].

The main clinical consequences of acromegaly are depicted in the Fig. 15.4.

Screening for acromegaly in hypertensive patients

When to suspect acromegaly in hypertensive patients

Screening for secondary causes of hypertension should be considered after confirming that BP is elevated with ABPM [104]. Secondary hypertension due to acromegaly (Fig. 15.2) should be suspected especially in those patients with acral enlargement and facial features. In patients without typical manifestations, the suspicion of acromegaly should be raised in hypertensive patients who have several of these associated conditions: sleep apnea syndrome, diabetes mellitus (type 2), debilitating arthritis, carpal tunnel syndrome, and hyperhidrosis [105]. Biochemical screening of every hypertensive patient systematically for acromegaly is not recommended.

A study that gathered 1,209 patients seen by the general practitioners with newly diagnosed hypertension with at least one comorbidity (chronic headache, diabetes mellitus, chronic diffuse arthralgia, carpal tunnel syndrome, and hyperhidrosis) in the absence of acral enlargement showed that 22 patients had elevated IGF-1. Of those, four had inadequate GH suppression after glucose load; however, MRI did not reveal any changes in the pituitary, nor did chest and abdominal contrast-enhanced computed tomography. At the time of the publication, patients were followed for up to 3 years. Though an ectopic source for GH was considered unlikely in the absence of imaging findings or disease progression, it was not ruled out as longer follow-up is needed [106]. It is well known that in some cases there is a discrepancy between IGF-1 and GH. This can be encountered in certain conditions such as hepatic and renal failure, hypothyroidism, malnutrition, severe infection, and poorly controlled diabetes mellitus where IGF-1 can be falsely elevated, normal, or low [105]. The degree of GH suppression depends on BMI, sex, and estrogen status in women [107]. Secondary hypertension in patients with acromegaly without enlargement of the extremities is rare; however, acromegaly remains underdiagnosed. Data from 324 patients with acromegaly presenting between 1981 and 2006 were retrospectively analyzed and results showed that the delay in diagnosis was an average of 5.3 ± 4 years [108], and patients typically visit on an average 3.4 physicians prior to diagnosis [109]. Delays of 15 or even 25 years have been reported in the diagnosis of acromegaly [31]. Patients with acromegaly may present with common signs and symptoms (including hypertension), but a long diagnostic delay among these patients could reflect a failure of healthcare professionals to recognize the disease earlier [109]. As such, an increased awareness of acromegaly among healthcare professionals is needed.

Patients with newly diagnosed acromegaly should be screened for hypertension, cardiovascular disease, sleep apnea, diabetes mellitus [105], and dyslipidaemia [73]. The diagnosis of hypertension should be based on repeated office-based BP measurements on more than one visit (except when hypertension is severe), or on out-of-office BP measurements (using ABPM). The latter has the advantage to identify white-coat and masked hypertension but can be expensive and has limited availability [104]. Cardiac ultrasound is recommended at diagnosis to evaluate the presence of cardiomyopathy [110]. If suggestive symptoms are present for cardiac rhythm abnormalities, a 12-lead electrocardiogram, or a 24-hour Holter monitoring could be used depending on the circumstances [73]. It is worth mentioning that additional screening is recommended in acromegaly for bone fractures (vertebral fracture assessment), colon neoplasia, and thyroid neoplasia if clinically indicated (palpable thyroid nodule) [105,110].

Treatment

Therapeutical options in acromegaly

Treatment options include transsphenoidal surgery (TSS), medical therapy, or radiotherapy. TSS is the primary treatment for most of the patients. Tumor size and invasiveness of surrounding structures, especially the cavernous sinus, are important determinants of surgical remission [36]. If the surgical resection is unlikely due to parasellar extension, surgical debulking to improve treatment response to medical therapy is recommended [105].

In case of persistent disease (patients who do not achieve biochemical control), medical therapy is recommended, although reoperation is also an option. For milder disease, a trial of dopamine agonists (cabergoline) is suggested, whereas for significant disease, somatostatin analogues (SSAs: lanreotide, octreotide, or pasireotide in some patients) or GH-receptor antagonists (pegvisomant) can be used. If the patient is a poor surgical candidate, medical treatment can be used as a first line. Radiotherapy is regarded as an adjuvant therapy when surgery and medical therapy have failed to control disease, although, it may be considered at any point after incomplete surgery [36,105].

The effect of disease activity on blood pressure

Successful treatment of acromegaly improves the BP in hypertensive patients in up to a third of the cases [111]. In one study, after 24 months of treatment for acromegaly, in those who had controlled disease, up to 70% also had controlled hypertension, whereas in those with inadequate control of acromegaly, hypertension had been controlled only in 24% of the cases [80]. Not all studies report an improvement in BP after acromegaly treatment [112]. Both first-line surgery and SSA treatment reduced the BP in a similar way [113], but when compared to pegvisomant, surgery was associated with a significant BP reduction [114]. A possible explanation for this latter result is the fact that most patients on pegvisomant treatment have more challenging acromegaly, and hence it is more difficult to control the disease and consequently the BP. Acromegaly treatment may impact differently the components of BP: a preferential decline in SBP [111,114,115] or DBP [83,113] or both [80,112] have been reported.

The impact of each treatment modality on BP is summarized in Table 15.2.

TABLE 15.2 Impact of acromegaly therapies treatment on BP.

No. of patients	Cohort description (pre-treatment)	Treatment	Controlled acromegaly	Poorly controlled	Reference
30 (15 CD vs. 15 UD)	HTN (40%); BP nondipper profile (35%)	TSS	↓24-h-SBP* ↑ 24-h-DBP BP circadian rhythm restored in 83%	↑ 24-h-SBP ↑ 24-h-DBP Persistent non-dipper pattern	[111]
31	HTN (n = 10) BP nondipper profile (n = 15)	TSS	↓24-h-SBP* ↔ 24-h-DBP HTN cured ~ 33% BP circadian rhythm restored in 80%		[115]
380	Systematic review; hypertensive cohort in 1 study	SSAs	(3 studies, n = 72) ↓ BP (14 studies, n = 308) ↔ BP		[112]
89 (56 first line SSAs vs. 33 first-line surgery)	For stage 1 HTN: 33.9 vs. 36.4% For stage 2 HTN: 25% vs. 18.2%	Surgery, SSAs	↔ SBP ↓ DBP* For stage 1 HTN: 25% vs. 27.3% For stage 2 HTN: 10.7% vs. 6.1%		[113]
96	HTN (n = 21)	Surgery, SSAs, PEGV	↓24-h-SBP* in HT; ↓24-h-SBP* surgery vs. PEGV		[114]
105 (76 CD vs. 29 UD)	All patients were HT	SSAs alone or as part of multimodal treatment in 103/105	↓SBP*,↓ DBP*; Controlled HTN in ~70%	↓ SBP, ↓ DBP Controlled HTN in ~24%	[80]
58 (28 NT vs.30 HT, of which 17 CD vs. 13 UD)	Surgically naïve patients; HT cohort	SSAs ± PEGV or PEGV alone	CD in 56.7% of HT vs. 53.6% of NT; ↓24-h-SBP and ↓24-h-DBP*	↑ 24-h-SBP*, ↓24-h-DBP Overt HTN in 46% of NT	[83]
2,090 (1,344 HT vs. 747 NT)	64% HT	PEGV alone or PEGV ± SSAs ± DAs	↓ SBP and ↓ DBP in HT and NT		[35]

BP, blood pressure; *CD*, controlled disease; *DAs*, dopamine agonists; *DBP*, diastolic blood pressure; *HT*, hypertensive; *HTN*, hypertension; *NT*, normotensive; *PEGV*, pegvisomant; *SBP*, systolic blood pressure; 24-h-BP represents data captured with ambulatory blood pressure monitoring (ABPM); *SSAs*, somatostatin analogues; *TSS*, transsphenoidal surgery; *UD*, uncontrolled disease; ↔, no change; *, statistically significant.

Hypertension management

In patients where acromegaly treatment did not improve the BP, standard antihypertensive drugs should be used [104]. There is not enough evidence for preferring any particular antihypertensive drug class over other classes for the treatment of hypertension in patients with acromegaly; however, given the enhanced activity of ENaC, treatment with amiloride could be more efficient in theory [116]. Currently, amiloride is reserved for cases when spironolactone is not tolerated [104].

Growth hormone deficiency and hypertension

Adult GH deficiency (AGHD) is a clinical entity that has been recognized as a syndrome three decades ago [117], and is characterized by a clustering of cardiovascular risk factors which overlap with the metabolic syndrome regarding visceral obesity, impaired glucose metabolism, dyslipidaemia, and hypertension [118]. AGHD is a relatively rare disease with an estimated prevalence of 2−3 per 10,000 population [119], and an average incidence rate of 1.65 per 100,000 [120].

Epidemiology

The reported prevalence of hypertension varies from less than 20%−66% [121,122], but it can reach up to 90% [123] in AGHD patients $\geq$65 years of age. Hypertension is more frequent in AGHD compared to controls or background population. In a cohort of patients ($n = 104$) with adulthood-onset of GHD without GH-replacement, but with adequate substitution for other pituitary hormone deficiencies, the prevalence of hypertension was 11.3% for men and 15.1% for women [121]. In a larger cohort ($n = 926$), the prevalence of hypertension was reported to be 22.6% for men and 21.7% for women [124]. In another large cohort ($n = 632$), hypertension was present in 18% of GHD patients [125]. In smaller cohorts, hypertension was present at study entry in 66% of patients with treatment-naïve AGHD ($n = 50$) [122]. More recently, the prevalence of hypertension at study entry was reported to be 90% ($n = 9$) in AGHD patients $\geq$65 years of age and 13.7% ($n = 4$) in AGHD patients below 65 years [123]. The prevalence of hypertension may vary due to different criteria to define hypertension or different background of the studied population, and different methods to assess BP. Additionally, given the relative rarity of the disease, the group of AGHD is very heterogeneous, and the presence of other pituitary deficiencies or certain etiologies that resulted in AGHD (craniopharyngioma, Cushing's disease or acromegaly) may represent an additional cardiovascular risk factor [118].

KIMS is a multinational, pharmacoepidemiological surveillance database that contains prospectively collected observational data from almost 16,000 adult patients with GHD from 31 countries [126,127]. The KIMS database provides subgroup analysis for naïve- (without GH treatment) and seminaïve AGHD patients (with GH replacement discontinued for at least 6 months before the enrollment in the study). The presence of multiple pituitary hormone deficiencies is suggested to be associated with a worse cardiovascular profile compared to isolated GHD [128]; however, hypertension was present in about 15% in both subgroups at study entry into KIMS [129].

The etiology of AGHD is heterogeneous, but the most frequent cause is a pituitary tumor (with the nonfunctioning pituitary adenoma being the most common subtype) followed by craniopharyngiomas. These two etiologies account for approximately 57% of the cases, whereas treated acromegaly or treated Cushing's disease account for 1.7% and 6.14%, respectively of AGHD cases [130].

Hypertension was slightly more common (9.4% vs. 8.7%) in patients with craniopharyngioma ($n = 351$) compared to patients with nonfunctioning pituitary adenomas ($n = 370$) but did not differ significantly between the groups at study entry [131]. The prevalence of hypertension did not differ (25% vs. 26%) between post-acromegaly GHD ($n = 115$) and GHD due to a nonfunctioning pituitary adenoma ($n = 142$) [132]. This was not the case for patients post-Cushing's disease GHD ($n = 135$), since the prevalence of hypertension was higher in this group compared to GHD due to other etiologies ($n = 1392$) including nonfunctioning pituitary tumors [133].

Childhood-onset of GHD (CO-GHD) represent approximately 22% of all AGHD [134]. Differences exist between CO-AGHD and adulthood-onset of GHD (AO-GHD) in terms of etiology and prevalence of hypertension. In CO-GHD idiopathic/congenital GHD is responsible for 30%−50% of the cases, and is followed by craniopharyngioma in 23% of the cases with GHD and multiple pituitary deficiencies, or by other sellar and extrasellar tumors in isolated GHD. Hypertension in CO-AGHD is less frequent than in AO-GHD (<5%) [129]. The prevalence of hypertension in AGHD is summarized in Table 15.3. The AGHD groups are mainly AO-GHD.

TABLE 15.3 The prevalence of hypertension in AGHD.

Country of study	No. of patients	AO-GHD or CO-GHD	GH-treatment naïve	Etiology for AGHD	HT prevalence		Reference
					AGHD	Controls or reference population	
Sweden	104 (66 M, 38 F)	AO-GHD	Naïve	Mixed	11.3% (men) 15.1% (women)	8% (men) 5.5% (women)	[121]
Spain	926 (441 M, 485 F)	AO-GHD	Naïve	Mixed	22.6% (men) 21.7% (women)	14.9% (ranging from 12.2% to 16.2%)	[124]
Germany	122 (79 M, 43 F)	N/A	Naïve	Mixed	18% (men) 19% (women)	16.5% (men)* 13.9% (women)*	[125]
The Netherlands	50 (48% M, 52% F)	AO-GHD	Naïve	Mixed	66%	35%	[122]
Italy	29 (10 EGHD patients, 29 AGHD)	N/A	Naïve	Mixed	90% EGHD 13.3% AGHD	50% EGHD 33.3% AGHD	[123]
International (KIMS data)	167 IGHD, 1992 MPHD	AO-GHD	Mixed (naïve and seminaïve)	Mixed	15% IGHD 15% MPHD		[129]
International (KIMS data)	351 CP patients (189 M and 162 F; vs. 370 NFPA (185 M, 185 F)	AO-GHD	Mixed (naïve and seminaïve)	CP and NFPA	9.4% CP 8.7% NFPA		[131]
International (KIMS)	115 adults Post-acro GHD (71 M, 74F); 142 NFPA (79 M, 63 F)	N/A	Mixed (naïve and seminaïve)	Post-acro GHD and NFPA	25% Post-acro GHD 26% NFPA		[132]
International (KIMS)	135 post-Cushing (78% F, 22% M)	AO-GHD	66% of patients had previously received GH therapy	Post-Cushing's AGHD	~25% (men) 30% (women)		[133]
International (KIMS)	1.395 AGHD <65yr; 170 AGHD >65yr	AO-GHD	Mixed (naïve and seminaïve)	Mixed	43.1% (>65yr) 13.6% (<65yr)		[135]

AGHD, adult growth hormone deficiency; *AO-GHD*, adulthood-onset of growth hormone deficiency; *CP*, craniopharyngioma; *EGHD*, elder growth hormone deficiency; *CO-GHD*, childhood-onset of growth hormone deficiency; *EGHD*, elder growth hormone deficiency; *F*, female; GH-treatment naïve, without previous GH replacement therapy; GH-treatment seminaïve, without GH replacement therapy in the past 6 months; *IGHD*, isolated growth hormone deficiency; *KIMS*, multinational pharmacoepidemiological surveillance database; *M*, male; *MPHD*, multiple pituitary growth hormone; *NFPA*, nonfunctioning pituitary adenoma; *N/A*, not available or not applicable; *Post-acro GHD*, growth hormone deficiency after cured acromegaly. * the prevalence for the reference population is available in another study [136].

Pathophysiology of hypertension in AGHD

The relationship between BP and IGF-1 can be described by a U-shaped curve, as both high levels and low levels of GH/IGF-1 are associated with hypertension [137,138]. One of the early explanations suggested for the higher prevalence of hypertension in AGHD patients is the fact that these patients have periodic health evaluations and, therefore, are more likely to have their high BP detected [121]. Although this argument is not totally acceptable, other mechanisms such as endothelial dysfunction and arterial stiffness [138], increased activity of the sympathetic nervous system [139], vitamin D deficiency [140], or insulin resistance are probably other accountable mechanisms for the pathophysiology of GHD-related hypertension. The proposed mechanisms are summarized in Fig. 15.5.

Endothelial dysfunction

Similar to acromegaly, AGHD is linked to endothelial dysfunction and decreased bioavailability of NO [141−143] that results in increased vascular smooth muscle tone and this affects peripheral arterial resistance [141] and large-artery elasticity [144]. Possible mechanisms to explain a diminished NO bioavailability include enhanced inactivation or impaired generation of NO. Patients with untreated AGHD were shown to have an enhanced oxidative environment [142,145] which inactivates NO, but in AGHD, NO is reduced primarily because of an impaired synthesis rather than enhanced inactivation. In one study, untreated AGHD patients ($n = 7$) had a blunted forearm blood flow response to endothelium-dependent vasodilator agent and reduced forearm release of nitrite, which is suggestive of a defect in NO generation. In addition, a blunted vasodilatory response was observed to sodium nitroprusside, an NO donor, which points toward an altered endothelial-independent vasodilatation, suggesting not only an impaired NO generation but also a reduced responsiveness of the vascular smooth muscle cells to NO [143]. GH/IGF-1 stimulates NO synthesis but may exert possible vasodilatory effects in the vascular smooth muscle cells through the K^+-ATP channel or Na^+/K^+-ATPase pump and this might explain the consequences of chronic GHD on the vascular smooth muscle cells in addition to endothelial dysfunction. Nonetheless, GH replacement therapy (GHRT) restores an adequate vascular function since patients with AGHD under GH substitution ($n = 8$) had normal response to both vasodilatory agents similar to normal subjects ($n = 10$) [143].

Increased sympathetic activity

An augmented sympathetic nerve activity of central origin together with diminished NO synthesis were suggested to be responsible for hypertension in patients with untreated AGHD. Muscle sympathetic nerve activity was recorded in AGHD

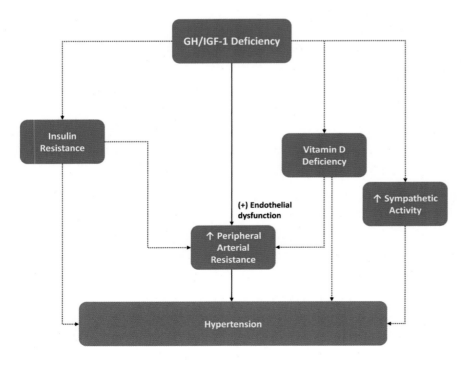

FIGURE 15.5 Possible mechanisms involved in adult growth-hormone deficiency-related hypertension Black *filled arrow*, indicates GH/IGF-1 direct mechanisms; *black dotted arrow*, indicates GH/IGF-1 indirect mechanisms; *GH*, growth hormone; *IGF-1*, insulin-like growth factor 1; (+), stimulatory effects; GH/IGF-1-promoting effects; ↑, increased.

patients ($n = 10$) and was markedly increased compared to controls ($n = 10$). In addition, the muscle sympathetic nerve activity negatively correlated with IGF-1 and positively with DBP. This augmented sympathetic discharge was suggested to be of central origin because norepinephrine is released to stimulate hypothalamic growth hormone-releasing hormone (GHRH) secretion, which in turn stimulates the release of GH; in the absence of GH/IGF-1, a positive feedback loop may arise which further stimulates central norepinephrine release [139].

Vitamin D deficiency

Poor vitamin D status was found to be a predictor of the prevalence of hypertension and additionally, it was linked to higher SBP [140,146]. GHD patients commonly have lower levels of vitamin D compared to controls, and some studies report that GH treatment improves vitamin D status [27]. The mutual relationship between GH/IGF-1 and vitamin D is complex and not fully understood. GH seems to modulate vitamin D metabolism by regulating renal 1 alpha-hydroxylase activity, and vitamin D in turn increases circulating IGF-I [27]. Vitamin D acts on extraskeletal sites including the vascular system since vitamin D receptors are expressed in the endothelial cells and in the vascular smooth muscle cells. The role of vitamin D includes NO generation in the endothelial cells and an antiproliferative activity in the vascular smooth muscle cells [147]. In addition, vitamin D was suggested to negatively regulate the RAAS in healthy humans [148]. The concept that vitamin D deficiency may impact BP is plausible, and proposed mechanisms include endothelial dysfunction, impairment of vascular compliance because of smooth muscle changes [149], or upregulation of RAAS [148]; however, RAAS seems less likely to be involved in the pathophysiology of hypertension in untreated AGHD because GHD patients have a low sodium and body water content [19] and this should normally trigger the RAAS. Renin levels were shown to be increased in AGHD patients but only after GHRT, whereas following placebo administration, renin levels did not change suggesting that GHD patients may have an impaired RAAS, and that GH substitution may improve this situation [150]. Treatment benefits from vitamin D supplementation on BP are not proven in the general population [151], yet it remains to be determined in AGHD patients.

Insulin resistance

In children and adolescents, GHD is associated with increased insulin sensitivity and reactive hypoglycaemia [152]. Insulin resistance is not part of the AGHD syndrome, it is rather a consequence of the metabolic syndrome that accompanies AGHD. Proposed mechanisms for hypertension due to insulin resistance include endothelial dysfunction with diminished bioavailable NO, or increased activity of the sympathetic nervous system [71]. In addition, changes in the BP circadian rhythm may be related to insulin resistance, since AGHD patients with a nondipping behavior were shown to have higher insulin levels and HOMA-IR (Homeostatic Model Assessment for Insulin Resistance) index than those with a normal circadian BP rhythm [153].

Phenotype of AGHD and characteristics of blood pressure profile

There is scarce data in the literature explicitly regarding hypertension in AGHD compared to acromegaly, and most of the data on BP abnormalities come from heterogeneous cohorts of AGHD.

Isolated GHD provides the ideal model to characterize GHD without the influence from other pituitary deficiencies or their treatment, but the prevalence for isolated GHD in adults is rather low (9.6%) [129]. In a cohort of 16 treatment-naïve AGHD patients with isolated GHD, SBP but not DBP was significantly higher than in controls [154].

Compared to those with multiple hormone deficiencies, patients with isolated GHD were younger [128,129], and were shown to have more frequently CO-GHD (38% vs. 26%) [128]. The mean SBP and DSP were significantly higher in patients with multiple hormone deficiencies, but this difference was lost after adjusting for age [128].

The clinical characteristics of patients depend on the underlying etiology for GHD. For example, in the KIMS study group, patients with craniopharyngioma had surgery more frequently by the transcranial route because of the tumor location which involves the hypothalamus and the pituitary stalk. As a consequence, these patients had more often multiple pituitary hormone deficiencies, and obesity with dyslipidaemia than patients with AGHD due to nonfunctioning pituitary adenomas. These aspects suggest that patients with craniopharyngioma carry a higher risk for cardiovascular disease; however, there was no difference between the groups for mean BP values [131]. In another subgroup analysis from the KIMS study group, AGHD patients previously treated for Cushing's disease had higher DBP values compared to those with nonfunctioning pituitary adenomas [155], whereas patients who were previously treated for acromegaly had a higher prevalence of stroke. In addition, a significant relationship between stroke and hypertension was found in post-acromegaly GHD patients [133].

Female patients with AGHD were suggested to carry a higher cardiovascular risk profile compared to controls [156], and increased cardiovascular mortality compared to men, possibly from oral estrogen replacement therapy [157]; however, when comparing the effects of GHD on the cardiovascular system according to gender in AO-GHD ($n = 36$) and in (gender-, age-, and BMI-matched) controls ($n = 36$), no gender differences were found between the groups for mean SBP or DBP values [158].

The clinical presentation of AGHD differs depending on the age of onset of GHD. Adults with CO-GHD are usually shorter, have a lower BMI, waist-hip ratio, and lean body mass along with a lesser impairment in lipid profile compared to adults with AO-GHD [159]. In addition, they are younger compared to patients with AO-GHD [129]. Increased DBP has been reported in patients with CO-GHD transitioning into AGHD who stopped growth hormone substitution [160], but not in adults with CO-AGHD where lower SBP [161] or a tendency toward low SBP and DBP [162] was reported.

A higher baseline DBP was reported in patients with AGHD post-Cushing's disease [155] or a preferential increase in DBP was observed in patients with AGHD above 65 years [135].

Vitamin D deficiency is considered an environmental risk factor for cardiovascular disease and has been associated with hypertension [163]. In treatment-naïve AGHD patients, vitamin D deficiency is more frequent compared to controls (51% vs. 14.6%), and is strongly associated with the presence of dyslipidaemia, hypertension, and metabolic syndrome [146]. In addition, a significant negative correlation was found between vitamin D levels and SBP in AGHD patients [140].

The analysis of BP behavior during a 24-hour period has been reported in few publications and the results are conflicting. The circadian rhythm of BP in treatment-naïve AGHD patient but with adequate substitution for the other pituitary deficiencies was reported to be abnormal by one group of study, with a nondipping behavior noted in 30%−37% of patients [153,162]. However, another group described a preserved circadian rhythm in a similar cohort of patients [164].

Despite a greater prevalence of hypertension in untreated AGHD patients [121,122,124,125], evidence from smaller case control studies report lower BP values in AGHD patients without treatment [165,166] or a tendency toward lower BP compared to controls [141,167]. A proposed mechanism that might explain why some of the patients may have lower BP in untreated AGHD is genetic variation in the genes that control renal tubular function. Polymorphism in *SLC12A3* gene (encodes thiazide-sensitive sodium-chloride Na$^+$:K$^+$:2Cl$^-$ cotransporter, also known as NKCC2; this gene is mutated in Gitelman syndrome) was associated with lower SBP and polymorphism in *SCNN1G* gene (encodes the gamma subunit of the amiloride-sensitive epithelial sodium channel, ENaC) was associated with lower DBP at baseline in 311 untreated AGHD patients [168].

The main characteristics and factors associated with BP in AGHD are summarized in Fig. 15.6.

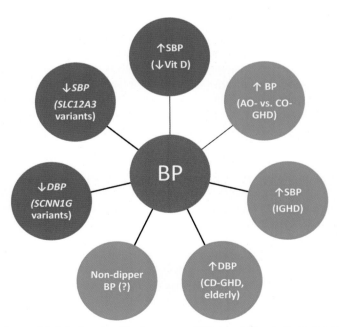

FIGURE 15.6 **Characteristics and associated factors for blood pressure (BP) in adult growth hormone deficiency** Darker green indicates correlated factors with blood pressure in adult growth hormone deficiency; lighter green indicates characteristics of blood pressure; (clockwise): *SBP*, systolic blood pressure; *Vit D*, vitamin D levels; *AO-GHD*, adulthood-onset of growth hormone deficiency; *CO-GHD*, childhood-onset of growth hormone deficiency; *IGHD*, isolated growth hormone deficiency; *DBP*, diastolic blood pressure; *CD-GHD*, Cushing's disease-related growth hormone deficiency; *SCNN1G* gene polymorphism, encodes amilorid-sensitive epithelial sodium channel in the aldosterone-sensitive distal nephron; *SLC12A3* gene encodes the thiazide-sensitive Na$^+$: K$^+$:2Cl$^-$ cotransporter in the thick ascending limb of Henle's loop; ↑, increased; ↓, decreased; (?), possible characteristic.

AGHD and comorbidities

Cardiac structure and performance

In healthy individuals, the GH/IGF-1 axis exerts a trophic effect on the cardiac muscle and maintains a normal cardiac performance. The importance of this axis on the cardiac structure and performance can be deducted from studies which focused on patients with GHD. Echocardiographic studies showed that untreated AGHD patients have lower left ventricular mass [169,170] and lower left ventricular systolic function [165] compared to controls. It was suggested that the consequences of GH on the heart are more marked in CO-GHD than in AO-GHD, because GH deficiency during the development of the heart results in a greater impairment in cardiac structure than GH deficiency acquired in adult life after the heart is fully developed [170]; however, cardiac performance was impaired in both CO- and AO-GHD compared to controls [161]. Cardiac MRI is a much more reliable technique for measuring myocardial mass and function, and by using this method, patients with untreated AGHD did not have significantly impaired systolic function or reduced left ventricular mass, although a tendency toward reduced cardiac mass compared to controls was observed [171]. Left ventricular hypertrophy in untreated AGHD is due to hypertension, and up to 40% of patients were shown to have left ventricular hypertrophy compared to 20% in the normotensive group, although this difference did not reach statistical significance [172].

Obesity

Characteristics of body composition of patients with GHD include excessive central pattern (visceral) of fat distribution and reduced lean tissue mass. Early studies showed that the fat mass is increased by 7% in GHD, whereas the lean body mass is decreased by 7%−8% compared with predicted values [117]. Excessive fat is considered the consequence of blunted lipolysis leading to accumulation of mainly visceral fat [163]. In addition, physical inactivity is part of the vicious circle in obesity since patients with GHD have reduced strength and exercise capacity [117]. Baseline data of 2,589 AGHD patients published by the KIMS study group showed that obesity was prominent since 32% had a BMI >30 kg/m^2 and only 4% had a BMI <20 kg/m^2. Waist circumference as a parameter which reflects visceral adiposity was above target in 40% of males (>102 cm) and in 56% of females (>88 cm). Factors that were associated with a higher BMI included adult onset of the disease, postmenopausal status, the presence of other hormone deficiencies, previous radiotherapy, and certain etiologies of GHD (e.g., craniopharyngioma). In addition, higher BMI was observed with increasing age, BP, and cholesterol [134].

Metabolic syndrome

The metabolic syndrome (MetS) is strongly associated with cardiovascular diseases in the general population [118] where its prevalence is between 20% and 30% [163]. The prevalence of MetS is reported to be higher in AGHD patients than in the general population; however, the prevalence varies depending on the definition used to score MetS or on the origin of the studied population. The National Cholesterol Education Program's Adult Treatment Panel III (NCEP) criteria [173] was used to define MetS in GHD patients [122], and with some adaptations in two large cohorts [174,175]. The components of MetS and cut-off values for each parameter that were defined by NCEP, and the adapted criteria used in the above-mentioned studies are summarized in Table 15.4.

AGHD patients ($n = 50$) were shown to have a 2-fold increase in the prevalence of MetS compared to controls (38.0 vs. 15.7%, $P < .0001$) [122]. In reports published by the KIMS study group [175] and by the Hypopituitary Control and Complications Study (HypoCCS) [174], patients had a similar overall prevalence for MetS (42% and 43% respectively); however it is worth to mention that the US cohort of AGHD had significantly higher age-adjusted prevalence of MetS compared to the European cohort of AGHD (51.8% vs. 28.6%, $P < .001$), and the differences in the background obesity prevalence as well as a lower proportion of CO-AGHD patients in the US cohort could explain the distinct results [174]. Patients with AGHD and MetS naïve to GH treatment had BP above the target (>130/85 mmHg) in a significantly larger proportion compared to those without MetS (60.9% vs. 19.6%). In addition, patients with MetS were shown to carry added cardiovascular and cerebrovascular morbidity besides the risk of diabetes mellitus [175].

Lipids

The changes seen in the lipid metabolism in AGHD patients is the results of GHD intertwined with abdominal obesity. Obesity-related changes in the lipid profile include hypertriglyceridemia, reduced HDL cholesterol, and increased numbers of small dense LDL particles. Increased LDL cholesterol is not a feature of the dyslipidemia seen with abdominal obesity [176]. Patients with AGHD were shown to present increments in LDL and total cholesterol levels in 40%−50% of the

TABLE 15.4 MetS components and cut-off values proposed by NCEP, and criteria used in the studies.

Risk factors for MetS	NCEP definition [173]	Adapted criteria in KIMS (n = 2479) [175]	Criteria adapted in HypoCCS, (n = 2531) [174]	Criteria used by Klaauw et al. (n = 50) [122]
Central obesity (waist circumference)	>102 cm for male >88 cm for female	≥102 cm for male ≥88 cm for female	≥102 cm for male ≥88 cm for female	>102 cm for male >88 cm for female
Fasting glucose	≥110 mg/dL	≥100 mg/dL or nonfasting plasma glucose ≥200 mg/dL or a serum HgbA1c ≥ 6.5% or a previous diagnosis of diabetes mellitus or the use of any antidiabetic drug	≥100 mg/dL or diabetes mellitus diagnosis or drug treatment for elevated glucose	≥110 mg/dL
Serum triglyceride concentration	≥150 mg/dL	≥150 mg/dL or the use of any lipid-lowering drug	≥150 mg/dL	≥150 mg/dL
HDL-cholesterol	<40 mg/dL for men <50 mg/dL for women	<40 mg/dL for men <50 mg/dL (<1.29 mmol/L) for women or the use of any lipid-lowering drug	<40 mg/dL for men <50 mg/dL for women	<40 mg/dL for men <50 mg/dL for women
Blood pressure	>130/85 mm Hg or on antihypertensive treatment	>130/85 mm Hg or on antihypertensive treatment	≥130/85 mm Hg or on antihypertensive treatment	≥130/85 mm Hg
Diagnosis	≥3 risk factors	≥3 risk factors	≥3 risk factors	≥3 risk factors

cases [117]. Some of the studies report increased triglyceride levels [122,146,177] and/or reduced HDL levels [146,156,178] compared to controls, but not all studies [154]. Hypertriglyceridemia seen with abdominal obesity, insulin resistance, and AGHD is the result of hepatic VLDL secretion enriched with triglycerides [176,179], whereas increased levels of LDL cholesterol is the consequence of GHD due to a decreased hepatic LDL receptor activity which can be reversed with GHRT [179]. One of the suggested mechanisms that lies behind a reduced HDL is the decreased activity of cholesterol ester transfer protein, the enzyme responsible for the exchange of triglycerides in VLDL for cholesterol esters in LDL and HDL particles [176]. The enzyme's activity is decreased in AGHD compared to controls, and if the transfer is impaired this may lead to lower HDL levels [179]. The particle size of LDL matters, because small dense LDL is considered a novel cardiovascular risk factor; however, studies of LDL fragments in AGHD are scarce and findings are inconsistent [163].

Impaired glucose metabolism

Patients with untreated GHD have been described to have a tendency toward hypoglycemia at least in children [152] whereas insulin resistance and diabetes mellitus are encountered in adults [163]; however, in treatment-naïve AGHD patients with isolated GHD, insulin levels and HOMA index were lower compared to controls [154]. These results suggest that other factors contribute to the insulin resistance among AGHD patients such as older age and increased fat mass [163], or the presence of other pituitary deficiencies and their specific hormonal replacement [154]. Diabetes mellitus is more prevalent in untreated patients with AGHD and MetS than in those without the MetS (16% vs. 3%) [175].

Atherosclerosis and mortality

Increased carotid intima media thickness is considered an early sign and marker of atherosclerosis as increased arterial thickness precedes hemodynamically important stenosis and it reflects changes elsewhere in the arterial tree [180]. AGHD is associated with premature atherosclerosis and untreated patients with AGHD have higher carotid intima media thickness than controls [180,181]. In addition, central aortic pulse pressure and aortic augmentation index are indirect markers for arterial stiffness. Patients with untreated AGHD ($n = 32$) were shown to have a higher augmentation index compared to controls [144]. These parameters suggest that similar to acromegaly, patients with AGHD may be at higher risk of atherosclerosis. The Framingham risk estimates were found to be higher in AGHD compared to controls at baseline in a study published by the KIMS study group. Treatment with GH reduced the risk by 50% after 2 years, and after 4 years of therapy the cardiovascular risk was normal in AGHD reflecting the beneficial effects of GH therapy on the cardiovascular risk factors [182]. Patients with hypopituitarism were found to have an excess mortality related to the cardiovascular and cerebrovascular diseases [101], and this was attributed to GHD; however, GHD does not equal hypopituitarism and in large cohort of 1,014 patients with hypopituitarism several factors other than GHD per se were shown to be associated with mortality such as younger age at hypopituitarism onset, craniopharyngioma, and radiotherapy [98]. Other factors such as GHD post-Cushing's disease, post-acromegaly, and female gender were associated with a higher mortality risk [130,132] suggesting that mortality among GHD patient is multifactorial. Results from a meta-analysis that gathered 19,153 patients with hypopituitarism with a follow-up duration of more than 99,000 person years showed that patients with hypopituitarism have an overall higher mortality risk but this becomes similar to the mortality risk of the background population in patients with GH substitution [157]. Treatment with GH improves some of the risk factors (lean and fat mass, total and LDL-cholesterol, and DBP) but not all [183]. Therefore, additional factors like close follow-up of patients, higher compliance and a tighter control of comorbidities might have an additive effect to GH therapy [182].

Screening for AGHD

The main AGHD-related comorbidities are summarized in Fig. 15.4.

When to suspect AGHD in hypertension?

The clinical suspicion of an acquired AGHD in patients with hypertension should be raised in patients with structural hypothalamic and/or pituitary disease, surgery/irradiation in these areas, head trauma, or evidence of other pituitary hormone deficiencies [184]. The presence of a low IGF-1 increases the likelihood of GHD [185]; however, around a fifth of AGHD patients may exhibit normal IGF-1 levels (particularly males) [102].

AGHD diagnosis

The diagnosis of AGHD relies on the reduced response of GH to dynamic stimulation tests [184]. Misinterpretation of test results can occur in central obesity because it attenuates both the spontaneous and stimulated secretion of GH [186]; therefore, BMI-related cut-offs for GH response should be applied [102]. In addition, thyroid [102] and glucocorticoid function [19] can also influence GH dynamics; therefore, central hypothyroidism and glucocorticoid deficiency should be treated before provocative tests are undertaken for sufficiency of GH secretion [102]. BP should be monitored every 6- to 12-month intervals; if it is clinically indicated, other investigations such as electrocardiography, echocardiography and carotid Doppler examination could be performed [187].

Treatment

One of the treatment goals of GHRT in AGHD includes normalization of cardiovascular risk factors [185]. Initially low dose GH replacement is preferred due to a dose-dependent fluid retention effect [102]. Dose escalation should be gradual, individualized, and guided by clinical and biochemical response. The age-adjusted IGF-1 level should be maintained below the upper limit of normal [102,185]. GHRT induces a certain degree of insulin resistance, and moderate elevation of fasting glucose and insulin levels are encountered despite improvement in the body composition [152]. In those patients at risk for diabetes mellitus (positive family history, obesity, or older age) careful monitoring is recommended [185]. Despite guideline recommendations, barriers to treatment still exit. Recently, results from an online survey gathered from 17 European countries (2139 AGHD patients) showed that GH replacement in AGHD is still not available or reimbursed in all European countries [188]. Regarding hypertension in AGHD, there is no specific treatment preference, and the current recommendations should be followed when choosing the antihypertensive drug classes for treatment [104].

Impact of AGHD management on blood pressure

Divergent results exist regarding the impact of GHRT on BP. Analysis of five observational studies with a duration of at least 2 years and with a maximum of 10 years showed that GH treatment had a neutral effect on SBP and DBP in four studies, whereas in one study only DBP was decreased during 7 years of treatment [122]. DBP was significantly decreased in AGHD patients post-Cushing's disease during 2 years of GH therapy [155], whereas in AGHD post-acromegaly or post–nonfunctioning pituitary tumor, BP did not change even after 5 years of treatment [132]. Results from a meta-analysis which included studies with rigorous design (blinded, randomized, placebo-controlled trials) showed that long-term GHRT (≥6 months of therapy) rather than short-term treatment had an effect on lowering the DBP. In addition, a greater beneficial effect of GH treatment was observed for DBP in AO-GHD compared to CO-GHD [183]. The systematic review analyzed 37 RCTs, of which only 10 trials ($n = 401$) mentioned BP as a measured outcome after GHRT, even though BP is monitored probably in all trials. This might suggest that GHRT had a neutral effect on BP in most of the studies [183]. The effects of GHRT were more recently analyzed from 11 clinical trials published in the recent decade. Similar to the previous meta-analysis, seven studies (of which two were RCTs) showed that GH treatment decreased only DBP [189]. In the elderly with AGHD (>60yr), there were no clear and consistent effects of GHRT on BP in the five studies that were analyzed: one study found no change, one a transient fall in BP and three found a reduction in DBP only [190]. Studies where ABPM was used to assess BP before and after 12 months of treatment showed that both SBP and DBP significantly decreased after treatment [164,191].

GH therapy could improve both SBP and DBP by modulating the endothelial function. This is achieved by promoting NO generation [142–144], and this in turn, is associated with a decrease in the central blood pressure [144], and the total peripheral resistance [141]. Given the fact that several studies report an improvement only in DBP, it was speculated that GHRT reduces BP in subgroups of AGHD patients possibly in those who have high DBP at baseline [192], such as patients with previous Cushing's disease [155] or elderly with GHD [135]. Another mechanism that could explain the individual differences in BP response after GHRT is genetic polymorphism. The calcium-sensing receptor gene encodes for a protein that inhibits the NKCC2 cotransporter, which decreases sodium and secondarily calcium reabsorption; a variant in this gene was associated with changes in SBP during GH therapy [168]. Fluid retention is seen during GH substitution; however, despite the volume expansion induced by GH therapy [150], frank hypertension is an uncommon event and is dose-dependent [166]. Attanasio et al. analyzed the MetS components before and after 3 years of GH therapy, and reported a significant increase in the prevalence of BP (from 59.8% to 69.7%) and fasting glucose after therapy. These findings were suggested to be related to ageing of the treated patients [174]. Contradictory results make it difficult to draw a firm conclusion regarding the effects of GH therapy but perhaps because of the rigorous study design, the meta-analysis of

TABLE 15.5 The impact of GH replacement therapy on BP.

Number of studies analyzed	Type of studies included in the analysis	No. of patients	Treatment duration	Impact on BP	Publication year for study	Reference
10	Meta-analysis of blinded, randomized, placebo-controlled trials	401	Short-term (<6 months) Long-term (≥6 months)	↔ SBP; ↓ DBP*	2004	[183]
5	Observational studies	218	48 –120 months	4 studies: ↔ SBP; ↔ DBP 1 study: ↔ SBP; ↓ DBP*	2007	[122]
5	Systematic review in AGHD (>60yr); 1 double-blinded RCT; 4 prospective open-label studies	379	6–12 months	3 studies: ↔ SBP; ↓ DBP* 1 study: ↔ SBP; ↔ DBP 1 study: transient ↓ BP	2011	[190]
7	Meta-analysis of interventional studies (1 double-blinded and 1 single-blinded RCT studies; 1 prospective longitudinal cohort study, 1 case–control study, 3 before-after controlled trials)	405	3–48 months	↔ SBP ↓ DBP*	2020	[189]

↔, no change; ↓, decrease; *, statistically significant; BP, blood pressure; DBP, diastolic blood pressure; SBP, systolic blood pressure.

RCTs provides stronger evidence. Different results might be considered given the heterogeneity of patients in terms of etiology, age, GH replacement dose, and even genetic variation. The impact of GHRT on BP from various studies is summarized in Table 15.5.

Summary and closing remarks

Acromegaly and GHD are two clinical entities in sharp contrast when it comes to GH/IGF-1 levels. Even though they are diametrically opposite diseases, hypertension occurs in both the situations. The curve that best describes the relationship between GH/IGF-1 and hypertension is a U-shaped one, as both GH/IGF-1 excess and GH/IGF-1 deficiency is related to hypertension. The case for acromegaly and hypertension is a solid one. There is less explicit literature regarding hypertension in AGHD and the effects of GH replacement therapy on BP show conflicting results. In addition, isolated GHD provides the ideal model to better understand the effects GHD on BP, but the majority of the AGHD cohorts are heterogeneous, and several other confounding factors are present making it more difficult to assess the direct consequences of GHD and subsequent changes in the blood pressure. Hypertension is also influenced by impaired glucose metabolism, dyslipidaemia, and endothelial dysfunction. Atherosclerosis and mortality are suggested to be higher in both conditions, but for different reasons. There is no specific treatment recommendation for the treatment of hypertension in acromegaly or AGHD patients and, therefore, the management should be according to the current guidelines.

Learning points

- Patients with acromegaly typically visit on average 3.4 physicians prior to diagnosis; therefore, an increased awareness of acromegaly among healthcare professionals is needed.
- Hypertension is a frequent complication of patients with acromegaly, but it represents a negligible percent of the global hypertension burden owing to the rarity of acromegaly.
- Successful treatment of acromegaly is associated with an improvement of hypertension in up to one-third of patients.
- GHD is a heterogeneous disease in terms of age of onset of the disease (CO-and AO-GHD), etiology of GHD (e.g., genetic forms of GHD, craniopharyngioma, Cushing's disease, acromegaly) or the presence/absence of additional pituitary hormone deficiencies, and these factors might explain, at least partly, the wide variation seen in the prevalence of hypertension.
- Screening for vitamin D deficiency and correction of the deficit in GHD might be advisable since vitamin D may also play a role in the pathophysiology of hypertension in patients with GHD.
- Despite guideline recommendations, GH replacement in GHD is not universally available or reimbursed in all European countries; therefore, the management of these patients needs improvement.

References

[1] Le Roith D, Bondy C, Yakar S, Liu JL, Butler A. The somatomedin hypothesis: 2001. Endocr Rev 2001;22:53−74.

[2] Sjogren K, Liu JL, Blad K, Skrtic S, Vidal O, Wallenius V, LeRoith D, Tornell J, Isaksson OG, Jansson JO, Ohlsson C. Liver-derived insulin-like growth factor I (IGF-I) is the principal source of IGF-I in blood but is not required for postnatal body growth in mice. Proc Natl Acad Sci USA 1999;96:7088−92.

[3] Fan Y, Menon RK, Cohen P, Hwang D, Clemens T, DiGirolamo DJ, Kopchick JJ, Le Roith D, Trucco M, Sperling MA. Liver-specific deletion of the growth hormone receptor reveals essential role of growth hormone signaling in hepatic lipid metabolism. J Biol Chem 2009;284:19937−44.

[4] Caicedo D, Diaz O, Devesa P, Devesa J. Growth hormone (GH) and cardiovascular system. Int J Mol Sci 2018;19:290.

[5] Napoli R, Guardasole V, Angelini V, D'Amico F, Zarra E, Matarazzo M, Sacca L. Acute effects of growth hormone on vascular function in human subjects. J Clin Endocrinol Metab 2003;88:2817−20.

[6] Copeland KC, Nair KS. Recombinant human insulin-like growth factor-I increases forearm blood flow. J Clin Endocrinol Metab 1994;79:230−2.

[7] Fryburg DA. NG-monomethyl-L-arginine inhibits the blood flow but not the insulin-like response of forearm muscle to IGF- I: possible role of nitric oxide in muscle protein synthesis. J Clin Invest 1996;97:1319−28.

[8] Wickman A, Jonsdottir IH, Bergstrom G, Hedin L. GH and IGF-I regulate the expression of endothelial nitric oxide synthase (eNOS) in cardiovascular tissues of hypophysectomized female rats. Eur J Endocrinol 2002;147:523−33.

[9] Tivesten A, Barlind A, Caidahl K, Klintland N, Cittadini A, Ohlsson C, Isgaard J. Growth hormone-induced blood pressure decrease is associated with increased mRNA levels of the vascular smooth muscle KATP channel. J Endocrinol 2004;183:195−202.

[10] Standley PR, Zhang F, Zayas RM, Muniyappa R, Walsh MF, Cragoe E, Sowers JR. IGF-I regulation of Na(+)-K(+)-ATPase in rat arterial smooth muscle. Am J Physiol 1997;273:E113−21.

[11] Rymaszewski Z, Cohen RM, Chomczynski P. Human growth hormone stimulates proliferation of human retinal microvascular endothelial cells in vitro. Proc Natl Acad Sci USA 1991;88:617−21.

[12] Back K, Islam R, Johansson GS, Chisalita SI, Arnqvist HJ. Insulin and IGF1 receptors in human cardiac microvascular endothelial cells: metabolic, mitogenic and anti-inflammatory effects. J Endocrinol 2012;215:89−96.

[13] Messias de Lima CF, Dos Santos Reis MD, da Silva Ramos FW, Ayres-Martins S, Smaniotto S. Growth hormone modulates in vitro endothelial cell migration and formation of capillary-like structures. Cell Biol Int 2017;41:577−84.

[14] Bondanelli M, Ambrosio MR, degli Uberti EC. Pathogenesis and prevalence of hypertension in acromegaly. Pituitary 2001;4:239−49.

[15] Ito H, Hiroe M, Hirata Y, Tsujino M, Adachi S, Shichiri M, Koike A, Nogami A, Marumo F. Insulin-like growth factor-I induces hypertrophy with enhanced expression of muscle specific genes in cultured rat cardiomyocytes. Circulation 1993;87:1715−21.

[16] von Lewinski D, Voss K, Hulsmann S, Kogler H, Pieske B. Insulin-like growth factor-1 exerts Ca2+-dependent positive inotropic effects in failing human myocardium. Circ Res 2003;92:169−76.

[17] Cittadini A, Ishiguro Y, Stromer H, Spindler M, Moses AC, Clark R, Douglas PS, Ingwall JS, Morgan JP. Insulin-like growth factor-1 but not growth hormone augments mammalian myocardial contractility by sensitizing the myofilament to Ca2+ through a wortmannin-sensitive pathway: studies in rat and ferret isolated muscles. Circ Res 1998;83:50−9.

[18] Houck WV, Pan LC, Kribbs SB, Clair MJ, McDaniel GM, Krombach RS, Merritt WM, Pirie C, Iannini JP, Mukherjee R, Spinale FG. Effects of growth hormone supplementation on left ventricular morphology and myocyte function with the development of congestive heart failure. Circulation 1999;100:2003−9.

[19] Kamenicky P, Mazziotti G, Lombes M, Giustina A, Chanson P. Growth hormone, insulin-like growth factor-1, and the kidney: pathophysiological and clinical implications. Endocr Rev 2014;35:234−81.

[20] Corvilain J, Abramow M, Bergans A. Some effects of human growth hormone on renal hemodynamics and on tubular phosphate transport in man. J Clin Invest 1962;41:1230−5.

[21] Gurevich E, Segev Y, Landau D. Growth hormone and IGF1 actions in kidney development and function. Cells 2021;10:3371.

[22] Teulon J, Wang W-H. Chapter 8 - studying Na+ and K+ channels in aldosterone-sensitive distal nephrons. In: Weimbs T, editor. Methods in cell biology, vol 153. Academic Press; 2019. p. 151−68.

[23] Tong Q, Gamper N, Medina JL, Shapiro MS, Stockand JD. Direct activation of the epithelial Na(+) channel by phosphatidylinositol 3,4,5-trisphosphate and phosphatidylinositol 3,4-bisphosphate produced by phosphoinositide 3-OH kinase. J Biol Chem 2004;279:22654−63.

[24] Gonzalez-Rodriguez E, Gaeggeler HP, Rossier BC. IGF-1 vs insulin: respective roles in modulating sodium transport via the PI-3 kinase/Sgk1 pathway in a cortical collecting duct cell line. Kidney Int 2007;71:116−25.

[25] Kamenicky P, Viengchareun S, Blanchard A, Meduri G, Zizzari P, Imbert-Teboul M, Doucet A, Chanson P, Lombes M. Epithelial sodium channel is a key mediator of growth hormone-induced sodium retention in acromegaly. Endocrinology 2008;149:3294−305.

[26] Kamenicky P, Blanchard A, Frank M, Salenave S, Letierce A, Azizi M, Lombes M, Chanson P. Body fluid expansion in acromegaly is related to enhanced epithelial sodium channel (ENaC) activity. J Clin Endocrinol Metab 2011;96:2127−35.

[27] Ciresi A, Giordano C. Vitamin D across growth hormone (GH) disorders: from GH deficiency to GH excess. Growth Hormone IGF Res 2017;33:35−42.

[28] Hansen TB, Brixen K, Vahl N, Jorgensen JO, Christiansen JS, Mosekilde L, Hagen C. Effects of 12 months of growth hormone (GH) treatment on calciotropic hormones, calcium homeostasis, and bone metabolism in adults with acquired GH deficiency: a double blind, randomized, placebo-controlled study. J Clin Endocrinol Metab 1996;81:3352−9.

[29] Kamenicky P, Blanchard A, Gauci C, Salenave S, Letierce A, Lombes M, Brailly-Tabard S, Azizi M, Prie D, Souberbielle JC, Chanson P. Pathophysiology of renal calcium handling in acromegaly: what lies behind hypercalciuria? J Clin Endocrinol Metab 2012;97:2124−33.

[30] NCD-Risk-Factor-Collaboration. Worldwide trends in hypertension prevalence and progress in treatment and control from 1990 to 2019: a pooled analysis of 1201 population-representative studies with 104 million participants. Lancet 2021;398:957−80.

[31] Lavrentaki A, Paluzzi A, Wass JA, Karavitaki N. Epidemiology of acromegaly: review of population studies. Pituitary 2017;20:4−9.

[32] Kasuki L, Rocha PDS, Lamback EB, Gadelha MR. Determinants of morbidities and mortality in acromegaly. Arch Endocrinol Metab 2019;63:630−7.

[33] Vitale G, Pivonello R, Auriemma RS, Guerra E, Milone F, Savastano S, Lombardi G, Colao A. Hypertension in acromegaly and in the normal population: prevalence and determinants. Clin Endocrinol (Oxf) 2005;63:470−6.

[34] Puglisi S, Terzolo M. Hypertension and acromegaly. Endocrinol Metab Clin North Am 2019;48:779−93.

[35] Vila G, Luger A, van der Lely AJ, Neggers S, Webb SM, Biller BMK, Valluri S, Hey-Hadavi J. Hypertension in acromegaly in relationship to biochemical control and mortality: global ACROSTUDY outcomes. Front Endocrinol (Lausanne) 2020;11:577173.

[36] Giustina A, Barkhoudarian G, Beckers A, Ben-Shlomo A, Biermasz N, Biller B, Boguszewski C, Bolanowski M, Bollerslev J, Bonert V, Bronstein MD, Buchfelder M, Casanueva F, Chanson P, Clemmons D, Fleseriu M, Formenti AM, Freda P, Gadelha M, Geer E, Gurnell M, Heaney AP, Ho KKY, Ioachimescu AG, Lamberts S, Laws E, Losa M, Maffei P, Mamelak A, Mercado M, Molitch M, Mortini P, Pereira AM, Petersenn S, Post K, Puig-Domingo M, Salvatori R, Samson SL, Shimon I, Strasburger C, Swearingen B, Trainer P, Vance ML, Wass J, Wierman ME, Yuen KCJ, Zatelli MC, Melmed S. Multidisciplinary management of acromegaly: a consensus. Rev Endocr Metab Disord 2020;21:667−78.

[37] Minniti G, Moroni C, Jaffrain-Rea ML, Bondanini F, Gulino A, Cassone R, Tamburrano G. Prevalence of hypertension in acromegalic patients: clinical measurement versus 24-hour ambulatory blood pressure monitoring. Clin Endocrinol (Oxf) 1998;48:149−52.

[38] Costenaro F, Martin A, Horn RF, Czepielewski MA, Rodrigues TC. Role of ambulatory blood pressure monitoring in patients with acromegaly. J Hypertens 2016;34:1357−63.

[39] Colao A, Pivonello R, Grasso LF, Auriemma RS, Galdiero M, Savastano S, Lombardi G. Determinants of cardiac disease in newly diagnosed patients with acromegaly: results of a 10 year survey study. Eur J Endocrinol 2011;165:713−21.

[40] Arosio M, Reimondo G, Malchiodi E, Berchialla P, Borraccino A, De Marinis L, Pivonello R, Grottoli S, Losa M, Cannavo S, Minuto F, Montini M, Bondanelli M, De Menis E, Martini C, Angeletti G, Velardo A, Peri A, Faustini-Fustini M, Tita P, Pigliaru F, Borretta G, Scaroni C, Bazzoni N, Bianchi A, Appetecchia M, Cavagnini F, Lombardi G, Ghigo E, Beck-Peccoz P, Colao A, Terzolo M, Italian Study Group of Acromegaly. Predictors of morbidity and mortality in acromegaly: an Italian survey. Eur J Endocrinol 2012;167:189−98.

[41] Dimke H, Flyvbjerg A, Bourgeois S, Thomsen K, Frokiaer J, Houillier P, Nielsen S, Frische S. Acute growth hormone administration induces antidiuretic and antinatriuretic effects and increases phosphorylation of NKCC2. Am J Physiol Renal Physiol 2007;292:F723−35.

[42] Viengchareun S, Le Menuet D, Martinerie L, Munier M, Pascual-Le Tallec L, Lombes M. The mineralocorticoid receptor: insights into its molecular and (patho)physiological biology. Nucl Recept Signal 2007;5:e012.

[43] Stein Jr JD, Bennett LL, Batts AA, Li CH. Sodium, potassium and chloride retention produced by growth hormone in the absence of the adrenals. Am J Physiol 1952;171:587−91.

[44] Moller J, Moller N, Frandsen E, Wolthers T, Jorgensen JO, Christiansen JS. Blockade of the renin-angiotensin-aldosterone system prevents growth hormone-induced fluid retention in humans. Am J Physiol 1997;272:E803−8.

[45] Bielohuby M, Roemmler J, Manolopoulou J, Johnsen I, Sawitzky M, Schopohl J, Reincke M, Wolf E, Hoeflich A, Bidlingmaier M. Chronic growth hormone excess is associated with increased aldosterone: a study in patients with acromegaly and in growth hormone transgenic mice. Exp Biol Med (Maywood) 2009;234:1002−9.

[46] McKnight JA, McCance DR, Hadden DR, Kennedy L, Roberts G, Sheridan B, Atkinson AB. Basal and saline-stimulated levels of plasma atrial natriuretic factor in acromegaly. Clin Endocrinol (Oxf) 1989;31:431−8.

[47] Deray G, Chanson P, Maistre G, Warnet A, Eurin J, Barthelemy C, Masson F, Martinez F, Lubetzki J, Legrand JC, et al. Atrial natriuretic factor in patients with acromegaly. Eur J Clin Pharmacol 1990;38:409−13.

[48] Colao A, Ferone D, Marzullo P, Lombardi G. Systemic complications of acromegaly: epidemiology, pathogenesis, and management. Endocr Rev 2004;25:102−52.

[49] Cryer PE. Plasma norepinephrine and epinephrine in acromegaly. J Clin Endocrinol Metab 1975;41:542−5.

[50] Bondanelli M, Ambrosio MR, Franceschetti P, Margutti A, Trasforini G, Degli Uberti EC. Diurnal rhythm of plasma catecholamines in acromegaly. J Clin Endocrinol Metab 1999;84:2458−67.

[51] Redon J, Lurbe E. Nocturnal blood pressure versus nondipping pattern: what do they mean? Hypertension 2008;51:41−2.

[52] Pietrobelli DJ, Akopian M, Olivieri AO, Renauld A, Garrido D, Artese R, Feldstein CA. Altered circadian blood pressure profile in patients with active acromegaly. Relationship with left ventricular mass and hormonal values. J Hum Hypertens 2001;15:601−5.

[53] Attal P, Chanson P. Endocrine aspects of obstructive sleep apnea. J Clin Endocrinol Metab 2010;95:483−95.

[54] Izzard AS, Rizzoni D, Agabiti-Rosei E, Heagerty AM. Small artery structure and hypertension: adaptive changes and target organ damage. J Hypertens 2005;23:247−50.

[55] Rizzoni D, Porteri E, Giustina A, De Ciuceis C, Sleiman I, Boari GE, Castellano M, Muiesan ML, Bonadonna S, Burattin A, Cerudelli B, Agabiti-Rosei E. Acromegalic patients show the presence of hypertrophic remodeling of subcutaneous small resistance arteries. Hypertension 2004;43:561−5.

[56] Schiffrin EL. Remodeling of resistance arteries in essential hypertension and effects of antihypertensive treatment. Am J Hypertens 2004;17:1192−200.

[57] Paisley AN, Izzard AS, Gemmell I, Cruickshank K, Trainer PJ, Heagerty AM. Small vessel remodeling and impaired endothelial-dependent dilatation in subcutaneous resistance arteries from patients with acromegaly. J Clin Endocrinol Metab 2009;94:1111−7.

[58] Gallo A, Chaigneau E, Jublanc C, Rosenbaum D, Mattina A, Paques M, Rossant F, Girerd X, Leban M, Bruckert E. IGF-1 is an independent predictor of retinal arterioles remodeling in subjects with uncontrolled acromegaly. Eur J Endocrinol 2020;182:375−83.

[59] Ahmad A, Dempsey SK, Daneva Z, Azam M, Li N, Li PL, Ritter JK. Role of nitric oxide in the cardiovascular and renal systems. Int J Mol Sci 2018;19:2605.

[60] Maison P, Demolis P, Young J, Schaison G, Giudicelli JF, Chanson P. Vascular reactivity in acromegalic patients: preliminary evidence for regional endothelial dysfunction and increased sympathetic vasoconstriction. Clin Endocrinol (Oxf) 2000;53:445−51.

[61] Ronconi V, Giacchetti G, Mariniello B, Camilletti A, Mantero F, Boscaro M, Vignini A, Mazzanti L. Reduced nitric oxide levels in acromegaly: cardiovascular implications. Blood Press 2005;14:227−32.

[62] Caicedo D, Devesa P, Alvarez CV, Devesa J. Why should growth hormone (GH) be considered a promising therapeutic agent for arteriogenesis? Insights from the GHAS trial. Cells 2020;9.

[63] Anagnostis P, Efstathiadou ZA, Gougoura S, Polyzos SA, Karathanasi E, Dritsa P, Kita M, Koukoulis GN. Oxidative stress and reduced anti-oxidative status, along with endothelial dysfunction in acromegaly. Horm Metab Res 2013;45:314−8.

[64] Yaron M, Izkhakov E, Sack J, Azzam I, Osher E, Tordjman K, Stern N, Greenman Y. Arterial properties in acromegaly: relation to disease activity and associated cardiovascular risk factors. Pituitary 2016;19:322−31.

[65] Moller N, Jorgensen JO. Effects of growth hormone on glucose, lipid, and protein metabolism in human subjects. Endocr Rev 2009;30:152−77.

[66] Vila G, Jorgensen JOL, Luger A, Stalla GK. Insulin resistance in patients with acromegaly. Front Endocrinol (Lausanne) 2019;10:509.

[67] Rizzoni D, Porteri E, Guelfi D, Muiesan ML, Valentini U, Cimino A, Girelli A, Rodella L, Bianchi R, Sleiman I, Rosei EA. Structural alterations in subcutaneous small arteries of normotensive and hypertensive patients with non-insulin-dependent diabetes mellitus. Circulation 2001;103:1238−44.

[68] Colao A, Baldelli R, Marzullo P, Ferretti E, Ferone D, Gargiulo P, Petretta M, Tamburrano G, Lombardi G, Liuzzi A. Systemic hypertension and impaired glucose tolerance are independently correlated to the severity of the acromegalic cardiomyopathy. J Clin Endocrinol Metab 2000;85:193−9.

[69] Jaffrain-Rea ML, Moroni C, Baldelli R, Battista C, Maffei P, Terzolo M, Correra M, Ghiggi MR, Ferretti E, Angeli A, Sicolo N, Trischitta V, Liuzzi A, Cassone R, Tamburrano G. Relationship between blood pressure and glucose tolerance in acromegaly. Clin Endocrinol (Oxf) 2001;54:189−95.

[70] Kamide K, Hori MT, Zhu JH, Takagawa Y, Barrett JD, Eggena P, Tuck ML. Insulin and insulin-like growth factor-I promotes angiotensinogen production and growth in vascular smooth muscle cells. J Hypertens 2000;18:1051−6.

[71] Muniyappa R, Montagnani M, Koh KK, Quon MJ. Cardiovascular actions of insulin. Endocr Rev 2007;28:463−91.

[72] National Institute for Health and Care Excellence (NICE). Obstructive sleep apnoea/hypopnoea syndrome and obesity hypoventilation syndrome in over 16s. 2021. https://www.nice.org.uk/guidance/ng202/chapter/1-Obstructive-sleep-apnoeahypopnoea-syndrome.

[73] Gadelha MR, Kasuki L, Lim DST, Fleseriu M. Systemic complications of acromegaly and the impact of the current treatment landscape: an update. Endocr Rev 2019;40:268−332.

[74] Wolters TLC, Netea MG, Riksen NP, Hermus A, Netea-Maier RT. Acromegaly, inflammation and cardiovascular disease: a review. Rev Endocr Metab Disord 2020;21:547−68.

[75] Seif F, Patel SR, Walia HK, Rueschman M, Bhatt DL, Blumenthal RS, Quan SF, Gottlieb DJ, Lewis EF, Patil SP, Punjabi NM, Babineau DC, Redline S, Mehra R. Obstructive sleep apnea and diurnal nondipping hemodynamic indices in patients at increased cardiovascular risk. J Hypertens 2014;32:267−75.

[76] Parolin M, Dassie F, Alessio L, Wennberg A, Rossato M, Vettor R, Maffei P, Pagano C. Obstructive sleep apnea in acromegaly and the effect of treatment: a systematic review and meta-analysis. J Clin Endocrinol Metab 2020;105:e23−31.

[77] Pengo MF, Soranna D, Giontella A, Perger E, Mattaliano P, Schwarz EI, Lombardi C, Bilo G, Zambon A, Steier J, Parati G, Minuz P, Fava C. Obstructive sleep apnoea treatment and blood pressure: which phenotypes predict a response? A systematic review and meta-analysis. Eur Respir J 2020;55:1901945.

[78] Sardella C, Cappellani D, Urbani C, Manetti L, Marconcini G, Tomisti L, Lupi I, Rossi G, Scattina I, Lombardi M, Di Bello V, Marcocci C, Martino E, Bogazzi F. Disease activity and lifestyle influence comorbidities and cardiovascular events in patients with acromegaly. Eur J Endocrinol 2016;175:443−53.

[79] Portocarrero-Ortiz LA, Vergara-Lopez A, Vidrio-Velazquez M, Uribe-Diaz AM, Garcia-Dominguez A, Reza-Albarran AA, Cuevas-Ramos D, Melgar V, Talavera J, Rivera-Hernandez AJ, Valencia-Mendez CV, Mercado M, Mexican Acromegaly Registry G. The Mexican Acromegaly Registry: clinical and biochemical characteristics at diagnosis and therapeutic outcomes. J Clin Endocrinol Metab 2016;101:3997−4004.

[80] Colao A, Terzolo M, Bondanelli M, Galderisi M, Vitale G, Reimondo G, Ambrosio MR, Pivonello R, Lombardi G, Angeli A, degli Uberti EC. GH and IGF-I excess control contributes to blood pressure control: results of an observational, retrospective, multicentre study in 105 hypertensive acromegalic patients on hypertensive treatment. Clin Endocrinol (Oxf) 2008;69:613−20.

[81] Dassie F, Grillo A, Carretta R, Fabris B, Macaluso L, Bardelli M, Martini C, Paoletta A, Vettor R, Sicolo N, Fallo F, Maffei P. Ambulatory arterial stiffness indexes in acromegaly. Eur J Endocrinol 2012;166:199−205.

[82] Berg C, Petersenn S, Lahner H, Herrmann BL, Buchfelder M, Droste M, Stalla GK, Strasburger CJ, Roggenbuck U, Lehmann N, Moebus S, Jockel KH, Mohlenkamp S, Erbel R, Saller B, Mann K. Investigative Group of the Heinz Nixdorf Recall Study and the German Pegvisomant Observational Study Board Investigators. Cardiovascular risk factors in patients with uncontrolled and long-term acromegaly: comparison with matched data from the general population and the effect of disease control. J Clin Endocrinol Metab 2010;95:3648−56.

[83] Sardella C, Urbani C, Lombardi M, Nuzzo A, Manetti L, Lupi I, Rossi G, Del Sarto S, Scattina I, Di Bello V, Martino E, Bogazzi F. The beneficial effect of acromegaly control on blood pressure values in normotensive patients. Clin Endocrinol (Oxf) 2014;81:573−81.

[84] Ramos-Levi AM, Marazuela M. Bringing cardiovascular comorbidities in acromegaly to an update. How should we diagnose and manage them? Front Endocrinol (Lausanne) 2019;10:120.

[85] Yang H, Tan H, Huang H, Li J. Advances in research on the cardiovascular complications of acromegaly. Front Oncol 2021;11:640999.

[86] dos Santos Silva CM, Gottlieb I, Volschan I, Kasuki L, Warszawski L, Balarini Lima GA, Xavier SS, Pedrosa RC, Neto LV, Gadelha MR. Low frequency of cardiomyopathy using cardiac magnetic resonance imaging in an acromegaly contemporary cohort. J Clin Endocrinol Metab 2015;100:4447−55.

[87] Colao A, Spinelli L, Marzullo P, Pivonello R, Petretta M, Di Somma C, Vitale G, Bonaduce D, Lombardi G. High prevalence of cardiac valve disease in acromegaly: an observational, analytical, case-control study. J Clin Endocrinol Metab 2003;88:3196−201.

[88] Pereira AM, van Thiel SW, Lindner JR, Roelfsema F, van der Wall EE, Morreau H, Smit JW, Romijn JA, Bax JJ. Increased prevalence of regurgitant valvular heart disease in acromegaly. J Clin Endocrinol Metab 2004;89:71−5.

[89] Casini AF, Neto LV, Fontes R, Franca RF, Xavier SS, Gadelha MR. Aortic root ectasia in patients with acromegaly: experience at a single center. Clin Endocrinol (Oxf) 2011;75:495−500.

[90] Wiper A, Eisenberger M, McPartlin A, El-Omar M. Gross aortic root dilation in a young woman with acromegaly. Exp Clin Cardiol 2012;17:257−9.

[91] Kahaly G, Olshausen KV, Mohr-Kahaly S, Erbel R, Boor S, Beyer J, Meyer J. Arrhythmia profile in acromegaly. Eur Heart J 1992;13:51−6.

[92] Warszawski L, Kasuki L, Sa R, Dos Santos Silva CM, Volschan I, Gottlieb I, Pedrosa RC, Gadelha MR. Low frequency of cardniac arrhythmias and lack of structural heart disease in medically-naive acromegaly patients: a prospective study at baseline and after 1 year of somatostatin analogs treatment. Pituitary 2016;19:582—9.

[93] Campos-Nonato I, Ramirez-Villalobos M, Flores-Coria A, Valdez A, Monterrubio-Flores E. Prevalence of previously diagnosed diabetes and glycemic control strategies in Mexican adults: ENSANUT-2016. PLoS One 2020;15:e0230752.

[94] Vilar L, Naves LA, Costa SS, Abdalla LF, Coelho CE, Casulari LA. Increase of classic and nonclassic cardiovascular risk factors in patients with acromegaly. Endocr Pract 2007;13:363—72.

[95] Parolin M, Dassie F, Martini C, Mioni R, Russo L, Fallo F, Rossato M, Vettor R, Maffei P, Pagano C. Preclinical markers of atherosclerosis in acromegaly: a systematic review and meta-analysis. Pituitary 2018;21:653—62.

[96] Dal J, Feldt-Rasmussen U, Andersen M, Kristensen LO, Laurberg P, Pedersen L, Dekkers OM, Sorensen HT, Jorgensen JO. Acromegaly incidence, prevalence, complications and long-term prognosis: a nationwide cohort study. Eur J Endocrinol 2016;175:181—90.

[97] Schofl C, Petroff D, Tonjes A, Grussendorf M, Droste M, Stalla G, Jaursch-Hancke C, Stormann S, Schopohl J. Incidence of myocardial infarction and stroke in acromegaly patients: results from the German Acromegaly Registry. Pituitary 2017;20:635—42.

[98] Tomlinson JW, Holden N, Hills RK, Wheatley K, Clayton RN, Bates AS, Sheppard MC, Stewart PM. Association between premature mortality and hypopituitarism. West Midlands Prospective Hypopituitary Study Group. Lancet 2001;357:425—31.

[99] Ayuk J, Clayton RN, Holder G, Sheppard MC, Stewart PM, Bates AS. Growth hormone and pituitary radiotherapy, but not serum insulin-like growth factor-I concentrations, predict excess mortality in patients with acromegaly. J Clin Endocrinol Metab 2004;89:1613—7.

[100] Bolfi F, Neves AF, Boguszewski CL, Nunes-Nogueira VS. Mortality in acromegaly decreased in the last decade: a systematic review and meta-analysis. Eur J Endocrinol 2018;179:59—71.

[101] Rosen T, Bengtsson BA. Premature mortality due to cardiovascular disease in hypopituitarism. Lancet 1990;336:285—8.

[102] Fleseriu M, Hashim IA, Karavitaki N, Melmed S, Murad MH, Salvatori R, Samuels MH. Hormonal replacement in hypopituitarism in adults: an endocrine society clinical practice guideline. J Clin Endocrinol Metab 2016;101:3888—921.

[103] Mazziotti G, Marzullo P, Doga M, Aimaretti G, Giustina A. Growth hormone deficiency in treated acromegaly. Trends Endocrinol Metab 2015;26:11—21.

[104] Williams B, Mancia G, Spiering W, Agabiti Rosei E, Azizi M, Burnier M, Clement DL, Coca A, de Simone G, Dominiczak A, Kahan T, Mahfoud F, Redon J, Ruilope L, Zanchetti A, Kerins M, Kjeldsen SE, Kreutz R, Laurent S, Lip GYH, McManus R, Narkiewicz K, Ruschitzka F, Schmieder RE, Shlyakhto E, Tsioufis C, Aboyans V, Desormais I, Authors/Task Force M. 2018 ESC/ESH guidelines for the management of arterial hypertension: the task force for the management of arterial hypertension of the European Society of Cardiology and the European Society of Hypertension: the task force for the management of arterial hypertension of the European Society of Cardiology and the European Society of Hypertension. J Hypertens 2018;36:1953—2041.

[105] Katznelson L, Laws Jr ER, Melmed S, Molitch ME, Murad MH, Utz A, Wass JA, Endocrine S. Acromegaly: an endocrine society clinical practice guideline. J Clin Endocrinol Metab 2014;99:3933—51.

[106] Rosario PW, Calsolari MR. Screening for acromegaly in adult patients not reporting enlargement of the extremities, but with arterial hypertension associated with another comorbidity of the disease. Arq Bras Endocrinol Metabol 2014;58:807—11.

[107] Schilbach K, Gar C, Lechner A, Nicolay SS, Schwerdt L, Haenelt M, Dal J, Jorgensen JL, Stormann S, Schopohl J, Bidlingmaier M. Determinants of the growth hormone nadir during oral glucose tolerance test in adults. Eur J Endocrinol 2019;181:55—67.

[108] Reid TJ, Post KD, Bruce JN, Nabi Kanibir M, Reyes-Vidal CM, Freda PU. Features at diagnosis of 324 patients with acromegaly did not change from 1981 to 2006: acromegaly remains under-recognized and under-diagnosed. Clin Endocrinol (Oxf) 2010;72:203—8.

[109] Kreitschmann-Andermahr I, Siegel S, Kleist B, Kohlmann J, Starz D, Buslei R, Koltowska-Haggstrom M, Strasburger CJ, Buchfelder M. Diagnosis and management of acromegaly: the patient's perspective. Pituitary 2016;19:268—76.

[110] Giustina A, Barkan A, Beckers A, Biermasz N, Biller BMK, Boguszewski C, Bolanowski M, Bonert V, Bronstein MD, Casanueva FF, Clemmons D, Colao A, Ferone D, Fleseriu M, Frara S, Gadelha MR, Ghigo E, Gurnell M, Heaney AP, Ho K, Ioachimescu A, Katznelson L, Kelestimur F, Kopchick J, Krsek M, Lamberts S, Losa M, Luger A, Maffei P, Marazuela M, Mazziotti G, Mercado M, Mortini P, Neggers S, Pereira AM, Petersenn S, Puig-Domingo M, Salvatori R, Shimon I, Strasburger C, Tsagarakis S, van der Lely AJ, Wass J, Zatelli MC, Melmed S. A consensus on the diagnosis and treatment of acromegaly comorbidities: an update. J Clin Endocrinol Metab 2020;105:e937—46.

[111] Minniti G, Moroni C, Jaffrain-Rea ML, Esposito V, Santoro A, Affricano C, Cantore G, Tamburrano G, Cassone R. Marked improvement in cardiovascular function after successful transsphenoidal surgery in acromegalic patients. Clin Endocrinol (Oxf) 2001;55:307—13.

[112] Heidarpour M, Shafie D, Aminorroaya A, Sarrafzadegan N, Farajzadegan Z, Nouri R, Najimi A, Dimopolou C, Stalla G. Effects of somatostatin analog treatment on cardiovascular parameters in patients with acromegaly: a systematic review. J Res Med Sci 2019;24:29.

[113] Colao A, Pivonello R, Galderisi M, Cappabianca P, Auriemma RS, Galdiero M, Cavallo LM, Esposito F, Lombardi G. Impact of treating acromegaly first with surgery or somatostatin analogs on cardiomyopathy. J Clin Endocrinol Metab 2008;93:2639—46.

[114] Briet C, Ilie MD, Kuhn E, Maione L, Brailly-Tabard S, Salenave S, Cariou B, Chanson P. Changes in metabolic parameters and cardiovascular risk factors after therapeutic control of acromegaly vary with the treatment modality. Data from the Bicetre cohort, and review of the literature. Endocrine 2019;63:348—60.

[115] Jaffrain-Rea ML, Minniti G, Moroni C, Esposito V, Ferretti E, Santoro A, Infusino T, Tamburrano G, Cantore G, Cassone R. Impact of successful transsphenoidal surgery on cardiovascular risk factors in acromegaly. Eur J Endocrinol 2003;148:193—201.

[116] Kamenicky P, Maione L, Chanson P. Cardiovascular complications of acromegaly. Ann Endocrinol (Paris) 2021;82:206—9.

[117] Cuneo RC, Salomon F, McGauley GA, Sonksen PH. The growth hormone deficiency syndrome in adults. Clin Endocrinol (Oxf) 1992;37:387—97.

[118] Gazzaruso C, Gola M, Karamouzis I, Giubbini R, Giustina A. Cardiovascular risk in adult patients with growth hormone (GH) deficiency and following substitution with GH–an update. J Clin Endocrinol Metab 2014;99:18−29.

[119] Feldt-Rasmussen U, Klose M. Adult growth hormone deficiency clinical management. In: Feingold KR, Anawalt B, Boyce A, Chrousos G, de Herder WW, Dhatariya K, Dungan K, Hershman JM, Hofland J, Kalra S, Kaltsas G, Koch C, Kopp P, Korbonits M, Kovacs CS, Kuohung W, Laferrere B, Levy M, McGee EA, McLachlan R, Morley JE, New M, Purnell J, Sahay R, Singer F, Sperling MA, Stratakis CA, Trence DL, Wilson DP, editors. Endotext. South Dartmouth (MA): MDText.com, Inc.; 2017.

[120] Stochholm K, Gravholt CH, Laursen T, Jorgensen JO, Laurberg P, Andersen M, Kristensen LO, Feldt-Rasmussen U, Christiansen JS, Frydenberg M, Green A. Incidence of GH deficiency - a nationwide study. Eur J Endocrinol 2006;155:61−71.

[121] Rosen T, Eden S, Larson G, Wilhelmsen L, Bengtsson BA. Cardiovascular risk factors in adult patients with growth hormone deficiency. Acta Endocrinol (Copenh) 1993;129:195−200.

[122] van der Klaauw AA, Biermasz NR, Feskens EJ, Bos MB, Smit JW, Roelfsema F, Corssmit EP, Pijl H, Romijn JA, Pereira AM. The prevalence of the metabolic syndrome is increased in patients with GH deficiency, irrespective of long-term substitution with recombinant human GH. Eur J Endocrinol 2007;156:455−62.

[123] Scarano E, Riccio E, Somma T, Arianna R, Romano F, Di Benedetto E, de Alteriis G, Colao A, Di Somma C. Impact of long-term growth hormone replacement therapy on metabolic and cardiovascular parameters in adult growth hormone deficiency: comparison between adult and elderly patients. Front Endocrinol (Lausanne) 2021;12:635983.

[124] Sanmarti A, Lucas A, Hawkins F, Webb SM, Ulied A. Observational study in adult hypopituitary patients with untreated growth hormone deficiency (ODA study). Socio-economic impact and health status. Collaborative ODA (Observational GH Deficiency in Adults) Group. Eur J Endocrinol 1999;141:481−9.

[125] Wuster C, Slenczka E, Ziegler R. Increased prevalence of osteoporosis and arteriosclerosis in conventionally substituted anterior pituitary insufficiency: need for additional growth hormone substitution? Klin Wochenschr 1991;69:769−73.

[126] Monson JP, Brooke AM, Akker S. Adult growth hormone deficiency. In: Feingold KR, Anawalt B, Boyce A, Chrousos G, de Herder WW, Dhatariya K, Dungan K, Hershman JM, Hofland J, Kalra S, Kaltsas G, Koch C, Kopp P, Korbonits M, Kovacs CS, Kuohung W, Laferrere B, Levy M, McGee EA, McLachlan R, Morley JE, New M, Purnell J, Sahay R, Singer F, Sperling MA, Stratakis CA, Trence DL, Wilson DP, editors. Endotext. South Dartmouth (MA): MDText.com, Inc.; 2015.

[127] Hoybye C, Burman P, Feldt-Rasmussen U, Hey-Hadavi J, Aydin F, Camacho-Hubner C, Mattsson AF. Change in baseline characteristics over 20 years of adults with growth hormone (GH) deficiency on GH replacement therapy. Eur J Endocrinol 2019;181:629−38.

[128] van Bunderen CC, van den Dries CJ, Heymans MW, Franken AA, Koppeschaar HP, van der Lely AJ, Drent ML. Effect of long-term GH replacement therapy on cardiovascular outcomes in isolated GH deficiency compared with multiple pituitary hormone deficiencies: a sub-analysis from the Dutch National Registry of Growth Hormone Treatment in Adults. Eur J Endocrinol 2014;171:151−60.

[129] Abs R, Mattsson AF, Bengtsson BA, Feldt-Rasmussen U, Goth MI, Koltowska-Haggstrom M, Monson JP, Verhelst J, Wilton P, Group KS. Isolated growth hormone (GH) deficiency in adult patients: baseline clinical characteristics and responses to GH replacement in comparison with hypopituitary patients. A sub-analysis of the KIMS database. Growth Hormone IGF Res 2005;15:349−59.

[130] Gaillard RC, Mattsson AF, Akerblad AC, Bengtsson BA, Cara J, Feldt-Rasmussen U, Koltowska-Haggstrom M, Monson JP, Saller B, Wilton P, Abs R. Overall and cause-specific mortality in GH-deficient adults on GH replacement. Eur J Endocrinol 2012;166:1069−77.

[131] Verhelst J, Kendall-Taylor P, Erfurth EM, Price DA, Geffner M, Koltowska-Haggstrom M, Jonsson PJ, Wilton P, Abs R. Baseline characteristics and response to 2 years of growth hormone (GH) replacement of hypopituitary patients with GH deficiency due to adult-onset craniopharyngioma in comparison with patients with nonfunctioning pituitary adenoma: data from KIMS (Pfizer International Metabolic Database). J Clin Endocrinol Metab 2005;90:4636−43.

[132] Tritos NA, Johannsson G, Korbonits M, Miller KK, Feldt-Rasmussen U, Yuen KC, King D, Mattsson AF, Jonsson PJ, Koltowska-Haggstrom M, Klibanski A, Biller BM. Effects of long-term growth hormone replacement in adults with growth hormone deficiency following cure of acromegaly: a KIMS analysis. J Clin Endocrinol Metab 2014;99:2018−29.

[133] Feldt-Rasmussen U, Abs R, Bengtsson BA, Bennmarker H, Bramnert M, Hernberg-Stahl E, Monson JP, Westberg B, Wilton P, Wuster C, Group KISBoKS. Growth hormone deficiency and replacement in hypopituitary patients previously treated for acromegaly or Cushing's disease. Eur J Endocrinol 2002;146:67−74.

[134] Abs R, Feldt-Rasmussen U, Mattsson AF, Monson JP, Bengtsson BA, Goth MI, Wilton P, Koltowska-Haggstrom M. Determinants of cardiovascular risk in 2589 hypopituitary GH-deficient adults - a KIMS database analysis. Eur J Endocrinol 2006;155:79−90.

[135] Monson JP, Jonsson P. Aspects of growth hormone (GH) replacement in elderly patients with GH deficiency: data from KIMS. Horm Res 2003;60:112−20.

[136] Assmann G, Schulte H. The Prospective Cardiovascular Munster (PROCAM) study: prevalence of hyperlipidemia in persons with hypertension and/or diabetes mellitus and the relationship to coronary heart disease. Am Heart J 1988;116:1713−24.

[137] Colao A, Di Somma C, Cascella T, Pivonello R, Vitale G, Grasso LF, Lombardi G, Savastano S. Relationships between serum IGF1 levels, blood pressure, and glucose tolerance: an observational, exploratory study in 404 subjects. Eur J Endocrinol 2008;159:389−97.

[138] Towie DHP, Merriam GR. Hypertension in growth hormone excess and deficiency. Endocrine Hypertension. Totowa: Humana Press; 2013. p. 151−79.

[139] Sverrisdottir YB, Elam M, Herlitz H, Bengtsson BA, Johannsson G. Intense sympathetic nerve activity in adults with hypopituitarism and untreated growth hormone deficiency. J Clin Endocrinol Metab 1998;83:1881−5.

[140] Uzunova I, Kirilov G, Zacharieva S, Zlatareva N, Kalinov K. Does vitamin D status correlate with cardiometabolic risk factors in adults with growth hormone deficiency? Horm Metab Res 2017;49:499−506.

[141] Boger RH, Skamira C, Bode-Boger SM, Brabant G, von zur Muhlen A, Frolich JC. Nitric oxide may mediate the hemodynamic effects of recombinant growth hormone in patients with acquired growth hormone deficiency. A double-blind, placebo-controlled study. J Clin Invest 1996;98:2706−13.

[142] Evans LM, Davies JS, Anderson RA, Ellis GR, Jackson SK, Lewis MJ, Frenneaux MP, Rees A, Scanlon MF. The effect of GH replacement therapy on endothelial function and oxidative stress in adult growth hormone deficiency. Eur J Endocrinol 2000;142:254−62.

[143] Capaldo B, Guardasole V, Pardo F, Matarazzo M, Di Rella F, Numis F, Merola B, Longobardi S, Sacca L. Abnormal vascular reactivity in growth hormone deficiency. Circulation 2001;103:520−4.

[144] Smith JC, Evans LM, Wilkinson I, Goodfellow J, Cockcroft JR, Scanlon MF, Davies JS. Effects of GH replacement on endothelial function and large-artery stiffness in GH-deficient adults: a randomized, double-blind, placebo-controlled study. Clin Endocrinol (Oxf) 2002;56:493−501.

[145] Suzuki K, Yanagi K, Shimizu M, Wakamatsu S, Niitani T, Hosonuma S, Sagara M, Aso Y. Effect of growth hormone replacement therapy on plasma diacron-reactive oxygen metabolites and endothelial function in Japanese patients: the GREAT clinical study. Endocr J 2018;65:101−11.

[146] Savanelli MC, Scarano E, Muscogiuri G, Barrea L, Vuolo L, Rubino M, Savastano S, Colao A, Di Somma C. Cardiovascular risk in adult hypopituitaric patients with growth hormone deficiency: is there a role for vitamin D? Endocrine 2016;52:111−9.

[147] Kassi E, Adamopoulos C, Basdra EK, Papavassiliou AG. Role of vitamin D in atherosclerosis. Circulation 2013;128:2517−31.

[148] Forman JP, Williams JS, Fisher ND. Plasma 25-hydroxyvitamin D and regulation of the renin-angiotensin system in humans. Hypertension 2010;55:1283−8.

[149] Rosen CJ, Adams JS, Bikle DD, Black DM, Demay MB, Manson JE, Murad MH, Kovacs CS. The nonskeletal effects of vitamin D: an Endocrine Society scientific statement. Endocr Rev 2012;33:456−92.

[150] Moller J, Fisker S, Rosenfalck AM, Frandsen E, Jorgensen JO, Hilsted J, Christiansen JS. Long-term effects of growth hormone (GH) on body fluid distribution in GH deficient adults: a four months double blind placebo controlled trial. Eur J Endocrinol 1999;140:11−6.

[151] Zhang D, Cheng C, Wang Y, Sun H, Yu S, Xue Y, Liu Y, Li W, Li X. Effect of vitamin D on blood pressure and hypertension in the general population: an update meta-analysis of cohort studies and randomized controlled trials. Prev Chronic Dis 2020;17:E03.

[152] Jorgensen JOL, Juul A. Therapy of endocrine disease: growth hormone replacement therapy in adults: 30 years of personal clinical experience. Eur J Endocrinol 2018;179:R47−56.

[153] Brasil RR, Soares DV, Spina LD, Lobo PM, da Silva EM, Mansur VA, Pinheiro MF, Conceicao FL, Vaisman M. Association of insulin resistance and nocturnal fall of blood pressure in GH-deficient adults during GH replacement. J Endocrinol Invest 2007;30:306−12.

[154] Barreto-Filho JA, Alcantara MR, Salvatori R, Barreto MA, Sousa AC, Bastos V, Souza AH, Pereira RM, Clayton PE, Gill MS, Aguiar-Oliveira MH. Familial isolated growth hormone deficiency is associated with increased systolic blood pressure, central obesity, and dyslipidemia. J Clin Endocrinol Metab 2002;87:2018−23.

[155] Johannsson G, Sunnerhagen KS, Svensson J. Baseline characteristics and the effects of two years of growth hormone replacement therapy in adults with growth hormone deficiency previously treated for Cushing's disease. Clin Endocrinol (Oxf) 2004;60:550−9.

[156] Bulow B, Hagmar L, Eskilsson J, Erfurth EM. Hypopituitary females have a high incidence of cardiovascular morbidity and an increased prevalence of cardiovascular risk factors. J Clin Endocrinol Metab 2000;85:574−84.

[157] Pappachan JM, Raskauskiene D, Kutty VR, Clayton RN. Excess mortality associated with hypopituitarism in adults: a meta-analysis of observational studies. J Clin Endocrinol Metab 2015;100:1405−11.

[158] Colao A, Di Somma C, Cuocolo A, Spinelli L, Acampa W, Spiezia S, Rota F, Savanelli MC, Lombardi G. Does a gender-related effect of growth hormone (GH) replacement exist on cardiovascular risk factors, cardiac morphology, and performance and atherosclerosis? Results of a two-year open, prospective study in young adult men and women with severe GH deficiency. J Clin Endocrinol Metab 2005;90:5146−55.

[159] Attanasio AF, Lamberts SW, Matranga AM, Birkett MA, Bates PC, Valk NK, Hilsted J, Bengtsson BA, Strasburger CJ. Adult growth hormone (GH)-deficient patients demonstrate heterogeneity between childhood onset and adult onset before and during human GH treatment. Adult Growth Hormone Deficiency Study Group. J Clin Endocrinol Metab 1997;82:82−8.

[160] Johannsson G, Albertsson-Wikland K, Bengtsson BA. Discontinuation of growth hormone (GH) treatment: metabolic effects in GH-deficient and GH-sufficient adolescent patients compared with control subjects. Swedish Study Group for Growth Hormone Treatment in Children. J Clin Endocrinol Metab 1999;84:4516−24.

[161] Longobardi S, Cuocolo A, Merola B, Di Rella F, Colao A, Nicolai E, Cardei S, Salvatore M, Lombardi G. Left ventricular function in young adults with childhood and adulthood onset growth hormone deficiency. Clin Endocrinol (Oxf) 1998;48:137−43.

[162] Conceicao FL, de Rooij Mansur VA, Brasil RR, Vaisman M. Ambulatory monitoring of blood pressure in growth hormone-deficient adults. Blood Press Monit 2002;7:89−94.

[163] Ratku B, Sebestyen V, Erdei A, Nagy EV, Szabo Z, Somodi S. Effects of adult growth hormone deficiency and replacement therapy on the cardiometabolic risk profile. Pituitary 2022;25:211−28.

[164] Ahmad AM, Hopkins MT, Weston PJ, Fraser WD, Vora JP. Effects of GH replacement on 24-h ambulatory blood pressure and its circadian rhythm in adult GH deficiency. Clin Endocrinol (Oxf) 2002;56:431−7.

[165] Cittadini A, Cuocolo A, Merola B, Fazio S, Sabatini D, Nicolai E, Colao A, Longobardi S, Lombardi G, Sacca L. Impaired cardiac performance in GH-deficient adults and its improvement after GH replacement. Am J Physiol 1994;267:E219−25.

[166] Thuesen L, Jorgensen JO, Muller JR, Kristensen BO, Skakkebaek NE, Vahl N, Christiansen JS. Short and long-term cardiovascular effects of growth hormone therapy in growth hormone deficient adults. Clin Endocrinol (Oxf) 1994;41:615−20.

[167] Johannsson G, Bengtsson BA, Andersson B, Isgaard J, Caidahl K. Long-term cardiovascular effects of growth hormone treatment in GH-deficient adults. Preliminary data in a small group of patients. Clin Endocrinol (Oxf) 1996;45:305—14.

[168] Barbosa EJ, Glad CA, Nilsson AG, Bosaeus N, Nystrom HF, Svensson PA, Bengtsson BA, Nilsson S, Bosaeus I, Boguszewski CL, Johannsson G. Extracellular water and blood pressure in adults with growth hormone (GH) deficiency: a genotype-phenotype association study. PLoS One 2014;9:e105754.

[169] Merola B, Cittadini A, Colao A, Longobardi S, Fazio S, Sabatini D, Sacca L, Lombardi G. Cardiac structural and functional abnormalities in adult patients with growth hormone deficiency. J Clin Endocrinol Metab 1993;77:1658—61.

[170] Sartorio A, Ferrero S, Conti A, Bragato R, Malfatto G, Leonetti G, Faglia G. Adults with childhood-onset growth hormone deficiency: effects of growth hormone treatment on cardiac structure. J Intern Med 1997;241:515—20.

[171] Thomas JD, Dattani A, Zemrak F, Burchell T, Akker SA, Gurnell M, Grossman AB, Davies LC, Korbonits M. Characterisation of myocardial structure and function in adult-onset growth hormone deficiency using cardiac magnetic resonance. Endocrine 2016;54:778—87.

[172] de Gregorio C, Curto L, Marini F, Ando G, Trio O, Trimarchi F, Coglitore S, Cannavo S. Systemic hypertension counteracts potential benefits of growth hormone replacement therapy on left ventricular remodeling in adults with growth hormone deficiency. J Endocrinol Invest 2013;36:243—8.

[173] Expert Panel on Detection Evaluation and Treatment of High Blood Cholesterol in Adults. Executive summary of the third report of the National Cholesterol Education Program (NCEP) expert Panel on detection, evaluation, and treatment of high blood cholesterol in adults (adult treatment Panel III). JAMA 2001;285:2486—97.

[174] Attanasio AF, Mo D, Erfurth EM, Tan M, Ho KY, Kleinberg D, Zimmermann AG, Chanson P, International Hypopituitary Control Complications Study Advisory B. Prevalence of metabolic syndrome in adult hypopituitary growth hormone (GH)-deficient patients before and after GH replacement. J Clin Endocrinol Metab 2010;95:74—81.

[175] Verhelst J, Mattsson AF, Luger A, Thunander M, Goth MI, Koltowska-Haggstrom M, Abs R. Prevalence and characteristics of the metabolic syndrome in 2479 hypopituitary patients with adult-onset GH deficiency before GH replacement: a KIMS analysis. Eur J Endocrinol 2011;165:881—9.

[176] Carr MC, Brunzell JD. Abdominal obesity and dyslipidemia in the metabolic syndrome: importance of type 2 diabetes and familial combined hyperlipidemia in coronary artery disease risk. J Clin Endocrinol Metab 2004;89:2601—7.

[177] Abdu TA, Neary R, Elhadd TA, Akber M, Clayton RN. Coronary risk in growth hormone deficient hypopituitary adults: increased predicted risk is due largely to lipid profile abnormalities. Clin Endocrinol((Oxf) 2001;55:209—16.

[178] Rosen T, Wilhelmsen L, Bengtsson BA. Altered lipid pattern explains increased cardiovascular mortality in hypopituitary patients with growth hormone deficiency. Clin Endocrinol (Oxf) 1998;48:525—6.

[179] Twickler TB, Cramer MJ, Dallinga-Thie GM, Chapman MJ, Erkelens DW, Koppeschaar HP. Adult-onset growth hormone deficiency: relation of postprandial dyslipidemia to premature atherosclerosis. J Clin Endocrinol Metab 2003;88:2479—88.

[180] Markussis V, Beshyah SA, Fisher C, Sharp P, Nicolaides AN, Johnston DG. Detection of premature atherosclerosis by high-resolution ultrasonography in symptom-free hypopituitary adults. Lancet 1992;340:1188—92.

[181] Colao A, Di Somma C, Spiezia S, Savastano S, Rota F, Savanelli MC, Lombardi G. Growth hormone treatment on atherosclerosis: results of a 5-year open, prospective, controlled study in male patients with severe growth hormone deficiency. J Clin Endocrinol Metab 2008;93:3416—24.

[182] Schneider HJ, Klotsche J, Wittchen HU, Stalla GK, Schopohl J, Kann PH, Kreitschmann-Andermahr I, Wallaschofski H, German Kb, of the Ds. Effects of growth hormone replacement within the KIMS survey on estimated cardiovascular risk and predictors of risk reduction in patients with growth hormone deficiency. Clin Endocrinol (Oxf) 2011;75:825—30.

[183] Maison P, Griffin S, Nicoue-Beglah M, Haddad N, Balkau B, Chanson P, Metaanalysis of Blinded RP-CT. Impact of growth hormone (GH) treatment on cardiovascular risk factors in GH-deficient adults: a metaanalysis of blinded, randomized, placebo-controlled trials. J Clin Endocrinol Metab 2004;89:2192—9.

[184] Molitch ME, Clemmons DR, Malozowski S, Merriam GR, Vance ML, Endocrine S. Evaluation and treatment of adult growth hormone deficiency: an Endocrine Society clinical practice guideline. J Clin Endocrinol Metab 2011;96:1587—609.

[185] Ho KK, GH Deficiency Consensus Workshop Participants. Consensus guidelines for the diagnosis and treatment of adults with GH deficiency II: a statement of the GH Research Society in association with the European Society for Pediatric Endocrinology, Lawson Wilkins Society, European Society of Endocrinology, Japan Endocrine Society, and Endocrine Society of Australia. Eur J Endocrinol 2007;157:695—700.

[186] Johannsson G. Central adiposity as an important confounder in the diagnosis of adult growth hormone deficiency. J Clin Endocrinol Metab 2008;93:4221—3.

[187] Yuen KCJ, Biller BMK, Radovick S, Carmichael JD, Jasim S, Pantalone KM, Hoffman AR. American Association of Clinical Endocrinologists and American College of Endocrinology guidelines for management of growth hormone deficiency in adults and patients transitioning from pediatric to adult care. Endocr Pract 2019;25:1191—232.

[188] Martel-Duguech LM, Jorgensen JOL, Korbonits M, Johannsson G, Webb SM, Amadidou F, Mintziori G, Arosio M, Giavoli C, Badiu C, Boschetti M, Ferone D, Ricci Bitti S, Brue T, Albarel F, Cannavo S, Cotta OR, Carvalho D, Salazar D, Christ E, Debono M, Dusek T, Garcia-Centeno R, Ghigo E, Gasco V, Goth MI, Olah D, Kovacs L, Hoybye C, Kocjan T, Mlekus Kozamernik K, Kuzma M, Payer J, Medic-Stojanoska M, Novak A, Milicevic T, Pekic S, Miljic D, Perez Luis J, Pico AM, Preda V, Raverot G, Borson-Chazot F, Rochira V, Monzani ML, Sandahl K, Tsagarakis S, Mitravela V, Zacharieva S, Zilaitiene B, Verkauskiene R. ESE audit on management of adult growth hormone deficiency in clinical practice. Eur J Endocrinol 2020;184:321—32.

[189] Zhang S, Li Z, Lv Y, Sun L, Xiao X, Gang X, Wang G. Cardiovascular effects of growth hormone (GH) treatment on GH-deficient adults: a meta-analysis update. Pituitary 2020;23:467−75.

[190] Kokshoorn NE, Biermasz NR, Roelfsema F, Smit JW, Pereira AM, Romijn JA. GH replacement therapy in elderly GH-deficient patients: a systematic review. Eur J Endocrinol 2011;164:657−65.

[191] Abdu TA, Elhadd TA, Buch H, Barton D, Neary R, Clayton RN. Recombinant GH replacement in hypopituitary adults improves endothelial cell function and reduces calculated absolute and relative coronary risk. Clin Endocrinol (Oxf) 2004;61:387−93.

[192] Isgaard J, Arcopinto M, Karason K, Cittadini A. GH and the cardiovascular system: an update on a topic at heart. Endocrine 2015;48:25−35.

Chapter 16

Hypertension in thyroid disease and primary hyperparathyroidism

Naomi Szwarcbard[1] and Duncan J. Topliss[1,2]

[1]Department of Endocrinology & Diabetes, Alfred Health, Melbourne, VIC, Australia; [2]Monash University, Melbourne, VIC, Australia

Visit the *Endocrine Hypertension: From Basic Science to Clinical Practice, First Edition* companion web site at: https://www.elsevier.com/books-and-journals/book-companion/9780323961202.

Graphical Abstract

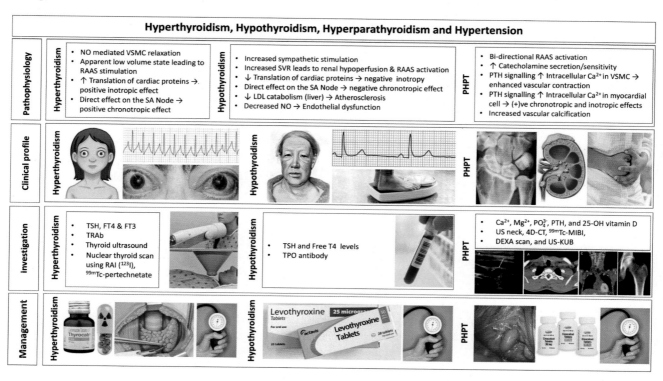

Endocrine Hypertension. https://doi.org/10.1016/B978-0-323-96120-2.00005-4

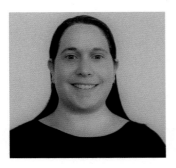

Naomi Szwarcbard

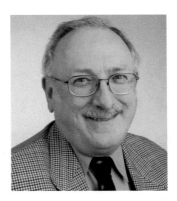

Duncan J. Topliss

Introduction

Although severe hypertension is uncommon among patients with thyroid disease and primary hyperparathyroidism, these endocrinopathies are identified as causes for endocrine hypertension. Free thyroid hormones are positively correlated to elevated blood pressure in subjects with normal thyroid function [1]. The three major determinants of hypertension are cardiac output, peripheral vascular resistance, and renal function. Thyroid hormones play a vital pathophysiological role in the development of hypertension by influencing the above three determinants [2]. Both overt and subclinical stages of thyroid dysfunction—hypothyroidism and hyperthyroidism—can be associated with hypertension [3]. Whereas hyperthyroidism is associated with elevated systolic blood pressure, hypothyroidism is associated with elevated diastolic blood pressure [2]. Primary hyperparathyroidism—both normocalcemic as well as hypercalcemic—is also associated with hypertension, and parathyroidectomy may be associated with improvement in systolic blood pressure and diastolic blood pressure, as well as normalization of biochemical parameters [4,5].

Thyroid disease

Physiology of hypothalamo–pituitary–thyroid axis and cardiovascular system

In response to thyroid stimulating hormone (TSH), the thyroid gland synthesizes, stores, and secretes two biologically active thyroid hormones: thyroxine (T4) and tri-iodothyronine (T3). Once released, 80% of the circulating T3 is derived from peripheral deiodination of T4. Free thyroid hormone levels exert direct negative feedback on the synthesis and secretion of the pituitary TSH, and an indirect negative effect on the synthesis and secretion of thyrotropin-releasing hormone through inhibition at the level of hypothalamus. Iodine is an essential component of the thyroid hormones; four iodine atoms and three iodine atoms are added to thyronines bound to thyroglobulin to create T4 and T3, respectively. Thyroid hormone is essential for the normal functioning of every cell, and in particular it influences protein, carbohydrate and fat metabolism, growth and development, catecholamine sensitivity, gut motility, and the overall basal metabolic rate [3,6]. Following thyroidal secretion, thyroid hormones are transported highly bound (>99%) to serum proteins predominantly thyroxine-binding globulin, albumin, and transthyretin in dynamic equilibrium with the free thyroid hormone fraction. Free thyroid hormone enters the peripheral cells via membrane-bound transporters [7] which do not act as a rate-limiting step in normal physiology. T4 is deiodinated to T3 in many tissues, most actively in the liver and kidney, but also in the skin and muscle. Cardiac myocytes have low intracellular deiodinase activity, and therefore are mostly responsive to circulating T3 levels [3,8]. T3 has higher affinity for the nuclear thyroid hormone receptors which control protein transcription regulation and is therefore more metabolically active than T4 [9,10]. While thyroid hormone activity is essential throughout the body, major sites of action include the brain, skeleton, and cardiovascular system.

Activation of cardiac-specific thyroid hormone receptors control the translation of various cardiac proteins including the sarcoplasmic reticulum calcium adenosine triphosphatase (SERCA or SR Ca^{2+}-ATPase), phospholamban, α-myosin heavy chain (α-MHC), β-myosin heavy chain (β-MHC), β1-adrenoceptors, atrial natriuretic hormone, sodium/potassium-ATPase (Na^+/K^+-ATPase), sodium-calcium exchanger (NCX), and voltage-gated potassium channels [8,11,12]. Excess or reduced thyroid hormone availability can, therefore, result in distinct changes in the production of these cardiac proteins leading to alterations in the numerous cardiovascular parameters they control.

Pathophysiology of hypertension in thyroid dysfunction

Blood pressure is regulated by cardiac output and systemic vascular resistance [13]. In healthy individuals, T3 activity reduces the vascular resistance, increases the cardiac contractility and chronotropy, and also alters the sensitivity to sympathetic stimulation [8,12,14,15]. Therefore, multiple systemic changes seen in hypo- and hyperthyroidism contribute to alterations in blood pressure.

Hyperthyroidism decreases the systemic vascular resistance due to nitric oxide-mediated vascular smooth muscle relaxation [8,16,17]. It also increases the cardiac contractility [8,15,18,19] and heart rate [8,12,18]. Stimulation of increased protein synthesis in cardiac myocytes in response to increased hemodynamic load (from increased contractility and heart rate) can lead to left ventricular hypertrophy, resulting in impaired diastolic filling [8,15,20]. As a result of decreased systemic vascular resistance, there is an apparent low-volume state, stimulating the release of renin and aldosterone. This stimulates sodium reabsorption from the kidney, increasing the blood volume and the resultant cardiac output [8,18,21]. Hyperthyroidism preferentially elevates the systolic blood pressure with a resultant widened pulse pressure [2,8,11,12]. Hyperthyroidism is also associated with pulmonary hypertension. It is postulated that the decreased systemic vascular resistance usually observed in response to excess T3 does not occur in the pulmonary vasculature. In association with a high cardiac output state, this can lead to right heart failure resulting in pulmonary hypertension [8]. The cardiac response to subclinical hyperthyroidism is less uniform. However, prolonged exposure to subclinical thyroid hormone excess can lead to increased heart rate, arrhythmias, and left ventricular hypertrophy, the common cardiac manifestations that can contribute to elevations in blood pressure [3,11,12]. The pathophysiological mechanisms leading to the development of hypertension in hyperthyroidism are depicted in Fig. 16.1.

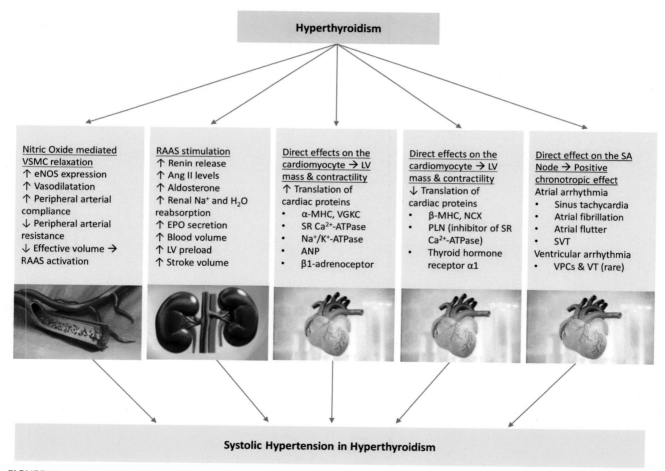

FIGURE 16.1 The pathophysiology of hypertension in hyperthyroidism. *Ang II*, angiotensin II, *ATP*, adinsine triphosphate; Ca^{2+}, calcium ion; *eNOS*, endothelial nitric oxide synthase; *EPO*, erythropoietin; H_2O, water; *LV*, left ventricle; *MHC*, myosin heavy chain; Na^+, sodium; *NCX*, Na^+/Ca^{2+} exchanger; *PLN*, phospholamban; *RAAS*, renin-angiotensin-aldosterone system; *SA*, sinoatrial; *SR*, sarcoplasmic reticulum; *SVT*, supraventricular tachycardia; *VGKC*, voltage gated potassium channel; *VPCs*, ventricular premature contractions; *VSMC*, vascular smooth muscle cell; *VT*, ventricular tachycardia.

Hypothyroidism results in increased systemic vascular resistance due to lowered arterial compliance [8,11,12,17,22], decreased cardiac contractility [12], decreased heart rate, cardiac output, and blood volume [8,11,12,18], and is associated with delayed ventricular diastolic relaxation [15]. In addition to left ventricular diastolic dysfunction, hypothyroidism has also been demonstrated to compromise longitudinal left ventricular systolic function [23]. Hypothyroidism is also associated with increased sympathetic stimulation and elevated catecholamine levels [15,24]. Increased systemic vascular resistance leads to renal hypoperfusion and reduced glomerular hydrostatic pressure. This results in activation of the macula densa and renin—angiotensin—aldosterone system (RAAS) stimulating further vasoconstriction and resulting in decreased total body water excretion [2,15,24]. In addition, a lack of regular antidiuretic hormone (ADH) suppression in the absence of sufficient thyroid hormone also leads to further total body water retention [24,25]. Weight gain associated with hypothyroidism may also contribute to the increased risk of hypertension [24]. Compared with hyperthyroidism, hypothyroidism preferentially increases diastolic blood pressure and results in a narrowed pulse pressure [2,8,11,12]. The evidence for hypertension associated with subclinical hypothyroidism is mixed. However, prolonged exposure to an elevated TSH is associated with elevation of surrogate cardiovascular risk factors, such as increased carotid intima-media thickness, and therefore is also likely to contribute to the cardiovascular alterations and hypertension [3,26].

The pathophysiological mechanisms associated with the development of hypertension in subjects with hypothyroidism are shown in Fig. 16.2.

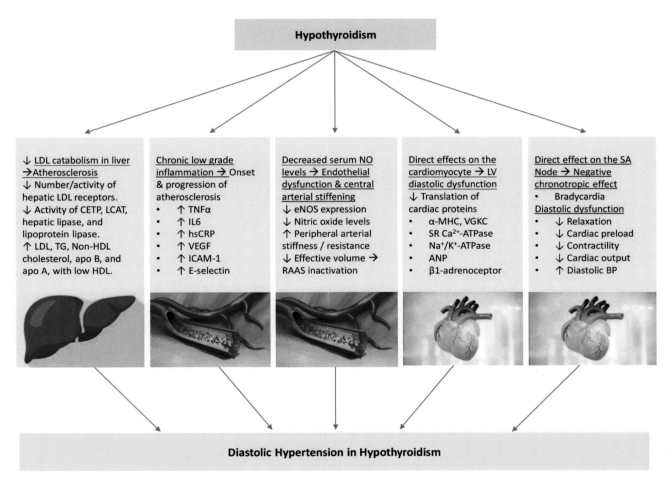

FIGURE 16.2 The pathophysiology of hypertension in hypothyroidism. *ANP*, atrial natriuretic peptide; *apo*, apolipoprotein; *ATP*, adinsine triphosphate; *BP*, blood pressure; *Ca²⁺*, calcium ion; *CTEP*, cholesterol ester transfer protein; *eNOS*, endothelial nitric oxide synthase; *HDL*, high density lipoprotein; *hsCRP*, highly sensitive c-reactive protein; *IL*, interleukin; *K⁺*, potassium; *LCAT*, lecithin-cholesterol acyltransferase; *LDL*, low density lipoprotein; *LV*, left ventricle; MHC, myosin heavy chain; Na+, sodium; NO, nitric oxide; *RAAS*, renin-angiotensin-aldosterone system; *SA*, sinoatrial; *SR*, sarcoplasmic reticulum; *TG*, triglyceride; *TNF*, tumor necrosis factor; *VEGF*, vascular endothelial growth factor; *VGKC*, voltage gated potassium channel.

Subclinical or overt hypothyroidism and associated hypertension

Epidemiology

Overt primary hypothyroidism is defined as an elevated TSH level and a low free T4 level, while subclinical hypothyroidism is defined as an elevated TSH level with a normal range free T4 level [27]. Secondary hypothyroidism will involve a low level of free T4, but with a normal or low level of TSH. The prevalence of overt hypothyroidism in the population ranges from 0.2% to 5.3%. Hypothyroidism preferentially affects women, its prevalence increases with advancing age, and is more common in Caucasian populations [27–31]. The prevalence of subclinical hypothyroidism ranges from 3.4% to 9.0% [28,30]. The prevalence of hypertension in patients with hypothyroidism varies widely with a reported range of 15% −43% [14]. The causes of primary hypothyroidism include chronic autoimmune lymphocytic thyroiditis (Hashimoto's), infectious or infiltrative thyroiditis (e.g., IgG4-associated, amyloidosis, hemochromatosis), iodine deficiency, radioactive iodine (RAI) therapy, thyroidectomy, external beam neck irradiation, and various drugs (e.g., lithium, amiodarone, and immune checkpoint inhibitors, i.e., CTLA4 inhibitors and PD-1 inhibitors). Secondary or central hypothyroidism results from various hypothalamic or pituitary diseases [3,27,31,32].

Clinical features

Symptoms of hypothyroidism are related to the severity and duration of hypothyroidism and include constipation, fatigue, weight gain, cold intolerance, muscle weakness and cramps, exertional dyspnea, changes in the menstrual cycle, cognitive dysfunction, and impaired memory [28]. Clinical features may include goiter, dry skin and hair, periorbital edema, hair loss, macroglossia, and delayed tendon reflex relaxation. Atrioventricular block, sinus bradycardia, prolonged QTc interval with the rare potential for *torsades de pointes,* and pleural and pericardial effusions are all features associated with hypothyroidism [12,15]. Diastolic hypertension is also a common feature. Moreover, hypothyroidism is associated with elevated cholesterol levels, in particular a marked increase in low-density lipoproteins (LDLs) and apolipoprotein B, mainly due to the reduced hepatic LDL clearance. This contributes to accelerated atherosclerosis, and when combined with additional coagulation protein changes, there is a significantly increased risk of coronary artery disease [3,8,12,28]. Excess free water retention can lead to dilutional hyponatremia associated with an elevated ADH level [24]. Severe hypothyroidism can result in myxedema coma, which is identified by decreased conscious state with significant hypothermia, bradycardia, hypoventilation, and hyponatremia. Clinical findings are subtle in subclinical hypothyroidism compared with overt hypothyroidism, with the majority of individuals remaining asymptomatic [12,28].

Investigation and management

Laboratory diagnosis of hypothyroidism requires measurement of serum TSH and T4 levels. Because autoimmune disease is a common cause, serum antibodies directed against thyroid peroxidase (TPO) and thyroglobulin are often elevated [33]. Management of hypothyroidism generally involves thyroid hormone replacement with levothyroxine. In primary hypothyroidism, levothyroxine dosing is adjusted to achieve a TSH level within the normal laboratory reference range which results in resolution of signs and symptoms of hypothyroidism. In secondary hypothyroidism, the dose of levothyroxine should be adjusted to achieve a mid- to high-normal free T4. The use of liothyronine (T3) is not routinely required in the vast majority of patients with hypothyroidism [34,35].

Impact of treatment of hypothyroidism on hypertension and cardiovascular disease

Treatment of hypothyroidism with exogenous levothyroxine administration reduces the systemic vascular resistance [16] as well as the other cardiovascular alterations seen in hypothyroidism [19,36]. Overall, this leads to improvements in blood pressure, and hypertension can abate without the need for additional antihypertensive agents [8,24,37]. The treatment benefit of subclinical hypothyroidism is not as well established, but there is evidence that levothyroxine replacement can improve the blood pressure control, and therefore overall cardiovascular risk reduction [38].

Subclinical or overt hyperthyroidism and associated hypertension

Epidemiology

Overt hyperthyroidism is defined as a low, usually suppressed, TSH level and an elevated T4 and/or T3 level. Subclinical hyperthyroidism is defined as a low TSH level with a normal T4 level, without interference from hypothalamic, pituitary, or nonthyroidal illness [31,39]. The prevalence of overt hyperthyroidism ranges from 0.1% to 0.5% of the population, and this preferentially affects women and non-White populations [28,30,39]. The prevalence of subclinical hyperthyroidism ranges from 0.5% to 2.1% [28,30]. The prevalence of hypertension in hyperthyroid patients is 20%–30%, but can be above 50% in those aged over 60 years [40]. The prevalence of pulmonary hypertension in patients with hyperthyroidism can range from 36% to 65%, though the majority of cases are mild [3]. The common causes of hyperthyroidism are Graves' disease, toxic multinodular goiter (MNG), autonomously functioning toxic nodules, and subacute thyroiditis. Excessive iodine intake or exposure can provoke hyperthyroidism if an underlying thyroid disease is present (e.g., euthyroid MNG). Amiodarone, as a source of excess iodine, can cause hyperthyroidism as in type 1 amiodarone-induced hyperthyroidism but is also a source of organified iodine that can cause thyroiditis as in type 2 amiodarone-induced hyperthyroidism. Excessive thyroid hormone replacement can cause factitious or iatrogenic hyperthyroidism [3,31,39].

Clinical features

Symptoms of hyperthyroidism include weight loss despite normal or increased appetite, fatigue, palpitations, exertional dyspnea, tremor, heat intolerance, muscle weakness, diplopia, anxiety, agitation, poor concentration, disrupted sleep, increased stool frequency, and changes in the menstrual cycle, usually oligomenorrhea [39,41,42]. Clinical features include hyperactivity, fine tremor, warm skin with increased perspiration, hair thinning, proximal myopathy, hyperreflexia, and the eye signs of lid retraction and lid lag. In Graves' disease, autoimmune thyroid eye disease can cause proptosis, conjunctival injection, and ophthalmoplegia, and autoimmune dermopathy usually manifests as pretibial myxedema [39,41,42]. Tachycardia is a common finding with an increased risk of atrial arrhythmias (atrial fibrillation and premature atrial complexes), as well as left ventricular hypertrophy, and heart failure [12,14,15,28,39,42]. Although hyperthyroidism does not adversely affect lipid metabolism, it can still lead to elevated coronary artery disease risk due to endothelial dysfunction [43]. Hyperthyroidism can cause hypercalcemia due to increased bone turnover, leading to decreased bone mineral density, and increased fracture risk [39,41,42]. A rare complication of hyperthyroidism is hypokalemic thyrotoxic periodic paralysis caused by acute potassium shifts into muscle cells due to mutations in the thyroid hormone-regulated potassium channels, most frequently seen in persons of Chinese ethnicity [42].

Investigation and management

Laboratory diagnosis of hyperthyroidism involves measurement of serum TSH, free T4, and free T3 levels. Antibodies against the TSH receptor (TRAb) are a hallmark of Graves' hyperthyroidism. The ratio of serum T3 to T4 may also indicate the underlying etiology of hyperthyroidism; a hyperactive thyroid gland will produce more T3 than T4, while a destructive thyroiditis will release more preformed T4 than T3. Nuclear thyroid imaging, usually with a technetium (^{99m}Tc) scan, can assist in determining the etiology of hyperthyroidism. Diffusely increased (homogenous) uptake is indicative of Graves' disease, focal uptake with suppressed uptake in the remainder of the thyroid indicates a toxic adenoma (autonomously functioning thyroid nodule), a toxic MNG is represented by multiple focal areas of increased and reduced uptake (nodular heterogenous uptake), while diffusely reduced or absent uptake indicates a destructive process such as subacute thyroiditis, postpartum thyroiditis, iodine overload, or factitious hyperthyroidism from exogenous thyroid hormone. Thyroid ultrasonography with color flow Doppler imaging can determine the presence of structural abnormalities as well as changes in thyroid vascularity. Increased vascularity is more consistent with a hyperactive gland (e.g., Graves' hyperthyroidism and type 1 amiodarone-induced hyperthyroidism), while decreased vascularity suggests a destructive thyroiditis (e.g., type 2 amiodarone-induced hyperthyroidism) [39,41].

Management of hyperthyroidism, irrespective of the underlying etiology, involves both acute interventions to render a patient euthyroid, as well as long-term definitive options to prevent further recurrences. Destructive thyroiditis is managed with ongoing monitoring, beta-adrenergic blockade for symptom benefit, and nonsteroidal antiinflammatory drugs, or glucocorticoids if required. Glucocorticoids are often necessary for type 2 amiodarone-induced hyperthyroidism. The thionamide antithyroid drugs (ATDs) are used to reduce the excessive thyroid hormone synthesis and secretion. These are methimazole and carbimazole, or propylthiouracil, which inhibit TPO activity, and thus reduce the iodide organification and thyroid hormone synthesis. Beta-adrenergic blockade, with a preference for nonselective agents, assists acutely with symptom control. High-dose beta-adrenergic blocker therapy can also reduce the peripheral deiodination of T4 to T3. Management of Graves' hyperthyroidism will often involve a prolonged 12–18-month course of ATDs to allow for immunological remission, whereas in toxic MNG, or in toxic adenoma, remission is unlikely, especially in the absence of excess iodine exposure. Hence, definitive (ablative) management with either RAI, or thyroidectomy should be considered after the ATD therapy has resulted in biochemical euthyroidism. Persistent or recurrent Graves' hyperthyroidism is usually treated by ablative therapy. Long-term management with low-dose ATDs may be appropriate in selected cases if ablative therapy is contraindicated. RAI therapy may be used in Graves' disease, toxic MNG, or toxic adenoma to achieve long-term euthyroidism. RAI is a less invasive treatment option, without anesthetic risk when compared with surgery. However, RAI may require more than one dose to achieve euthyroidism and carries a risk of early or late hypothyroidism, requiring surveillance to detect. RAI should be avoided in patients with active Graves' ophthalmopathy and women of child-bearing age planning pregnancy within 6 months. Thyroidectomy may be the preferred option in the setting of women planning pregnancy in less than 6 months, large symptomatic goiters, in thyroids with insufficient uptake for RAI administration, and in the presence of large nodules with increased malignancy risk (e.g., greater than 4 cm diameter). However, it involves an invasive surgical procedure which carries both surgical and anesthetic risk, as well as requirement for life-long levo-thyroxine replacement [39,41].

Impact of treatment of hyperthyroidism on hypertension and cardiovascular disease

Treatment of the underlying hyperthyroidism leads to reversal of the cardiac manifestations that contribute to hypertension and may result in normalization of blood pressure without the requirement for additional antihypertensive treatment [8,14].

When to suspect hypothyroidism and hyperthyroidism in hypertensive subjects?

Endocrine causes of hypertension are important, although thyroid disorders are less prominent than pheochromocytoma, primary aldosteronism, and Cushing's syndrome [3]. However, disorders of thyroid function are relatively common in the general population and very easily treatable. Therefore, clinical assessment for thyroid disease and use of TSH measurement for case finding in hypertensive patients is an easy adjunct, and therefore recommended [24].

Parathyroid disease

Physiology of parathyroid hormone action

The four parathyroid glands in human beings lie posterior to the thyroid gland in the neck. Parathyroid chief cells produce the precursor molecule preproparathyroid hormone (prepro-PTH), which is then degraded to the active 84 amino acid PTH prior to release. PTH regulates calcium and phosphate homeostasis in conjunction with calcium monitoring via the G protein-coupled calcium-sensing receptors (CaSRs). In response to a reduction in serum calcium level, PTH is secreted from the parathyroid glands and acts on the bone and the kidneys to activate the PTH cell surface receptors. PTH increases serum calcium levels via a number of distinct mechanisms. PTH directly stimulates the osteoclastic activity, and inhibits the osteoblastic activity in the skeletal system, resulting in bone breakdown and release of calcium into the blood stream. PTH directly stimulates the increased reabsorption of calcium from the distal convoluted tubules in the kidneys. Phosphate reabsorption is inhibited in the proximal and distal tubules by PTH, leading to a concurrent increase in renal phosphate excretion. PTH also stimulates the release of the active form of vitamin D_3 [$1,25(OH)_2D_3$] from the renal tubules. $1,25(OH)_2D_3$, in turn, stimulates the increased dietary calcium absorption from the intestines via its intracellular nuclear receptor. The increase in serum calcium and increase in $1,25(OH)_2D_3$ levels provide a negative feedback to the parathyroid glands to suppress further PTH production [44].

Pathophysiology of hypertension in primary hyperparathyroidism

The prevalence of hypertension in patients with primary hyperparathyroidism ranges from 40% to 65%, compared with the global prevalence of hypertension in adults of 32% and 34% in women and men, respectively [45−47]. Patients with primary hyperparathyroidism also have concurrently higher rates of metabolic syndrome and its associated disorders including obesity, dyslipidemia, and diabetes mellitus. This may further contribute to the elevated rates of hypertension seen in these patients [46−48]. The increased risk of metabolic syndrome has been demonstrated in patients with hypercalcemic as well as normocalcemic hyperparathyroidism, suggesting a direct relationship with PTH action, rather than the absolute serum calcium level [49]. In fact, hyperparathyroidism associated with moderate or severe elevations in PTH may have a greater impact on calcium and bone metabolism, whereas those associated with mild elevations in PTH presenting with normocalcemia or only mild hypercalcemia are more often associated with an elevated metabolic syndrome prevalence and an increased cardiovascular disease risk [47].

In addition to its actions on calcium homeostasis, PTH works directly on the cells of the cardiovascular system with multifactorial contributions to hypertension, though debate remains regarding the exact underlying mechanisms. Elevated serum calcium levels can lead to increased vascular calcification, driven by either endothelial or intimal dysfunction, with resultant reduced vascular reactivity, and impaired vasodilation [50−52]. PTH also stimulates cyclic adenosine monophosphate (cAMP)-driven Ca^{2+} influx into the vascular smooth muscle cells leading to enhanced vascular contraction, and increased peripheral vascular resistance [51,53], as well as independent markers of increased arterial stiffness [54,55]. Elevated PTH levels have also been associated with elevated secretion and sensitivity to circulating catecholamines, in particular noradrenaline, leading to further vasoconstriction [56,57]. In addition, PTH activates G protein-coupled L-type Ca^{2+} channels in adult cardiac myocytes, leading to increased influx of extracellular Ca^{2+}, and increased cardiac myocyte contractility [51,53]. PTH can also lead to positive chronotropic effects by activation of cAMP and cardiac L-type Ca^{2+} channels leading to an influx of Ca^{2+} intracellularly [51,53]. Finally, PTH can mediate stimulation of protein synthesis and proliferation of cardiac myocytes via activation of protein kinase C, resulting in ventricular hypertrophy [51,53].

Bidirectional relation between renin—angiotensin—aldosterone system and PTH

RAAS contributes to the control of blood pressure via its effects on electrolytes, fluid balance, and systemic vascular resistance. Angiotensinogen is cleaved to angiotensin I (Ang I) by the enzyme renin. Renin is released from the juxtaglomerular cells of the kidney when the afferent arteriole is stimulated by reduced renal arteriolar perfusion pressure resulting from a decreased systemic arterial perfusion (via increased circulating catecholamines). Renin is also stimulated by reduced Na^+ and Cl^- delivery to the macula densa. The Ang I is then cleaved to form angiotensin II (Ang II) by the angiotensin-converting enzyme (ACE). Ang II activates the Ang II type 1 (AT1) receptors, which triggers vasoconstriction of the peripheral arteries and arterioles, increases sympathetic release and catecholamine sensitivity, and increases aldosterone production from the adrenal zona glomerulosa. Aldosterone increases Na^+ resorption from the tubular fluid via epithelial sodium channels in exchange for K^+ and H^+ ion secretion into the filtrate. Water movement follows the Na^+ gradient, leading to fluid retention, and expansion of the plasma volume. These multifactorial mechanisms lead to mineralocorticoid-induced hypertension [44].

Release and activity of PTH and RAAS demonstrate a bidirectional relationship in the elevation of blood pressure. Aldosterone-secreting adenoma cells express type 1 PTH receptors and primary aldosteronism is associated with concurrent elevations in PTH levels that improve following adrenalectomy or RAAS blockade [58,59]. It is thought that the Ang II and aldosterone have a direct stimulatory effect on PTH release via the AT1 receptors that are also found on parathyroid cells [60]. Several studies have also postulated that elevated PTH levels seen in primary aldosteronism are via an indirect mechanism due to RAAS-driven hypertension altering renal Ca^{2+} handling, leading to decreased serum Ca^{2+} with a resultant elevation in PTH level [61]. An additional mechanism is the loss of the diurnal decrease in renin and aldosterone secretion that may be mediated by the hypercalcemia of primary hyperparathyroidism [62].

Parathyroid cells also express mineralocorticoid receptors [63], and an increase in renin secretion can also be seen in cases of primary hyperparathyroidism, which improves following parathyroidectomy [64]. PTH activates cAMP, phospholipase C, and protein kinase-C second messenger signaling, as well as increasing intracellular Ca^{2+} entry via L-type Ca^{2+} channels. Intracellular Ca^{2+} availability is essential for the mitochondrial matrix, a vital step for CYP11B2-driven steroidogenesis, and resultant mineralocorticoid formation [63]. PTH-induced increase in intracellular Ca^{2+} is also thought to directly stimulate aldosterone release [65]. It appears that excess levels of both PTH and aldosterone can activate further release of each other, leading to parallel summative positive effects on blood pressure elevation.

Putative mechanisms in the development of hypertension in patients with primary hyperparathyroidism are shown in Fig. 16.3.

Epidemiology of PHPT

Primary hyperparathyroidism is the most common cause of hypercalcemia. The prevalence of primary hyperparathyroidism is higher in women compared to men, with a ratio of 3—4:1, and the prevalence increases with age. The prevalence varies between countries and races; however, the current prevalence in the general population is ~0.86%. The vast majority of these cases are due to an adenoma in a single parathyroid gland (80%—85%), with a smaller proportion due to disease in multiple parathyroid glands or parathyroid hyperplasia (15%—20%). Multigland parathyroid hyperplasia is more common in patients with Multiple Endocrine Neoplasia 1 (MEN1). Parathyroid carcinoma is a very rare malignant cancer that makes up <1% of all primary hyperparathyroidism cases. It should be considered as a possibility, particularly in younger patients (less than 40 years) with very high calcium and PTH levels. Most cases of primary hyperparathyroidism are sporadic. However, potential contributing environmental factors include ionizing radiation exposure, chronically low dietary calcium, elevated BMI, and chronic lithium therapy. Inherited forms from genetic mutations are responsible for up

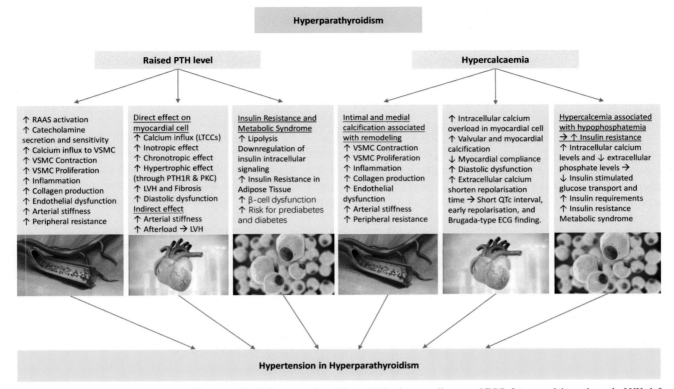

FIGURE 16.3 The pathophysiology of hypertension in hyperparathyroidism. *ECG*, electrocardiogram; *LTCC*, L-type calcium channel; *LVH*, left ventricular hypertrophy; *PKC*, protein kinase C, *PTH1R* , parathyroid hormone 1 receptor; *RAAS*, renin-angiotensin-aldosterone system; *VSMC*, vascular smooth muscle cell.

to 10% of primary hyperparathyroidism and include MEN1 (*MEN1* gene), MEN2A (*RET*), and hyperparathyroidism—jaw tumor syndrome (*CDC73*) [66,67].

Differential diagnoses for hypercalcemia other than primary hyperparathyroidism include malignancy (due to either lytic skeletal lesions or tumor secretion of PTH-related peptide), granulomatous disease (e.g., sarcoidosis, tuberculosis, fungal infections), increasing levels of $1,25(OH)_2D_3$, medications (e.g., thiazide, lithium), familial hypocalciuric hypercalcemia, endocrine conditions (e.g., hyperthyroidism, pheochromocytoma, and hypoadrenalism), exogenous hypervitaminosis D, or prolonged immobilization. Secondary hyperparathyroidism can be due to either chronic kidney disease, 25-OH vitamin D deficiency, low dietary calcium, or medications (e.g., diuretics, denosumab, and bisphosphonates) [66,67].

Clinical features of primary hyperparathyroidism

The clinical features of primary hyperparathyroidism are mainly related to the severity of resultant hypercalcemia, which can range from asymptomatic normocalcemia to severe symptomatic hypercalcemia. Symptoms of hypercalcemia include polyuria, polydipsia, dehydration, constipation, anorexia, vomiting, bone pain, fatigue, confusion, and altered mental state. Low bone mineral density (in particular in the peripheral skeleton, such as the distal third of the radius), fragility fractures, and skeletal deformities result from PTH-driven increased bone turnover. Hypercalcemia can also cause cardiac dysrhythmias, a shortened QT interval, the presence of a J wave, and ventricular arrhythmias. Renal manifestations include renal calculi, nephrocalcinosis, and renal impairment [66,67]. Normocalcemic primary hyperparathyroidism is a more recently recognized entity that is characterized by elevated PTH but persistently normal serum calcium levels. Despite normal calcium levels, a proportion of patients will still eventually develop complications such as reduced bone mineral density, and increased cardiovascular risk factors, and a small proportion will also eventually develop hypercalcemia [49,68].

Investigation and management

Biochemical investigations to establish a diagnosis of primary hyperparathyroidism, and to exclude other causes of hypercalcemia, include measurement of serum calcium (total and/or ionized), serum phosphate, alkaline phosphatase (ALP), PTH, creatinine, 25-OH vitamin D, thyroid function, and serum protein electrophoresis. Primary hyperparathyroidism is characterized by hypercalcemia accompanied by inappropriately normal or elevated PTH levels. Raised 24-hour urinary calcium excretion with an elevated calcium—creatinine ratio differentiates hyperparathyroidism from familial hypocalciuric hypercalcemia. Localization imaging studies include neck ultrasonography, ^{99m}Tc-sestamibi radionuclide scan, and four-dimensional neck CT scanning. Parathyroid tumor localization by two distinct forms of imaging modality enhances operative localization success. Preoperative parathyroid gland fine needle aspirate is not routinely required. Neck magnetic resonance imaging and selective venous sampling should only be considered in cases involving difficult preoperative localization, or after a prior failed neck exploration. Screening for complications of hyperparathyroidism includes bone mineral density via dual-energy X-ray absorptiometry (DEXA) scan, vertebral spine radiography, and abdominal imaging via ultrasound, or CT scan for detection of renal calculi or nephrocalcinosis. Genetic testing should be performed in patients with a positive family history, aged under 40 years, or with multigland disease, to rule out a familial hyperparathyroidism syndrome, such as MEN, or hyperparathyroidism—jaw tumor syndrome [66,67].

Parathyroidectomy is considered to be the only definitive treatment option to manage primary hyperparathyroidism and is therefore the preferred treatment for all symptomatic patients, especially those aged under 60 years. Minimally invasive parathyroidectomy is the preferred approach in patients with single gland involvement on preoperative imaging as it is associated with a smaller incision, faster recovery, and lower rates of complications when compared with bilateral neck exploration. Current consensus guideline indications to consider parathyroidectomy in patients aged over 60 years include elevation of serum calcium by 1 mg/dL (0.25 mmol/L) above the upper limit of normal, evidence of osteoporosis (T-score < −2.5 or fragility fracture), or neurocognitive/psychiatric symptoms of hypercalcemia. Parathyroidectomy is also indicated with evidence of definitive renal involvement, including hypercalciuria (24-hour urine calcium level >400 mg/day or 10 mmol/day), renal impairment (creatinine clearance <60 mL/min), renal calculi, or nephrocalcinosis [66,67]. Consensus discussion from the 2014 Fourth International Workshop on Asymptomatic Primary Hyperparathyroidism concluded that treatment of primary hyperparathyroidism for the benefit of cardiovascular outcomes was not a significant indication for parathyroidectomy [68]. However, more recent guidelines released in 2016 from the American Association of Endocrine Surgeons do consider cardiovascular outcome benefits as a weak indication to consider intervention with parathyroidectomy; however, this excludes isolated hypertension [67].

Medical management is less effective than surgical treatment but may be required in patients unwilling or unable to undergo surgical intervention who have a persistently elevated serum calcium and/or symptoms of hypercalcemia. Treatment with intravenous bisphosphonate, subcutaneous denosumab, or the calcimimetic agent cinacalcet can all be considered. The CaSR agonist cinacalcet can be used alone or in combination with either a bisphosphonate or denosumab to improve the bone mineral density in addition to lowering serum calcium levels [66,67].

Impact of parathyroidectomy in hypertension and cardiovascular disease

Successful parathyroidectomy is accompanied by rapid improvement in biochemistry as well as bone mineral density and a significant reduction in renal calculi risk. Renal impairment and nephrocalcinosis, however, are not reversed post-parathyroidectomy [66,67,69,70]. Improvements in the neurocognitive symptoms of primary hyperparathyroidism have been more difficult to demonstrate. However, some studies have suggested that postparathyroidectomy, patients can have improved cognition, sleep disturbance, and quality of life [71—73]. Findings for cardiovascular benefit post-parathyroidectomy are not consistent. Recent studies have demonstrated improvement in cardiovascular and metabolic factors, including systolic and diastolic blood pressure, following parathyroidectomy [57,74—76]. However, other studies have found no improvement in cardiovascular risk factors post-parathyroidectomy [77].

When to suspect PHPT in hypertensive subjects?

Clearly, if symptoms suggestive of hypercalcemia are present, or if renal impairment, nephrocalcinosis, or a history of renal calculi accompany a diagnosis of hypertension, then primary hyperparathyroidism should be excluded. In a practical sense, all hypertensive patients should have hypercalcemia excluded in the course of evaluation of their hypertension.

Summary and conclusions

Thyroid and parathyroid dysfunction are relatively common endocrine disorders; however, they are rare causes of secondary hypertension. Hyperthyroidism, hypothyroidism, and primary hyperparathyroidism exert pathophysiological effects on the cardiovascular system and can contribute to hypertension through a variety of mechanisms. Assessment of thyroid and parathyroid function is therefore warranted in patients with hypertension, given the simplicity of investigation. Treatment of overt thyroid and parathyroid disease should be undertaken and can potentially reverse hypertension without the need for further antihypertensive therapy. Treatment of subclinical thyroid disease should be considered, but its influence on the treatment of hypertension remains uncertain.

Learning points

- Hyperthyroidism is associated with systolic hypertension and pulmonary hypertension, while hypothyroidism is associated with diastolic hypertension.
- Measurement of serum TSH level is a reliable case-finding tool.
- Treatment of overt hyperthyroidism and hypothyroidism is effective for the improvement of associated hypertension.
- The role of subclinical hyperthyroidism and hypothyroidism in hypertension is less well defined, but cardiovascular benefit may result from treatment.
- Primary hyperparathyroidism contributes to hypertension via intracellular calcium signaling and activation of the renin—angiotensin—aldosterone system, which can be irrespective of serum calcium levels.
- Treatment of overt primary hyperparathyroidism by parathyroidectomy is the standard of care resulting in biochemical improvement and may provide additional cardiovascular benefit.

References

[1] Gu Y, Zheng L, Zhang Q, Liu L, Meng G, Yao Z, et al. Relationship between thyroid function and elevated blood pressure in euthyroid adults. J Clin Hypertens (Greenwich). 2018;20(10):1541—9.

[2] Jankauskas SS, Morelli MB, Gambardella J, Lombardi A, Santulli G. Thyroid hormones regulate both cardiovascular and renal mechanisms underlying hypertension. J Clin Hypertens (Greenwich). 2021;23(2):373—81.

[3] Berta E, Lengyel I, Halmi S, Zrinyi M, Erdei A, Harangi M, et al. Hypertension in thyroid disorders. Front Endocrinol (Lausanne) 2019;10:482.

[4] Fisher SB, Perrier ND. Primary hyperparathyroidism and hypertension. Gland Surg 2020;9(1):142—9.

[5] Nelson JA, Alsayed M, Milas M. The role of parathyroidectomy in treating hypertension and other cardiac manifestations of primary hyperparathyroidism. Gland Surg 2020;9(1):136—41.

[6] Shoback DGD. Greenspan's basic & clinical endocrinology. 8th ed. McGraw Hill; 2007.

[7] Hennemann G, Docter R, Friesema EC, de Jong M, Krenning EP, Visser TJ. Plasma membrane transport of thyroid hormones and its role in thyroid hormone metabolism and bioavailability. Endocr Rev 2001;22(4):451—76.

[8] Klein I, Danzi S. Thyroid disease and the heart. Circulation 2007;116(15):1725—35.

[9] Giammanco M, Di Liegro CM, Schiera G, Di Liegro I. Genomic and non-genomic mechanisms of action of thyroid hormones and their catabolite 3,5-diiodo-L-thyronine in mammals. Int J Mol Sci 2020;21(11):4140.

[10] Anyetei-Anum CS, Roggero VR, Allison LA. Thyroid hormone receptor localization in target tissues. J Endocrinol 2018;237(1):R19—r34.

[11] Kahaly GJ, Dillmann WH. Thyroid hormone action in the heart. Endocr Rev 2005;26(5):704—28.

[12] Klein I, Ojamaa K. Thyroid hormone and the cardiovascular system. N Engl J Med 2001;344(7):501—9.

[13] Klabunde RE. Cardiovascular physiology concepts. 2nd ed., xi. Philadelphia, PA: Lippincott Williams & Wilkins/Wolters Kluwer; 2012. 243 p.

[14] Danzi S, Klein I. Thyroid hormone and blood pressure regulation. Curr Hypertens Rep 2003;5(6):513—20.

[15] Polikar R, Burger AG, Scherrer U, Nicod P. The thyroid and the heart. Circulation 1993;87(5):1435—41.

[16] Ojamaa K, Klemperer JD, Klein I. Acute effects of thyroid hormone on vascular smooth muscle. Thyroid 1996;6(5):505—12.

[17] Park KW, Dai HB, Ojamaa K, Lowenstein E, Klein I, Sellke FW. The direct vasomotor effect of thyroid hormones on rat skeletal muscle resistance arteries. Anesth Analg 1997;85(4):734—8.

[18] KIO I. Thyroid hormone and blood pressure regulation. In: Hypertension: pathophyisology, diagnosis and management. New York: Raven Press; 1995.

[19] Klein I. Thyroid hormone and the cardiovascular system. Am J Med 1990;88(6):631—7.

[20] Biondi B, Palmieri EA, Lombardi G, Fazio S. Effects of thyroid hormone on cardiac function: the relative importance of heart rate, loading conditions, and myocardial contractility in the regulation of cardiac performance in human hyperthyroidism. J Clin Endocrinol Metab 2002;87(3):968—74.

[21] Resnick LM, Laragh JH. PLasma renin activity in syndromes of thyroid hormone excess and deficiency. Life Sci 1982;30(7—8):585—6.

[22] Obuobie K, Smith J, Evans LM, John R, Davies JS, Lazarus JH. Increased central arterial stiffness in hypothyroidism. J Clin Endocrinol Metab 2002;87(10):4662—6.

[23] Tafarshiku R, Henein MY, Berisha-Muharremi V, Bytyci I, Ibrahimi P, Poniku A, et al. Left ventricular diastolic and systolic functions in patients with hypothyroidism. Medicina (Kaunas). 2020;56(10):524.

[24] Fletcher AK, Weetman AP. Hypertension and hypothyroidism. J Hum Hypertens 1998;12(2):79—82.

[25] Hanna FW, Scanlon MF. Hyponatraemia, hypothyroidism, and role of arginine-vasopressin. Lancet 1997;350(9080):755—6.

[26] Kwon Y, Kim HJ, Park S, Park Y-G, Cho K-H. Body mass index-related mortality in patients with type 2 diabetes and heterogeneity in obesity paradox studies: a dose-response meta-analysis. PLoS One 2017;12(1):e0168247—.

[27] Okosieme O, Gilbert J, Abraham P, Boelaert K, Dayan C, Gurnell M, et al. Management of primary hypothyroidism: statement by the British Thyroid Association Executive Committee. Clin Endocrinol (Oxf). 2016;84(6):799—808.

[28] Canaris GJ, Manowitz NR, Mayor G, Ridgway EC. The Colorado thyroid disease prevalence study. Arch Intern Med 2000;160(4):526—34.

[29] Taylor PN, Albrecht D, Scholz A, Gutierrez-Buey G, Lazarus JH, Dayan CM, et al. Global epidemiology of hyperthyroidism and hypothyroidism. Nat Rev Endocrinol 2018;14(5):301—16.

[30] Aoki Y, Belin RM, Clickner R, Jeffries R, Phillips L, Mahaffey KR. Serum TSH and total T4 in the United States population and their association with participant characteristics: National Health and Nutrition Examination Survey (NHANES 1999—2002). Thyroid 2007;17(12):1211—23.

[31] Vanderpump MP. The epidemiology of thyroid disease. Br Med Bull 2011;99:39—51.

[32] Zimmermann MB, Boelaert K. Iodine deficiency and thyroid disorders. Lancet Diabetes Endocrinol 2015;3(4):286—95.

[33] Mariotti S, Caturegli P, Piccolo P, Barbesino G, Pinchera A. Antithyroid peroxidase autoantibodies in thyroid diseases. J Clin Endocrinol Metab 1990;71(3):661—9.

[34] Jonklaas J, Bianco AC, Bauer AJ, Burman KD, Cappola AR, Celi FS, et al. Guidelines for the treatment of hypothyroidism: prepared by the American Thyroid Association task force on thyroid hormone replacement. Thyroid 2014;24(12):1670—751.

[35] Wiersinga WM, Duntas L, Fadeyev V, Nygaard B, Vanderpump MPJ. 2012 ETA guidelines: the use of L-T4 + L-T3 in the treatment of hypothyroidism. Eur Thyroid J 2012;1(2):55—71.

[36] Crowley WF, Ridgway EC, Bough EW, Francis GS, Daniels GH, Kourides IA, et al. Noninvasive evaluation of cardiac function in hypothyroidism. N Engl J Med 1977;296(1):1—6.

[37] Saito I, Saruta T. Hypertension in thyroid disorders. Endocrinol Metab Clin North Am 1994;23(2):379—86.

[38] He W, Li S, Zhang JA, Zhang J, Mu K, Li XM. Effect of levothyroxine on blood pressure in patients with subclinical hypothyroidism: a systematic review and meta-analysis. Front Endocrinol (Lausanne) 2018;9:454.

[39] RossDouglas S, BurchHenry B, CooperDavid S, Carol G, Luiza M, RivkeesScott A, et al. 2016 American Thyroid Association guidelines for diagnosis and management of hyperthyroidism and other causes of thyrotoxicosis. Thyroid 2016;26(10):1343—421.

[40] Prisant LM, Gujral JS, Mulloy AL. Hyperthyroidism: a secondary cause of isolated systolic hypertension. J Clin Hypertens (Greenwich, Conn) 2006;8(8):596—9.

[41] Kahaly GJ, Bartalena L, Hegedus L, Leenhardt L, Poppe K, Pearce SH. 2018 European Thyroid Association guideline for the management of Graves' hyperthyroidism. Eur Thyroid J 2018;7(4):167—86.

[42] De Leo S, Lee SY, Braverman LE. Hyperthyroidism. Lancet 2016;388(10047):906—18.

[43] Coban E, Aydemir M, Yazicioglu G, Ozdogan M. Endothelial dysfunction in subjects with subclinical hyperthyroidism. J Endocrinol Invest 2006;29(3):197—200.

[44] Kronenberg H, Williams RH. Williams textbook of endocrinology. 11th ed., xix. Philadelphia: Saunders/Elsevier; 2008. 1911 p. p.

[45] Zhou B, Carrillo-Larco RM, Danaei G, Riley LM, Paciorek CJ, Stevens GA, et al. Worldwide trends in hypertension prevalence and progress in treatment and control from 1990 to 2019: a pooled analysis of 1201 population-representative studies with 104 million participants. Lancet 2021;398(10304):957—80.

[46] Pepe J, Cipriani C, Sonato C, Raimo O, Biamonte F, Minisola S. Cardiovascular manifestations of primary hyperparathyroidism: a narrative review. Eur J Endocrinol 2017;177(6):R297—308.

[47] Han D, Trooskin S, Wang X. Prevalence of cardiovascular risk factors in male and female patients with primary hyperparathyroidism. J Endocrinol Invest 2012;35(6):548—52.

[48] Snijder MB, Lips P, Seidell JC, Visser M, Deeg DJ, Dekker JM, et al. Vitamin D status and parathyroid hormone levels in relation to blood pressure: a population-based study in older men and women. J Intern Med 2007;261(6):558—65.

[49] Yener Ozturk F, Erol S, Canat MM, Karatas S, Kuzu I, Dogan Cakir S, et al. Patients with normocalcemic primary hyperparathyroidism may have similar metabolic profile as hypercalcemic patients. Endocr J 2016;63(2):111—8.

[50] Garcia de la Torre N, Wass JAH, Turner HE. Parathyroid adenomas and cardiovascular risk. Endocr Relat Cancer 2003;10(2):309—22.

[51] Fitzpatrick LA, Bilezikian JP, Silverberg SJ. Parathyroid hormone and the cardiovascular system. Curr Osteoporos Rep 2008;6(2):77—83.

[52] Tuna MM, Dogan BA, Arduc A, Imga NN, Tutuncu Y, Berker D, et al. Impaired endothelial function in patients with mild primary hyperparathyroidism improves after parathyroidectomy. Clin Endocrinol (Oxf). 2015;83(6):951—6.

[53] Schlüter KD, Piper HM. Cardiovascular actions of parathyroid hormone and parathyroid hormone-related peptide. Cardiovasc Res 1998;37(1):34—41.

[54] Rubin MR, Maurer MS, McMahon DJ, Bilezikian JP, Silverberg SJ. Arterial stiffness in mild primary hyperparathyroidism. J Clin Endocrinol Metab 2005;90(6):3326—30.

[55] Oinonen L, Tikkakoski A, Koskela J, Eräranta A, Kähönen M, Niemelä O, et al. Parathyroid hormone may play a role in the pathophysiology of primary hypertension. Endocr Connect 2021;10(1):54—65.

[56] Schiffl H, Sitter T, Lang SM. Noradrenergic blood pressure dysregulation and cytosolic calcium in primary hyperparathyroidism. Kidney Blood Press Res 1997;20(5):290−6.

[57] Schiffl H, Lang SM. Hypertension secondary to PHPT: cause or coincidence? Int J Endocrinol 2011;2011:974647.

[58] Maniero C, Fassina A, Seccia TM, Toniato A, Iacobone M, Plebani M, et al. Mild hyperparathyroidism: a novel surgically correctable feature of primary aldosteronism. J Hypertens 2012;30(2):390−5.

[59] Brown J, de Boer IH, Robinson-Cohen C, Siscovick DS, Kestenbaum B, Allison M, et al. Aldosterone, parathyroid hormone, and the use of renin-angiotensin-aldosterone system inhibitors: the multi-ethnic study of atherosclerosis. J Clin Endocrinol Metab 2015;100(2):490−9.

[60] Brown JM, Williams JS, Luther JM, Garg R, Garza AE, Pojoga LH, et al. Human interventions to characterize novel relationships between the renin-angiotensin-aldosterone system and parathyroid hormone. Hypertension 2014;63(2):273−80.

[61] Zheng MH, Li FX, Xu F, Lin X, Wang Y, Xu QS, et al. The interplay between the renin-angiotensin-aldosterone system and parathyroid hormone. Front Endocrinol (Lausanne). 2020;11:539.

[62] Porter L, Conlin PR, Scott J, Brown EM, El-Hajj Fuleihan G. Calcium modulation of the renin-aldosterone axis. J Endocrinol Invest 1999;22(2):115−21.

[63] Seccia TM, Caroccia B, Gomez-Sanchez EP, Gomez-Sanchez CE, Rossi GP. The biology of normal zona glomerulosa and aldosterone-producing adenoma: pathological implications. Endocr Rev 2018;39(6):1029−56.

[64] Gennari C, Nami R, Gonnelli S. Hypertension and primary hyperparathyroidism: the role of adrenergic and renin-angiotensin-aldosterone systems. Miner Electrolyte Metab 1995;21(1−3):77−81.

[65] Olgaard K, Lewin E, Bro S, Daugaard H, Egfjord M, Pless V. Enhancement of the stimulatory effect of calcium on aldosterone secretion by parathyroid hormone. Miner Electrolyte Metab 1994;20(5):309−14.

[66] Bilezikian JP. Primary hyperparathyroidism. J Clin Endocrinol Metab 2018;103(11):3993−4004.

[67] Wilhelm SM, Wang TS, Ruan DT, Lee JA, Asa SL, Duh QY, et al. The American Association of Endocrine Surgeons guidelines for definitive management of primary hyperparathyroidism. JAMA Surg 2016;151(10):959−68.

[68] Bilezikian JP, Brandi ML, Eastell R, Silverberg SJ, Udelsman R, Marcocci C, et al. Guidelines for the management of asymptomatic primary hyperparathyroidism: summary statement from the Fourth International Workshop. J Clin Endocrinol Metab 2014;99(10):3561−9.

[69] Mollerup CL, Vestergaard P, Frøkjaer VG, Mosekilde L, Christiansen P, Blichert-Toft M. Risk of renal stone events in primary hyperparathyroidism before and after parathyroid surgery: controlled retrospective follow up study. BMJ 2002;325(7368):807.

[70] Zhu CY, Nguyen DT, Yeh MW. Who benefits from treatment of primary hyperparathyroidism? Surg Clin North Am 2019;99(4):667−79.

[71] Mittendorf EA, Wefel JS, Meyers CA, Doherty D, Shapiro SE, Lee JE, et al. Improvement of sleep disturbance and neurocognitive function after parathyroidectomy in patients with primary hyperparathyroidism. Endocr Pract 2007;13(4):338−44.

[72] Quiros RM, Alef MJ, Wilhelm SM, Djuricin G, Loviscek K, Prinz RA. Health-related quality of life in hyperparathyroidism measurably improves after parathyroidectomy. Surgery 2003;134(4):675−81. discussion 81-3.

[73] Prager G, Kalaschek A, Kaczirek K, Passler C, Scheuba C, Sonneck G, et al. Parathyroidectomy improves concentration and retentiveness in patients with primary hyperparathyroidism. Surgery 2002;132(6):930−5. discussion 5−6.

[74] Heyliger A, Tangpricha V, Weber C, Sharma J. Parathyroidectomy decreases systolic and diastolic blood pressure in hypertensive patients with primary hyperparathyroidism. Surgery 2009;146(6):1042−7.

[75] Luigi P, Chiara FM, Laura Z, Cristiano M, Giuseppina C, Luciano C, et al. Arterial hypertension, metabolic syndrome and subclinical cardiovascular organ damage in patients with asymptomatic primary hyperparathyroidism before and after parathyroidectomy: preliminary results. Int J Endocrinol 2012;2012:408295.

[76] Beysel S, Caliskan M, Kizilgul M, Apaydin M, Kan S, Ozbek M, et al. Parathyroidectomy improves cardiovascular risk factors in normocalcemic and hypercalcemic primary hyperparathyroidism. BMC Cardiovasc Disord 2019;19(1):106.

[77] Bollerslev J, Rosen T, Mollerup CL, Nordenström J, Baranowski M, Franco C, et al. Effect of surgery on cardiovascular risk factors in mild primary hyperparathyroidism. J Clin Endocrinol Metab 2009;94(7):2255−61.

Chapter 17

Obesity, insulin resistance, and obstructive sleep apnea

Dominic Oduro-Donkor[1,2] and Thomas M. Barber[1,2]

[1]Warwickshire Institute for the Study of Diabetes, Endocrinology and Metabolism, University Hospitals Coventry and Warwickshire, Coventry, United Kingdom; [2]Division of Biomedical Sciences, Warwick Medical School, University of Warwick, Coventry, United Kingdom

Visit the *Endocrine Hypertension: From Basic Science to Clinical Practice*, *First Edition* companion web site at: https://www.elsevier.com/books-and-journals/book-companion/9780323961202.

Graphical Abstract

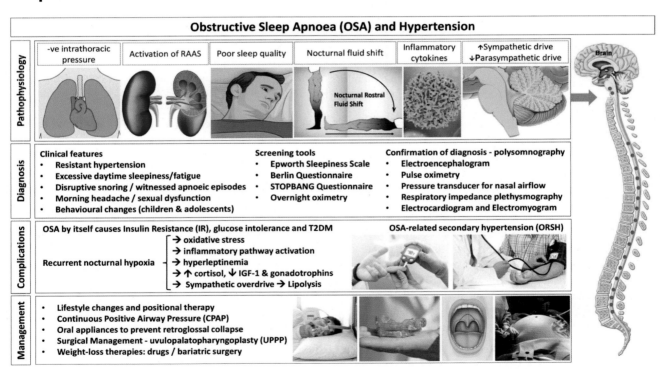

Endocrine Hypertension. https://doi.org/10.1016/B978-0-323-96120-2.00012-1

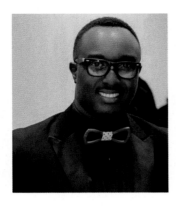

Dominic Oduro-Donkor

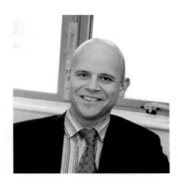

Thomas M. Barber

Introduction

Over the last half century, increasing rates of obesity globally have contributed toward a tsunami of more than 50 obesity-related conditions that collectively represent one of the most important threats to human health and well-being. In the United Kingdom, obesity now affects one in four adults, and overweight/obesity has become the norm, affecting the majority of the adult population, 68% of men and 60% of women [1]. Obesity-related sequelae have a variety of complex and bidirectional etiologies that incorporate biomechanics, oncogenesis, reproductive, and psycho-social functioning. An important subgroup, with the umbrella term, "Metabolic Syndrome," has insulin resistance as a central unifying factor that mediates the pathogenic effects of obesity (particularly visceral adiposity) commensurately on numerous facets of metabolic function. This includes primary hypertension, an important contributor to cardiovascular disease. In the United States, among the adult population, primary hypertension affects 40% with obesity, 25% with overweight, and 15% of normal-weight people [2]. The Framingham Heart Study estimated obesity-related primary hypertension to affect 78% and 65% of men and women, respectively [3]. Furthermore, maintaining a normal body weight appears to be an effective strategy to prevent hypertension, and current evidence suggests that weight loss reduces blood pressure in most people with hypertension [4,5].

The effects of obesity on the development of insulin resistance and primary hypertension become complicated in the context of Obstructive sleep apnea (OSA), another obesity-related condition, and the commonest form of sleep-disordered breathing [6]. In addition to obesity contributing toward the development of OSA, there are also complex bidirectional pathogenic pathways that pertain. Severe OSA is associated with increased cardiovascular morbidity and mortality [7]. OSA itself is also an independent risk factor for the development of insulin resistance. Therefore, in people with obesity who also develop OSA, a metabolic "double-whammy" exists in which obesity-related insulin resistance is intensified by the independent effects of OSA. Insulin resistance-mediated metabolic dysfunction, in turn, tends to have a more severe phenotype in those obese people who also develop OSA. In the case of hypertension, there are additional complexities that implicate recurrent nocturnal sympathetic overdrive and activation of the renin—angiotensin—aldosterone system (RAAS), each of which typifies OSA. Such effects further drive heightened blood pressure and contribute toward the development of OSA-related secondary hypertension (ORSH), which is often resistant to therapies [8—11]. Indeed, up to 70% of people with obesity and OSA manifest ORSH, the prevalence of which increases with the severity of OSA [12].

This chapter outlines the epidemiology, diagnosis, and management strategies for OSA and explores the complex interlinks that underlie obesity-related insulin resistance, OSA and ORSH.

Epidemiology of OSA

OSA is common and affects between 15% and 24% of all adults [13]. However, the true prevalence of OSA is likely to be even greater given that OSA can remain unnoticed, relatively asymptomatic, and therefore underdiagnosed [14]. Furthermore, the prevalence of OSA will likely increase with the growth of global populations with obesity. Rates of OSA vary according to the population studied and key demographics such as age and sex. In one systematic review of the current literature, there was an overall population prevalence of OSA (defined as at least five apneic episodes per hour) between 9% and 38%, with rates skewed toward men [15]. Furthermore, in older populations (more than 60 years of age), the prevalence of OSA was up to 90% and 78% in men and women, respectively [15]. For more severe OSA (defined as at least 15 apneic episodes per hour), there was an overall population prevalence of between 6% and 17%, and up to 49% in those of older age [15]. To conclude, OSA is common among the adult population and remains underdiagnosed. Being male, older age, and the development of obesity are important risk factors.

OSA and obesity

The most important driver of OSA prevalence is global obesity [16]. There is a close association between body weight and the development and severity of OSA, with a 10% increase in body weight elevating sixfold the risk of OSA development. Conversely, in those with OSA, its severity (measured by Apnea Hypopnea Index [AHI]) reduces commensurately with weight loss [17]. The question then is why obesity is such an important risk factor for OSA development, and why body weight appears to predict the severity of OSA.

Essentially, weight gain and obesity (particularly in men) is associated with fat deposition in subcutaneous depots in the neck and around the upper airway [18]. This results in narrowing and enhanced collapsibility of the upper airway (from reduced pharyngeal dilator muscle tone), with an increased propensity for apneic episodes during sleep [19]. To compound the situation, obesity is also associated with excessive truncal fat deposition with reduced respiratory compliance (including expiratory reserve volume, forced vital capacity, forced expiratory volume, and maximum voluntary ventilation) and a corresponding reduction in alveolar—arterial oxygen gradient (even in the context of intubation and mechanical ventilation [20]). Importantly, these obesity-associated impairments of respiratory function worsen in a person lying supine, thereby contributing toward hypoxia during sleep [21]. Therefore, increased neck and truncal body fat in the context of sleeping in a supine position create a perfect storm in which there is increased upper airway collapsibility and impaired respiratory function. This forms the quintessence of OSA, manifesting with repetitive episodes of nocturnal apnea [22,23] driving recurrent hypoxia, hypercapnia, and surges of sympathetic overactivity associated with endothelial dysfunction, and hypercoagulability [24]. On waking, the pharyngeal airway patency is temporarily restored until sleep resumes, and the cycle recurs numerous times each night.

The sex differences in the propensity for OSA with a ratio of about 4:1 in men versus premenopausal women [25] merit further discussion. Crucially, on gaining weight, men tend to deposit fat in central/truncal locations (including abdomen, chest, and neck), differing from the typical deposition of fat in the thighs and buttocks in premenopausal women—the classical apple versus pear patterns of sex-related fat deposition [26]. Furthermore, a longer airway in men, independent of body height, compared to that in women may contribute toward sex differences in upper airway collapsibility [27]. Finally, the male pharyngeal airway, independent of Body Mass Index (BMI) and obesity, appears to be inherently more collapsible than in women due to sex-related anatomical differences, thereby further contributing toward male susceptibility to OSA [28]. The aging process diminishes the elastic recoil, collagen content, and tethering within the upper airway [28]. Other risk factors for OSA include ethnic origin, genetic factors, craniofacial abnormalities, and smoking (the latter due to increased inflammation of the upper airway and reduced airway sensitization affecting the arousal threshold during sleep) [28].

Given the known changes in female body habitus, with a propensity for android fat deposition at the time of menopause, an important question relates to the risk of OSA in older postmenopausal women. Interestingly, the use of hormone replacement therapy (HRT) in postmenopausal women appears to have a protective effect with the risk for OSA similar to that in their premenopausal counterparts. Such effects of HRT may be mediated through the estrogen- and progesterone-related redistribution of fat to a more gynoid habitus [29,30]. Conversely, the absence of HRT usage in postmenopausal women appears to increase the risk of OSA, although the overall risk remains substantially lower than in age- and BMI-matched men [25]. Regardless of menopausal status or HRT usage, obesity remains the overriding risk factor for OSA in both men and women of all ages.

To conclude this section, OSA associates strongly with obesity. Men are particularly susceptible to OSA development due to their propensity to deposit fat centrally and around the neck and to their inherent upper airway collapsibility (stemming from a longer trachea and anatomical differences compared with women). The aging process augments upper airway collapsibility. Other factors like smoking may further increase the risk of developing OSA. It should be noted that the pathogenesis of OSA is complex and remains incompletely understood. Although the biomechanical factors that underlie OSA (as outlined here) are easily understood, there are likely multiple other factors (including some that act centrally) that may contribute towards disturbed sleep in OSA and its association with obesity, which should form a focus for future research.

Diagnosis of OSA

The effective diagnosis of OSA is notoriously challenging and usually requires a proactive approach by the healthcare professional. The person suffering from OSA rarely seeks medical attention themselves, primarily because they may be unaware of their nocturnal experiences. Indeed, the main clinical features of OSA (other than resistant hypertension) include excessive daytime sleepiness and fatigue, which may have been attributed to other factors like stress. Often, it will be the partner of the person with OSA who will alert a healthcare professional to the disruptive snoring and/or witnessed apneic episodes.

The clinical assessment of OSA includes a detailed history and examination; investigations to exclude other conditions such as heart failure; accurate measurements of body weight, height (with calculated BMI), blood pressure, waist circumference, and neck circumference; and assessment for the presence of macroglossia and a crowded oropharynx. Aside from the daytime somnolence, other features of OSA may include morning headaches, sexual dysfunction, and behavioral changes (the latter particularly in children and adolescents). As a measure of daytime sleepiness, various scoring criteria are used, such as Epworth Sleepiness Scale, Berlin Questionnaire, and STOPBANG Questionnaire [31].

The gold standard diagnostic test for OSA is polysomnography, although overnight oximetry can be used as a screener. During polysomnography, patients are monitored with an electroencephalogram (EEG), pulse oximetry, temperature, and pressure sensors for the measurement of nasal airflow (using pressure transducer), respiratory impedance plethysmography with resistance belts around the chest and abdomen to detect motion, electrocardiogram, and electromyogram sensors to detect muscle contraction in the chin, chest, and legs [31]. Polysomnography generates substantial data. Of particular relevance to OSA are data on apnea which is defined as the absence of breathing for ≥ 10 s, and hypopnea which is defined as a decrease in airflow of $\geq 30\%$ for ≥ 10 s, associated with $\geq 3\%$ drop in oxygen saturations and/or detection of sleep arousal on the EEG [32]. Such data are used to form the AHI, which determines the diagnosis and severity of OSA. The AHI simply refers to the mean average number of apneic or hypopnea episodes that occur per hour of sleep [33], with the grading of severity shown in Table 17.1.

Pathophysiology of OSA-related secondary hypertension

Having established the prevalence and the diagnostic criteria for OSA, its association with the obesity, and population-based risk factors, it is important to explore the pathophysiology of ORSH. Our current understanding implicates five separate processes, outlined in Fig. 17.1. These include the following: (i) nocturnal sympathetic overdrive; (ii) chronic inflammation and oxidative stress driven by hypoxia; (iii) nocturnal fluid shifts; (iv) cardiac effects of nocturnal negative intrathoracic pressure; and (v) activation of the RAAS.

Nocturnal sympathetic overdrive

Restful sleep is usually characterized by parasympathetic overdrive, associated with a reduction in sympathetic nervous system output. This scenario occurs particularly during the nonrapid eye movement (NREM) sleep, the duration of which accounts for the greatest proportion of the sleep cycle [17]. This sleep-induced parasympathetic dominance usually ensures that resting heart rate and blood pressure both drop during the entire duration of sleep. Interspersed between NREM sleep is the rapid eye movement (REM) sleep, with cycles of NREM and REM sleep typically occurring multiple times each night (with a cyclical duration of around 90-minutes). REM sleep is characterized by a generalized loss of skeletal muscle tone.

TABLE 17.1 Grading of severity of obstructive sleep apnea (OSA) according to apnea hypopnea index (AHI).

Grading of OSA severity	AHI
Mild OSA	≥ 5 and <15
Moderate OSA	≥ 15 and <30
Severe OSA	≥ 30

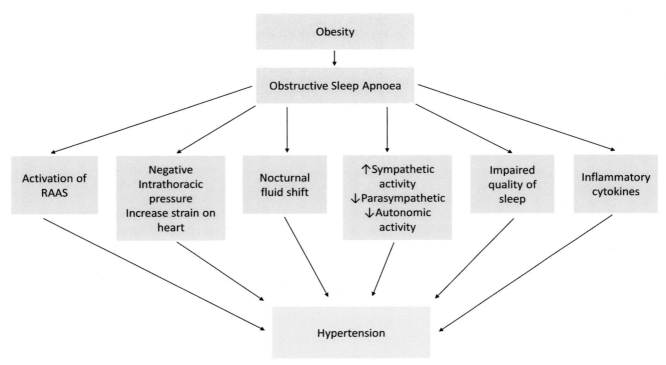

FIGURE 17.1   Overview of the pathophysiology of OSA-related secondary hypertension (ORSH).

In normal physiology and in people without OSA, such loss of muscle tone does not lead to any interference with the airway.

However, in people with OSA, this loss of muscle tone during the REM sleep contributes toward the collapse of the pharyngeal airway with resultant recurrent apneic episodes, hypoxia, hypercapnia, stimulation of carotid body chemoreceptors, and reflex sympathetic overdrive [34]. The OSA-related sympathetic overdrive stimulates the cardiovascular system with increased heart rate and blood pressure, thereby contributing to the development and worsening of hypertension. Therefore, rather than the usual physiological drop of around 10%−15% in blood pressure that occurs during NREM sleep, in people with OSA there is typically a rise in blood pressure during sleep, with spikes in blood pressure correlating with hypoxic episodes [35]. Importantly, in subjects with OSA, the sympathetic overdrive-mediated rise in nocturnal blood pressure that occurs following airway obstruction is sustained due to a surge in serum catecholamines [36]. Over time, this leads to the development of ORSH [13].

Chronic inflammation and oxidative stress driven by hypoxia

In OSA, recurrent nocturnal apnea-associated hypoxia and hypercapnia results in stimulation of inflammatory pathways and enhanced oxidative stress [37]. This includes the release of reactive oxygen species, inflammatory cytokines, and vasoactive substances such as highly sensitive C-reactive protein (hs-CRP), interleukins (IL-1, IL-6, and IL-8), and tumor necrosis factor-α (TNF-α) [38]. This heightened inflammatory response and the oxidative stress worsens the insulin resistance that in turn contributes toward development and worsening of hypertension and increased overall cardiovascular risk [39]. Moreover, the inflammatory response and the oxidative stress are associated with enhanced endothelin-1 and reduced nitric oxide levels resulting in vasoconstriction and endothelial dysfunction [40].

Nocturnal fluid shifts

People with OSA tend to have relative fluid overload compared to those without OSA, resulting from activation of the RAAS and overproduction of aldosterone [41]. During the day, the interstitial fluid usually accumulates in the legs through gravitational effects. During the night, while supine, there is a fluid redistribution from the legs into the rest of the body, including the torso and neck. The fluid that redistributes to the neck during the night can contribute toward the narrowing of the pharyngeal airway, thereby worsening the severity of OSA [42]. In addition, nocturnal fluid redistribution from the interstitium of the legs while supine can increase the intravascular volume load and therefore also contribute toward ORSH. These effects are particularly evident in fluid-retaining conditions like heart failure, in which nocturnal fluid redistribution can also result in venous engorgement and mucosal fluid accumulation within the neck, and further enhancing the tissue pressure around the airway [43,44].

Cardiac effects of nocturnal negative intrathoracic pressure

During apneic episodes in people with OSA, there is an increased inspiratory effort. When this occurs in the context of a blocked upper airway, there is enhanced negative intrathoracic pressure with associated increased venous return and right ventricular preload. The concurrent apnea-induced hypoxia induces pulmonary venous constriction and increased right ventricular afterload [23,45]. Apnea-induced sympathetic overdrive causes a surge in catecholamine release that has further cardiac effects through both inotropic and chronotropic mechanisms. Over time, these effects may lead to left ventricular hypertrophy, impairment in left ventricular diastolic filling, reduced stroke volume, atrial remodeling, and arrhythmias that ultimately increase the risk for the development of heart failure [23]. The cardiac effects of apnea-induced negative intrathoracic pressure outlined here contribute toward the development of ORSH.

Activation of the RAAS

Evidence from the literature, including meta-analyses, reveals a clear association between OSA and its associated apneic episodes with the activation of RAAS, resulting in overproduction of aldosterone. In people with OSA, there are changes in the expression of the angiotensin-converting enzyme (ACE) gene, increasing susceptibility to hypertension via RAAS activation [46]. A meta-analysis showed that people with OSA have elevated serum angiotensin II levels compared to controls, and those with ORSH have increased serum levels of aldosterone [47]. Activation of the RAAS contributes toward the pathogenesis of ORSH through enhanced sodium and water retention, vasoconstriction, and cardiac inotropic effects [47,48]. The overproduction of aldosterone contributes to sarcopenia characterized by decreased skeletal muscle mass and function, leading to upper airway dilator dysfunction and worsening of OSA [49].

The nocturnal hypoxia also results in accelerated loss of kidney function [50] through hypoxia-induced tubulointerstitial injury [51,52]. Furthermore, impairment of renal function appears to increase the risk of OSA, with every 10 mL/min/1.73m^2 reduction in eGFR increasing the odds of developing OSA by around 42%, following adjustment for confounders [53]. Primary aldosteronism also needs to be considered as OSA may coexist with primary aldosteronism in as many as 70%, and serum aldosterone levels may correlate with the severity of OSA [54]. Therefore, it is useful to screen patients with primary aldosteronism for OSA. Although the complex bidirectional links between OSA and renal dysfunction remain incompletely understood, it is likely that the RAAS and blood pressure play important mediating roles.

OSA and insulin resistance

As outlined in the last section, the pathophysiology of ORSH implicates numerous mechanisms that stem from a diverse range of factors that include recurrent nocturnal hypoxia, enhanced negative intrathoracic pressure, and the supine habitus of sleeping. These factors all contribute to the development of ORSH. However, beyond blood pressure effects, OSA also contributes toward metabolic dysfunction more generally through its associated enhancement of insulin resistance as summarized in Fig. 17.2. This includes increased risk for the development of conditions like type 2 diabetes mellitus (T2DM) [55−58] and polycystic ovary syndrome (PCOS) [59−62], and atherosclerotic cardiovascular sequelae like myocardial infarction and stroke.

Although obesity is the main contributor to the development of insulin resistance, it is important to note that OSA worsens insulin resistance independent of any obesity-related effects. It is likely that hypoxia-induced inflammation and oxidative stress mediate this process, with observations of hypoxia-associated increase in fasting insulin levels and homeostasis model assessment of insulin resistance (HOMA-IR) [57]. OSA-related sympathetic overdrive typically increases the levels of circulating free fatty acids and other metabolites like ceramides, diacylglycerol, and acyl-CoA via the stimulation of lipolysis [63]. This process activates the serine kinase cascade that in turn impairs the insulin signaling and glucose transport, thereby further promoting insulin resistance [64].

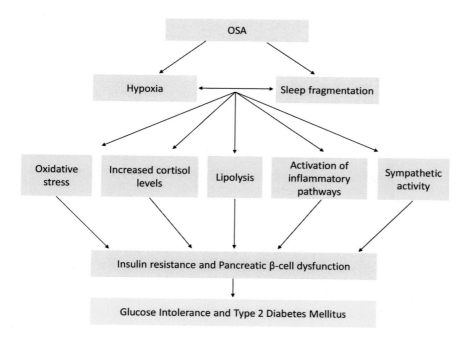

FIGURE 17.2 Mechanisms by which OSA associates with insulin resistance.

Furthermore, leptin may play complex bidirectional pathogenic roles mediating OSA and obesity with insulin resistance [65]. It is known that hyperleptinemia and obesity-related leptin resistance are associated with insulin resistance and metabolic dysfunction [66]. OSA appears to worsen the hyperleptinemia independent of obesity-related effects, possibly through recurrent nocturnal hypoxia [67], with a correlation between serum levels of leptin and the severity of OSA [68]. To further complicate the picture, the severity of OSA and associated insulin resistance can be worsened in the context of diabetic autonomic neuropathy due to the impairment of key respiratory neurons, diminished chemoreception, blunted hypercapnic, and hypoxic ventilatory responses [69,70].

Other than the effects on insulin and leptin levels and on the sympathetic overdrive, recurrent nocturnal hypoxia in OSA also impacts on other endocrine systems, which in turn may contribute toward its association with insulin resistance [71]. Of particular relevance is the elevated serum adrenocorticotrophic hormone (ACTH) and cortisol levels in response to hypoxia-induced activation of the hypothalamic—pituitary—adrenal (HPA) axis [72,73] and its reversal in response to therapy with continuous positive airway pressure (CPAP) [74,75]. In addition to the effects of prolonged elevation of serum cortisol levels on the promotion of insulin resistance, elevated ACTH levels also stimulate the adrenal production of aldosterone that in turn contributes toward the development of ORSH [76].

Coupled with activation of the HPA axis, hypoxia also suppresses the somatotrophin axis, with an inverse correlation between the severity of OSA and serum levels of insulin-like growth factor 1 (IGF-1) [77]. As with hypoxia-related changes in serum cortisol, the changes in serum IGF-1 are also reversed with CPAP therapy [78,79]. Finally, OSA is associated with suppression of the gonadal axis and the development of hypogonadotropic hypogonadism [71]. Suppressed serum levels of both IGF-1 and gonadal hormones contribute toward the development of insulin resistance.

To summarize this section, there are numerous and diverse effects of OSA on the development of insulin resistance. This includes neuronal effects from sympathetic overactivity, hormone effects of leptin and insulin, and changes in the hypothalamic—pituitary regulation of the HPA, somatotrophin, and gonadal axes. These neuro-hormonal aberrations appear to be related to hypoxia. Accordingly, correction of hypoxia with CPAP facilitates improved insulin sensitivity. This is a useful segue to switch our focus from epidemiology, diagnostics, and pathophysiology to the final section of our chapter on management strategies for OSA.

Management of OSA

The effective management of OSA involves the establishment of improved airflow to overcome the airway narrowing and the collapsibility during sleep. Prior to this, it is important to exclude other conditions that may cause upper airway narrowing including hypothyroidism and congestive heart failure that may require separate management. Broadly, the approaches to the management of OSA include conservative management approaches; augmenting the airway patency during sleep using CPAP or oral appliances; permanent anatomical changes to the upper airway through surgery; and weight loss therapies including bariatric surgery.

Conservative management

This includes lifestyle changes to optimize the severity of OSA, such as avoidance of respiratory depressants like alcohol and opioids to limit nocturnal apneic episodes [28]. Furthermore, avoidance of the supine position while sleeping may also help to relieve the gravitational effects on the tongue and the upper airway that is associated with increased risk of occlusion, and the increased effort of breathing while sleeping in a supine position [80]. Such positional therapy for OSA includes encouragement of sleeping in a lateral position. High-resistance inspiratory muscle strength training, a form of physical training, has shown sustained improvements in blood pressure, arterial stiffness, endothelial dysfunction, and cardiovascular health in middle-aged and older adults with raised blood pressure [81,82].

The effective management of ORSH is important. Antihypertensive therapies may be required [34]. Given the association of OSA with activation of the RAAS and sympathetic overactivity, ACE inhibitors, angiotensin receptor blockers, mineralocorticoid receptor blockers (spironolactone, eplerenone, finerenone), and beta blockers have a theoretical advantage over other classes of antihypertensive drugs. The mineralocorticoid receptor blockers may reduce leg to neck fluid redistribution and improve AHI; spironolactone has been shown to reduce blood pressure in patients with OSA-associated resistant hypertension reducing oxygen desaturation index, plasma aldosterone levels, AHI, hypopnea, and both clinical and ambulatory BP in one single center study [83]. Other benefits from mineralocorticoid receptor blockers such as eplerenone include reduced neck circumference, aortic pulse wave velocity, and arterial wall stiffness [84]. Diuretics have also been shown to have a role in the reduction of fluid displacement from the lower extremities to the neck and may have a synergistic effect with combined usage with mineralocorticoid receptor blockers [85].

CPAP

CPAP is the gold standard management strategy for OSA [34], which demonstrated long-term survival benefits [86] and resolution of symptoms through diligent and continuous usage [31], although symptoms of OSA can recur within 1−3 days of interruption of CPAP therapy [22]. CPAP is typically used during sleep and acts as a splint; with the continuous positive pressure, it provides maintenance of airway patency and prevents the collapse of the upper airway, with immediately improved sleep and minimal side effects [87]. The positive pressure required for upper airway patency varies between patients and according to the severity of OSA [22]. In addition to maintaining upper airway patency, CPAP has multiple beneficial effects, including reduction of sympathetic overactivity, blood pressure [88], free radicals, and inflammatory cytokine production [89]. CPAP also increases serum levels of nitric oxide, a potent vasodilator essential for the regulation of vascular tone and inflammatory cascades [90,91], and downregulates the RAAS and renal hemodynamics, thereby contributing toward reduced blood pressure [52] and glomerular pressure [92]. CPAP therapy helps to improve insulin sensitivity and reduces vascular risk in patients with metabolic syndrome [93], including reduced mortality from stroke by up to 8%, and from ischemic heart disease by up to 5% [94,95].

Prior to the introduction of CPAP therapy, it is important to counsel patients regarding the primary purpose of CPAP—to alleviate the symptoms of OSA. Furthermore, educational support should help to improve the adherence to CPAP, particularly in those patients with nasal difficulties. In this subgroup, strategies include the addition of nasal decongestants, heated humidification, and the use of alternative masks after exploring patient preferences (including nasal mask, a full mask, or a nasal pillow device) [28]. Adherence to CPAP therapy is 50%−80%, with relatively few side effects, being mainly mask related (pressure-related discomfort and nasal congestion) [28].

In addition to its longer-term usage in patients with OSA, CPAP therapy can also be used in certain acute scenarios. One example is in the perioperative management of patients with OSA, particularly in relation to the use of anesthesia and/or opioids, in which close monitoring is required due to an increased risk of reduced pharyngeal muscle tone and airway collapse. Since most surgical procedures are performed with the patient in the supine position, this may further aggravate the potential for perioperative apnea [21]. Preoperative assessment should identify those patients who will require postoperative CPAP therapy, to improve ventilation and oxygenation and to reduce the development of respiratory complications such as atelectasis and pneumonia. CPAP therapy may also help in the management of hemodynamic fluctuations that co-occur with airway collapse [96].

Oral appliances

Oral appliances are an alternative to CPAP therapy in people with mild and moderate OSA [97]. A variety of oral devices exist, although the aim of each is to prevent retroglossal collapse by applying pressure to the jaw. One of the main challenges of oral devices is that several dental visits may be required over a period of time for gradual adjustment of the device, and satisfactory outcomes may take up to 9 months to occur [28]. However, when used successfully, oral devices confer beneficial effects on reducing the systolic and diastolic blood pressure, and mean arterial pressure [97].

Surgical management

Surgical management of OSA is usually considered in those who do not adhere to, comply with, or tolerate CPAP therapy [98]. The main surgical approach is uvulopalatopharyngoplasty (UPPP) which is often effective at reducing the AHI [99,100]. Tonsillectomy with UPPP has also been shown to improve symptoms of OSA [101]. It should be noted that any surgical approach to the management of OSA may also require the reintroduction of CPAP therapy as surgery may improve, but not actually eliminate the upper airway collapse due to nonanatomical factors such as pharyngeal muscle tonicity [100,102]. Although the reintroduction of CPAP may seem problematic postsurgery, procedures like modified UPPP reduce retropalatal obstruction, preserving the palate and velopharyngeal sphincter functions, thereby minimizing any potential complications of CPAP therapy [103]. Other surgical approaches to the management of OSA include maxillomandibular advancement where both upper and lower jaws are advanced surgically to increase the space in the oropharynx, though this procedure may be less successful in patients with larger necks [31]. In extreme cases of OSA, treatment with a tracheostomy may be required to bypass the oropharyngeal obstruction [31].

Weight loss therapies

The most effective management strategy for OSA is through effective and sustained weight loss. It is beyond the scope of this chapter to provide a detailed exposition of the management of obesity. In summary, this consists of lifestyle therapies including dietary modification combined with physical activity; pharmacotherapies; and bariatric surgery; often coordinated through a multidisciplinary approach. In addition to a reduction in fat tissue around the neck and therefore improved upper airway patency, effective weight loss will also reduce adiposity around the trunk and chest, therefore reducing the effort of breathing, particularly when supine [21].

Perhaps the most effective long-term strategy for the management of OSA is through bariatric surgery. In one meta-analysis, it was shown that bariatric surgery results in the resolution of OSA in around 85% of patients overall [104]. Of course, morbid obesity with OSA often occurs in the context of multiple other metabolic dysfunctions [104]. In this common scenario, bariatric surgery, through achieving substantial and sustained weight loss, often represents an excellent treatment option for metabolic dysfunction. In addition to the metabolic benefits of weight loss, resolution of OSA will also independently benefit metabolic status due to its independent effects on insulin resistance as outlined earlier. Finally, effective reduction of adiposity from the abdominal region following bariatric surgery reduces pressure on the inferior vena cava, thereby improving the venous return and reducing activation of the RAAS, thereby improving blood pressure and microalbuminuria.

Conclusions

Within the realm of obesity-related conditions, OSA occupies an important position. Its development often goes unnoticed, with nonspecific features of tiredness and fatiguability which may be attributed to other factors such as stress. This highlights the importance of the healthcare professional taking a proactive role in the screening and diagnosis of OSA, and the importance of gaining insight from sleeping partners, regarding witnessed snoring and apneic episodes. In short, as healthcare professionals we need to heighten our suspicions when it comes to OSA given its elusiveness and underdiagnosis, its association with dysmetabolic and cardio-respiratory dysfunction, and the potential benefits from effective treatment. Screening for OSA through questionnaires like Epworth Sleepiness Scale takes very little effort and time and can be repeated easily at annual clinical assessments and well-being checks, especially in those patients at increased risk, including obesity and other dysmetabolic conditions. Those identified to be at high risk of OSA from screening need referral for polysomnography.

OSA contributes toward metabolic dysfunction, including ORSH and insulin resistance through obesity-independent effects, likely implicating hypoxia. This is important given that those with obesity who also develop OSA have a metabolic double-whammy that requires focused effort from healthcare professionals regarding close monitoring for the development of metabolic dysfunction (such as regular measurements of blood pressure, HbA1C, and serum lipid profile), and the early institution of effective management strategies. As outlined, there are numerous factors that mediate links between obesity and OSA with ORSH and insulin resistance that include diverse neuro-endocrine pathways.

Aside from the importance of proactivity in our approach to the screening and diagnosis of OSA, a key learning point from this chapter is that OSA is eminently treatable. Given its association with obesity, it is no surprise to learn that effective and sustained weight loss, especially following bariatric surgery, represents the best management strategy for OSA. However, numerous other treatment strategies are available, including the use of CPAP therapy. Our aims when managing OSA are to improve overall well-being including reduced tiredness and fatiguability, but also to improve future cardiovascular risk, and to optimize cardiac, respiratory, renal, and vascular functionality. A management strategy that includes a focus on successful and sustained weight loss will provide further health benefits that extend well beyond merely treating OSA per se.

Finally, when managing OSA, we should always be mindful that behind every diagnosis there is a person, with the possibility of a partner, a family, job, friends, and inner and outer social groups. The implications of OSA on that person and the people and institutions associated with them should be considered carefully and empathically on an individual basis. Their management should be tailored accordingly. Although the effective management of OSA can be challenging, it is also one of the most satisfying conditions to treat across the whole realm of medicine, with the possibility of literally transforming someone's life (and that of partners and families, etc.). This message of hope should act as our guiding light to motivate us to do what is right for our patients in the timely and effective diagnosis and management of OSA.

Learning points

- OSA is a common obesity-related condition that is likely underdiagnosed.
- OSA associates independently with worsening insulin resistance and is a risk factor for metabolic dysfunction including hypertension through multiple pathophysiological mechanisms implicating nocturnal sympathetic overdrive, inflammation-mediated effects of hypoxia, nocturnal fluid shifts, cardiac effects, and activation of the RAAS.
- Given its strong association with metabolic dysfunction and its eminent treatability, prompt diagnosis of OSA is important through simple questionnaire screening tests and polysomnography.
- Among the multiple management strategies for OSA incorporating conservative and surgical approaches and CPAP, effective and sustained weight loss remains key.

Acknowledgments

We acknowledge the many patients, relatives, nurses, and physicians who contributed to the ascertainment of the various clinical samples reported on in this chapter.

References

[1] 1 England H hH, Health Survey for England, 2 Health Survey for England 2019 [NS]. NHS digital. NHS Digital; 2021. Available from: https://digital.nhs.uk/data-and-information/publications/statistical/health-survey-for-england/2019#.

[2] Landsberg L, Aronne LJ, Beilin LJ, Burke V, Igel LI, Lloyd-Jones D, et al. Obesity-related hypertension: pathogenesis, cardiovascular risk, and treatment—a position paper of the the Obesity Society and the American Society of Hypertension. Obesity 2013;21(1):8—24.

[3] Garrison RJ, Kannel WB, Stokes III J, Castelli WP. Incidence and precursors of hypertension in young adults: the Framingham Offspring Study. Prev Med 1987;16(2):235—51.

[4] Jones DW, Miller ME, Wofford MR, Anderson DC, Cameron ME, Willoughby DL, et al. The effect of weight loss intervention on antihypertensive medication requirements in the Hypertension Optimal Treatment (HOT) study. Am J hypertens 1999;12(12):1175—80.

[5] Stevens VJ, Obarzanek E, Cook NR, Lee I-M, Appel LJ, Smith West D, et al. Long-term weight loss and changes in blood pressure: results of the Trials of Hypertension Prevention, phase II. Ann Intern Med 2001;134(1):1—11.

[6] Malhotra A, White DP. Obstructive sleep apnoea. Lancet 2002;360(9328):237—45.

[7] Benjamin EJ, Muntner P, Alonso A, Bittencourt MS, Callaway CW, Carson AP, et al. Heart disease and stroke statistics—2019 update: a report from the American Heart Association. Circulation 2019;139(10):e56—528.

[8] Marin JM, Agusti A, Villar I, Forner M, Nieto D, Carrizo SJ, et al. Association between treated and untreated obstructive sleep apnea and risk of hypertension. JAMA 2012;307(20):2169—76.

[9] Valaiyapathi B, Calhoun DA. Role of mineralocorticoid receptors in obstructive sleep apnea and metabolic syndrome. Curr Hypertens Rep 2018;20(3):1—6.

[10] Prejbisz A, Kołodziejczyk-Kruk S, Lenders JW, Januszewicz A. Primary aldosteronism and obstructive sleep apnea: is this a bidirectional relationship? Horm Metab Res 2017;49(12):969−76.

[11] Pedrosa RP, Drager LF, Gonzaga CC, Sousa MG, de Paula LK, Amaro AC, et al. Obstructive sleep apnea: the most common secondary cause of hypertension associated with resistant hypertension. Hypertension 2011;58(5):811−7.

[12] Gonçalves SC, Martinez D, Gus M, de Abreu-Silva EO, Bertoluci C, Dutra I, et al. Obstructive sleep apnea and resistant hypertension: a case-control study. Chest 2007;132(6):1858−62.

[13] Patel AR, Patel AR, Singh S, Singh S, Khawaja I. The association of obstructive sleep apnea and hypertension. Cureus 2019;11(6):e4858.

[14] Silverberg DS, Oksenberg A. Are sleep-related breathing disorders important contributing factors to the production of essential hypertension? Curr Hypertens Rep 2001;3(3):209−15.

[15] Senaratna CV, Perret JL, Lodge CJ, Lowe AJ, Campbell BE, Matheson MC, et al. Prevalence of obstructive sleep apnea in the general population: a systematic review. Sleep Med Rev 2017;34:70−81.

[16] Young T, Peppard PE, Gottlieb DJ. Epidemiology of obstructive sleep apnea: a population health perspective. Am J Respir Crit Care Med 2002;165(9):1217−39.

[17] Peppard PE, Young T, Palta M, Dempsey J, Skatrud J. Longitudinal study of moderate weight change and sleep-disordered breathing. JAMA 2000;284(23):3015−21.

[18] Mortimore I, Marshall I, Wraith P, Sellar R, Douglas N. Neck and total body fat deposition in nonobese and obese patients with sleep apnea compared with that in control subjects. Am J Respir Crit Care Med 1998;157(1):280−3.

[19] Schwartz AR, Gold AR, Schubert N, Stryzak A. Effect of weight loss on upper airway collapsibility in obstructive sleep apnea1-3. Am Rev Respir Dis 1991;144(3 pt. 1):494−8.

[20] Pelosi P, Croci M, Ravagnan I, Vicardi P, Gattinoni L. Total respiratory system, lung, and chest wall mechanics in sedated-paralyzed postoperative morbidly obese patients. Chest 1996;109(1):144−51.

[21] De Sousa A, Cercato C, Mancini M, Halpern A. Obesity and obstructive sleep apnea-hypopnea syndrome. Obes Rev 2008;9(4):340−54.

[22] Spicuzza L, Caruso D, Di Maria G. Obstructive sleep apnoea syndrome and its management. Ther Adv Chronic Dis 2015;6(5):273−85.

[23] Bradley TD, Floras JS. Obstructive sleep apnoea and its cardiovascular consequences. Lancet 2009;373(9657):82−93.

[24] Abboud F, Kumar R. Obstructive sleep apnea and insight into mechanisms of sympathetic overactivity. J Clin Invest 2014;124(4):1454−7.

[25] Bixler EO, Vgontzas AN, Lin H-M, Ten Have T, Rein J, Vela-Bueno A, et al. Prevalence of sleep-disordered breathing in women: effects of gender. Am J Respir Crit Care Med 2001;163(3):608−13.

[26] Whittle AT, Marshall I, Mortimore IL, Wraith PK, Sellar RJ, Douglas NJ. Neck soft tissue and fat distribution: comparison between normal men and women by magnetic resonance imaging. Thorax 1999;54(4):323−8.

[27] Malhotra A, Huang Y, Fogel RB, Pillar G, Edwards JK, Kikinis R, et al. The male predisposition to pharyngeal collapse: importance of airway length. Am J Respir Crit Care Med 2002;166(10):1388−95.

[28] Jordan AS, McSharry DG, Malhotra A. Adult obstructive sleep apnoea. Lancet 2014;383(9918):736−47.

[29] Shahar E, Redline S, Young T, Boland LL, Baldwin CM, Nieto FJ, et al. Hormone replacement therapy and sleep-disordered breathing. Am J Respir Crit Care Med 2003;167(9):1186−92.

[30] Gambacciani M, Ciaponi M, Cappagli B, De Simone L, Orlandi R, Genazzani A. Prospective evaluation of body weight and body fat distribution in early postmenopausal women with and without hormonal replacement therapy. Maturitas 2001;39(2):125−32.

[31] Slowik JM, Collen JF. Obstructive sleep apnea. In: StatPearls [Internet]. Treasure Island (FL): StatPearls Publishing; 20222022 Jan.

[32] Berry RB, Budhiraja R, Gottlieb DJ, Gozal D, Iber C, Kapur VK, et al. Rules for scoring respiratory events in sleep: update of the 2007 AASM manual for the scoring of sleep and associated events: deliberations of the sleep apnea definitions task force of the American Academy of Sleep Medicine. J Clin Sleep Med 2012;8(5):597−619.

[33] Pevernagie DA, Gnidovec-Strazisar B, Grote L, Heinzer R, McNicholas WT, Penzel T, et al. On the rise and fall of the apnea− hypopnea index: a historical review and critical appraisal. J Sleep Res 2020;29(4):e13066.

[34] Ahmad M, Makati D, Akbar S. Review of and updates on hypertension in obstructive sleep apnea. Int J Hypertens 2017;2017:1848375.

[35] Staessen J, Bulpitt CJ, O'Brien E, Cox J, Fagard R, Stanton A, et al. The diurnal blood pressure profile: a population study. Am J hypertens 1992;5(6_Pt_1):386−92.

[36] Almeneessier AS, Alshahrani M, Aleissi S, Hammad OS, Olaish AH, BaHammam AS. Comparison between blood pressure during obstructive respiratory events in REM and NREM sleep using pulse transit time. Sci Rep 2020;10(1):1−10.

[37] Konecny T, Kara T, Somers VK. Obstructive sleep apnea and hypertension: an update. Hypertension 2014;63(2):203−9.

[38] McNicholas WT. Obstructive sleep apnea and inflammation. Prog Cardiovasc Dis 2009;51(5):392−9.

[39] Shahar E, Whitney CW, Redline S, Lee ET, Newman AB, Javier Nieto F, et al. Sleep-disordered breathing and cardiovascular disease: cross-sectional results of the Sleep Heart Health Study. Am J Respir Crit Care Med 2001;163(1):19−25.

[40] Atkeson A, Yeh SY, Malhotra A, Jelic S. Endothelial function in obstructive sleep apnea. Prog Cardiovasc Dis 2009;51(5):351−62.

[41] Ding N, Lin W, Zhang X-L, Ding W-X, Gu B, Ni B-Q, et al. Overnight fluid shifts in subjects with and without obstructive sleep apnea. J Thorac Dis 2014;6(12):1736.

[42] White LH, Bradley TD. Role of nocturnal rostral fluid shift in the pathogenesis of obstructive and central sleep apnoea. J Physiol 2013;591(5):1179−93.

[43] Redolfi S, Bradley DT, Tantucci C. Role of overnight caudo-rostral fluid shift in the pathogenesis of sleep apnea. Shortness Breath 2013;2(1):10−8.

[44] Silva BC, Kasai T, Coelho FM, Zatz R, Elias RM. Fluid redistribution in sleep apnea: therapeutic implications in Edematous states. Front Med 2018;4:256.

[45] Stoohs R, Guilleminault C. Cardiovascular changes associated with obstructive sleep apnea syndrome. J Appl Physiol 1992;72(2):583−9.

[46] Boström KB, Hedner J, Melander O, Grote L, Gullberg B, Råstam L, et al. Interaction between the angiotensin-converting enzyme gene insertion/deletion polymorphism and obstructive sleep apnoea as a mechanism for hypertension. J Hypertens 2007;25(4):779−83.

[47] Jin Z-N, Wei Y-X. Meta-analysis of effects of obstructive sleep apnea on the renin-angiotensin-aldosterone system. J Geriatr Cardiol 2016;13(4):333.

[48] Sim JJ, Yan EH, Liu ILA, Rasgon SA, Kalantar-Zadeh K, Calhoun DA, et al. Positive relationship of sleep apnea to hyperaldosteronism in an ethnically diverse population. J Hypertens 2011;29(8):1553−9.

[49] Wang Y, Li CX, Lin YN, Zhang LY, Li SQ, Zhang L, et al. The role of aldosterone in OSA and OSA-related hypertension. Front Endocrinol 2021;12.

[50] Ahmed SB, Ronksley PE, Hemmelgarn BR, Tsai WH, Manns BJ, Tonelli M, et al. Nocturnal hypoxia and loss of kidney function. PLoS One 2011;6(4):e19029.

[51] Nangaku M. Chronic hypoxia and tubulointerstitial injury: a final common pathway to end-stage renal failure. J Am Soc Nephrol 2006;17(1):17−25.

[52] Nicholl DD, Hanly PJ, Poulin MJ, Handley GB, Hemmelgarn BR, Sola DY, et al. Evaluation of continuous positive airway pressure therapy on renin−angiotensin system activity in obstructive sleep apnea. Am J Respir Crit Care Med 2014;190(5):572−80.

[53] Sakaguchi Y, Shoji T, Kawabata H, Niihata K, Suzuki A, Kaneko T, et al. High prevalence of obstructive sleep apnea and its association with renal function among nondialysis chronic kidney disease patients in Japan: a cross-sectional study. Clin J Am Soc Nephrol 2011;6(5):995−1000.

[54] Buffolo F, Li Q, Monticone S, Heinrich DA, Mattei A, Pieroni J, et al. Primary aldosteronism and obstructive sleep apnea: a cross-sectional multiethnic study. Hypertension 2019;74(6):1532−40.

[55] Punjabi NM, Shahar E, Redline S, Gottlieb DJ, Givelber R, Resnick HE. Sleep-disordered breathing, glucose intolerance, and insulin resistance: the Sleep Heart Health Study. Am J Epidemiol 2004;160(6):521−30.

[56] Archontogeorgis K, Papanas N, Nena E, Tzouvelekis A, Tsigalou C, Voulgaris A, et al. Insulin sensitivity and insulin resistance in non-diabetic middle-aged patients with obstructive sleep apnoea syndrome. Open Cardiovasc Med J 2017;11:159.

[57] Ip MS, Lam B, Ng MM, Lam WK, Tsang KW, Lam KS. Obstructive sleep apnea is independently associated with insulin resistance. Am J Respir Crit Care Med 2002;165(5):670−6.

[58] Rajan P, Greenberg H. Obstructive sleep apnea as a risk factor for type 2 diabetes mellitus. Nat Sci Sleep 2015;7:113.

[59] Gopal M, Duntley S, Uhles M, Attarian H. The role of obesity in the increased prevalence of obstructive sleep apnea syndrome in patients with polycystic ovarian syndrome. Sleep Med 2002;3(5):401−4.

[60] Vgontzas AN, Bixler E, Chrousos G. Metabolic disturbances in obesity versus sleep apnoea: the importance of visceral obesity and insulin resistance. J Intern Med 2003;254(1):32−44.

[61] Vgontzas AN, Legro RS, Bixler EO, Grayev A, Kales A, Chrousos GP. Polycystic ovary syndrome is associated with obstructive sleep apnea and daytime sleepiness: role of insulin resistance. J Clin Endocrinol Metab 2001;86(2):517−20.

[62] Butt M, Dwivedi G, Khair O, Lip GY. Obstructive sleep apnea and cardiovascular disease. Int J Cardiol 2010;139(1):7−16.

[63] Björntorp P. Metabolic implications of body fat distribution. Diabetes Care 1991;14(12):1132−43.

[64] Delarue J, Magnan C. Free fatty acids and insulin resistance. Curr Opin Clin Nutr Metab Care 2007;10(2):142−8.

[65] Myers Jr MG, Leibel RL, Seeley RJ, Schwartz MW. Obesity and leptin resistance: distinguishing cause from effect. Trends Endocrinol Metabol 2010;21(11):643−51.

[66] Blüher S, Mantzoros CS. Leptin in humans: lessons from translational research. Am J Clin Nutr 2009;89(3):991S-7S.

[67] Tatsumi K, Kasahara Y, Kurosu K, Tanabe N, Takiguchi Y, Kuriyama T. Sleep oxygen desaturation and circulating leptin in obstructive sleep apnea-hypopnea syndrome. Chest 2005;127(3):716−21.

[68] Tokuda F, Sando Y, Matsui H, Koike H, Yokoyama T. Serum levels of adipocytokines, adiponectin and leptin, in patients with obstructive sleep apnea syndrome. Intern Med 2008;47(21):1843−9.

[69] Javaheri S, Colangelo G, Lacey W, Gartside PS. Chronic hypercapnia in obstructive sleep apnea-hypopnea syndrome. Sleep 1994;17(5):416−23.

[70] Rasche K, Keller T, Tautz B, Hader C, Hergenc G, Antosiewicz J, et al. Obstructive sleep apnea and type 2 diabetes. Eur J Med Res 2010;15(2):1−5.

[71] Lanfranco F, Motta G, Minetto MA, Baldi M, Balbo M, Ghigo E, et al. Neuroendocrine alterations in obese patients with sleep apnea syndrome. Int J Endocrinol 2010;2010:474518.

[72] Ekstedt M, Åkerstedt T, Söderström M. Microarousals during sleep are associated with increased levels of lipids, cortisol, and blood pressure. Psychosom Med 2004;66(6):925−31.

[73] Spiegel K, Leproult R, Van Cauter E. Impact of sleep debt on metabolic and endocrine function. Lancet 1999;354(9188):1435−9.

[74] Schmoller A, Eberhardt F, Jauch-Chara K, Schweiger U, Zabel P, Peters A, et al. Continuous positive airway pressure therapy decreases evening cortisol concentrations in patients with severe obstructive sleep apnea. Metabolism 2009;58(6):848−53.

[75] Vgontzas AN, Pejovic S, Zoumakis E, Lin H-M, Bentley C, Bixler E, et al. Hypothalamic-pituitary-adrenal axis activity in obese men with and without sleep apnea: effects of continuous positive airway pressure therapy. J Clin Endocrinol Metab 2007;92(11):4199−207.

[76] Buckley TM, Schatzberg AF. On the interactions of the hypothalamic-pituitary-adrenal (HPA) axis and sleep: normal HPA axis activity and circadian rhythm, exemplary sleep disorders. J Clin Endocrinol Metab 2005;90(5):3106−14.

[77] Ursavas A, Karadag M, Ilcol YO, Ercan I, Burgazlioglu B, Coskun F, et al. Low level of IGF-1 in obesity may be related to obstructive sleep apnea syndrome. Lung 2007;185(5):309–14.

[78] Saini J, Krieger J, Brandenberger G, Wittersheim G, Simon C, Follenius M. Continuous positive airway pressure treatment. Horm Metab Res 1993;25(07):375–81.

[79] Grunstein RR, Handelsman DJ, Lawrence SJ, Blackwell C, Caterson ID, Sullivan CE. Neuroendocrine dysfunction in sleep apnea: reversal by continuous positive airways pressure therapy. J Clin Endocrinol Metab 1989;68(2):352–8.

[80] Chahal CAA, Somers III VK. Secondary hypertension D. Obstructive sleep apnea. J Am Soc Hypertens 2015;9(3):244.

[81] Craighead DH, Heinbockel TC, Freeberg KA, Rossman MJ, Jackman RA, Jankowski LR, et al. Time-efficient inspiratory muscle strength training lowers blood pressure and improves endothelial function, NO bioavailability, and oxidative stress in midlife/older adults with above-normal blood pressure. J Am Heart Assoc 2021;10(13):e020980.

[82] Tavoian D, Ramos-Barrera LE, Craighead DH, Seals DR, Bedrick EJ, Alpert JS, et al. Six months of inspiratory muscle training to lower blood pressure and improve endothelial function in middle-aged and older adults with above-normal blood pressure and obstructive sleep apnea: protocol for the CHART clinical trial. Front Cardiovasc Med 2021;8.

[83] Yang L, Zhang H, Cai M, Zou Y, Jiang X, Song L, et al. Effect of spironolactone on patients with resistant hypertension and obstructive sleep apnea. Clin Exp Hypertens 2016;38(5):464–8.

[84] Krasinska B, Miazga A, Cofta S, Szczepaniak-Chichel L, Trafas T, Krasinski Z, et al. Effect of eplerenone on the severity of obstructive sleep apnea and arterial stiffness in patients with resistant arterial hypertension. Pol Arch Med Wewn 2016;126(5):330–9.

[85] Kasai T, Bradley TD, Friedman O, Logan AG. Effect of intensified diuretic therapy on overnight rostral fluid shift and obstructive sleep apnoea in patients with uncontrolled hypertension. J Hypertens 2014;32(3):673–80.

[86] He J, Kryger MH, Zorick FJ, Conway W, Roth T. Mortality and apnea index in obstructive sleep apnea: experience in 385 male patients. Chest 1988;94(1):9–14.

[87] Gami AS, Caples SM, Somers VK. Obesity and obstructive sleep apnea. Endocrinol Metab Clin 2003;32(4):869–94.

[88] Somers VK, Dyken ME, Clary MP, Abboud FM. Sympathetic neural mechanisms in obstructive sleep apnea. J Clin Invest 1995;96(4):1897–904.

[89] Schulz R, Mahmoudi S, Hattar K, Sibelius U, Olschewski H, Mayer K, et al. Enhanced release of superoxide from polymorphonuclear neutrophils in obstructive sleep apnea: impact of continuous positive airway pressure therapy. Am J Respir Crit Care Med 2000;162(2):566–70.

[90] Ip MS, Lam B, Chan L-y, Zheng L, Tsang KW, Fung PC, et al. Circulating nitric oxide is suppressed in obstructive sleep apnea and is reversed by nasal continuous positive airway pressure. Am J Respir Crit Care Med 2000;162(6):2166–71.

[91] Wennmalm A. Endothelial nitric oxide and cardiovascular disease. J Intern Med 1994;235(4):317–27.

[92] Kinebuchi S-i, Kazama JJ, Satoh M, Sakai K, Nakayama H, Yoshizawa H, et al. Short-term use of continuous positive airway pressure ameliorates glomerular hyperfiltration in patients with obstructive sleep apnoea syndrome. Clin Sci 2004;107(3):317–22.

[93] Yee B, Liu P, Phillips C, Grunstein R. Neuroendocrine changes in sleep apnea. Curr Opin Pulm Med 2004;10(6):475–81.

[94] Lenfant C, Chobanian AV, Jones DW, Roccella EJ. Seventh report of the Joint National Committee on the Prevention, Detection, Evaluation, and Treatment of High Blood Pressure (JNC 7) resetting the hypertension sails. Am Heart Assoc 2003:1178–9.

[95] Turnbull F. Blood Pressure Lowering Treatment Trialists' Collaboration: effects of different blood-pressure-lowering regimens on major cardiovascular events: results of prospectively-designed overviews of randomised trials. Lancet 2003;362:1527–35.

[96] Reeder M, Goldman M, Loh L, Muir A, Casey K, Gitlin D. Postoperative obstructive sleep apnoea: haemodynamic effects of treatment with nasal CPAP. Anaesthesia 1991;46(10):849–53.

[97] Iftikhar IH, Hays ER, Iverson M-A, Magalang UJ, Maas AK. Effect of oral appliances on blood pressure in obstructive sleep apnea: a systematic review and meta-analysis. J Clin Sleep Med 2013;9(2):165–74.

[98] Weaver TE, Grunstein RR. Adherence to continuous positive airway pressure therapy: the challenge to effective treatment. Proc Am Thorac Soc 2008;5(2):173–8.

[99] Browaldh N, Nerfeldt P, Lysdahl M, Bring J, Friberg D. SKUP3 randomised controlled trial: polysomnographic results after uvulopalatopharyngoplasty in selected patients with obstructive sleep apnoea. Thorax 2013;68(9):846–53.

[100] MacKay S, Carney AS, Catcheside PG, Chai-Coetzer CL, Chia M, Cistulli PA, et al. Effect of multilevel upper airway surgery vs medical management on the apnea-hypopnea index and patient-reported daytime sleepiness among patients with moderate or severe obstructive sleep apnea: the SAMS randomized clinical trial. JAMA 2020;324(12):1168–79.

[101] Sommer JU, Heiser C, Gahleitner C, Herr RM, Hörmann K, Maurer JT, et al. Tonsillectomy with uvulopalatopharyngoplasty in obstructive sleep apnea: a two-center randomized controlled trial. Deutsches Ärzteblatt International 2016;113(1–2):1.

[102] Eckert DJ, White DP, Jordan AS, Malhotra A, Wellman A. Defining phenotypic causes of obstructive sleep apnea. Identification of novel therapeutic targets. Am J Respir Crit Care Med 2013;188(8):996–1004.

[103] Khan A, Ramar K, Maddirala S, Friedman O, Pallanch JF, Olson EJ. Uvulopalatopharyngoplasty in the management of obstructive sleep apnea: the mayo clinic experience. Mayo Clin Proc 2009;84(9):795–800.

[104] Buchwald H, Avidor Y, Braunwald E, Jensen MD, Pories W, Fahrbach K, et al. Bariatric surgery: a systematic review and meta-analysis. JAMA 2004;292(14):1724–37.

Chapter 18

Endocrine hypertension in children

Badhma Valaiyapathi[1] and Ambika P. Ashraf[2]

[1]University of Alabama at Birmingham, Birmingham, AL, United States; [2]Director, Division of Pediatric Endocrinology and Diabetes, University of Alabama at Birmingham, Birmingham, AL, United States

Visit the *Endocrine Hypertension: From Basic Science to Clinical Practice, First Edition* companion web site at: https://www.elsevier.com/books-and-journals/book-companion/9780323961202.

Graphical Abstract

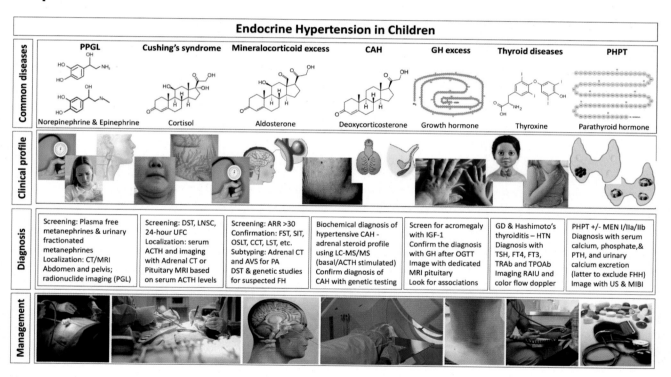

Endocrine Hypertension. https://doi.org/10.1016/B978-0-323-96120-2.00008-X

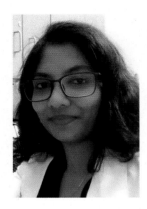

Badhma Valaiyapathi

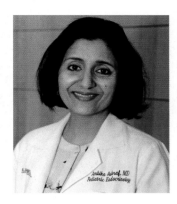

Ambika P. Ashraf

Introduction

The prevalence of childhood hypertension has seen an upward trend in the past 2 decades. In a recent systematic review and meta-analysis conducted by Song et al. the global prevalence of hypertension in children younger than 19 years was estimated to be 4%. In addition, the global prevalence of prehypertension in children was estimated to be 9.67% [1]. The prevalence of hypertension in children is increasing likely related to the rise in prevalence of obesity. The prevalence has significantly increased from 1.26% in the 1990s to 6.02% in 2015 and has followed a trend very similar to that of global obesity prevalence among adults. As mentioned earlier, the increase in the body mass index (BMI) showed a proportionate increase in the blood pressure (BP), with the prevalence of hypertension being 15.27% among obese children, and 4.99% among overweight children, compared to only 1.90% in children who are normal weight. Similarly, puberty has a significant influence on the BP trajectory, with the prevalence increasing at the age of puberty, reaching a peak at the end of puberty, and finally starting to decline steadily until early adulthood. In 2015, the hypertension prevalence was found to be 4.32% at age 6 years, peaking at 7.89% around puberty at the age of 14 years and 3.28% among those aged 19 years [1]. An elevated BP in childhood progresses to hypertension in young adulthood with the progression occurring at 5.9% over a 2-year period [2].

Definition of hypertension: Hypertension in pediatric patients is defined as a blood pressure that is greater than the 95th percentile for age, gender, and height. A new criterion for the diagnosis of hypertension in children has been proposed by the recent Hypertension Canada (2020) guideline, where a BP threshold of 120/80 mmHg were suggested for children aged 6–11 years and a threshold of 130/85 mmHg for children aged 12–17 years [3]. In addition to these static cut offs, the Hypertension Canada guideline continued to follow the blood pressure percentile cut offs proposed by previous [4] and current guidelines (systolic or diastolic blood pressure greater than or equal to the 95th percentile for age, sex, and height) [5]. However, they simplified the staging of hypertension in children, and classified hypertension in children as stage 1 if the blood pressure is lesser than 95th centile plus 12 mmHg; and stage 2 if it is greater than 95th centile plus 12 mmHg [3]. Prior to this, the American Academy of Pediatrics (AAP, 2017) guideline has proposed a static cut off 130/80 mmHg in children more than 13 years regardless of gender and height [6,7]. However, the AAP 2017 guideline has led to more children being classified as having hypertension when compared with alternative definitions [8].

The longitudinal data suggested an improved identification and risk stratification of those children at increased risk for adult cardiovascular disease [9,10]. The United States Preventive Services Task Force stated that the current evidence is insufficient to recommend screening asymptomatic children and adolescents for essential hypertension [11]. However, the recent Canadian and French guidelines recommend to regularly measure BP in children greater than 3 years [3,5]. Investigations for secondary hypertension should be done in children regardless of the age at presentation, as nearly two-thirds of the hypertension in this age group has secondary hypertension of renal or cardiac origin.

Primary versus secondary hypertension in children

Hypertension can be either primary or secondary. Primary hypertension is generally associated with obesity in genetically predisposed individuals [12].

Among children presenting with a diagnosis of hypertension, more than 60% have a secondary cause. Renal and renovascular diseases are the leading causes of secondary hypertension in children with renal causes accounting for 34% −79% and renovascular diseases contributing to 12%−13% of childhood hypertension [13,14]. Endocrine causes are relatively rare and contribute to the etiology of pediatric hypertension at a rate of 0.05%−6% [5].

Secondary hypertension presents more commonly among young children compared to adolescents and adults. Secondary forms of hypertension in children present as severe hypertension and are mostly treatable when the underlying cause is identified. Table 18.1 summarizes the myriad of disease conditions responsible for secondary hypertension in the pediatric age group [15]. Unlike primary hypertension which peaks at puberty, secondary hypertension can either peak at the first 6 years of life due to congenital abnormalities or respiratory abnormalities due to premature birth and again peaks at an older age due to acquired conditions [15].

Endocrine hypertension in children

Endocrine hypertension could be due to an excessive production or enhanced responsiveness to hormones including catecholamines, mineralocorticoids, cortisol, and parathyroid hormones. Thyroid hormones and growth hormone disorders can lead to secondary hypertension when in excess or deficient. Other predominant cause of secondary hypertension is insulin resistance [16]. Early identification and treatment of the underlying hormonal abnormality could prevent progression to organ damage from endocrine hypertension. A majority of cases of endocrine hypertension is related to adrenal gland pathology and an abnormal synthesis of adrenal hormones.

TABLE 18.1 Etiology of secondary hypertension in children and adolescents.

Organ system	Disease conditions
Renal	Glomerulonephritis, congenital anomalies, nephrotic syndrome, hydronephrosis, nephropathy, renal artery stenosis, renal dysplasia, Wilms' tumor, polycystic kidney disease, hemolytic uremic syndrome, nephrolithiasis, henoch-schonlein purpura, renal trauma
Respiratory	Chronic lung disease, bronchopulmonary dysplasia
Cardiac	Coarctation of aorta, patent ductus arteriosus
Vascular	Renal artery stenosis, renal vein thrombosis, arteriovenous fistula
Endocrine	Disorders of adrenal gland and abnormal synthesis of adrenal hormones: Cushing's syndrome, pheochromocytoma, aldosterone producing adenoma, familial hyperaldosteronism, primary glucocorticoid resistance, adrenal neuroblastoma, congenital adrenal hyperplasia due to 17α-hydroxylase deficiency and 11β-hydroxylase deficiency, Liddle syndrome Others: Thyroid and parathyroid disorders (hyperthyroidism, hypothyroidism and primary hyperparathyroidism), excessive growth hormone secretion, diabetes mellitus, hypercalcemia
Autoimmune	Systemic lupus erythematosus, juvenile ankylosing spondylitis, antineutrophil cytoplasmic antibody-associated vasculitis
Hematological	Sickle cell disease
Gastrointestinal	Gastroschisis
Neurological	Severe intraventricular hemorrhage, brain tumor, hydrocephalus, atrioventricular malformation, neural tube defect, Arnold Chiari malformation, Guillain-Barre syndrome
Sleep disorders	Obstructive sleep apnea, narcolepsy
Medications	Steroids, adrenocorticotropic hormone (ACTH), oral contraceptives, anabolic steroids, nicotine, caffeine, sympathomimetics
Others	Williams syndrome, Turner syndrome, Leigh syndrome, heavy metal exposure including cadmium, lead, and phthalates, following orthopedic procedures

Clinical presentation of endocrine hypertension in children

Catecholamine producing tumors

Pheochromocytomas and paragangliomas in children

Catecholamine secreting tumors arising from chromaffin cells of the adrenal medulla are termed pheochromocytomas, whereas tumors arising outside the adrenals are called paragangliomas (PGLs) and they are usually grouped together as pheochromocytomas and paragangliomas (PPGL). Pheochromocytomas are the more common than PGLs. PGLs may arise anywhere along the sympathetic chain, near the aorta at the level of inferior mesenteric artery, peripheral adrenal area, urinary bladder, ureteral walls, thoracic cavity, or rarely in the cervical region. PPGLs are rare with an annual incidence of ~ 1 in 300,000, and 20% of these cases occur in children and are more likely to be malignant [17,18]. PPGL accounts for $\sim 1\%$ of pediatric hypertension.

Unlike adults who present with paroxysmal hypertension, children with PPGL usually present with sustained severe hypertension, which is seen in 60%–90% of cases [19]. With markedly elevated BP, children often present with symptoms of hypertensive encephalopathy. Symptoms usually vary based on the type of catecholamine hormone secreted by the tumor. The classic triad of symptoms includes palpitations, diaphoresis, and headaches, which can be episodic in nature. Common symptoms include headache, palpitation, sweating, pallor, nausea, flushing, anxiety, weight loss, polyuria, polydipsia, and visual disturbance. In addition to these, children with epinephrine secreting tumors may present with hyperglycemia and hypertensive crisis due to catecholamine excess. Dopamine secreting tumors may be asymptomatic except for the mass effect. Head and neck PGLs can lead to dysphagia, hoarseness, and hearing disturbances from mass effect [19] and are rarely associated with hypertension.

Germline mutations are found in 70% of children <10 years of age and 51% of children between ages 11–20 years [20,21]. PPGLs are commonly familial with 30%–40% of cases having a hereditary background with a multifocal origin involving mutations in several susceptibility genes which are divided into two cluster groups. Cluster group 1 include a noradrenergic phenotype (secreting norepinephrine and is associated with an increase in plasma or urinary normetanephrine), mostly located in extraadrenal areas and includes 2 subclusters: Cluster 1 A has gene mutations in the Krebs cycle related genes including mutations of the genes encoding the succinate dehydrogenase (SDH) complex including *SDHA, SDHB, SDHC* and *SDHD*, malate dehydrogenase 2 (*MDH2*), fumarate hydratase (*FH*), and others [21]. Cluster 1B is due to gene mutations in the hypoxia signaling pathway including Von Hippel-Lindau (*VHL*) tumor suppressor, Egl-9 prolyl hydroxylase one and 2 (*EGLN1/2*), hypoxia-inducible factor 2 alpha (*HIF2A*), and others. Cluster group 2 includes an adrenergic phenotype (secreting epinephrine and is associated with an increase in plasma or urinary metanephrines) and comprises mutations in the rearranged-during-transfection (*RET*) proto-oncogene, neurofibromatosis type 1 tumor suppressor gene (*NF1*), genes encoding transmembrane protein 127 (*TMEM127*), MYC-associated factor X (*MAX*), and Harvey rat sarcoma viral oncogene homolog (*HRAS*), which leads to activation of tyrosine kinase associated signaling pathways. Genetic testing for the most common mutations should be considered to determine accurate diagnosis and prognosis.

Pheochromocytomas are commonly associated with von Hippel-Lindau disease (10%–20%), multiple endocrine neoplasia (MEN) syndromes (MEN-2A and MEN-2B), and rarely associated with other diseases like tuberous sclerosis, Sturge-Weber syndrome, ataxia-telangiectasia, and neurofibromatosis. Paragangliomas are commonly associated with Carney dyad and Carney triad syndromes where they are associated with gastrointestinal stromal tumors. The Carney triad and Carney dyad associations have heterogeneous genetic etiology and majority of patients with Carney dyad syndrome have mutations of the *SDH* complex. Mutations of the *SDH* complex are associated with paragangliomas as well as pheochromocytomas. Familial PGL syndromes are usually due to inactivating mutations in *SDHx*, leading to dysfunction of complex II in the electron transport chain. Germline mutations especially involving *VHL* and *SDHB* genes have been reported in majority of pediatric pheochromocytoma cases [18,19], and usually present with multifocal, recurrent, and malignant disease [18]. VHL- and SDHx-associated tumors are typically noradrenergic, whereas those associated with MEN2, NF1, and sporadic tumors are often adrenergic.

Diagnosis

Twenty-four-hour urinary fractionated metanephrines (normetanephrine and metanephrine) and catecholamines (norepinephrine, epinephrine, and dopamine): Most patients with pheochromocytoma or paraganglioma have increased urinary excretion of these substances. False-negative results are rare, and hence, this is the first-line investigation to exclude pheochromocytomas and catecholamine-secreting paragangliomas. The 24-h urine sample measurements are usually more stable. It is essential to measure the urinary creatinine in the sample to verify a complete 24-h urine collection [22]. False-positive results can occur with use of medications such as acetominophen, α- and β-adrenergic blockers, tricyclic antidepressants, monoamine oxidase inhibitors, and sympathomimetic agents (nicotine, ephedrine, pseudoephedrine, cocaine).

Plasma fractionated metanephrines: This diagnostic test is helpful and convenient for patients with strong risk factors for a catecholamine-secreting tumor (i.e., those with known pathogenic variants for familial pheochromocytoma). This test is slightly more sensitive than 24-h urinary fractionated metanephrines, however, has a false-positive rate of 15%. It is ideal to draw the blood sample from an intravenous catheter with the patient supine for 30 min before the blood test, calm and relaxed, fasted and not had caffeine or strenuous physical activity for at least 8–12 h before testing.

Radiologic evaluation to locate the tumor: Once a biochemical diagnosis of pheochromocytoma or catecholamine-secreting paraganglioma is established, imaging is essential. Further evaluation by computed tomography (CT) or magnetic resonance imaging (MRI) of the abdomen and pelvis is recommended. Abdominal ultrasound is not recommended due to lack of imaging sensitivity to localize pheochromocytoma or paraganglioma. In those with positive biochemical tests, but with a negative CT or MRI scan of the abdomen and pelvis, radionuclide imaging (i.e., ^{123}I-MIBG or PET/CT or ^{68}Ga-DOTATOC scan) is indicated to evaluate for paragangliomas or those children with catecholamine-secreting extra-adrenal tumors.

Genetic testing is also recommended in children, since 40%–50% of pheochromocytomas and catecholamine-secreting paragangliomas are associated with underlying genetic abnormalities. Open surgery, or laparoscopic adrenalectomy is the treatment of choice for children with PPGLs. Preoperative correction of tachycardia with β-blockers following adequate α-blockade to control hypertension is required. For further reading on PPGL, please refer Chapter 11 and 12.

Cushing's syndrome in children

Cushing's syndrome results from excessive plasma cortisol due to exogenous sources or endogenous secretion, and is uncommon in pediatric clinical practice. Excessive production of cortisol from endogenous causes includes ACTH secreting pituitary adenoma causing Cushing's disease (CD); adrenal lesions (adenoma, carcinoma, or bilateral adrenal hyperplasia) causing adrenal Cushing's syndrome; ectopic ACTH secretion (EAS) from bronchial or thymic carcinoid, other neuroendocrine tumors of pancreas and gut; small cell carcinoma of lung, medullary carcinomas of thyroid, and pheochromocytoma [20]. Exogenous administration of glucocorticoids for a prolonged period is the most common cause of Cushing's syndrome [23,24].

In children less than 7 years, adrenal Cushing's syndrome is the common cause, whereas in children more than 7 years, Cushing's disease is the common cause (accounting for nearly 75% of cases). EAS caused by ACTH secretion from nonpituitary tissues is an unusual diagnosis in children. It accounts for less than 1% of all the Cushing's syndrome cases in adolescent age group [25].

EAS is more commonly associated with hypertension in the pediatric age group compared to other forms of endogenous hypercortisolemia. Almost half of the affected children present with hypertension with occasional progression to heart failure. Prolonged hypercortisolism results in increased plasma volume, increased peripheral vascular resistance, increased cardiac output, and increased pressor response to epinephrine and angiotensin II, resulting in hypertension. Glucocorticoids activate renin–angiotensin–aldosterone system (RAAS), leading to enhanced mineralocorticoid activity, excessive activation of vasoactive substances, and suppression of vasodilation. Markedly increased cortisol levels can activate the mineralocorticoid receptor (MR) directly as cortisol binds to, and activates the MR, and can increase the deoxycorticosterone synthesis. The increased cardiac output due to hypercortisolemic response results predominantly in an increase in systolic BP [26]. Hypertension can also be caused by a central nervous system (CNS) dysregulation via glucocorticoid and mineralocorticoid receptors [27]. Biochemically, hypernatremia and hypokalemic metabolic alkalosis can occur.

Clinical presentation of Cushing's syndrome is more pronounced in infants than in older children [25,28,29]. In growing children, one of the hallmarks of Cushing's syndrome is the excessive weight gain accompanied by poor linear growth. Children with Cushing's syndrome or Cushing's disease present with round and flushed face with prominent cheeks (moon like face) and truncal obesity. Other clinical features are precipitous weight gain, muscle weakness, fatigue, immune suppression, irregular menses, depression, anxiety, osteoporosis, hyperglycemia, and headaches.

Almost 65% of Cushing's syndrome in younger children are caused by an adrenal tumor, mostly due to adrenal carcinomas [25]. Tumors may secrete androgens and mineralocorticoids in addition to cortisol, which manifest with virilization. Children with adrenal tumors can present with acne, hirsutism, pubic hair, deepening voice (in boys) and enlarged clitoris (in girls). Adrenal carcinomas often have rapid progression, while adenomas have an insidious course.

Diagnostic evaluations

An accurate and timely diagnosis is important for initiating appropriate treatment for patients with Cushing's syndrome. Children with a normal hypothalamic-pituitary-adrenal (HPA) axis exhibits a normal diurnal profile for cortisol, i.e., higher levels of cortisol are seen early in the morning and lower levels in the evening. In contrast, patients with CS demonstrate an altered rhythm of HPA axis with a disrupted diurnal cortisol profile. Thus, lack of reduction in serum cortisol in the late evening is a diagnostic marker for CS in children. A midnight serum cortisol value >7 mcg/dL has a high sensitivity and specificity for diagnosis of CS, but not preferred due to the requirement for an inpatient stay.

Initial screening: Initial screening poses a significant clinical challenge, and is aimed at establishing hypercortisolism. The three recommended screening tests are, obtaining at least two urine collections for urinary free cortisol (UFC), or two salivary collections for late night salivary cortisol, and/or an overnight dexamethasone-suppression test (DST) [30].

Urine free cortisol: A value greater than 4 times the upper limit of normal is typically associated with Cushing's syndrome. UFC measurements are cumbersome with issues related to proper sampling and confounding factors such as variations in fluid intake and renal function. False-positive UFC can occur due to pseudo-Cushing states (e.g., stress, severe obesity, chronic exercise, depression, poor diabetes control, anorexia, narcotic use, anxiety, malnutrition, and high-water intake etc.). False-negatives can result due to inadequate sample collection of urine.

Salivary cortisol: Late-night salivary cortisol (two measurements) is an accepted initial screening test in adults with CS with excellent diagnostic sensitivity and specificity comparable to urine free cortisol. In children age- and gender-specific reference values for late night salivary cortisol and cortisone are lacking. A recent study has reported [31] a bedtime salivary cortisol above 2.4 nmol/L (measured by LC-MS/MS) can be considered as a positive screening test for CS in children and does not require age- and gender-specific cut-off levels. According to Lodish et al. a salivary cortisol of >0.13 mcg/dL is considered a positive screening test [30].

Overnight dexamethasone-suppression test (ODST): ODST involves administering 1 mg of dexamethasone overnight (at 11 p.m.) and drawing a blood sample for cortisol measurement at 8 a.m. Patients with Cushing's syndrome will demonstrate inadequate cortisol suppression (i.e., 8 a.m. serum cortisol >1.8 mcg/dL).

Once the diagnosis of hypercortisolism is confirmed, the next step is to distinguish ACTH-dependent from the ACTH-independent disease. A morning plasma ACTH ≥29 pg/mL in children may indicate ACTH-dependent CS with a sensitivity of 70% [30].

A high-dose dexamethasone suppression test is recommended to differentiate CD from ectopic ACTH secretion and adrenal causes of CS. Plasma cortisol is measured at 9 a.m. the morning before, followed by dexamethasone 120 μg/kg (maximum dose 8 mg) is administered at 11 p.m., and thereafter the plasma cortisol is again measured at 9 a.m. the morning following the dexamethasone. Patients with ectopic Cushing's disease will not have ACTH suppression response to high-dose dexamethasone in contrast to patients with CD. In children, a 20% cortisol suppression from baseline had a sensitivity and specificity of 97.5% and 100% for differentiating CD from adrenal CS [30]. Even though an ovine CRH stimulation test can also be used for the differentiation of CD from ectopic ACTH secretion, these are only available in specialized tertiary care centers [30].

Patients with certain conditions such as depression, obesity, or poorly controlled diabetes can present with pseudo-Cushing's syndrome characterized by some of the symptoms and mildly abnormal cortisol levels that overlap with those seen in Cushing's syndrome [25]. With increasing prevalence of obesity, diagnosis of Cushing's syndrome poses challenges as most patients with obesity present very similar to Cushing's phenotype [32]. Cushing's syndrome should be suspected in children who have hypertension, poor linear growth, obesity, and purplish striae [23,24].

Once the biochemical workup is confirmatory for hypercortisolism, the next step is localization of the tumor by diagnostic imaging: Adrenal CT scan is used in localizing adrenal causes of Cushing's syndrome. In the case of CD, pituitary MRI in thin sections (1–2 mm) with high resolution, and with contrast (gadolinium) is performed. Bilateral inferior petrosal sinus sampling (IPSS) has been used for the localization of a pituitary source of hypercortisolism, especially in cases where a lesion is not visible on pituitary MRI. High-resolution flourodeoxy glucose positron emission tomography (FDG PET) can be used for locating small functioning corticotroph adenomas. In the case of ectopic CS, a CT or MRI scan of the neck, chest, abdomen, and pelvis may be needed. Labeled octreotide scanning, positron-emission tomography (PET), and/or ^{68}Ga-DOTATATE PET/CT are used in specialized centers for localization of an ectopic ACTH source.

Transsphenoidal surgery (TSS) of the pituitary adenoma remains the treatment of choice for CD. These children are at risk for complications involving syndrome of inappropriate antidiuretic hormone secretion, hypopituitarism (i.e., diabetes insipidus, central hypothyroidism, hypogonadism, growth hormone deficiency), bleeding, infection, and pituitary apoplexy. Hence, it is essential to consult a surgeon with experience in management of these potential postoperative complications. Medical therapy after an unsuccessful pituitary surgery for CD is very limited in children and involves off label use of some drugs. Children with adrenal Cushing's syndrome often require surgical resection of the adrenal lesion.

However, children with Cushing's syndrome often run a risk of residual hypertension even after a significant improvement following surgical correction. For further reading on Cushing's syndrome, please refer Chapter 13 & 14.

Biochemical phenotype of mineralocorticoid excess in children

The RAAS plays an essential role in maintaining normal blood pressure. Renin is released from the juxtaglomerular apparatus in response to hypovolemia and hyponatremia, subsequently resulting in angiotensin II-mediated secretion of aldosterone from the zona glomerulosa of the adrenal gland. Aldosterone secretion can be regulated by the RAAS or directly by a rise in serum potassium. Aldosterone binds to the MR and activates specific amiloride-sensitive epithelial sodium channels (ENaC) and the sodium-potassium ATPase pump (Na^+-K^+-ATPase) to promote the sodium reabsorption, water retention, increased intravascular volume, and potassium excretion. Therefore, the phenotypic presentation of mineralocorticoid excess can result from overproduction of mineralocorticoids, overstimulation of mineralocorticoid receptors, or overactivity of the epithelial sodium channels.

See Table 18.2 for an approach to interpreting renin and aldosterone levels. Patients can present with low-renin and high-aldosterone hypertension, the main differential diagnoses include primary aldosteronism caused by aldosterone-

---

TABLE 18.2 Stepwise approach in the evaluation of pediatric hypertension.

Phase 1:
Ensure the diagnosis of true hypertension by ruling out white coat hypertension

- Repeat home blood pressure monitoring
- Ambulatory blood pressure monitoring (ABPM)
- Blood pressure measurement in school setting by trained nurses

PHASE 2:
Screen for appropriate underlying cause, end-organ damage, and associated comorbidities

- History of presenting symptoms, family history, medication history, birth history and past medical history
- Physical examination—BP in arms/legs, fundoscopy, auscultation for abdominal bruit
- Biochemical tests—urinalysis, blood tests for renal function, lipid profile, glucose; High BUN and creatinine—may imply renal parenchymal disease; hypokalemia—likely from high aldosterone
- ECG, echo, renal Doppler, fundoscopy, urine protein evaluation, polysomnography

PHASE 3:
Define/identify the abnormalities identified in phase 2 with extensive and focused evaluation

Abdominal CT scan or ultrasound—if clinical presentation warrants

If suspected secondary hypertension: Do FT4, and TSH. Do evaluation of the RAAS by renin level or plasma renin activity, and aldosterone concentration in patients with resistant hypertension and hypokalemic alkalosis
1. Conditions with suppressed plasma aldosterone and renin:
   - Liddle syndrome, glucocorticoid remediable aldosteronism (GRA), apparent mineralocorticoid excess (AME), Geller syndrome, Cushing's syndrome, CAH, primary generalized glucocorticoid resistance (Chrousos syndrome) and low renin essential hypertension
2. Conditions with normal plasma aldosterone and low renin:
   - Pseudohypoaldosteronism type II (Gordon syndrome)
3. Conditions with high plasma aldosterone and low renin:
   - Primary aldosteronism—adenoma, or hyperplasia; familial hyperaldosteronism type 1, 2, 3, and 4
4. Conditions with elevated plasma aldosterone and renin:
   - Secondary hypertension involving RAAS, that is, renin-secreting juxtaglomerular cell tumors (JGCTs), renal artery stenosis, renal parenchymal disease
5. Conditions with normal plasma aldosterone and renin:
   - Familial pheochromocytoma and paragangliomas

Catecholamine assessment if clinical presentation warrants: Plasma-free metanephrines and/or urinary fractionated metanephrines

Noninvasive renal imaging: VCUG, renovascular CT or MRA

PHASE 4:
Arrive at a definitive diagnosis to offer medical and/or surgical cure

Renal biopsy, renal angiography, genetic testing for specific mutation, MIBG scan, renal vein renin collection - depending on the condition

CT, computed tomography; *FT4*, free thyroxine; *MIBG*, metaiodobenzylguanidine; *MRA*, magnetic resonance angiography; *TSH*, thyroid stimulating hormone; *VCUG*, voiding cystourethrogram.

producing adenomas and familial aldosteronism as in glucocorticoid-remediable aldosteronism (GRA). Patients can also present with low-renin and low-aldosterone hypertension, the main differential diagnoses include apparent mineralocorticoid excess, primary generalized glucocorticoid resistance (Chrousos syndrome), Liddle syndrome, Geller syndrome, and congenital adrenal hyperplasia (CAH) due to 17α-hydroxylase and 11β-hydroxylase deficiency [33,34]. In the case of Gordon syndrome, patients can present with normal plasma aldosterone and low renin.

Primary aldosteronism

Primary aldosteronism is the most common form of endocrine hypertension with a preponderance toward female children and is caused by excessive production of aldosterone independent of the RAAS. Aldosterone secreting adenomas (which occur in younger children as young as 3.5 years), glucocorticoid-remediable aldosteronism and micronodular adrenal hyperplasia (which presents in older children) are the common causes of primary aldosteronism, in addition to the genetic causes, adrenal carcinomas, and idiopathic hyperaldosteronism [23,35,36]. Suppressed renin is the hallmark of primary aldosteronism and serves to distinguish it from secondary hyper-reninemic forms of hyperaldosteronism. Clinical features are: hypertension, hypokalemia, undetectable plasma renin activity (PRA), elevated Plasma Aldosterone Concentration (PAC), hypernatremia, and metabolic alkalosis. Children may present with headache, visual disturbance, and dizziness. In case of chronic hypokalemia, children may have muscle weakness, stunted growth, fatigue, and intermittent paralysis.

Laboratory work up should include testing paired samples of plasma aldosterone and plasma renin taken in the morning. In primary aldosteronism, the PRA is typically less than 1 ng/mL per hour and the Plasma Renin Concentration is undetectable. The ratio of plasma aldosterone to renin activity (aldosterone-to-renin ratio or ARR) is usually more than 30–50, compared to that of essential hypertension (ratio of 4–10). Other helpful tests include a 24-h urinary aldosterone excretion greater than 200 mEq (200 mmol/L) and urine aldosterone excretion greater than 12 µg/24 h after a 3-day oral sodium loading.

Differential diagnosis includes secondary hyperaldosteronism where both the PAC and PRA are increased, and the ARR is <10. This can be seen in renin-producing tumors, activation of the RAAS seen in renal artery stenosis, fibromuscular hyperplasia, or atherosclerosis of the renal arteries. Excess aldosterone and renin secretion can also occur in conditions with decreased effective circulating blood volume, that is, congestive heart failure, cirrhosis, dehydration, and chronic diuretic use.

Glucocorticoid-remediable aldosteronism (GRA)

GRA, also known as familial hyperaldosteronism type 1, is an autosomal dominant condition that accounts for 1% of primary aldosteronism [37]. It is the most common monogenic form of hypertension. The family history is remarkable for onset of hypertension before 20 years of age, stroke, or cerebral hemorrhage, and the hypertension is not very responsive to conventional antihypertensive medications. Typically, hypertension manifests before 13 years of age, even though a small percentage may continue to be normotensive until adulthood [38]. Biochemical characteristics include elevated ARR (>30) and suppressed PRA. Hypokalemia may occur. GRA is due a chimeric gene duplication that results from unequal crossing over of the 11β-hydroxylase (*CYP11B1*) and aldosterone synthase (*CYP11B2*) genes, which leads to transcription of aldosterone synthase in the zona fasciculata under the control of ACTH (rather than angiotensin II). The characteristic laboratory features include elevated PAC, suppressed PRA, and elevated urinary 18-hydroxycortisol and 18-oxocortisol, which will be suppressed in response to dexamethasone [39]. In addition to cardiovascular complications, children with GRA also develop cerebrovascular complications at an early age. Genetic testing is available and is 100% sensitive and specific.

The treatment options for patients with GRA are smallest effective dose of glucocorticoid (hydrocortisone/dexamethasone), spironolactone (competitive antagonist of aldosterone at the mineralocorticoid receptor) or eplerenone (second generation mineralocorticoid receptor antagonist with greater mineralocorticoid receptor specificity). Children with GRA achieve resolution of hypertension within 2 weeks of initiation of treatment with glucocorticoids. Hydrocortisone is the preferred drug of choice in children. If hypertension is not controlled with glucocorticoids, the addition of spironolactone will suffice. Low sodium diet should be recommended for correction of the salt-sensitive volume expansion. Some cases of GRA with bilateral enlarged adrenals presenting with severe hypertension at childhood may require bilateral adrenalectomy for correction of the hypertension.

Primary generalized glucocorticoid resistance (Chrousos syndrome)

This is a rare condition which could be sporadic or inherited in an autosomal dominant manner due to an inactivating mutation in the human glucocorticoid receptor gene (*NR3C1*) [40,41]. Affected individuals have reduced tissue sensitivity to glucocorticoids including resistance of the HPA axis. The cortisol and ACTH levels are elevated in these patients. The clinical presentation widely varies. Those with hypertension exhibit high cortisol levels (serum as well as 24-h UFC excretion) in the absence of cushingoid features (due to glucocorticoid resistance). Cortisol levels fail to suppress with overnight and low-dose dexamethasone suppression tests. Glucocorticoid resistance leads to elevated adrenal androgens including dehydroepiandrosterone (DHEA), dehydroepiandrosterone sulfate (DHEAS), and androstenedione; elevated steroid precursors that possess mineralocorticoid activity including deoxycorticosterone, and corticosterone. Glucocorticoid resistance is associated with low PRA and low PAC (low-renin low-aldosterone hypertension). Hyperandrogenism results in ambiguous genitalia and menstrual abnormalities in girls, oligospermia in boys, precocious puberty, acne, hirsutism, and infertility in both genders. The excessive cortisol levels overwhelm the Mineralocorticoid Receptor (MR) resulting in hypertension. Such MR activation can present as hypokalemia. Chrousos syndrome should be suspected in children with hyperandrogenism and hypertension of unknown cause [42,43]. Treatment of hypertension from Chrousos syndrome requires a mineralocorticoid receptor antagonist such as spironolactone or ACTH suppression with high doses of mineralocorticoid-sparing synthetic glucocorticoids, such as dexamethasone aimed at suppressing the increased production of adrenal steroids [42].

Apparent mineralocorticoid excess (AME)

AME is an autosomal recessive disease due to mutations in the *HSD11B2* gene that leads to impaired 11β-hydroxysteroid type 2 (11βHSD2) activity [44]. This results in defective conversion of cortisol to its inactive metabolite cortisone in the distal convoluted tubules and cortical collecting ducts. Cortisol circulates at 100 to 1000-fold higher concentrations than aldosterone and binds with equal affinity to the MR [45]. Excessive cortisol at the level of the aldosterone receptor displaces aldosterone at the MR leading to overstimulation of mineralocorticoid receptors causing a low-renin low-aldosterone severe hypertension, hypokalemic alkalosis, failure to thrive, polydipsia, and volume expansion [46]. They can be born small for gestational age and can also develop hypercalciuria, nephrocalcinosis, and renal insufficiency. Defective cortisol (F) to cortisone (E) conversion can be assessed by measuring the significantly elevated 24-h urine tetrahydrocortisol (THF) plus 5α-tetrahydrocortisol (5αTHF) to tetrahydrocortisone (THE) ratio (THF+5αTHF/THE) [47,48]. The 5α-tetrahydrocortisol is also abbreviated as allo-THF. Genetic testing is used to confirm the diagnosis. Multiple mutations leading to AME have been identified over the last few years [45,49]. Treatment of choice for children who have AME includes high doses of spironolactone, which blocks the MR. Dietary sodium restriction and potassium supplements are also recommended. Dexamethasone can also be used to suppress ACTH and cortisol. Successful renal transplant has also been performed in patients with AME.

Chronic ingestion of large amounts of liquorice can lead to low-renin low-aldosterone hypertension associated with hypokalemic alkalosis and is caused by its active ingredients carbenoxolone and glycyrrhetinic acid. Carbenoxolone and glycyrrhetinic acid are potent inhibitors of the enzyme 11βHSD2 causing an acquired form of AME [50].

Liddle syndrome

Liddle syndrome is a rare form of monogenic hypertension with an autosomal dominant inheritance resulting in low renin, low aldosterone hypertension associated with volume expansion. This results from a gain of function mutation in the epithelial sodium channels (ENaC) that are responsible for sodium reabsorption in the epithelial cells, resulting in excess sodium reabsorption in the distal tubules by prolonging the half-life of ENaCs as well as increasing the channel numbers. Patients present with early onset severe salt sensitive hypertension, metabolic alkalosis, low plasma aldosterone, suppressed PRA, and hypokalemia. ENaC blockers including triamterene and amiloride are the mainstay of treatment for controlling hypertension in patients with Liddle syndrome [51,52]. An important point to remember is that the hypertension resulting from Liddle syndrome does not respond to spironolactone.

Pseudohypoaldosteronism type II (Gordon syndrome)

Gordon syndrome is also known as pseudohypoaldosteronism type II or familial hyperkalemic hypertension. It is an autosomal dominant disorder characterized by hypertension presenting from childhood, hyperkalemia from birth, and metabolic acidosis. Patients usually have suppressed PRA and normal aldosterone. They can also have hyperchloremia. This results from mutations in the *WNK1, WNK4, KLHL3,* and *CUL3* genes [53,54]. The patients have an increased sensitivity of sodium reabsorption to thiazide diuretics, due to the involvement of the thiazide-sensitive sodium—chloride cotransporter (NCC) and hence they respond to thiazides.

Geller syndrome

Geller syndrome is a rare monogenic cause of hypertension due to constitutive activation of the mineralocorticoid receptor [55]. This autosomal dominant condition results from a gain-of-function mutation on chromosome 4q31, leading to altered specificities to the steroid hormones including progesterone which can stimulate the mineralocorticoid receptor in this condition. Even though the onset is in childhood, during pregnancy the patients develop severe hypertension due to elevated progesterone levels. The laboratory evaluation will reveal metabolic alkalosis and suppressed aldosterone and renin. Potassium levels are normal or low. Definitive diagnosis requires a targeted mutation analysis. There is no optimal management identified. Spironolactone is contraindicated in this condition. In most situations, delivery will reduce the high blood pressure.

Congenital adrenal hyperplasia and hypertension in children

Congenital adrenal hyperplasia (CAH) is a disorder of adrenal steroidogenesis comprising of a group of autosomal recessive disorders. Rare causes of CAH namely 17α-hydroxylase and 11β-hydroxylase deficiency can develop hypertension due to mineralocorticoid excess and are characterized by low levels of aldosterone and significant hypokalemia. Independent of the severity of blood pressure, mineralocorticoid excess can lead to a greater degree of end organ damage and metabolic disorders which may occasionally necessitate bilateral adrenalectomy [23,56].

Patients with **11β-hydroxylase deficiency** have mutations in the *CYP11B1* gene located on 8q24 chromosome. 11β-hydroxylase is involved in the last steps in aldosterone and cortisol synthesis resulting in inadequate conversion of deoxycorticosterone (DOC) to corticosterone and of 11-deoxycortisol to cortisol. Low cortisol feedback leads to increased ACTH, which results in overproduction of androgen precursors proximal to the enzyme blockade. Biochemical abnormalities include elevated deoxycorticosterone, androstenedione, and testosterone levels associated with low PRA. Elevated DOC leads to hypokalemia and hypertension. Girls with classic 11β-hydroxylase deficiency are born with virilized genitalia due to elevated adrenal androgens in the prenatal period. Boys can present with precocious puberty. Children with nonclassical 11β-hydroxylase deficiency may present with amenorrhea, infertility, and hypertension. Other clinical presentations include hyperpigmentation, acne, hirsutism, precocious puberty, and accelerated growth with reduced height. Hypertension presents later in childhood and is present in more than 50% of cases. Intracranial aneurysms may also occur occasionally [23,56].

17α-Hydroxylase/17,20-lyase deficiency due to *CYP17A1* gene mutations is another form of low-renin hypertension. Biochemical features include elevated deoxycorticosterone (DOC), corticosterone, and aldosterone. Inadequate production of androgens and estrogens secondary to deficient production of 17α-hydroxylase can lead to compensatory elevation of gonadotropins. Patients can also present with hypokalemic alkalosis. Affected girls (46 XX) appear phenotypically normal, but may not enter puberty spontaneously, while affected male (46 XY) neonates are typically born with undervirilized genitalia. The 46 XY patients can present with ambiguous genitalia with intraabdominal or inguinal testes and a blind vaginal pouch. The clinical presentation depends on how much enzyme activity is present. Some 46 XX patients can present as an ovarian hyperstimulation syndrome later in life with lack of estrogen and primary amenorrhea. The elevated LH and FSH can hyperstimulate ovary and can lead to huge ovarian cysts.

Androgen excess distinguishes 11β-hydroxylase deficiency from 17α-hydroxylase deficiency. Plasma concentrations of cortisol, 17-hydroxyprogesterone, deoxycorticosterone, 11-deoxycortisone, androstenedione, and dehydroepiandrosterone sulfate should be done in patients suspected to have 11β-hydroxylase deficiency (androgen excess) and 17α-hydroxylase deficiency (decreased production of sex steroids). Appropriate genetic testing for the culprit genes can prove the diagnosis with high sensitivity and specificity in patients with CAH and hypertension. CAH is treated with glucocorticoid replacement which corrects the hypertension, and plasma renin/deoxycorticosterone levels. In addition, children with CAH may also need appropriate sex steroid replacement concordant with sex of rearing at puberty. For detailed further reading, please refer Chapter 9.

Excessive growth hormone production

Excessive growth hormone from a growth hormone producing pituitary tumor results in gigantism in growing children and acromegaly after fusion of the epiphyses in the youth. Since GH-secreting pituitary adenomas are rare in children, other conditions such as McCune-Albright syndrome, multiple endocrine neoplasia type 1 and type 4, Carney complex due to mutations in the gene encoding *PRKAR1A*, familial isolated pituitary adenomas (FIPA), and X-linked acro-gigantism (XLAG) need to be considered in the differential diagnosis. Typically, these children exhibit height +3 to +4 standard deviations above normal (>99.9th percentile).

Patients present with hypertension due to sodium retention and extracellular volume expansion. Children also present with soft tissue and acral overgrowth, dental malocclusion, degenerative arthritis due to chondral and synovial tissue overgrowth, sweaty and oily skin, cardiac dysfunctions, and nerve entrapment such as carpal tunnel syndrome.

Insulin like growth factor 1 (IGF-1) and growth hormone levels should be measured with appropriate dynamic testing to elicit the lack of growth hormone suppression for establishing the biochemical diagnosis. Therapy for pituitary gigantism is individualized. TSS is the treatment of choice. However, in cases where surgical cure is not possible, diuretic therapy should be initiated to treat hypertension [57]. Even though radiation therapy is not preferred, cranial radiation may be used as an adjunctive therapy in rare situations. Pharmacologic agents such as bromocriptine, octreotide, lanreotide, pegvisomant, and other novel drugs may also be considered depending on the clinical scenario. Please refer Chapter 15 for detailed reading on growth hormone excess and hypertension.

Thyroid and parathyroid disorders and hypertension in children

Systolic hypertension is a common presentation in children who have thyrotoxicosis [58]. Grave's disease and Hashimoto's thyroiditis are autoimmune diseases which can commonly result in thyrotoxicosis. Grave's disease is caused by thyroid stimulating antibodies (Thyroid Stimulating Hormone [TSH] Receptor antibodies) which by interacting with the TSH receptor acts like the thyroid stimulating hormone. Thyrotoxicosis due to Grave's disease is uncommon in infants, but the prevalence increases with increasing age. Hashimoto's thyroiditis most often causes hypothyroidism. However, during the thyrotoxicosis phase of the disease, thyroxine (T4) and triiodothyronine (T3) are released due to the destruction of thyroid cells by the cytotoxic lymphocytes resulting in transient thyrotoxicosis. Children with hyperthyroidism can present with weight loss, systolic hypertension, wide pulse pressure, tachycardia, palpable thyroid enlargement with a bruit over the gland, tremors, nervousness, irritability, excessive crying, and emotional lability with poor school performance. Additionally, children with Grave's disease may also have ptosis, proptosis (exophthalmos), conjunctival injection, and puffy eyelids [23,59]. Evaluation of TSH and free T4, T3, TSH Receptor antibodies (TRAb), thyroid stimulating immunoglobulins (TSI), and thyroid peroxidase (TPO) antibodies can establish the underlying diagnosis. Beta-blockers should be used to treat hypertension, tachycardia and tremors followed by more cause specific treatment to treat hyperthyroidism.

Hypercalcemia due to primary hyperparathyroidism is associated with an increased frequency of hypertension. Primary hyperparathyroidism is the most common endocrine cause of hypercalcemia. Patients are usually asymptomatic but may present with symptoms relevant to chronic hypercalcemia including constipation, osteoporosis, polyuria, polydipsia, renal stones, and peptic ulcer disease in addition to hypertension. Laboratory picture of primary hyperparathyroidism include hypercalcemia, hypophosphatemia, elevated serum alkaline phosphatase, hypercalciuria with increased urinary calcium/creatinine ratio, and elevated serum parathyroid hormone (PTH) level. Parathyroidectomy is the primary treatment for hypertension that results from primary hyperparathyroidism [57]. For further reading on hypertension in thyroid disease and primary hyperparathyrodism, please refer Chapter 16.

Obesity, insulin resistance, and obstructive sleep apnea (OSA) associated with hypertension in children

Hypertension in the pediatric age group was thought to be due to secondary causes while essential hypertension was more commonly seen in adults. The last 2 decades have seen a drastic increase in the incidence of childhood obesity and a parallel increase in childhood hypertension attributed to obesity, which more often persists into hypertension in adulthood resulting in significant cardiovascular morbidity and mortality [60]. Hypertension is four times higher in morbidly obese children compared to nonobese children and the prevalence is also higher in obese children with a family history of hypertension and obesity [61]. Several studies conducted in the last several years have shown that obesity is an important predictor for hypertension irrespective of the age. With every 10% increase in BMI there is a 3.9 mmHg increase in systolic blood pressure [24,62]. Obese children with essential hypertension usually present with stage 1 hypertension, whereas stage 2 hypertension is more common in those with secondary hypertension. However, this does not rule out a diagnosis of secondary hypertension in children with stage 1 hypertension and obesity [63,64]. Moreover, isolated systolic hypertension is more common in obese children. Multiple factors are involved in the association of obesity and hypertension including overactivity of the sympathetic nervous system, altered balance between the sympathetic and the parasympathetic activity, activation of the RAAS, impaired natriuresis, insulin resistance, endothelial dysfunction, vascular changes, increased levels of leptin and decreased levels of adiponectin. There is usually a combination of these factors involved in the development of hypertension in obese children [64].

Insulin resistance results in vasoconstriction of the arterial bed due to an increase in the sympathetic nervous system activity which in turn results in reduced blood flow. Similarly, vasoconstriction of the renal blood vessels results in the production of renin and activation of the RAAS, and an ensuing elevated BP from salt retention. Hyperinsulinemia in obese children can also result in proliferation of the vascular smooth muscle cells of the resistance vessels resulting in increased peripheral vascular resistance. Insulin resistance, obesity, and elevated BP are all components of the metabolic syndrome which is defined by a constellation of symptoms including the above-mentioned factors along with dyslipidemia [64,65]. Each of the components of the metabolic syndrome poses a cardiovascular risk with the presence of multiple aggregating factors exponentially increasing the risk of developing cardiovascular comorbidities and organ damage in early adulthood.

There is a scarcity in research studies evaluating the association between OSA and hypertension in children as opposed to the well-established relationship in the adults. However, due to the high prevalence of drug resistant hypertension in population who are left with untreated OSA for a prolonged period, it is recommended to screen obese and hypertensive children for OSA. Obesity, hypertension, and OSA are all inter-related, and have a strong association with an influence of BMI on the relationship between OSA and hypertension. In addition, there is an independent relationship exerted on one in the absence of the other [7,66]. Children with OSA present with snoring (which is commonly mild), along with periods of apnea, frequent movements, sleep awakenings, and thoracoabdominal asynchrony during the rapid eye movement (REM) phase of the sleep. Elevated night-time and daytime diastolic blood pressure has been observed in children with OSA with the degree of hypertension directly proportional to the severity of OSA and obesity. Similarly, studies also found an elevation in daytime and night-time BP among prepubertal children independent of their BMI. Obese children with moderate to severe OSA had a significant increase in blood pressure compared to those with mild OSA indicating the relationship between hypertension and severity of OSA. Polysomnography should be considered in children who are obese and have snoring with or without hypertension [66–68]. For further reading on OSA and hypertension, please refer Chapter 17.

The Endocrine Society guideline recommends that all patients with OSA should be screened for primary aldosteronism [69]. However, the prevalence of primary aldosteronism in children affected by OSA has not been established at this time and there is no typical phenotype for primary aldosteronism in children. Hence, while this is an important recommendation in adults, it is not clear in children.

Diagnostic approach to endocrine hypertension in children

Hypertension could be the first clinical presentation in most cases of endocrine problems in children. Hence, appropriate and timely diagnosis of hypertension in children is essential for initiating treatment to prevent progression to adult hypertension and the ensuing end-organ damage. Secondary hypertension is more common in children and the adolescent. Hypertension in children younger than 6 years of age is more often due to secondary causes unless proven otherwise. Even though hypertension in older children is commonly due to secondary causes, the rising childhood obesity epidemic has resulted in the development of primary hypertension in this age group necessitating a thorough evaluation for the underlying causes. Hypertension is a silent condition, and if left undiagnosed can result in significant cardiovascular health problems in children. Almost 40% of children present with left ventricular hypertrophy at the time of diagnosis of hypertension which delineates the importance of measuring blood pressure at a younger age to capture the diagnosis early at its development. In addition, end organ damage due to hypertension can be reversed with initiation of treatment and having blood pressure under control. The American Academy of Pediatrics suggests that children should be evaluated for hypertension starting at the age of 3 years, during routine clinic visits, irrespective of whether they are symptomatic or asymptomatic, but this guideline is not routinely practiced. Fig. 18.1 illustrates an algorithm for the initial approach to elevated blood pressure in children. Underdiagnosis of hypertension is also a serious problem which needs to be addressed [70].

A four-phase evaluation of hypertension in a stepwise manner is suggested for ensuring an appropriate diagnosis as well as for avoiding unnecessary expensive and invasive diagnostic procedures [71]. Table 18.2 summarizes the phases of evaluation of hypertension which would apply for children and adults [14].

BP should be measured at least on three different occasions with three readings performed 2 min apart on each occasion before arriving at the diagnosis of hypertension among children. Ensuring the use of an appropriate cuff size, proper placement of the cuff, measuring techniques by allowing the patient to relax for at least 5 min before measuring,

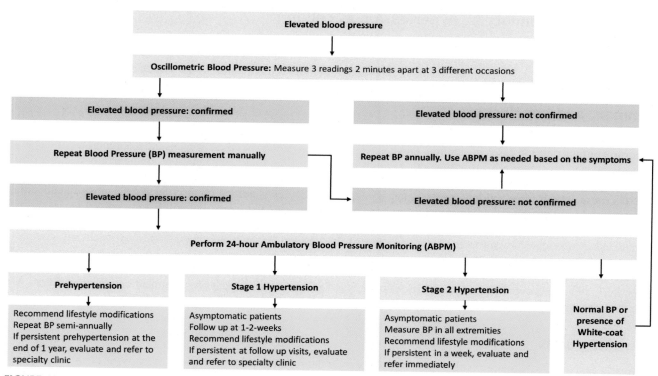

FIGURE 18.1 Initial evaluation algorithm for hypertension in children. *ABPM*, ambulatory blood pressure monitoring; *BP*, blood pressure; *HTN*, hypertension.

measurement taken in the right arm at the level of the heart, avoiding talking and crossing of the legs during the reading is important to prevent inappropriate readings. During initial evaluation, if children have high BP with an oscillometric device, it is advised to perform repeat measurements manually since oscillometric devices tend to overestimate BP in children. White coat hypertension and masked hypertension should be ruled out by the appropriate use of either home BP monitoring by self, Ambulatory Blood Pressure Monitoring (ABPM) or BP measurement performed by a trained school nurse. The BP monitor should be validated periodically. ABPM is a programmable device which can measure BP periodically usually over a period of 24 h. ABPM helps in identifying ambulatory day time BP, night-time BP, dipping, and nondipping patterns during sleep and BP load, all of which are helpful in predicting cardiovascular adverse outcomes [14,70,72].

It is essential to perform thyroid function tests and renal function in all cases of hypertension. The next diagnostic investigation has to be tailored according to the symptomatology and biochemical abnormality. Evaluation of the RAAS is essential to identify the common endocrine causes of hypertension. Excess secretion of aldosterone due to inappropriate activation of RAAS (high-renin high-aldosterone state) or renin-independent secretion from the adrenal glands (low-renin high-aldosterone state) can result in hypertension. Low renin and high aldosterone scenarios may include aldosterone producing adenoma or familial hyperaldosteronism type 1 (GRA). Biochemical testing based on the clinical presentation should be done to justify performing expensive imaging procedures. Individuals with a known germline mutation should have repeated biochemical testing in a periodic manner to avoid missing an early diagnosis, as this could be potentially life threatening especially in conditions such as PPGLs. Clinicians should consider screening patients with early onset hypertension who have a family history of young hemorrhagic stroke for primary or familial aldosteronism, and suggest treatment against aldosterone excess once found, as this cures the hypertension in more than 50% of cases, while resulting in significant improvement in the rest [57]. Children with hypertension, low levels of aldosterone and renin, and spontaneous hypokalemia should be evaluated for 11β-hydroxylase deficiency, 17α-hydroxylase deficiency, AME, Cushing's syndrome, Liddle syndrome and primary glucocorticoid resistance. Liddle syndrome is more likely in patients who have hypokalemia with a family history of hypertension. Obesity and Cushing's syndrome can have a similar clinical presentation and dexamethasone-suppression test should be considered to evaluate and distinguish the two conditions especially if there is a clinical suspicion of Cushing's Syndrome [57,73].

Management of endocrine hypertension in children

Children who are suspected to have endocrine hypertension should be referred to the endocrinologist for the timely diagnosis and management. The specific management has been described under each condition. Lifestyle modification and weight loss in obese children result in decreased blood pressure due to a reduction in the sympathetic overactivity [64].

Summary and conclusions

Even though the endocrine causes of hypertension listed in this chapter are uncommon/rare and account for only a small proportion of hypertension cases in children, the diagnosis and management at an early age is indeed important as they are often severe, and progression is faster than other causes of hypertension. Endocrine hypertension generally resolves once the underlying condition is identified and treated. This is especially challenging since history and examination will point toward a cause only in some children, while a more streamlined approach is needed for arriving at a diagnosis of endocrine hypertension in asymptomatic children. A lot has been learnt in the past few years and still being evolved regarding the etiology, pathogenesis, diagnosis, indications for treatment and management options of endocrine hypertension in children. We still need to bridge the gap in our understanding of the genetic determinants of endocrine hypertension, complex relationship between obesity, diabetes, sleep apnea, and metabolic syndrome on blood pressure. The evaluation of blood pressure using ABPM is promising to prevent end organ damage but remains underexplored in children due to the need for validation at this age group. There is also a lack of understanding and research regarding treatment options in children. All these indicate the importance of conducting more streamlined research in pediatric endocrine hypertension.

Learning points

- Nearly two-thirds of children with hypertension has secondary hypertension and a vast majority of them have hypertension secondary to renal or cardiac disease.
- Endocrinopathies account for only 0.05%−6% of cases of pediatric hypertension.
- There is a proportionate increase in the prevalence of hypertension with higher BMI among children.
- Though catecholamine producing tumors, endogenous hypercortisolism, and conditions associated with mineralocorticoid abnormalities are the common causes of endocrine hypertension in children, other conditions such as congenital adrenal hyperplasia, abnormalities of growth hormone, thyroid and parathyroid disease, insulin resistance and obstructive sleep apnea are sometimes associated with the disease in children.
- Early identification of the disorder causing endocrine hypertension and prompt treatment may improve blood pressure and the hypertensive complications in children.

References

[1] Song P, et al. Global prevalence of hypertension in children: a systematic review and meta-analysis. JAMA Pediatr 2019;173(12):1154−63.

[2] Falkner B, Lurbe E. Primordial prevention of high blood pressure in childhood: an opportunity not to be missed. Hypertension 2020;75(5):1142−50.

[3] Rabi DM, et al. Hypertension Canada's 2020 comprehensive guidelines for the prevention, diagnosis, risk assessment, and treatment of hypertension in adults and children. Can J Cardiol 2020;36(5):596−624.

[4] National high blood pressure education program working group on high blood pressure in, C. And adolescents, the fourth report on the diagnosis, evaluation, and treatment of high blood pressure in children and adolescents. Pediatrics 2004;114(2 Suppl. 4th Report):555−76.

[5] Bouhanick B, et al. Hypertension in children and adolescents: a position statement from a panel of multidisciplinary experts coordinated by the French society of hypertension. Front Pediatr 2021;9:680803.

[6] Genovesi S, et al. How to apply European and American guidelines on high blood pressure in children and adolescents. A position paper endorsed by the Italian society of hypertension and the Italian society of pediatrics. High Blood Pres Cardiovasc Prev 2020;27(3):183−93.

[7] Flynn JT, et al. Clinical practice guideline for screening and management of high blood pressure in children and adolescents. Pediatrics 2017;140(3).

[8] Yang L, et al. Impact of the 2017 American Academy of pediatrics guideline on hypertension prevalence compared with the fourth report in an international cohort. Hypertension 2019;74(6):1343−8.

[9] Condren M, et al. The impact of new guidelines on the prevalence of hypertension in children: a cross-sectional evaluation. J Clin Hypertens 2019;21(4):510−5.

[10] Brady TM, Altemose K, Urbina EM. Impact of the 2017 American Academy of pediatrics' clinical practice guideline on the identification and risk stratification of youth at increased cardiovascular disease risk. Hypertension 2021;77(6):1815−24.

[11] Gartlehner G, et al. Screening for hypertension in children and adolescents: updated evidence report and systematic review for the US preventive services task force. JAMA 2020;324(18):1884−95.

[12] Rao G. Diagnosis, epidemiology, and management of hypertension in children. Pediatrics 2016;138(2).

[13] Koch C, Papadopoulou-Marketou N, Chrousos GP. Overview of endocrine hypertension. In: Feingold KR, et al., editors. Endotext; 2000 [South Dartmouth (MA)].

[14] Goknar N, Caliskan S. New guidelines for the diagnosis, evaluation, and treatment of pediatric hypertension. Turk Pediatri Ars 2020;55(1):11−22.

[15] Gupta-Malhotra M, et al. Essential hypertension vs. secondary hypertension among children. Am J Hypertens 2015;28(1):73−80.

[16] Koch CA. Stress: aspects of endocrine hypertension. Dtsch Arztebl Int 2012;109(17):312. author reply 313-4.

[17] Seamon ML, Yamaguchi I. Hypertension in pheochromocytoma and paraganglioma: evaluation and management in pediatric patients. Curr Hypertens Rep 2021;23(5):32.

[18] Pamporaki C, et al. Characteristics of pediatric vs adult pheochromocytomas and paragangliomas. J Clin Endocrinol Metab April 1, 2017;102(4):1122−32. https://doi.org/10.1210/jc.2016-3829. PMID: 28324046.

[19] Bholah R, Bunchman TE. Review of pediatric pheochromocytoma and paraganglioma. Front Pediatr 2017;5:155.

[20] Neumann HPH, Young Jr WF, Eng C. Pheochromocytoma and paraganglioma. N Engl J Med August 8, 2019;381(6):552−65. https://doi.org/10.1056/NEJMra1806651. PMID: 31390501.

[21] Nölting S, Bechmann N, Taieb D, Beuschlein F, Fassnacht M, Kroiss M, et al. Personalized management of pheochromocytoma and paraganglioma. Endocr Rev March 2022;43(2):199−239. https://doi.org/10.1210/endrev/bnab019. Erratum in: Endocr Rev. 2021 Dec 14;: Erratum in: Endocr Rev. 2021 Dec 14;: PMID: 34147030.

[22] Perry CG, Sawka AM, Singh R, Thabane L, Bajnarek J, Young Jr WF. The diagnostic efficacy of urinary fractionated metanephrines measured by tandem mass spectrometry in detection of pheochromocytoma. Clin Endocrinol May 2007;66(5):703−8. https://doi.org/10.1111/j.1365-2265.2007.02805.x. PMID: 17388796.

[23] White PC. Endocrine hypertension. In: Pediatric hypertension. Totowa, NJ: Humana Press; 2013. p. 379−94.

[24] Sharma S, Meyers KE, Vidi SR. Secondary forms of hypertension in children: overview. Pediatric hypertension 2018:431−49.

[25] Stratakis CA. Cushing syndrome in pediatrics. Endocrinol Metab Clin N Am December 2012;41(4):793−803. https://doi.org/10.1016/j.ecl.2012.08.002. PMID: 23099271.

[26] Magiakou MA, et al. Blood pressure in children and adolescents with Cushing's syndrome before and after surgical care. J Clin Endocrinol Metab 1997;82(6):1734−8.

[27] Findling JW, Raff H. Cushing's Syndrome: important issues in diagnosis and management. J Clin Endocrinol Metab 2006;91(10):3746−53.

[28] Holst JM, et al. Cushing's syndrome in children and adolescents: a Danish nationwide population-based cohort study. Eur J Endocrinol 2017;176(5):567−74.

[29] Ferrigno R, et al. Paediatric Cushing's disease: epidemiology, pathogenesis, clinical management, and outcome. Rev Endocr Metab Disord 2021;22(4):817−35.

[30] Lodish MB, Keil MF, Stratakis CA. Cushing's syndrome in pediatrics: an update. Endocrinol Metab Clin N Am 2018;47(2):451−62.

[31] Ueland GA, et al. Bedtime salivary cortisol as a screening test for cushing syndrome in children. J Endocr Soc 2021;5(5):bvab033.

[32] Kleinendorst L, et al. Identifying underlying medical causes of pediatric obesity: results of a systematic diagnostic approach in a pediatric obesity center. PLoS One 2020;15(5):e0232990.

[33] Lu YT, et al. Overview of monogenic forms of hypertension combined with hypokalemia. Front Pediatr 2020;8:543309.

[34] Khandelwal P, Deinum J. Monogenic forms of low-renin hypertension: clinical and molecular insights. Pediatr Nephrol 2022;37(7):1495−509. https://doi.org/10.1007/s00467-021-05246-x.

[35] He X, Modi Z, Else T. Hereditary causes of primary aldosteronism and other disorders of apparent excess mineralocorticoid activity. Gland Surg 2020;9(1):150−8.

[36] Zennaro MC, Boulkroun S, Fernandes-Rosa FL. Pathogenesis and treatment of primary aldosteronism. Nat Rev Endocrinol 2020;16(10):578−89.

[37] Ehret GB, Caulfield MJ. Genes for blood pressure: an opportunity to understand hypertension. Eur Heart J 2013;34(13):951−61.

[38] Lenzini L, et al. Saga of familial hyperaldosteronism: yet a new channel. Hypertension 2018;71(6):1010−4.

[39] Halperin F, Dluhy RG. Glucocorticoid-remediable aldosteronism. Endocrinol Metab Clin N Am 2011;40(2):333−41 [viii].

[40] Vitellius G, Lombes M. Genetics in endocrinology: glucocorticoid resistance syndrome. Eur J Endocrinol 2020;182(2):R15−27.

[41] Nicolaides NC, Charmandari E. Primary generalized glucocorticoid resistance and hypersensitivity syndromes: a 2021 update. Int J Mol Sci 2021;22(19).

[42] Nicolaides NC, Charmandari E. Chrousos syndrome: from molecular pathogenesis to therapeutic management. Eur J Clin Invest 2015;45(5):504−14.

[43] Charmandari E, Kino T, Chrousos GP. Primary generalized familial and sporadic glucocorticoid resistance (Chrousos syndrome) and hypersensitivity. Endocr Dev 2013;24:67−85.

[44] Mangos GJ, et al. Glucocorticoids and the kidney. Nephrology 2003;8(6):267−73.

[45] Yau M, et al. Clinical, genetic, and structural basis of apparent mineralocorticoid excess due to 11beta-hydroxysteroid dehydrogenase type 2 deficiency. Proc Natl Acad Sci U S A 2017;114(52):E11248−56.

[46] Morineau G, et al. Apparent mineralocorticoid excess: report of six new cases and extensive personal experience. J Am Soc Nephrol 2006;17(11):3176−84.

[47] De Santis D, et al. Detection of urinary exosomal HSD11B2 mRNA expression: a useful novel tool for the diagnostic approach of dysfunctional 11beta-HSD2-related hypertension. Front Endocrinol 2021;12:681974.

[48] Lucas-Herald AK, et al. The pitfalls associated with urinary steroid metabolite ratios in children undergoing investigations for suspected disorders of steroid synthesis. Int J Pediatr Endocrinol 2015;2015(1):10.

[49] Ingelfinger JR. Monogenic and polygenic contributions to hypertension. In: Pediatric hypertension. Totowa, NJ: Humana Press; 2013. p. 83—101.

[50] Edwards CR, et al. Congenital and acquired syndromes of apparent mineralocorticoid excess. J Steroid Biochem Mol Biol 1993;45(1—3):1—5.

[51] Tetti M, et al. Liddle syndrome: review of the literature and description of a new case. Int J Mol Sci 2018;19(3).

[52] Cui Y, et al. Liddle syndrome: clinical and genetic profiles. J Clin Hypertens 2017;19(5):524—9.

[53] Brooks AM, et al. Pseudohypoaldosteronism type 2 presenting with hypertension and hyperkalaemia due to a novel mutation in the WNK4 gene. QJM 2012;105(8):791—4.

[54] Shibata S, et al. Kelch-like 3 and Cullin 3 regulate electrolyte homeostasis via ubiquitination and degradation of WNK4. Proc Natl Acad Sci U S A 2013;110(19):7838—43.

[55] Raina R, et al. Overview of monogenic or mendelian forms of hypertension. Front Pediatr 2019;7:263.

[56] Hinz L, Pacaud D, Kline G. Congenital adrenal hyperplasia causing hypertension: an illustrative review. J Hum Hypertens 2018;32(2):150—7.

[57] Young WF, Calhoun DA, Lenders JWM, Stowasser M, Textor SC. Screening for endocrine hypertension: an endocrine society scientific statement. Endocr Rev 2017;38(2):103—22.

[58] Berta E, et al. Hypertension in thyroid disorders. Front Endocrinol 2019;10:482.

[59] Raza J, Hindmarsh PC, Brook CG. Thyrotoxicosis in children: thirty years' experience. Acta Paediatr 1999;88(9):937—41.

[60] Sorof J, Daniels S. Obesity hypertension in children: a problem of epidemic proportions. Hypertension 2002;40(4):441—7.

[61] Brady TM. Obesity-related hypertension in children. Front Pediatr 2017;5:197.

[62] Parker ED, et al. Change in weight status and development of hypertension. Pediatrics 2016;137(3):e20151662.

[63] Kapur G, et al. Secondary hypertension in overweight and stage 1 hypertensive children: a midwest pediatric nephrology consortium report. J Clin Hypertens 2010;12(1):34—9.

[64] Batisky DL. Obesity hypertension: clinical aspects. In: Pediatric hypertension. 4th ed. Switzerland: Springer International Publishing; 2017. p. 1—19.

[65] Halpern A, et al. Metabolic syndrome, dyslipidemia, hypertension and type 2 diabetes in youth: from diagnosis to treatment. Diabetol Metab Syndrome 2010;2:55.

[66] Marcus CL, Greene MG, Carroll JL. Blood pressure in children with obstructive sleep apnea. Am J Respir Crit Care Med 1998;157(4 Pt 1):1098—103.

[67] Narang I, Mathew JL. Childhood obesity and obstructive sleep apnea. J Nutr Metab 2012;2012:134202.

[68] Leung LC, et al. Twenty-four-hour ambulatory BP in snoring children with obstructive sleep apnea syndrome. Chest 2006;130(4):1009—17.

[69] Funder JW, et al. The management of primary aldosteronism: case detection, diagnosis, and treatment: an endocrine society clinical practice guideline. J Clin Endocrinol Metab 2016;101(5):1889—916.

[70] Dionne JM. Hypertension diagnosis and management in children and adolescents: important updates. Curr Pediatrics Rep 2018;6(4):269—77.

[71] Swinford RD, Portman RJ. Diagnostic evaluation of pediatric hypertension. In: Pediatric hypertension. Humana Pr; 2004. p. 405—20.

[72] Hermida RC, et al. [2013 ambulatory blood pressure monitoring recommendations for the diagnosis of adult hypertension, assessment of cardiovascular and other hypertension-associated risk, and attainment of therapeutic goals (summary). Joint recommendations from the international society for chronobiology (ISC), American association of medical chronobiology and chronotherapeutics (AAMCC), Spanish society of applied chronobiology, chronotherapy, and vascular risk (SECAC), Spanish society of atherosclerosis (SEA), and Romanian society of internal medicine (RSIM)]. Clín Invest Arterioscler 2013;25(2):74—82.

[73] Bhavani N. Pediatric endocrine hypertension. Indian J Endocrinol Metab 2011;15(4):S361—6.

Chapter 19

Endocrine hypertension in pregnancy

Felix Jebasingh and Nihal Thomas
Christian Medical College Vellore, India

Visit the *Endocrine Hypertension: From Basic Science to Clinical Practice, First Edition* companion web site at: https://www.elsevier.com/books-and-journals/book-companion/9780323961202.

Graphical Abstract

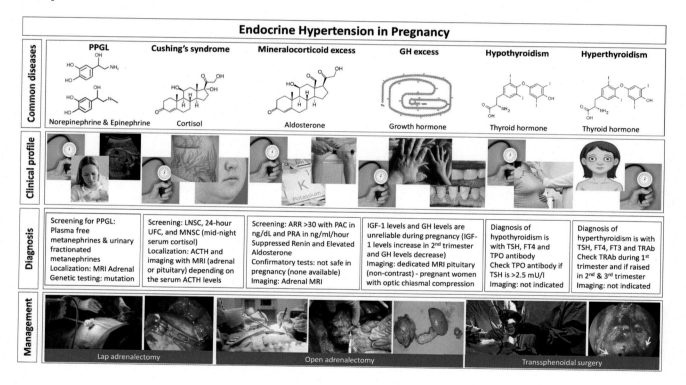

Endocrine Hypertension. https://doi.org/10.1016/B978-0-323-96120-2.00004-2

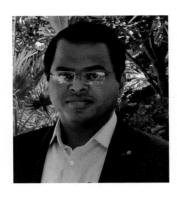

Felix Jebasingh

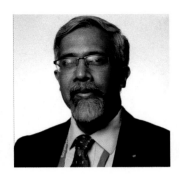

Nihal Thomas

Introduction

Endocrine disorders in pregnancy which may precipitate hypertension, such as primary aldosteronism (PA), pheochromocytoma, or Cushing syndrome (CS), are uncommon [1]. Causes which are much less frequently observed may include primary hyperparathyroidism and acromegaly. However, these disorders are associated with a rather significant quantum of maternal and fetal morbidity and mortality. Both in the general population as well as among pregnant women, the diagnosis of hypertension is being made with greater frequency than in the past [2].

Pregnancy is associated with physiological changes in the hypothalamo-pituitary-adrenal (HPA) axis with a resultant increase in cortisol, renin, and aldosterone levels but with no alteration in the catecholamine levels. This makes the diagnosis of primary hyperaldosteronism and CS challenging during pregnancy. On the other hand, it may be relatively more straightforward to make a diagnosis of pheochromocytoma during pregnancy, if a high index of clinical suspicion is maintained [3,4]. This chapter details the clinical, diagnostic, and therapeutic approaches to endocrine hypertension in pregnancy.

Primary hyperaldosteronism in pregnancy

In a pregnant woman presenting with resistant hypertension or hypertension with low serum potassium levels without vomiting, primary hyperaldosteronism should be considered as one of the differential diagnoses in addition to gestation-related hypertension. However, one should remember that more than half of all patients with primary hyperaldosteronism might present with normal serum potassium levels [5]. Therefore, resistant hypertension with normokalaemia in a young patient warrants an evaluation for primary hyperaldosteronism.

During pregnancy, there is a significant physiological alteration in the blood volume due to an increase in renin and aldosterone levels as well as atrial natriuretic peptide levels. However, hypokalemia does not occur despite having high renin and aldosterone levels [6,7]

Renin and aldosterone levels rise in pregnancy, causing an alteration in the aldosterone and renin ratio (ARR). This change was observed as early as the sixth week of gestation. During pregnancy, renin is generated in the kidney and placenta. The factors that regulate renin from the placenta are not clearly understood. Though there is an increased level of angiotensin II, this is countered by a reduction in responsiveness to angiotensin II. Moreover, aldosterone levels may increase up to 10 times greater than the normal limit, toward the end of gestation [8]. Despite all these hormonal alterations, an intact renin-angiotensin-aldosterone system (RAAS) is maintained during pregnancy. Progesterone plays an important role in potassium homeostasis, which acts as a competitive aldosterone inhibitor on the mineralocorticoid receptor, thereby maintaining normal plasma potassium levels in pregnant women despite having activated the RAAS [9].

A previous history of periodic paralysis that has been associated with hypertension also helps in suspecting the clinical diagnosis of primary hyperaldosteronism. A lowered serum potassium with an elevated bicarbonate level, without an associated gastrointestinal loss of potassium, provides clues to the diagnosis [10]. Since there is a physiological alteration in the angiotensin—renin—aldosterone axis, a biochemical diagnosis of primary hyperaldosteronism should be done diligently following serial evaluation.

A challenge that may be encountered in elucidating the diagnosis is that there are no large-scale studies that clearly define the ARR cutoff values in pregnant women with primary hyperaldosteronism. Studies have shown that the

TABLE-19.1 Displaying the antihypertensives and the safety categorization on their use in pregnancy.

Medications	Category	Dose (as divided doses)	Dosage intervals
Alpha methyldopa	B	500 mg–3 g	Twice to thrice daily
Labetalol	C	200–1200 mg	Twice to thrice daily
Nifedipine	C	30–120 mg	Twice to thrice daily
Hydralazine	C	50–300 mg	Twice to thrice daily
Beta blocker	C	Dosage depends on the drug	Once (sustained-release) to twice daily
Hydrochlorothiazide	C	12.5–50 mg	Once daily

nonpregnant reference interval for the diagnosis of primary hyperaldosteronism in itself is adequate for the diagnoses of primary hyperaldosteronism [10].

Definitive diagnostic tests such as the saline loading test, captopril test, or fludrocortisone test may not be appropriate to conduct in pregnant women, as they have not been clearly studied and there are certainly concerns with their safety during pregnancy. Once the diagnosis is confirmed, the subsequent challenge is to choose the appropriate imaging modalities to confirm the diagnosis of primary hyperaldosteronism [11]. Due to the lack of radiation risk, magnetic resonance imaging (MRI) of the abdomen may be preferred over a computed tomography (CT) scan during pregnancy. In pregnancy, the prevalence of an adrenal adenoma is far more common than that of bilateral adrenal hyperplasia [12]. The therapy of hyperaldosteronism due to bilateral adrenal hyperplasia involves the usage of mineralocorticoid receptor antagonists such as spironolactone or eplerenone. However, spironolactone may potentially cause feminization of the male fetus [13].

Therefore, therapy with calcium channel blockers such as verapamil may be a safe alternative for blood pressure control along with oral potassium supplements in patients with primary hyperaldosteronism. By and large, none of the antihypertensive agents which are commonly used, may be categorized as safe in pregnancy, particularly with reference to the first trimester. The medications that may be of use during pregnancy are shown in Table 19.1.

During the second trimester, patients may be given eplerenone, which is a safe alternative for spironolactone owing to its selective mineralocorticoid receptor antagonist property without a feminisation effect [11]. However, in situations wherein inadvertent usage of spironolactone has been reported, feminization of the male fetus has not been observed.

Patients with Conn's syndrome having a definite adrenal adenoma may need surgical excision during the latter half of the second trimester. Adrenal adenomas that are diagnosed during early pregnancy should be treated with antihypertensives and potassium supplements until the end of the second trimester by which time surgery may be relatively safe for mother and fetus [14].

During the postoperative phase, nearly 5% of patients have mineralocorticoid deficiency, and therefore close monitoring of these patients with serum sodium and potassium is required after surgery. Persistent hypotension during the postoperative period is a marker for mineralocorticoid deficiency. These patients might require a short duration of mineralocorticoid replacement [15].

A few may require antihypertensive agents even after surgery, particularly if they have end-organ damage in the form of proteinuria, severe hypertensive retinopathy, or left ventricular hypertrophy. Therefore, evaluation for end-organ damage will provide predictive clues for the persistence of hypertension following adrenalectomy [16].

An algorithm for evaluation and management of primary hyperaldosteronism is shown in Figure 19. 1

Retroperitoneal approach through laparoscopy is considered to be safe in pregnancy for the resection of adrenal tumours [17-19].

For more detailed reading on primary hyperaldosteronism, please refer Chapters 7, 8, and 21.

Cushing syndrome in pregnancy

Patients with CS may have associated suppression of gonadotrophins, and thereby they often have menstrual irregularities which may subsequently result in anovulation [20]. Therefore, infertility is common among patients with CS. However, patients with CS may present for the first time with isolated severe hypertension during pregnancy.

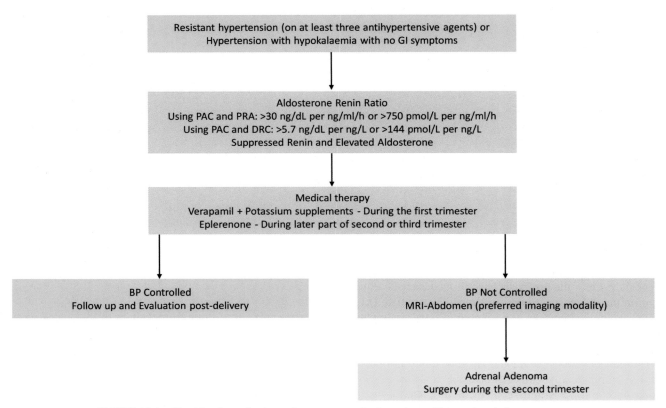

FIGURE 19.1 Algorithm for evaluation and management of primary hyperaldosteronism during pregnancy.

Untreated CS increases the risk of spontaneous abortion, perinatal death, premature birth, intrauterine growth retardation, hypertension, preeclampsia, and diabetes mellitus [21]. Adrenal adenomas are the causes of CS in up to 50% of pregnant women with endogenous CS, in contrast to only 15% of endogenous CS in nonpregnant women [22].

Unlike patients with primary hyperaldosteronism, patients with endogenous CS may have specific clinical features such as weight gain, hirsutism, emotional lability, and acne which may also be occasionally seen in normal pregnant women. However, a triad of hypertension, ecchymosis, and proximal muscle weakness in a pregnant woman should raise the suspicion of CS [23].

Once clinically suspected, the diagnosis may include a confirmation of altered circadian rhythm with a mid-night sleeping serum cortisol of more than 1.8 mcg/dL (50 nmol/L) or awake serum cortisol of more than 7.5 mcg/dL (207 nmol/L). Often, the effect of one milligram overnight dexamethasone suppression test response on the 8.00 am serum cortisol may be blunted and is therefore largely unreliable. This effect may be commonly observed during the second and third trimesters of pregnancy [24,25]. Moreover, the 24-hour urine free cortisol may be also misleading, as it may be up to threefold high among normal pregnant women resulting from an increase in the circulating cortisol. The high-dose dexamethasone suppression test also usually shows a variable result [26].

However, a quadrupling of elevated urinary free cortisol levels may be used alongside other confirmatory tests for the diagnosis of CS in pregnancy. In addition, the ACTH levels can be non-suppressed even in patients with an adrenal adenoma due to the impact of placental CRH on the maternal pituitary gland [27]. Recent evidence suggests that threefold the upper limit of normal late-night salivary cortisol or LNSC (>12 nmol/L; the normal upper limit of late-night salivary cortisol being 145 ng/dL or 4 nmol/L) has a 100% sensitivity and specificity for the diagnosis of overt CS in nonpregnant subjects [28]. Another recent study has shown that the same late-night cortisol cutoffs as healthy women can be used in pregnant women and women on oral contraceptives [29]. The LNSC threshold values for each trimester of pregnancy has been defined: <6.9 nmol/L for the first trimester, <7.2 nmol/L for the second trimester, and <9.1 nmol/L for the third trimester [30]. The LNSC is considered the most robust criterion for a positive diagnosis of CS during pregnancy [23]. More sophisticated evaluation with the statistical tools such as ROC curves, and likelihood ratios are not available for these tests during pregnancy.

An MRI without gadolinium is the most appropriate imaging modality for the localization of hypercortisolism in pregnancy [31]. However, an MRI pituitary without gadolinium might not detect a microadenoma. Moreover, the size of the pituitary increases during pregnancy, and the radiological difference between a pathological lesion and physiological enlargement may not be clearly discernible [32]. If an adrenal adenoma is suspected, an MRI of the abdomen is the imaging modality of choice to localize the lesion.

In patients with a proven hypercortisolemic state, medical or surgical therapy should be individualized to reduce the risk of fetal loss. Treating the other comorbidities such as diabetes and hypokalaemia is also important. Hypertension in patients with CS and pregnancy is treated with calcium channel blockers such as nifedipine or amlodipine, or a centrally acting medication such as methyldopa [33].

Typically, the timing of surgery for both adrenal adenomas and pituitary microadenomas should be delayed to the later part of the second trimester. Though there is no wide experience or case series available in this regard, a first-trimester surgical intervention is better avoided, as it may result in pregnancy loss [26].

If CS is diagnosed during early pregnancy, metyrapone (250−750 mg given in three divided doses per day), an inhibitor of 11β-hydroxylase in the steroidogenesis pathway of the adrenal cortex, is the medication of choice in reducing the serum cortisol to the acceptable levels for pregnancy. Metyrapone may cross the placenta, but its effect on fetal steroid production is rather negligible. Metyrapone may also cause hypertension and hypokalemia at higher doses owing to the accumulation of 11 deoxycorticosterone. Very occasionally hypocortisolemia may occur with the prolonged usage of metyrapone [34]. Therapy with ketoconazole is limited for use in patients with severe hypercortisolemia, due to its theoretical effect on potentially causing feminization of a male fetus, and maternal hepatotoxicity. However, in practice, feminization does not occur [35]. Other drugs such as mitotane, etomidate, and mifepristone that are used for hypercortisolism have severe teratogenic effects and are not studied extensively among pregnant women [36].

If metyrapone is continued throughout pregnancy, it should be temporarily withdrawn prior to labour, to maintain normal cortisol production. The therapies for the hypercortisolemic state should be restarted following childbirth. In addition, all patients on medical management, as well as those who achieve surgical remission should receive intravenous hydrocortisone during the intrapartum phase. Hydrocortisone can be gradually tapered and subsequently stopped [36].

An algorithm for diagnosis and management of CS during pregnancy is shown in Fig. 19.2.

For further reading on CS, please refer Chapters 13, 14, and 21.

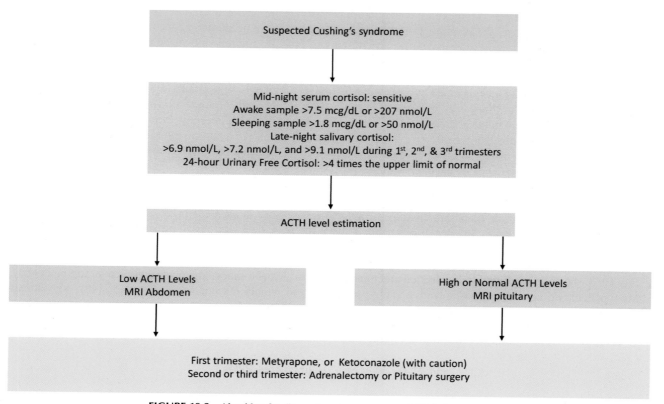

FIGURE 19.2 Algorithm for diagnosis and management of CS during pregnancy.

Pheochromocytoma and paraganglioma (PPGL) in pregnancy

Though unusual, pheochromocytoma may be a cause of secondary hypertension in pregnant women presenting with hypertension. Often, catecholamine secreting tumours cause typical paroxysmal symptoms of palpitations, impending doom, headache, tremors, and diaphoresis. However, both eclampsia and preeclampsia can raise the catecholamine levels, which could be a confounder in biochemical screening for PPGLs [37]

Episodic hypertension is a good clinical indicator in differentiating pheochromocytoma from other causes of secondary hypertension. There are several genetic mutations that are associated with PPGLs [38]. Untreated pheochromocytoma induces an increased risk for both the mother and the fetus due to uncontrolled hypertension and not due to elevated maternal catecholamine levels. Repeated cycles of episodic hypertension associated with rebound normotensive episodes may cause placental abruption, and severe hypoxia, thereby resulting in severe fetal distress [39].

The diagnosis in pregnant patients is often missed, as symptoms due to pheochromocytomas can mimic gestational hypertension or preeclampsia. However, preeclampsia is associated with proteinuria and pedal oedema, as well as sudden weight gain with associated biochemical (liver) or coagulation abnormalities. Moreover, obesity is an important risk factor that may contribute to preeclampsia. The differential diagnosis of a catecholamine secreting tumour should be considered in a pregnant woman presenting with a history of labile hypertension, headaches, palpitation, and the failure to respond to conventional antihypertensive agents. New-onset orthostatic hypotension is considered to be an important symptom in pregnant women with a pheochromocytoma. Other notable symptoms are related to cardiovascular manifestations, such as arrhythmias, acute heart failure, and cardiogenic shock [40].

Elevated 24-hour urinary fractionated metanephrine levels may suggest the diagnosis of PPGL and warrant an imaging evaluation. Plasma-free metanephrine levels may be performed in certain centres [41]. However, due to the unstable nature of metanephrines in usual laboratory conditions, it is not been frequently utilized at present in smaller centers [42,43]. An ultrasonography (USG) of the abdomen may be an initial screening modality; however, an enlarged uterus might make intraabdominal structures difficult to visualize in the case of an adrenal or a small extra-adrenal lesion. MRI of the abdomen is the most suitable imaging modality for localizing an adrenal or extra-adrenal mass during pregnancy.

Once a diagnosis is confirmed, the patient should be adequately hydrated (with at least 4—5 L of fluids per day), and salt loaded (with 8—12 g of NaCl a day) along with selective alpha-adrenoceptor blockade with drugs like prazosin or doxazosin for a period of 10—14 days. A nonselective alpha-blocker such as phenoxybenzamine might also be used; however, it should be reserved for life-threatening hypertension, as phenoxybenzamine may cross the placenta and could cause hypotension in the neonate. Moreover, it could induce perinatal depression in the mother. Prazosin and doxazocin are both safe alternatives to phenoxybenzamine. Beta-adrenergic blockers should be started preoperatively following adequate alpha-adrenergic blockade to prevent perioperative arrhythmia risk [44]. Beta-adrenergic blockers should be initiated prior to surgery to keep the heart rate less than 90/min. Esmolol, a cardio-selective β1 adrenergic receptor antagonist, or metoprolol (category-C) can be used as a beta-adrenergic blocking agent. Some studies also suggested that labetalol, a mixed α and β receptor antagonist, is a safe alternative owing to its short duration of action. In patients with preeclampsia, magnesium sulphate is a safe medication and is of value in preventing further progression to eclampsia. Magnesium sulphate inhibits the catecholamine release, induces the peripheral catecholamine receptor level blockade, and is a direct vasodilator. Other medications that are effective in the setting of a hypertensive crisis are hydralazine, nitroglycerine, and sodium nitroprusside. Due to the short-acting nature of esmolol and labetalol, both these medications can be used in hypertensive crises in the presence of tachyarrhythmias [45].

Surgery is the definitive treatment for a pheochromocytoma. There are no definitive guidelines for the timing of surgery in pregnancy. However, the timing depends on the gestational age, the accessibility of the tumour, and the presence of foetal distress. According to the literature, the tumour removal can be done in early pregnancy following adequate alpha- and beta-adrenoceptor blockade [46]. If the diagnosis is made after 24 weeks of gestation, surgical excision is recommended along with a caesarean section. Normal vaginal delivery has been shown to be associated with a higher maternal mortality rate in comparison with a caesarean section [47].

Fig. 19. 3. shows an algorithm for evaluation and management of pheochromocytoma/paraganglioma during pregnancy.

Most patients do not require postoperative antihypertensives and remain normotensive afterwards [48]. All patients with pheochromocytomas should be screened for genetic causes for PPGL syndromes such as multiple endocrine neoplasia 2a and 2b (MEN2a/MEN2b), von Hippel-Lindau (VHL), or *SDH* mutation related syndromes. Moreover, patients with a PPGL syndrome should be followed up periodically for the tumour recurrence as well as other manifestations of the genetic mutations.

Please refer to Chapters 2, 10, 11, and 21 for additional reading about PPGLs

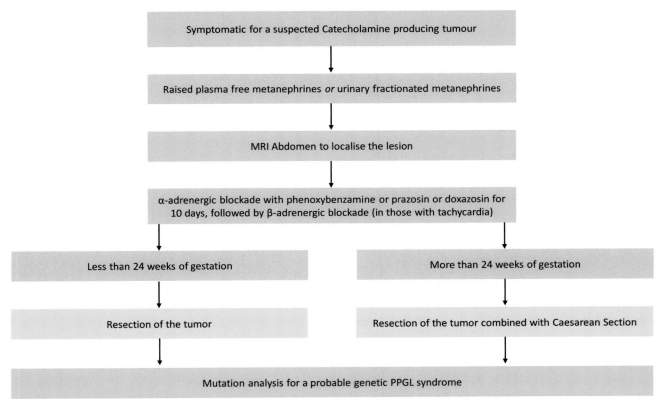

FIGURE 19.3 Algorithm for evaluation and management of pheochromocytoma/paraganglioma in pregnancy.

Primary hyperparathyroidism

Primary hyperparathyroidism very rarely presents with hypertension as an initial manifestation in pregnant women with a reported prevalence of ~0.9% in the general population. The calcium requirement for the developing fetus increases to a peak level toward the end of the third trimester. During the initial two trimesters, due to hemodilution and decrease in the albumin concentration, the serum calcium levels drop to low normal levels, but with no change in the ionised calcium or phosphate levels. An increase in calcium requirements during the third trimester is augmented by an increase in the parathyroid hormone related polypeptide (PTHrP) levels which may be secreted by various maternal organs. The calcium levels in the developing fetus are maintained by maternal as well as its own circulating serum calcium [49].

The maternal complications associated with hypercalcemia include nephrolithiasis, pancreatitis, and pre-eclampsia. Severe hypercalcemia may also cause vomiting and dehydration, thereby aggravating hyperemesis gravidarum. The fetal complications due to hypercalcemia include intrauterine growth restriction, preterm delivery, low birth weight, neonatal hypocalcemia, tetany, and an increased risk of miscarriage. Patients with primary hyperparathyroidism in pregnancy, in general have a past history suggestive of fractures or renal stones, if the hypercalcemia is very severe [50]. A minority of pregnant women with primary hyperparathyroidism may have worsening hypercalcemia during pregnancy due to the effect of PTHrP, and this could potentially precipitate a hypercalcemic crisis [51]. Significant hypertension associated with primary hyperparathyroidism is rather uncommon or rare, and is generally not severe. Biochemical diagnosis of hyperparathyroidism may be associated with hypercalcemia, hypercalciuria, and phosphaturia with elevated parathormone levels. Ultrasonography of neck is the imaging modality of choice for the localization of a parathyroid adenoma. Nuclear scans such as parathyroid scintigraphy and other imaging modalities like 4D CT are contraindicated in pregnancy [52].

The conservative management may largely encompass hydration and avoiding calcium supplementation. The level of calcium at which surgery should most certainly be advocated is still not clear due to a paucity of data [49]. Bisphosphonates should be avoided due to their teratogenic effects on the fetus [53]. Limited evidence suggests that cinacalcet and other calcimimetic agents may be used with caution in cases of severe hypercalcemia [54]. The Second trimester is the most appropriate time to plan for parathyroidectomy [52,55]. Postoperative transient hypocalcemia should be managed with at most care, as it may precipitate hypercalcemia in the fetus. Hence, therapy with calcium and activated vitamin D should be initiated if postoperative hypocalcemia is detected.

Though a majority of patients with primary hyperparathyroidism (up to 90%) occur sporadically, the remaining patients may have an associated genetic cause for parathyroid adenoma, that includes MEN1, MEN2A, MEN4, hyperparathyroidism jaw tumour (HPT-JT) syndrome, and familial isolated primary hyperparathyroidism (FIPH) [42]. Therefore, genetic testing in pregnant women should be considered for syndromic causes for primary hyperparathyroidism as most patients present at an early age with hypercalcemia [56].

Please refer Chapters 16 and 21 for additional reading on this topic.

Hyperthyroidism and hypothyroidism in pregnancy

Pregnancy and its impact on the thyroid have been well studied [57]. The fetal thyroid gland functions from 18 to 20 weeks of gestation, and until then the fetus mostly depends on maternal thyroxine. Physiological changes of pregnancy such as an increase in the concentration of thyroxine−binding globulin (TBG) due to a hyper-estrogenic state, increased urinary iodide clearance, and an increase in thyroxine degradation by type 3 deiodinase in the placenta occur during pregnancy. However, higher concentrations of human chorionic gonadotropin (hCG), which is a weak agonist of the TSH receptor, induces an increase in thyroxine production [58].

Thyroid hormone-related disorders are common in pregnancy. However, those disorders which present as hypertension in pregnancy are very rare. Poorly controlled or untreated thyrotoxicosis precipitates miscarriages, gestational hypertension, prematurity, low birth weight, intrauterine growth retardation in the fetus, and thyroid storm as well as congestive heart failure in the mother. Studies have shown that uncontrolled thyrotoxicosis during pregnancy increases the risk of preterm delivery and severe pre-eclampsia by 16 and 5 fold, respectively [59-61].

The diagnosis of over hyperthyroidism includes suppressed TSH and elevated free and total thyroxine levels. One should keep in mind that the pregnant women can have TSH in the low normal range and total thyroxine up to 1.5 times the upper limit of normal owing to the physiological changes that have already been described [62]. The therapy for hyperthyroidism includes therapy with beta-adrenergic blockers for sympathetic overactivity and controlling hyperthyroxinemia with antithyroid medications [62].

Antithyroid drugs such as methimazole or propylthiouracil are both associated with very occasional adverse effects when used in the early gestational period. Propylthiouracil may rarely be associated with maternal liver injury. The fetal effects include birth defects, such as preauricular sinuses and hydronephrosis. In addition, methimazole or carbimazole may be associated with maternal agranulocytosis and foetal malformations such as choanal atresia, aplasia cutis, and omphalocele [63]. Both these effects are generally idiosyncratic and could be dose-dependent, and often noticed when used at higher doses. These adverse effects can be avoided by using the lowest possible dose of antithyroid drugs. Using "block and replace" therapy in the form of antithyroid drugs and levothyroxine is not a good option for pregnant women with hyperthyroidism [63,64].

All patients treated with antithyroid drugs should be followed up at least once in 2−3 weeks initially to keep the free thyroxine level (FT4) close to the upper limit of normal. Most often, toward the third trimester, the dose of antithyroid medications need to be reduced to the lowest possible dose or may need to be withdrawn due to associated immune tolerance in the fetus. Large scale studies have shown that the use of propylthiouracil during the first trimester is associated with a lower risk of fetal adverse effects compared to carbimazole. Therefore, switching over to propylthiouracil is needed in women who are already on methimazole. Once the 16-week critical period of organogenesis has been crossed, the patients may be switched over to methimazole. Radio-iodine ablation is contraindicated in pregnant women [65].

A persistently high TSH receptor antibody (TRab) of more than three times the upper limit of normal during the third trimester is associated with an increased risk of fetal hyperthyroidism [66]. Therefore, for all the patients with newly detected hyperthyroidism as well as those who have already been treated with antithyroid drugs or are in remission, TRAb should be checked. Patients can be kept on follow-up if the maternal TRAb levels are low or undetectable during the first trimester.

If TRAb is high, TRAb should be repeated between 18 and 22 weeks. Of those with more than 3 times the upper limit, TRAb should be rechecked between 28 and 34 weeks as this poses a high risk for fetal hyperthyroidism [66].

Thyroidectomy should be reserved for those who are not tolerating antithyroid drugs or requiring a very high dose for control of hyperthyroid symptoms, or have an allergy to antithyroid medications, or those with a large goitre. An algorithm for evaluation and management of hyperthyroidism in pregnancy is shown in Fig. 19.4.

Untreated hypothyroidism can cause predominantly diastolic hypertension due to increased peripheral vascular resistance. The symptoms of hypothyroidism are highly variable and can be asymptomatic too. Universal screening for

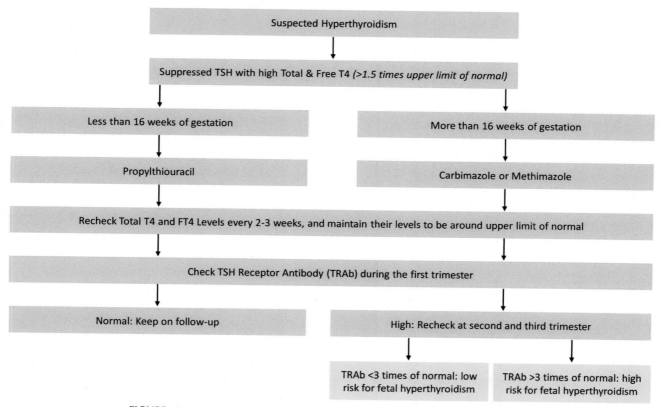

FIGURE 19.4 Algorithm for evaluation and management of hyperthyroidism in pregnancy.

hypothyroidism evaluation is not indicated in pregnancy. Because of the physiological changes in pregnancy, the reference range of thyroid hormone differs from that of the general population. The therapy for hypothyroidism involves replacement with thyroxine. Subclinical hypothyroidism (SCH) is more common in pregnancy, and hypertension is not a common clinical feature of SCH [67]. However, studies have demonstrated that patients with SCH detected during pregnancy may have a higher risk for preeclampsia (odds ratio—1.6) when compared to euthyroid women [68]. Following is an algorithm for evaluation and management of hypothyroidism in pregnancy (Fig. 19.5)

Please refer Chapters 16 for further reading on thyroid disease and hypertension.

Acromegaly in pregnancy

Hypertension is seen in more than 50% of patients diagnosed with acromegaly [69]. There are several mechanisms behind the occurrence of hypertension in patients with acromegaly. Untreated or partially treated acromegaly may cause hypertension during pregnancy [70].

In pregnancy, Human Placental Growth Hormone Variant (HGH-V) and Human Placental Lactogen (hPL), the latter also known as Human Chorionic Somatomammotropin are produced by the placenta. The pituitary gland increases in height during pregnancy to up to 12 mm. The increase in size is due to the increase in the number of lactotrophs secondary to the hyper-estrogenic state. During normal pregnancy, the somatotrophs are suppressed due to an increase in maternal insulin-like growth factor-1 (IGF-1) secondary to an enhanced production of HGH-V from the syncytiotrophoblast. The maternal IGF-1 level is suppressed during the first half of the pregnancy and increased during the second half of pregnancy due to placental HGH-V as well as hPL. Hence, with the impact of elevated IGF-1 concentration during the second half of pregnancy, the maternal HGH level is suppressed. However, placental HGH-V does not cross-react with the currently available commercial HGH assays [58]. Caron and colleagues have shown that amongst those with acromegaly, around 14% of women developed hypertension, and 7% developed diabetes mellitus during pregnancy [70].

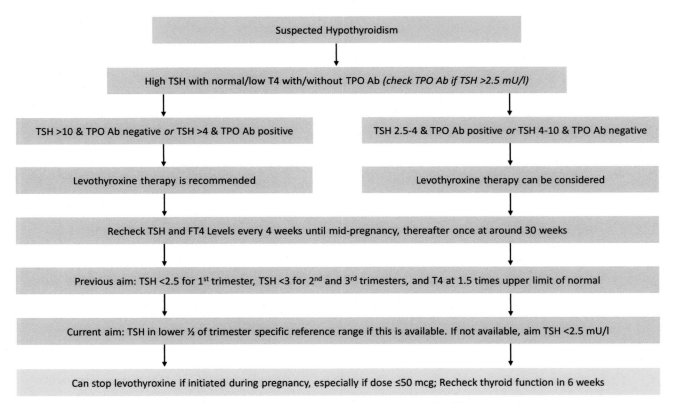

FIGURE 19.5 Algorithm for evaluation and management of hypothyroidism in pregnancy.

An untreated or partially treated growth hormone-producing tumor is a cause for infertility due to the suppression of gonadotropin as well as associated hyperprolactinemia. Growth hormone-producing pituitary macroadenomas theoretically increase in size. However, studies have shown that only around 10% of patients with acromegaly and a residual tumor increased in size during the pregnancy [71].

GH levels are elevated in patients with untreated or partially treated acromegaly. IGF1 levels are higher than anticipated in pregnant women with acromegaly due to the physiological alterations that occur during pregnancy. If the patients were on medical therapy for acromegaly, the therapy should be discontinued once pregnancy is confirmed. Available literature suggests that patients with less than 1 cm tumour or residue could be followed by trimester intervals for visual symptoms, as these do not increase in size. Residual or untreated tumour size more than 1 cm, or those on medical treatment for less than a year before conception should be followed monthly for visual defects or with visual field assessment. In those with clinical features of optic chiasmal compression, MRI pituitary without gadolinium contrast can be performed to see the extent of the tumour. Further treatment for acromegaly depends on the gestational age. The medical treatment with the dopamine agonists cabergoline should be advocated in case of worsening symptoms during the first trimester. In case of cabergoline failure, pituitary surgery is performed in the second trimester [72].

Somatostatin analogues are found to cross the placenta, and hence should be avoided, but can be used with caution as there are no safety profile concerns available on octreotide or lanreotide [73]. Use of cabergoline during pregnancy is associated with fetal macrosomia with no other major congenital anomalies [74]. Hence, the use of cabergoline should be limited only for patients with visual symptoms. Other pituitary hormones should be evaluated in pregnancy and should be replaced accordingly. An algorithm for evaluation and management of acromegaly during pregnancy is shown in Fig. 19.6.

For detailed additional reading about acromegaly, please refer Chapter 15.

Rare causes of endocrine hypertension in pregnancy

Other rarer causes of endocrine hypertension include adrenal cortical carcinomas (ACC), Deoxycorticosterone-secreting adrenal tumors, Liddle syndrome, and familial hyperaldosteronism.

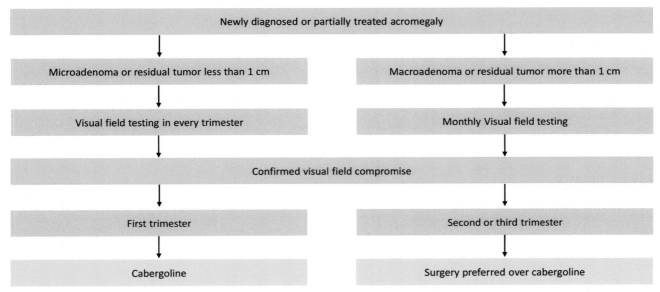

FIGURE 19.6 An algorithm for evaluation and management of acromegaly during pregnancy.

Adrenal cortical carcinoma/deoxycorticosterone-secreting adrenal tumor

ACC is an extremely rare cause of hypertension. If the ACC produces androgens, it generally causes virilization, and therefore infertility. An adrenocortical carcinoma might present with features of CS (as discussed previously) without skin hyperpigmentation. The laboratory assessment includes demonstration of hypercortisolemia with suppressed ACTH levels. The fetus may express the ill effects of hypercortisolemia as discussed previously. An MRI of the abdomen is the imaging modality for patients with suspected ACC. The second trimester is the appropriate time for intervention in pregnant women.

A deoxycorticosterone-secreting adrenal tumour is the tumour which secretes deoxycorticosterone, and predominantly causes hypertension and hypokalemia along with metabolic alkalosis. The specific biochemical findings include suppressed renin activity with normal to low aldosterone and elevated deoxycorticosterone (DOC) with normal cortisol, deoxycortisol, testosterone, and dehydroepiandrosterone (DHEA). As CT abdomen is contraindicated in pregnancy and MRI abdomen is the imaging choice for localizing the tumour [75].

Liddle's syndrome

Another rare cause of hypertension and metabolic alkalosis is Liddle's syndrome. Liddle syndrome is due to the mutation that encodes ENaC (Epithelial Sodium channels) wherein aldosterone acts in the collecting tubule. The biochemical profile includes hypokalemic metabolic alkalosis, suppressed renin, and aldosterone levels. The treatment for Liddle's syndrome is with amiloride or triamterene. Inhibitors of ENaC such as amiloride (category B) are preferred in pregnancy over triamterene (category C) due to its effect on folic acid metabolism. Treatment with amiloride usually resolves hypertension and hypokalemia [76]. For additional reading about Liddle syndrome, please refer Chapters 6, 10, and 21.

Very rare causes of hypertension during pregnancy also includes hypopituitarism as well as familial hyperaldosteronism [77].

Hypopituitarism

In hypopituitarism, patients generally have primary infertility. However, due to the other hormonal deficiencies, hypertension can be a feature during pregnancy. Treatment of other hormonal axes particularly thyroxine and glucocorticoid replacement are important since they pose a greater risk for maternal and fetal morbidity as well as mortality [78]. For additional reading, please refer Chapters 15.

Familial hyperaldosteronism

Familial hyperaldosteronism (FH) is another extremely rare cause of endocrine hypertension in pregnant women. An important indicator for the suspicion is the family history of young-onset stroke, aortic dissection, and severe uncontrolled hypertension. These patients can have paradoxical normalisation of blood pressure due to the increase in progesterone and its antagonistic effect on mineralocorticoid receptors [79]. Also, progesterone has been shown to inhibit the chimeric form of aldosterone synthase activity in vitro among patients with FH-I, the most common form of FH [80]. The biochemical profile bears similarity to that of primary hyperaldosteronism. However, the treatment of choice for this disorder is low-dose dexamethasone (0.25–0.5mg/day) [81]. However, chronic use of dexamethasone during pregnancy precipitates preterm labor, and intrauterine growth retardation [82]. For further reading, please refer Chapters 7, 8, and 21.

Geller syndrome

Geller syndrome is an uncommon autosomal dominant disorder due to gain-of-function mutations in the mineralocorticoid receptors allowing atypical stimulation by other steroids. This is a familial syndrome of hypertension (HTN) and hypokalemia, that is exacerbated by pregnancy due to the effect of progesterone on the mutated mineralocorticoid receptors. One of the close differential diagnoses for Geller syndrome is Liddle's syndrome. These patients have low serum renin and low aldosterone levels. Amiloride is the drug of choice for patients with this mutation which ameliorates hypertension as well as the serum potassium levels [83,84]. For additional reading, please refer Chapters 6 and 10.

Summary and conclusions

Hypertension is a common disorder that complicates pregnancy, and its prevalence has increased multifold in the recent times. There are several causes of endocrine-related hypertension. A detailed history, particularly involving a family history and a diligent clinical examination may help in clinching the endocrine diagnosis. Moreover, due to physiological changes involving a multitude of hormonal axes occurring during pregnancy, there can be alterations in the usual laboratory picture that must be duly considered. Therefore, a physician should keep this fact in mind while interpreting the biochemical and hormonal investigations. Moreover, specific therapy of the underlying endocrine disorder, along with customized usage of antihypertensive medications, improve subsequent fetal and maternal outcomes.

Learning points

- Hypertension is common during pregnancy
- Mild to severe hypertension may be due to an underlying endocrine disorder
- Biochemical results may be altered due to the physiological changes associated with pregnancy.
- MRI is the preferred imaging modality during gestation over CT because of the radiation risk.
- Some fetal complications could be due to suboptimal control of blood pressure, the underlying endocrine condition, or a result of the associated therapeutic agents being used.

References

[1] Affinati AH, Auchus RJ. Endocrine causes of hypertension in pregnancy. Gland Surg 2020 Feb;9(1):69−79.

[2] Ananth CV, Duzyj CM, Yadava S, Schwebel M, Tita ATN, Joseph KS. Changes in the prevalence of chronic hypertension in pregnancy, United States, 1970 to 2010. Hypertension 2019;74(5):1089−95.

[3] Ross JJ, Desai AS, Chutkow WA, Economy KE, Dec GW. Interactive medical case. A crisis in late pregnancy. N Engl J Med 2009 Nov 12;361(20):e45.

[4] Desai AS, Chutkow WA, Edelman E, Economy KE, Dec GW. Clinical problem-solving. A crisis in late pregnancy. N Engl J Med 2009 Dec 3;361(23):2271−7.

[5] Rossi GP, Bernini G, Caliumi C, Desideri G, Fabris B, Ferri C, et al. A prospective study of the prevalence of primary aldosteronism in 1,125 hypertensive patients. J Am Coll Cardiol 2006 Dec 5;48(11):2293−300.

[6] August P, Mueller FB, Sealey JE, Edersheim TG. Role of renin-angiotensin system in blood pressure regulation in pregnancy. Lancet Lond Engl 1995 Apr 8;345(8954):896−7.

[7] Broughton Pipkin F, Symonds EM, Lamming GD, Jadoul FA. Renin and aldosterone concentrations in pregnant essential hypertensives - a prospective study. Clin Exp Hypertens B 1983;2(2):255−69.

[8] Landau E, Amar L. Primary aldosteronism and pregnancy. Ann Endocrinol 2016 Jun;77(2):148−60.

[9] Karlberg BE, Rydén G, Wichman K. Changes in the renin-angiotensin-aldosterone and kallikrein-kinin systems during normal and hypertensive pregnancy. Acta Obstet Gynecol Scand Suppl 1984;118:17–24.

[10] Lewandowski KC, Tadros-Zins M, Horzelski W, Grzesiak M, Lewinski A. Establishing reference ranges for aldosterone, renin and aldosterone-to-renin ratio for women in the third-trimester of pregnancy. Exp Clin Endocrinol Diabetes 2022;130(4):210–6.

[11] Vidyasagar S, Kumar S, Morton A. Screening for primary aldosteronism in pregnancy. Pregnancy Hypertens 2021 Aug;25:171–4.

[12] Morton A. Primary aldosteronism and pregnancy. Pregnancy Hypertens 2015 Oct;5(4):259–62.

[13] Liszewski W, Boull C. Lack of evidence for feminization of males exposed to spironolactone in utero: a systematic review. J Am Acad Dermatol 2019 Apr 1;80(4):1147–8.

[14] Shekhar S, Haykal R, Kamilaris C, Stratakis CA, Hannah-Shmouni F. Curative resection of an aldosteronoma causing primary aldosteronism in the second trimester of pregnancy. Endocrinol Diabetes Metab Case Rep 2020 Aug 4;2020:20–0043.

[15] Yorke E, Stafford S, Holmes D, Sheth S, Melck A. Aldosterone deficiency after unilateral adrenalectomy for Conn's syndrome: a case report and literature review. Int J Surg Case Rep 2015 Jan 10;7:141–4.

[16] Savard S, Amar L, Plouin P-F, Steichen O. Cardiovascular complications associated with primary aldosteronism. Hypertension 2013 Aug 1;62(2):331–6.

[17] Kosaka K, Onoda N, Ishikawa T, Iwanaga N, Yamamasu S, Tahara H, et al. Laparoscopic adrenalectomy on a patient with primary aldosteronism during pregnancy. Endocr J 2006 Aug;53(4):461–6.

[18] Eschler DC, Kogekar N, Pessah-Pollack R. Management of adrenal tumors in pregnancy. Endocrinol Metab Clin North Am 2015 Jun;44(2):381–97.

[19] Parasiliti-Caprino M, Bioletto F, Ceccato F, Lopez C, Bollati M, Voltan G, et al. The diagnostic accuracy of adjusted unconventional indices for adrenal vein sampling in the diagnosis of primary aldosteronism subtypes. J Hypertens 2021 May 1;39(5):1025–33.

[20] Aron DC, Schnall AM, Sheeler LR. Cushing's syndrome and pregnancy. Am J Obstet Gynecol 1990 Jan 1;162(1):244–52.

[21] Gellner K, Emonts P, Hamoir E, Beckers A, Valdes-Socin H. Cushing's syndrome during pregnancy: diagnostic and therapeutic difficulties. Rev Med Liege 2018 Dec;73(12):603–9.

[22] Lo CY, Lo CM, Lam KY. Cushing's syndrome secondary to adrenal adenoma during pregnancy. Surg Endosc 2002 Jan;16(1):219–20.

[23] Brue T, Amodru V, Castinetti F. Management of endocrine disease: management of Cushing's syndrome during pregnancy: solved and unsolved questions. Eur J Endocrinol 2018 Jun;178(6):R259–66.

[24] Odagiri E, Ishiwatari N, Abe Y, Jibiki K, Adachi T, Demura R, et al. Hypercortisolism and the resistance to dexamethasone suppression during gestation. Endocrinol Jpn 1988 Oct;35(5):685–90.

[25] Grammatopoulos DK. Placental corticotrophin-releasing hormone and its receptors in human pregnancy and labour: still a scientific enigma. J Neuroendocrinol 2008 Apr;20(4):432–8.

[26] Ildefonso-Najarro SP, Plasencia-Dueñas EA, Benites-Moya CJ, Carrion-Rojas J, Concepción-Zavaleta MJ. Pregnancy during the course of Cushing's syndrome: a case report and literature review. Endocrinol Diabetes Metab Case Rep 2020 Apr 12;2020:20–0022.

[27] Duthie L, Reynolds RM. Changes in the maternal hypothalamic-pituitary-adrenal axis in pregnancy and postpartum: influences on maternal and fetal outcomes. Neuroendocrinology 2013;98(2):106–15.

[28] Nunes M-L, Vattaut S, Corcuff J-B, Rault A, Loiseau H, Gatta B, et al. Late-night salivary cortisol for diagnosis of overt and subclinical Cushing's syndrome in hospitalized and ambulatory patients. J Clin Endocrinol Metab 2009 Feb;94(2):456–62.

[29] Ambroziak U, Kondracka A, Bartoszewicz Z, Krasnodebska-Kiljańska M, Bednarczuk T. The morning and late-night salivary cortisol ranges for healthy women may be used in pregnancy. Clin Endocrinol (Oxf). 2015 Dec;83(6):774–8.

[30] Lopes LML, Francisco RPV, Galletta MAK, Bronstein MD. Determination of nighttime salivary cortisol during pregnancy: comparison with values in non-pregnancy and Cushing's disease. Pituitary 2016 Feb;19(1):30–8.

[31] Karaca Z, Tanriverdi F, Unluhizarci K, Kelestimur F. Pregnancy and pituitary disorders. Eur J Endocrinol 2010 Mar 1;162(3):453–75.

[32] Elster AD, Sanders TG, Vines FS, Chen MY. Size and shape of the pituitary gland during pregnancy and post partum: measurement with MR imaging. Radiology 1991 Nov 1;181(2):531–5.

[33] Azzola A, Eastabrook G, Matsui D, Berberich A, Tirona RG, Gray D, et al. Adrenal Cushing syndrome diagnosed during pregnancy: successful medical management with metyrapone. J Endocr Soc 2020 2020 Nov 5;5(1):bvaa167.

[34] Blanco C, Maqueda E, Rubio JA, Rodriguez A. Cushing's syndrome during pregnancy secondary to adrenal adenoma: metyrapone treatment and laparoscopic adrenalectomy. J Endocrinol Invest 2006 Feb;29(2):164–7.

[35] Berwaerts J, Verhelst J, Mahler C, Abs R. Cushing's syndrome in pregnancy treated by ketoconazole: case report and review of the literature. Gynecol Endocrinol Off J Int Soc Gynecol Endocrinol 1999 Jun;13(3):175–82.

[36] Nieman LK, Biller BM, Findling JW, Murad MH, Newell-Price J, Savage MO, Tabarin A, Endocrine Society. Treatment of Cushing's syndrome: An endocrine society clinical practice guideline. J Clin Endocrinol Metab 2015 Aug;100(8):2807–31.

[37] Oian P, Kjeldsen SE, Eide I, Maltau JM. Increased arterial catecholamines in pre-eclampsia. Acta Obstet Gynecol Scand 1986;65(6):613–7.

[38] Alrezk R, Suarez A, Tena I, Pacak K. Update of pheochromocytoma syndromes: Genetics, biochemical evaluation, and imaging. Front Endocrinol (Lausanne) 2018 Nov 27;9:515.

[39] Gruber LM, Young WF, Bancos I. Pheochromocytoma and paraganglioma in pregnancy: a new era. Curr Cardiol Rep 2021 May 7;23(6):60.

[40] Gu YW, Poste J, Kunal M, Schwarcz M, Weiss I. Cardiovascular manifestations of pheochromocytoma. Cardiol Rev 2017 Sep/Oct;25(5):215–22.

[41] Lenders JWM, Langton K, Langenhuijsen JF, Eisenhofer G. Pheochromocytoma and pregnancy. Endocrinol Metab Clin North Am 2019 Sep;48(3):605–17.

[42] Grouzmann E, Fathi M, Gillet M, de Torrenté A, Cavadas C, Brunner H, et al. Disappearance rate of catecholamines, total metanephrines, and neuropeptide Y from the plasma of patients after resection of pheochromocytoma. Clin Chem 2001 Jun;47(6):1075−82.

[43] Kudva YC, Sawka AM, Young Jr WF. The laboratory diagnosis of adrenal pheochromocytoma: the Mayo Clinic experience. J Clin Endocrinol Metab 2003 Oct 1;88(10):4533−9.

[44] Lenders JWM. Pheochromocytoma and pregnancy: a deceptive connection. Eur J Endocrinol 2012 Feb;166(2):143−50.

[45] Prete A, Paragliola RM, Salvatori R, Corsello SM. Management of catecholamine-secreting tumors in pregnancy: a review. Endocr Pract Off J Am Coll Endocrinol Am Assoc Clin Endocrinol 2016 Mar;22(3):357−70.

[46] Lenders JW, Duh QY, Eisenhofer G, Gimenez-Roqueplo AP, Grebe SK, Murad MH, Naruse M, Pacak K, Young Jr WF, Endocrine Society. Pheochromocytoma and paraganglioma: an endocrine society clinical practice guideline. J Clin Endocrinol Metab 2014 Jun;99(6):1915−42.

[47] Ahlawat SK, Jain S, Kumari S, Varma S, Sharma BK. Pheochromocytoma associated with pregnancy: case report and review of the literature. Obstet Gynecol Surv 1999 Nov;54(11):728−37.

[48] Prakash P, Kulshrestha V, Ramachandran R, Kumar R. Successful pregnancy outcomes after laparoscopic management of pheochromocytoma. J Endourol Case Rep 2020 Sep 1;6(3):170−3.

[49] McCarthy A, Howarth S, Khoo S, Hale J, Oddy S, Halsall D, et al. Management of primary hyperparathyroidism in pregnancy: a case series. Endocrinol Diabetes Metab Case Rep 2019 May 16;2019:19−0039.

[50] DiMarco AN, Meeran K, Christakis I, Sodhi V, Nelson-Piercy C, Tolley NS, et al. Seventeen cases of primary hyperparathyroidism in pregnancy: a call for management guidelines. J Endocr Soc 2019 May 1;3(5):1009−21.

[51] Khan AA, Clarke B, Rejnmark L, Brandi ML. Management of Endocrine Disease: Hypoparathyroidism in pregnancy: review and evidence-based recommendations for management. Eur J Endocrinol 2019 Feb 1;180(2):R37−44.

[52] McMullen TP, Learoyd DL, Williams DC, Sywak MS, Sidhu SB, Delbridge LW. Hyperparathyroidism in pregnancy: options for localization and surgical therapy. World J Surg 2010 Aug;34(8):1811−6.

[53] Djokanovic N, Klieger-Grossmann C, Koren G. Does treatment with bisphosphonates endanger the human pregnancy? J Obstet Gynaecol Can JOGC J Obstet Gynecol Can JOGC 2008 Dec;30(12):1146−8.

[54] Nadarasa K, Bailey M, Chahal H, Raja O, Bhat R, Gayle C, et al. The use of cinacalcet in pregnancy to treat a complex case of parathyroid carcinoma. Endocrinol Diabetes Metab Case Rep 2014;2014:140056.

[55] Ali DS, Dandurand K, Khan AA. Primary hyperparathyroidism in pregnancy: literature review of the diagnosis and management. J Clin Med 2021 Jun 30;10(13):2956.

[56] Jiao H-N, Sun L-H, Liu Y, Zhou J-Q, Chen X, Liu J-M, et al. Multidisciplinary team efforts to improve the pregnancy outcome of pregnancy complicated with primary hyperparathyroidism: case series from a single hospital. BMC Pregnancy Childbirth 2021 Aug 22;21(1):576.

[57] Korevaar TIM, Medici M, Visser TJ, Peeters RP. Thyroid disease in pregnancy: new insights in diagnosis and clinical management. Nat Rev Endocrinol 2017 Oct;13(10):610−22.

[58] Hershman JM. The role of human chorionic gonadotropin as a thyroid stimulator in normal pregnancy. J Clin Endocrinol Metab 2008 Sep;93(9):3305−6.

[59] Lazarus J, Brown RS, Daumerie C, Hubalewska-Dydejczyk A, Negro R, Vaidya B. 2014 European thyroid association guidelines for the management of subclinical hypothyroidism in pregnancy and in children. Eur Thyroid J 2014 Jun;3(2):76−94.

[60] Alemu A, Terefe B, Abebe M, Biadgo B. Thyroid hormone dysfunction during pregnancy: a review. Int J Reprod Biomed 2016 Nov;14(11):677−86.

[61] Korevaar TIM, Steegers EAP, Chaker L, Medici M, Jaddoe VWV, Visser TJ, et al. The risk of preeclampsia according to high thyroid function in pregnancy differs by hCG concentration. J Clin Endocrinol Metab 2016 Dec;101(12):5037−43.

[62] Alexander EK, Pearce EN, Brent GA, Brown RS, Chen H, Dosiou C, et al. 2017 Guidelines of the American Thyroid Association for the diagnosis and management of thyroid disease during pregnancy and the postpartum. Thyroid 2017 Mar;27(3):315−89.

[63] Francis T, Francis N, Lazarus JH, Okosieme OE. Safety of antithyroid drugs in pregnancy: update and therapy implications. Expert Opin Drug Saf 2020 May;19(5):565−76.

[64] Azizi F, Amouzegar A. Management of hyperthyroidism during pregnancy and lactation. Eur J Endocrinol 2011 Jun;164(6):871−6.

[65] Andersen SL, Andersen S. Antithyroid drugs and birth defects. Thyroid Res 2020 Jun 27;13(1):11.

[66] Bucci I, Giuliani C, Napolitano G. Thyroid-stimulating hormone receptor antibodies in pregnancy: clinical relevance. Front Endocrinol 2017 Jun 30;8:137.

[67] Lai H, Zhan ZY, Liu H. Association between thyroid hormone parameters during early pregnancy and gestational hypertension: a prospective cohort study. J Int Med Res 2020 Feb;48(2). 300060520904814.

[68] Wilson KL, Casey BM, McIntire DD, Halvorson LM, Cunningham FG. Subclinical thyroid disease and the incidence of hypertension in pregnancy. Obstet Gynecol 2012 Feb;119(2 Pt 1):315−20.

[69] Bondanelli M, Ambrosio MR, degli Uberti EC. Pathogenesis and prevalence of hypertension in acromegaly. Pituitary 2001 Sep;4(4):239−49.

[70] Caron P, Broussaud S, Bertherat J, Borson-Chazot F, Brue T, Cortet-Rudelli C, Chanson P. Acromegaly and pregnancy: A retrospective multicenter study of 59 pregnancies in 46 women. J Clin Endocrinol Metab 2010 Oct;95(10):4680−7.

[71] Petersenn S, Christ-Crain M, Droste M, Finke R, Flitsch J, Kreitschmann-Andermahr I, et al. Pituitary disease in pregnancy: special aspects of diagnosis and treatment? Geburtshilfe Frauenheilkd 2019 Apr;79(4):365−74.

[72] Chanson P, Vialon M, Caron P. An update on clinical care for pregnant women with acromegaly. Expert Rev Endocrinol Metab 2019 Mar;14(2):85−96.

[73] Hannon AM, Frizelle I, Kaar G, Hunter SJ, Sherlock M, Thompson CJ, et al. Octreotide use for rescue of vision in a pregnant patient with acromegaly. Endocrinol Diabetes Metab Case Rep 2019 May 20;2019. 19−0019.

[74] Lebbe M, Hubinont C, Bernard P, Maiter D. Outcome of 100 pregnancies initiated under treatment with cabergoline in hyperprolactinaemic women. Clin Endocrinol (Oxf) 2010 Aug;73(2):236−42.

[75] Marques P, Tufton N, Bhattacharya S, Caulfield M, Akker SA. Hypertension due to a deoxycorticosterone-secreting adrenal tumour diagnosed during pregnancy. Endocrinol Diabetes Metab Case Rep 2019 May 3;2019:18−0164.

[76] Awadalla M, Patwardhan M, Alsamsam A, Imran N. Management of Liddle syndrome in pregnancy: a case report and literature review. Case Rep Obstet Gynecol 2017;2017:6279460.

[77] Laway BA, Mir SA. Pregnancy and pituitary disorders: challenges in diagnosis and management. Indian J Endocrinol Metab 2013;17(6):996−1004.

[78] Du X, Yuan Q, Yao Y, Li Z, Zhang H. Hypopituitarism and successful pregnancy. Int J Clin Exp Med 2014 Dec 15;7(12):4660−5.

[79] Campino C, Trejo P, Carvajal CA, Vecchiola A, Valdivia C, Fuentes CA, et al. Pregnancy normalized familial hyperaldosteronism type I: a novel role for progesterone? J Hum Hypertens 2015 Feb;29(2):138−9.

[80] Vecchiola A, Lagos CF, Fuentes CA, Allende F, Campino C, Valdivia C, et al. Different effects of progesterone and estradiol on chimeric and wild type aldosterone synthase in vitro. Reprod Biol Endocrinol RBE 2013 Aug 13;11:76.

[81] Sanga V, Lenzini L, Seccia TM, Rossi GP. Familial hyperaldosteronism type 1 and pregnancy: successful treatment with low dose dexamethasone. Blood Press 2021 Apr;30(2):133−7.

[82] Elsnosy E, Shaaban OM, Abbas AM, Gaber HH, Darwish A. Effects of antenatal dexamethasone administration on fetal and uteroplacental Doppler waveforms in women at risk for spontaneous preterm birth. Middle East Fertil Soc J 2017 Mar 1;22(1):13−7.

[83] Geller DS, Farhi A, Pinkerton N, Fradley M, Moritz M, Spitzer A, et al. Activating mineralocorticoid receptor mutation in hypertension exacerbated by pregnancy. Science 2000 Jul 7;289(5476):119−23.

[84] Pintavorn P, Munie S. A case report of recurrent hypokalemia during pregnancies associated with nonaldosterone-mediated renal potassium loss. Can J Kidney Health Dis 2021 May 28;8. 20543581211017424.

Further reading

[1] Management of Primary aldosteronism: case detection, diagnosis, and treatment: an endocrine society clinical practice guideline I the journal of clinical endocrinology & metabolism I Oxford Academic [Internet]. [cited 2022 Feb 5]. Available from: https://academic.oup.com/jcem/article/101/5/1889/2804729.

Chapter 20

Imaging for patients with endocrine hypertension

Katherine Ordidge[1] and Anju Sahdev[2]

[1]Consultant Radiologist, Department of Imaging, St Bartholomew's Hospital, Barts Health NHS Trust, London, United Kingdom; [2]Consultant Radiologist, Department of Imaging, St Bartholomew's Hospital, Barts Health NHS Trust and Clinical Professor of Diagnostic Imaging, Barts Cancer Institute, Queen Mary University Hospital, London, United Kingdom

Visit the *Endocrine Hypertension: From Basic Science to Clinical Practice, First Edition* companion web site at: https://www.elsevier.com/books-and-journals/book-companion/9780323961202.

Graphical Abstract

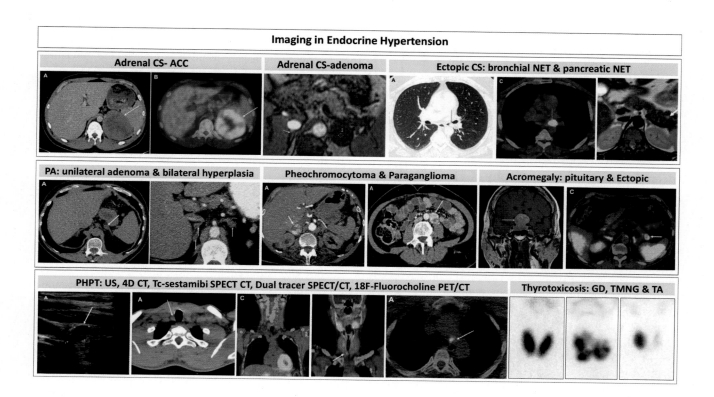

Endocrine Hypertension. https://doi.org/10.1016/B978-0-323-96120-2.00013-3

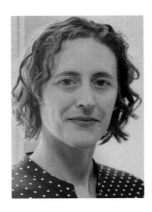

Katherine Ordidge

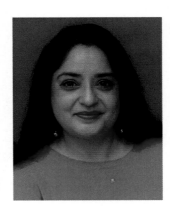

Anju Sahdev

Introduction

Among adults with hypertension, nearly 85% have idiopathic (essential) hypertension, the rest have secondary hypertension. Hypertension secondary to endocrine disease accounts for about 5%–10% among the adult population with high blood pressure [1]. The common causes for endocrine hypertension include excessive production of mineralocorticoids (primary hyperaldosteronism), glucocorticoids (Cushing's syndrome [CS]), and catecholamines (pheochromocytoma [PCC]) [2,3]. Less frequent causes of endocrine hypertension include primary hyperparathyroidism (PHPT), hypothyroidism, hyperthyroidism, acromegaly, and Adult Growth Hormone Deficiency (AGHD).

Imaging studies are an important supplement to the diagnosis of diseases associated with endocrine hypertension. The role of anatomical and functional imaging studies includes localization of the lesions, surgical planning, assessment of treatment response, and surveillance following treatment. In patients with endocrine hypertension, the cause when detected is usually clear and can be treated surgically in most cases. Surgical intervention may result in complete cure, obviating lifelong antihypertensive treatment or significantly decrease the number or dosage of medical treatments required to control the hypertension. Computed tomography (CT), magnetic resonance imaging (MRI), ultrasonography (US), and several nuclear medicine imaging techniques are used to evaluate the adrenal, thyroid, and pituitary gland. This chapter discusses the relevant imaging modalities, their advantages, and disadvantages in the diagnostic work up of patients with endocrine hypertension.

Adrenal computed tomography (CT)

Advantages of CT imaging include its high throughput, comparative low cost, and good spatial resolution crucial for the detection of small lesions. On CT imaging, the normal adrenal gland appears as an inverted "Y"- or "V"-shaped organ surrounded by retroperitoneal fat and lies superior to the upper pole of the kidneys. CT imaging with a 3-phase protocol is used to characterize adrenal lesions based on their density and contrast enhancement properties. However, it cannot differentiate functioning from nonfunctioning adenomas. A standard adrenal CT protocol includes an unenhanced non-contrast phase, portal venous (PV) contrast enhanced phase 60 seconds after intravenous contrast injection, and a delayed phase 15 minutes after intravenous contrast injection. Adrenal adenomas are identified as well-defined homogenous nodules. On non-contrast CT if the density is less than 10 Hounsfield units (HU), an adrenal nodule can be confidently diagnosed as a lipid-rich adenoma with 71% sensitivity and 98% specificity (Fig. 20.1) [4]. This low density is due to the presence of intracellular fat, and no further imaging for the diagnosis of an adenoma is needed. 70% of adenomas are lipid rich [5]. If the non-contrast CT density is above 10HU, the lesion is equivocal, and the patient can proceed to contrast enhanced imaging to measure contrast washout properties of the lesion. Approximately one-third of adenomas are lipid-poor and do not contain enough intracellular fat to have a density below 10HU on unenhanced CT. However, they will show rapid washout of contrast on delayed phase imaging, compared to other adrenal lesions such as PCCs, malignant lesions and metastases, where washout is typically slower. The equations below are used to calculate absolute and relative washout. Absolute washout greater than 60% and relative washout greater than 40% is in keeping with an adenoma (Fig. 20.2) [6]. Lesions that do not meet the washout criteria remain indeterminate on CT and may proceed to further imaging or surveillance.

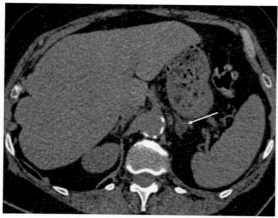

FIGURE 20.1   Axial-unenhanced CT image showing a lipid-rich adenoma, 6HU, in the left adrenal gland (*arrow*) in a patient with cortisol excess.

$$\text{Absolute washout}(\%) = \frac{PV(HU) - delayed(HU)}{PV(HU) - unenhanced(HU)} \times 100$$

$$\text{Relative washout }(\%) = \frac{PV(HU) - delayed(HU)}{PV(HU)} \times 100$$

Adrenal magnetic resonance imaging (MRI)

Lipid-poor and lipid-rich adenomas can also be diagnosed on MRI which is a useful alternative in patients who cannot have contrast enhanced CT, for example those with contrast allergy, or in patients with equivocal CT findings. The most useful MRI sequence is chemical shift imaging (CSI) that takes advantage of the different resonant frequencies of fat and water within the lesion. This is a dual-echo gradient echo sequence where both echoes are performed in a single breath-hold. It relies on the admixture of water and intracellular fat within the adenoma causing a signal dropout on the out of phase imaging compared with in phase images. This signal dropout can be visually observed or measured using a region of

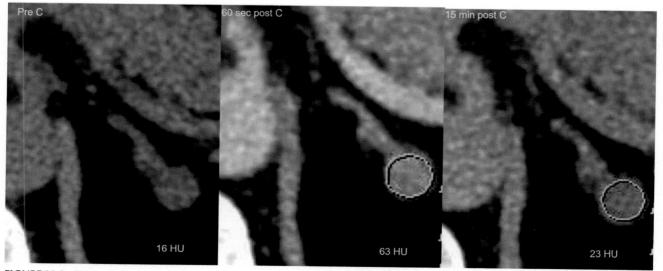

FIGURE 20.2   Triple phase adrenal CT for contrast washout demonstrating a lipid poor adenoma. A) Precontrast CT showing a left adrenal nodule with an attenuation of 16HU. This is a lipid-poor lesion and requires further characterization. B) Postcontrast CT at 60 sec shows the nodule enhances in keeping with a solid lesion and measures 63HU. C) Delayed 15 minute CT shows a reduction in attenuation to 23HU. The lesion has an absolute contrast washout of 85% and relative washout of 58% in keeping with a lipid poor adenoma.

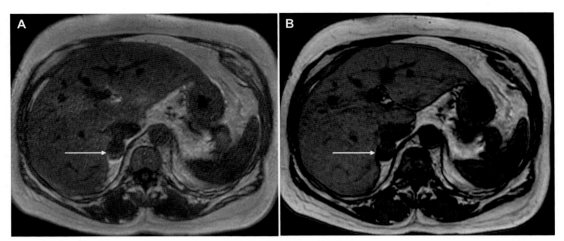

FIGURE 20.3   Adrenal MRI of a 2 cm right adrenal adenoma. A) In-phase image. B) Out-of-phase, showing visual signal drop out (*arrow*).

interest. The sensitivity and specificity of CSI in diagnosing adenomas are higher than CT at 81%−100% and 94%−100%, respectively (Fig. 20.3) [7]. To distinguish between intracellular fat seen in adenomas and the macroscopic fat seen in lipomas and myelolipomas, a fat-suppressed sequence is included in the imaging protocol as well as standard anatomical sequences. Contrast enhancement can be assessed using gadolinium-based contrast agents which assist in distinguishing from nonenhancing adrenal cysts.

Both CT and MRI techniques and protocols are designed to confirm benignity in an adrenal lesion. Therefore, they are best placed and have a high specificity (>98%) to confirm cysts, myelolipomas, and adenomas [4,8]. Conversely, techniques such as FDG PET/CT have a higher sensitivity for malignant disease although the specificity is poor due to metabolically active benign lesions [9].

Adrenal venous sampling (AVS)

In cases of mineralocorticoid excess states where there are bilateral adrenal nodules, this could be due to bilateral adrenal hyperplasia (BAH), or unilateral aldosterone secreting adrenocortical adenoma (ACA) with a contralateral incidental nonfunctioning adenoma. To differentiate unilateral from bilateral aldosterone production, AVS is the gold standard diagnostic technique. It is an invasive angiographic procedure involving cannulation of the adrenal veins and venous blood sampling for measurement of aldosterone and cortisol in the adrenal veins and IVC. Cannulation of the right adrenal vein is technically challenging with a high failure rate (because of its small size and anatomical variations) [10]. However, in specialist centers, the success rate of the procedure is up to 96% [11,12], with diagnostic laterlization in 45.5% [13]. This procedure is offered only in a limited number of tertiary referral centers, is expensive, and may lead to complications such as bleeding, infection, and catheter-induced adrenal vein thrombosis, with success rates as low as 8%−10% in low-volume centers [14].

Imaging for mineralocorticoid excess states

Mineralocorticoids are secreted by the zona glomerulosa of the adrenal cortex and regulate body fluid volume and electrolyte balance. The principal mineralocorticoid, aldosterone, plays a crucial role in potassium and blood pressure hemostasis, and excess production of this hormone can lead to hypokalemia, sodium and water retention, and hypertension. Primary aldosteronism is a common cause of secondary hypertension accounting for around 10% cases attending the hypertension clinics, and in a significant number of these patients there is an aldosterone secreting ACA, which can be resected to achieve surgical cure. The remaining is caused by BAH, which is often treated medically.

The role of imaging is to differentiate between ACA (Fig. 20.4) and BAH (Fig. 20.5) to allow appropriate treatment between medical therapy and surgery, respectively. Aldosterone secreting adenomas are usually small with a mean size of 1.6−2.2 cm but can be as small as 5mm, and hence, can be difficult to locate [15]. The sensitivity of detection with CT is 87%−93% with a specificity of 82%−85% [15]. Adrenal hyperplasia appears on CT imaging as enlarged medial and lateral limbs of one or both adrenal glands, which can be smooth or nodular in appearance and measure greater than 10 mm in diameter. The clinical picture can be complicated by the presence of multiple incidental nonfunctioning nodules, and

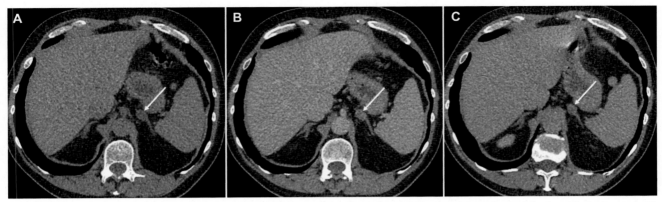

FIGURE 20.4 A young patient with hypertension and raised aldosterone with a 16 mm lipid-poor adenoma in the left adrenal body (*arrows*). A) Unenhanced phase CT image demonstrating an adrenal nodule with an attenuation value of 20HU. B) Portal venous phase CT image with the adrenal nodule enhancing to an attenuation value of 64HU. C) Delayed phase with the adrenal nodule attenuation value of 26HU, providing an absolute contrast washout of 86% in keeping with a lipid-poor adenoma. Note the right adrenal is normal.

bilateral nodules that have increased incidence with age and hypertension. These nonfunctioning bilateral nodules can mask an ACA and falsely provide a picture of BAH. Equally, a dominant nodule in one adrenal and undetected micronodular disease in the contralateral gland provides a false impression of an ACA with resultant failure of hypertension control following surgery. The use of CT or MRI findings and AVS has been proposed as part of a clinical prediction score (CPS) to correctly identify patients with unilateral disease suitable for adrenalectomy. Applying the CPS to this group of patients produced a sensitivity of 38·8% and a specificity of 88·5% of correctly identifying unilateral aldosterone production [16]. In the presence of a unilateral adenoma on CT with a normal contralateral adrenal, unilateral adrenalectomy has a 96% efficiency of achieving cure (46.2%) or improvement (50%) of hypertension [17].

Imaging for glucocorticoid excess states

Glucocorticoids are secreted by the zona fasciculata of the adrenal cortex, and the principal glucocorticoid is cortisol. Excess cortisol has been linked to hypertension with a linear dose relationship and is a feature of endogenous CS as well as iatrogenic CS caused by synthetic glucocorticoids. Most of the cases of endogenous CS are adrenocorticotrophin (ACTH) dependent (80%−85%). Among patients with ACTH dependent CS, majority (82%−91%) are caused by an ACTH secreting pituitary adenoma [18]. Less commonly, an ectopic source of ACTH production may be the cause (9%−18% of all ACTH dependent CS) [19]. In patients with ACTH secreting pituitary adenoma, an MRI pituitary should be performed (see acromegaly section).

CS with suppressed ACTH levels indicates an adrenal source of cortisol overproduction. In an adult with adrenal CS (ACTH independent CS), which represents 15%−20% of all endogenous CS, nearly 95% are secondary to an adrenal adenoma or carcinoma (Figs. 20.6 and 20.7). On CT and MRI, adrenal adenomas causing CS are usually greater than 2.0 cm and have the properties of lipid rich adenomas [15].

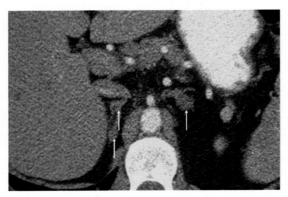

FIGURE 20.5 Postcontrast CT of a patient with hypertension and biochemically proven Conn's syndrome. Multiple bilateral nodules are demonstrated in the adrenals (*arrows*), imaging suggestive of BAH.

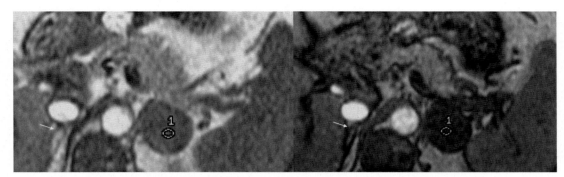

FIGURE 20.6 Cushing's adenoma. A) In-phase chemical shift MRI image. B) Out-of-phase chemical shift MRI image. A large left adrenal adenoma (numbered 1) with signal drop out on the out-of-phase image in keeping with an adenoma in a patient with biochemical ACTH-independent Cushing's syndrome. The contralateral right adrenal (*arrowed*) is atrophic and poorly visualized.

Adrenal carcinomas are rare with a reported incidence of 0.7–2.0 cases per 1,000,000 per year, and approximately 60% are functional, with CS being the most common hormone excess [20]. Adrenal carcinomas are also associated with Carney complex (CNC), Li Fraumeni syndrome (LFS), Beckwith-Wiedemann syndrome (BWS), Lynch syndrome, Familial Adenomatous Polyposis (FAP), Multiple Endocrine Neoplasia type 1 (MEN 1), Neurofibromatosis type 1 and Werner's syndrome [19–23]. In the rare instance of a functioning adrenocortical carcinoma, it can usually be distinguished from an adenoma by virtue of its size (usually more than 6 cm), heterogeneity and the presence of local invasion, and tumor extension into the inferior vena cava. These tumours tend to appear necrotic with regions of hemorrhage and show peripheral enhancement with little washout in the delayed phase imaging. Smaller ACCs can be distinguished from adenoma as they have imaging properties of lipid poor lesions with absolute and relative contrast washout of less than 60% and 40% respectively.

Macronodular BHA (seen in older adults) in association with Massive Macronodular Adrenocortical Disease (MMAD), and Primary Bilateral Macronodular Adrenocortical Hyperplasia (PBMAH) (Fig. 20.8), and micronodular BHA (seen in

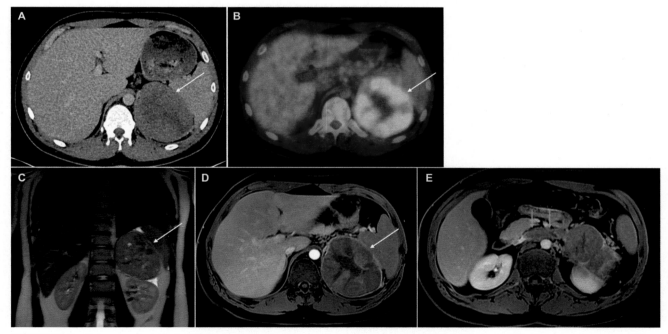

FIGURE 20.7 A young male patient with Cushing's syndrome and a left adrenal mass. A) Axial CT image in PV phase showing a large 10 cm heterogeneously enhancing suprarenal mass with central low density suggestive of necrosis. B) Axial image from the patient's FDG PET CT showing intense tracer uptake peripherally with central necrosis. C) Coronal T2 image showing the suprarenal location with mass effect on the left kidney and spleen. D) Axial images from contrast-enhanced T1 fat-saturated image sequence (LAVA) showing the large left adrenal mass with heterogeneous enhancement and vascular invasion of the adrenal vein into the left renal vein (*blue arrows*). Imaging findings are of an adrenocortical carcinoma.

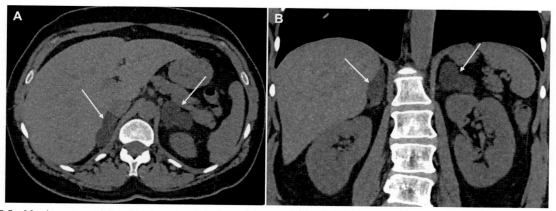

FIGURE 20.8   Massive macronodular adrenal hyperplasia. A) axial and B) coronal-unenhanced CT images of a patient with bilateral enlargement of the adrenals with preservation of the adreniform contour in the context of mild Cushing's syndrome (*arrows*).

children and younger adults) in association with Primary Pigmented Nodular Adrenal Hyperplasia (PPNAD), and isolated Micronodular Adrenocortical Disease (iMAD), are rarer causes of adrenal CS [24].

Ectopic production of ACTH, for example, from bronchial and thymic carcinoids, pancreatic neuroendocrine tumours (pNETs), small cell lung cancer (SCLC), medullary thyroid cancer, or a PPGL (PCC/paraganglioma) counts for 9%—18% of ACTH dependent CS [19]. If an ectopic source of ACTH is suspected, CT imaging of the thorax, abdomen and pelvis with contrast is recommended. The tumour is most likely to be within the lungs (48%), with bronchial carcinoids being the most likely tumor (30%), followed by SCLC (18%) (Figs. 20.9 and 20.10) [25,26]. However, these tumors can be small and difficult to localize, and the sensitivity of lesion detection with CT is only 66% in patients with ectopic ACTH secretion [27], though the number of unidentified ACTH secreting lesions has improved to 10%—30% in recent years with the improvement of CT technology, the use of thin-slice CT with arterial phase contrast enhancement, and with an increasing awareness among radiologists [19].

Positron-emission tomography (PET)/CT to localize an ectopic source of ACTH secretion

[68]Gallium DOTATATE is a radiolabelled somatostatin receptor 2 (SSTR2) analogue used for the radiological localization of ectopic ACTH secretion, as these receptors are overexpressed by neuroendocrine tumors. It has been shown to be significantly more sensitive than previous techniques such as metaiodobenzylguanidine (MIBG) scintigraphy and [111]Indium octreotide scan and is now the functional imaging method of choice for the diagnosis and staging of neuroendocrine tumours. With a benchtop [68]Germanium/[68]Gallium eluting generator, this radiotracer can be made on site or at a local facility and has a short half-life of 68 minutes resulting in a lower effective dose to the patient. It is chelated with 1,4,7,10-tetraazacyclododecane-1,4,7,10-tetraacetic acid (DOTA) to the peptide Octreotate, that specifically binds to SSTR2. For detecting and staging neuroendocrine tumors ^{68}Ga DOTATATE PET/CT is now the imaging method of choice, with a sensitivity of 93% and a specificity of 95% [28].

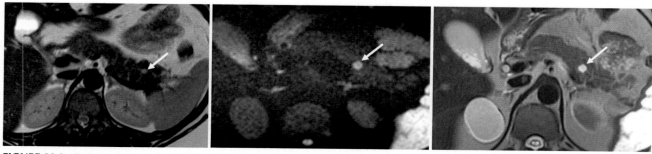

FIGURE 20.9   Patient with ACTH-dependent Cushing's syndrome and a normal pituitary MRI and AVS. A) T2-weighted sequence showing a tiny indeterminate lesion in the pancreas, suspicious, but not diagnostic of a NET. B) Diffusion-weighted image (b = 800) demonstrating the same lesion with greater conspicuity. C) DOTATATE PET MRI confirming the lesion as a NET. Resection of this lesion was curative for the Cushing's syndrome.

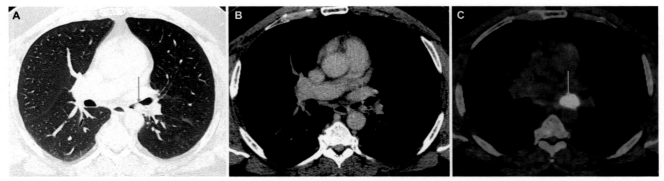

FIGURE 20.10 A middle-aged male patient with ectopic ACTH secretion. A) Axial lung window image showing an endobronchial nodule (*arrows*). B) Axial soft tissue window image of the mediastinum confirms a solid a left main bronchus lesion. C) Axial fused image from the ^{68}Ga-DOTATATE PET/CT—the lesion demonstrates intense tracer uptake in keeping with a bronchial carcinoid.

Imaging for catecholamine excess states

The adrenal medulla consists of chromaffin cells, derived from embryonic neural crest cells, and secretes the catecholamines—epinephrine and norepinephrine—in response to stimulation by sympathetic preganglionic neurons. Chromaffin-cell tumors of the adrenal medulla are known as PCCs, those originating from the extra-adrenal autonomic ganglia as paragangliomas (PGLs), and collectively they are termed as PPGLs. PCCs account for 80%—85% of all PPGLs, whereas PGLs account for the remaining 15%—20% [29]. PCCs and sympathetic PGLs (of the thorax, abdomen, and pelvis) are functional tumors that secrete hormones, whereas nearly 2/3rd of the parasympathetic PGLs (of the head and neck) are nonfunctional tumors [29]. Nearly 50% of the PCCs has an adrenergic phenotype, and predominantly secrete epinephrine, but with varying amounts of norepinephrine [30]. The remainder of the PCCs and all the sympathetic PGLs predominantly or exclusively secrete norepinephrine (noradrenergic phenotype), but some secrete significant amounts of dopamine (dopaminergic phenotype). A functioning PPGL can also secrete other hormones such as parathyroid hormone, calcitonin, gastrin, serotonin, and ACTH [15].

Up to 70% of PPGLs are genetically determined by either germline a mutation (30%—35%), thereby hereditary, or by somatic mutation (35%—40%) in one of the known susceptibility genes [31]. Increasing frequency of PPGLs is seen in various neuroectodermal syndromes such as neurofibromatosis type 1 (NF1), von Hippel-Lindau (VHL) disease, tuberous sclerosis, and multiple neuroendocrine neoplasia types 2A and 2B (MEN2A/2B). In general, 15%—17% of all PPGLs are metastatic, where metastasis (defined as the presence of chromaffin tissue in nonchromaffin organs including lymph nodes, liver, lungs, and bone) is reported in 2%—25% of PCCs and 2.4%—60% of PGLs [29]. The metastatic potential varies depending on presence or absence mutations. The highest rate of metastatic potential is noted for PPGL associated with *SDHB* mutation (30%—70%), whereas that for *NF1* is 10%, and that for MEN2/2B, *VHL*, and *SDHD* is <5% [29]. Similarly, the rate of bilaterality is highest for MEN2A/2B (50%—60%), followed by VHL (40%—50%), and NF1 (20%). PPGLs with *SDH* mutations have a very low rate of bilaterality.

PCC and PGL are rare causes for hypertension, accounting for 0.2%—0.6% of cases [30]. Hypertension is present in nearly 95% of PPGL patients, with sustained hypertension in 55% and episodic hypertension in 45% [32]. Hypertension in these patients is often refractory to medical therapy. Clinical symptoms also include headache, sweats, blurred vision, palpitations, and tachycardia. About 10%—49% of the PPGLs are found as adrenal incidentalomas and about 4%—8% of the adrenal incidentalomas are PCCs.

The common sites for PGLs are the para-aortic region at the level of the renal hila, the organ of Zuckerkandl at the aortic bifurcation or origin of the inferior mesenteric artery, thoracic paraspinal region, urinary bladder, and head and neck [33]. Carotid body tumors and glomus jugulare tumors account for nearly 80% of the head and neck PGL, whereas glomus vagale tumors are less common (2.5%—4.5%) [34].

The diagnosis of PPGL is made by detecting increased catecholamines or their metabolites in blood or urine samples. Imaging studies are vital to locate the tumour and plan surgical resection. PCCs detected in association with neuro-ectodermal syndromes, where patients are periodically screened, are often small, whilst sporadic PCCs are usually larger and more easily detected by imaging studies.

A contrast enhanced CT is used as the initial modality for tumor localization and has a sensitivity of 97% and a specificity of 67% for differentiating PCC from ACA [35]. PCCs have a varied appearance on imaging. A typical lesion will demonstrate a density >10HU on unenhanced images, with a sensitivity of 99% [36]. Speckled calcification and

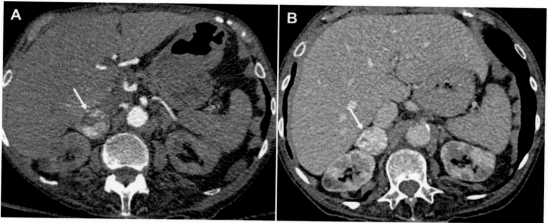

FIGURE 20.11   Typical appearances of pheochromocytomas on CT. A) Arterial phase with the pheochromocytoma demonstrating avid enhancement. B) Portal venous phase imaging of a right pheochromocytoma showing persistent enhancement with no significant washout in the portal venous phase.

central necrosis are seen in around 12%, and the majority will enhance avidly [15]. Imaging the neck, thorax, abdomen, and pelvis with CT scan allows detection of over 95% of adrenal and extra adrenal PPGLs along with associated tumors in the neuroectodermal syndromes (Fig. 20.11).

On MR imaging, PCCs are classically hyperintense on T2-weighted images, giving a "light bulb" appearance and are iso- or hypointense to the liver on T1 weighted images, with high T1 signal of hemorrhage in up to 20%. Diffusion weighted imaging increases the lesion conspicuity and aids the detection of small lesions in patients being screened for PCCs (Fig. 20.12). Larger tumors are usually more heterogeneous with areas of necrosis, hemorrhage and/or calcification (Fig. 20.13). There is typically no signal drop out on out-of-phase CSI to suggest intracellular fat content. Without the presence of vascular and adjacent organ invasion or metastatic disease, imaging is unable to distinguish between benign and malignant PCCs. ^{68}Ga DOTATATE PET/CT is useful in detecting and characterizing occult extra-adrenal tumors, multifocal lesions, or metastatic disease (Fig. 20.14).

Imaging for primary hyperparathyroidism

Primary hyperparathyroidism is associated with hypertension in 40%—65% of patients [37], and observational studies show an increased prevalence of hypertension and cardiovascular disease among these patients, although the precise biochemical mechanism is currently unclear. The available literature to date suggests that hypertension improves after parathyroidectomy, although large prospective studies have not been performed. After biochemical confirmation of primary hyperparathyroidism (PHPT), imaging is an essential tool for localizing the hyperfunctioning parathyroid gland or

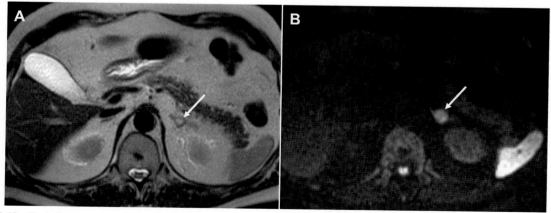

FIGURE 20.12   Typical appearances of pheochromocytomas on MRI. A) T2-weighted MRI image showing a high signal intensity 12 mm left adrenal pheochromocytoma in a patient with raised plasma metanephrines. B) This demonstrates marked restricted diffusion on diffusion-weighted imaging and the high signal contrasts with the surrounding organ signal paucity, making the pheochromocytoma more conspicuous.

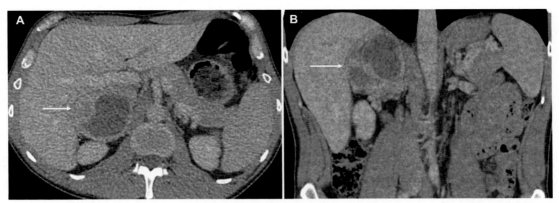

FIGURE 20.13   Large atypical pheochromocytoma. A) Axial and B) coronal-reconstructed CT images of an atypical pheochromocytoma with a large cystic component. This could easily be misdiagnosed on imaging as an adrenocortical carcinoma due to its irregular shape and internal necrosis.

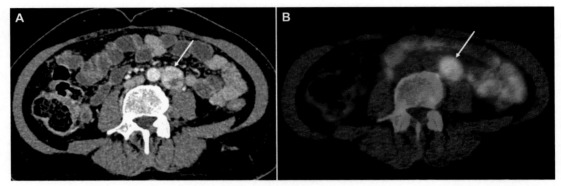

FIGURE 20.14   Left para-aortic paraganglioma. A) Axial CT image in the portal venous phase of a patient with hypertension, showing a hyper-enhancing left para-aortic mass. B) The mass is intensely avid on the ^{68}Ga DOTATATE PET/CT, in keeping with a paraganglioma.

glands, and to plan parathyroidectomy that usually cures the disease and possibly hypertension. PHPT is most often caused by a single parathyroid adenoma, accounting for approximately 80%—85% of cases, with 4% of patients having multiple adenomas [38]. Parathyroid hyperplasia accounts of 10%—15% cases and parathyroid carcinoma is the rarest accounting for less than 1% [38]. Since successful treatment requires removal of the hyperfunctioning gland(s), with few options for medical management, accurate preoperative anatomical localization using imaging is crucial to obtain cure. This allows selective minimally invasive parathyroidectomy rather than a full 4-gland exploration, reducing operating theatre time, patient morbidity, and recovery time. Pre-operative imaging often takes a multi-modality approach, starting with simple, cost-effective methods such as neck ultrasound (US), and moving on to more advanced imaging techniques, if the gland cannot be easily located.

Neck ultrasound

Neck US is the first-line preoperative imaging technique for localization of parathyroid adenoma(s) with the advantages of low cost and no ionising radiation. This should be performed by an experienced specialist head and neck sonographer or radiologist. In expert hands, the sensitivity of neck US in locating a lone parathyroid adenoma is in the region of 69%—79% [39,40]. This drops to 35% in multi-gland disease, with a positive predictive value of 87%. The sensitivity is further reduced in ectopic glands due to the limitations of US in assessing the mediastinum, where the sound waves are reflected by bony structures. On US, the enlarged gland is identified as an oval hypoechoic nodule, generally well encapsulated, compared with the more hyperechoic anterior thyroid gland (Fig. 20.15). Typically, Doppler imaging may show a small feeding artery. Imaging with US is usually combined with another modality to aid diagnostic confidence.

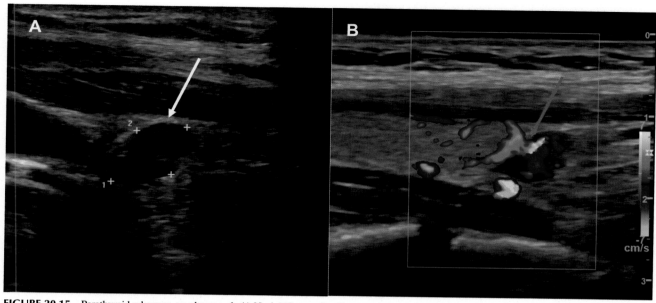

FIGURE 20.15   Parathyroid adenoma on ultrasound. A) Neck US scan showing a small, well-encapsulated hypoechoic nodule inferior to the thyroid pole (*arrow*). B) Color Doppler US shows a feeding vessel (*red arrow*).

4D computed tomography (CT)

CT using iodinated intravenous contrast media is performed in three dimensions—with axial, sagittal and coronal reformats to aid lesion detection. The scan is usually also performed in three phases of contrast enhancement (fourth dimension)—unenhanced, arterial phase, and delayed phase, looking for an arterially enhancing parathyroid gland that is low attenuation in the unenhanced images and displays washout of contrast media (and hence a reduction in density) in the delayed phase (Fig. 20.16). The advantages of CT are that it allows excellent anatomical localization, and the scan should include the full neck and extend to the mediastinum to search for potential ectopic glands. The sensitivity of 4D CT is only marginally better than US, at 76.5% for localization to the correct anatomical quadrant with a specificity of 91.5% [41]. The disadvantages are a higher cost and the high radiation burden from the CT performed in multiple phases [42].

SPECT/CT imaging with 99mTc-sestamibi

99mTechnetium-sestamibi (99mTc-MIBI) SPECT/CT is a functional nuclear medicine imaging technique combining SPECT imaging of radiotracer accumulation in the target tissue with anatomical imaging using CT. 99mTc-MIBI is the most widely used radio-pharmaceutical for parathyroid imaging. It is usually used in conjunction with neck US as a second modality to

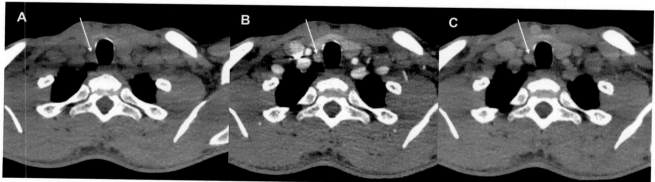

FIGURE 20.16   Axial slices of a 4D CT scan at the thoracic inlet with a parathyroid adenoma. A) Unenhanced phase with a small 10 mm nodule right paratracheal lesion located posterior to the right thyroid inferior pole (*arrow*). B) Arterial phase showing marked enhancement in the nodule (*arrow*). C) Delayed phase with washout within the nodule (*arrow*).

increase diagnostic confidence. ^{99m}Tc has the advantage that it can be produced relatively cheaply from a benchtop eluting generator and has an ideal half-life of 6 hours allowing adequate time for dose preparation, injection of the patient, uptake time, and imaging. Hyperfunctioning parathyroid glands demonstrate uptake of sestamibi which is related to increased number of mitochondria in the oxophil-rich cells [43]. ^{99m}Tc-MIBI washes rapidly out of the thyroid gland, and slowly from the hyperfunctioning parathyroid. This allows dual-time-point tracer imaging with early and delayed phase imaging. Early phase imaging demonstrates tracer uptake in both thyroid and parathyroid glands, whilst late imaging shows continuing tracer accumulation in the parathyroid glands but washout from the thyroid gland, highlighting the hyperfunctioning parathyroid gland(s). The CT component is used for attenuation correction and anatomical localization, increasing the diagnostic performance of this technique when compared with planar imaging alone (Fig. 20.17). In a meta-analysis of 1236 patients, the detection rate of ^{99m}Tc-MIBI was 88% on a per patient and per lesion-base analysis [44] and has been shown to have 88% sensitivity for solitary adenomas [39].

Alternatively dual tracer SPECT/CT imaging can be used, where in addition to ^{99m}Tc-MIBI, ^{99m}Tc-pertechnetate is used to image the thyroid gland, after which the image is subtracted to reveal the parathyroid glands (Fig. 20.18). This technique is helpful in patients with thyroid disease such as nodules, which may retain sestamibi, mimicking parathyroid glands leading to inaccurate results [45,46]. However, this carries a higher radiation burden to the patient, and is more expensive [43].

PET/CT with 18-fluorine labeled choline analogues

Choline is a marker of cell membrane proliferation that is incorporated into phospholipids of the cell membrane in rapidly dividing cells [47]. Its utility in parathyroid imaging was discovered accidentally while imaging patients with prostate cancer during which incidental parathyroid adenomas were detected [48,49]. It is now in use at tertiary referral centers as

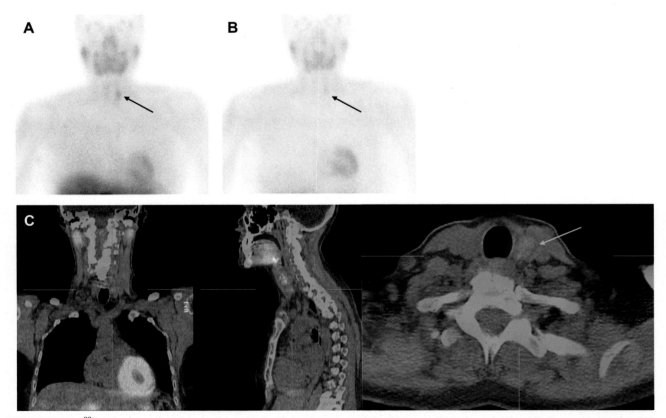

FIGURE 20.17 ^{99m}Technetium-sestamibi scan in a patient with hyperparathyroidism with no candidate for a parathyroid adenoma identified on US neck. A) Early phase planar imaging with the location of the lesion *arrowed*. B) Delayed phase planar imaging shows a focal region of increased tracer uptake at the inferior left thyroid pole. C) Multiplanar SPECT CT imaging shows the exact position of the nodule adjacent to the inferior pole of the thyroid confirming a parathyroid adenoma.

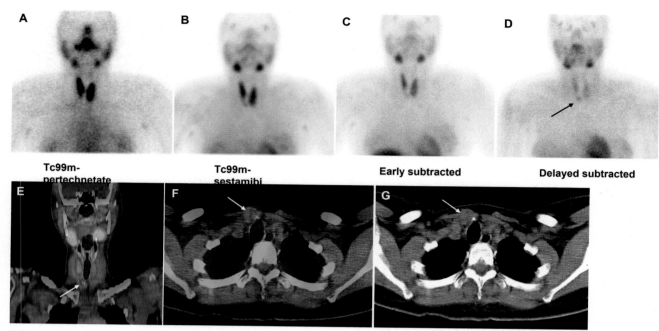

FIGURE 20.18 Dual tracer SPECT/CT imaging of a right parathyroid adenoma (*arrows*). A) ^{99m}Tc-pertechnetate coronal planar image showing thyroid uptake. B) ^{99m}Tc-sestamibi planar coronal image showing uptake in the thyroid as well as a small focus of tracer uptake adjacent to the inferior right lobe of the thyroid. C) This focal region appears separate to the thyroid on the early phase subtraction imaging, and D) becomes more apparent in the delayed phase subtraction images. E) Coronal fused SPECT CT imaging shows the anatomical location of the lesion. F) Axial fused SPECT/CT imaging and G) Axial-unenhanced CT image at the same anatomical location showing a 19 mm hypodense, well-encapsulated nodule inferior to the right lower lobe of the thyroid.

the second-line imaging of choice for preoperative localization, where standard imaging techniques have failed to localize an adenoma. Further studies are ongoing to evaluate its use as a first-line imaging technique.

The most commonly used radiopharmaceutical is ^{18}F-fluorocholine and the advantages of this technique include the superior spatial resolution and sensitivity of PET/CT, as well as a lower radiation dose, and shorter acquisition time compared to ^{99m}Tc-MIBI SPECT/CT, with the disadvantage that it is more expensive (Fig. 20.19).

In a meta-analysis of 517 patients imaged with radiolabelled choline PET/CT, the sensitivity of detecting hyper-functioning parathyroid glands was 95% with a PPV of 97% [50], and the sensitivity of detection has been shown to be

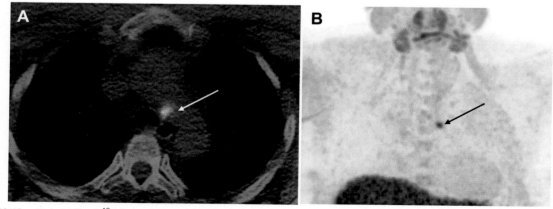

FIGURE 20.19 A) Axial fused ^{18}F-fluorocholine PET/CT image. B) Maximum intensity projection (MIP) image of ^{18}F-fluorocholine PET/CT in a patient with hyperparathyroidism, recurrent renal calculi, and previous four-gland removal. Previous US neck, 4D CT, and ^{99m}Tc-sestamibi scans were negative. There is focal tracer uptake in an ectopic mediastinal parathyroid adenoma in the aortopulmonary window. The PTH fell from 25 to 2.8 following thoracoscopic parathyroidectomy.

significantly higher than ^{99m}Tc-MIBI SPECT/CT [51]. A comparison of various imaging modalities, their costs, radiation doses, sensitivity, specificty and the usefulness for localization of ectopic parathyroid adenomas is shown in Table 20.1.

Imaging for hyperthyroidism and hypothyroidism

Both hypo- and hyperthyroidism are associated with hypertension. Approximately 30% of patients with clinical hypothyroidism have hypertension; however, this is predominantly caused by autoimmune thyroiditis and can be confirmed with thyroid peroxidase antibody assay, with little role for imaging except to evaluate a palpable nodule. In hyperthyroid patients, excess T3 is well known to cause increased heart rate and cardiac output with a high output state with resultant systolic hypertension. Pulmonary hypertension is also a common complication in hyperthyroid patients due to Graves' disease or toxic multinodular goiter. In hyperthyroid patients, thyroid US provides important diagnostic information on the possible cause, size, echogenicity, and vascularization of the gland, as well as identifying thyroid nodules. A radionuclide thyroid scan can diagnose Graves' disease (in thyrotrophin receptor antibody [TRAb] negative patients) and distinguish autonomously functioning surgically resectable nodules from toxic multinodular goiter. The hypertension in approximately one-third of patients with hyperthyroidism usually resolves after achieving euthyroidism.

Thyroiditis of any etiology often demonstrates classical appearances on imaging, with anatomical changes such as gland enlargement, and hyper/hypo-vascularity, and functional changes in radiopharmaceutical uptake patterns. For these reasons, thyroid scintigraphy, and ultrasound play central roles in the imaging of thyroid pathology and have been in routine clinical use for many decades.

Thyroid ultrasound

On ultrasound, the normal thyroid gland is homogeneously hyperechoic with a smooth margin, and has well-defined normal values for its dimensions, such as a craniocaudal length of 4—7 cm for each lobe. There are several widely used scoring systems to risk stratify detected nodules based on their US appearances. Nodules rated as indeterminate, suspicious, or malignant on US will usually undergo fine needle aspiration at the time of scanning with a view to curative resection (Fig. 20.20). Thyroiditis on US can be apparent if there is significant gland enlargement and hypervascularity on color Doppler imaging.

Planar scintigraphy

Functional imaging using radioisotopes that accumulate in the thyroid gland can be used to classify hyperfunctioning thyroid nodules, assess thyroid function, and in some cases find ectopic hyperfunctioning thyroid tissue. Commonly used radiopharmaceuticals for thyroid scintigraphy include ^{99m}Tc-pertechnetate, ^{123}Iodine, and ^{131}Iodine. Thyroid follicular cells trap both iodine and ^{99m}Tc, where the latter is a pharmacologic mimic of iodine. However only iodine can be incorporated into the organ and stored as thyroglobulin within the cell, whereas ^{99m}Tc will washout after approximately

TABLE 20.1 Comparison of imaging modalities for parathyroid adenoma localization.

Imaging modality	Cost	Average radiation dose	Sensitivity	Specificity	Sensitivity in ectopic adenomas
US neck	£52	Nil	57%—72%	96%	17%
4D CT	£105	8.5 mSv	76%	92%	
^{99m}Tc-sestamibi SPECT/CT	£285	10.3 mSv	88%	79%	
Dual tracer SPECT/CT	£1531	10.5 mSv	93%	90%	
^{18}F-fluorocholine PET/CT	£300	6—8 mSv	91%—95% in difficult cases, up to 100% otherwise	100%	100%

4D CT, four-dimension computed tomography; *SPECT/CT,* single photon emission computed tomography; *US,* ultrasound.

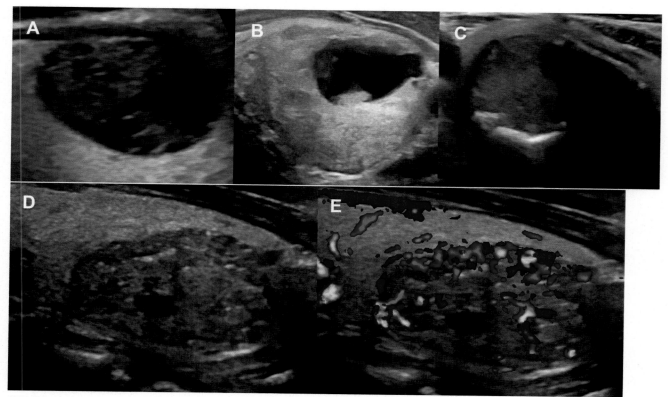

FIGURE 20.20 Examples of images from multiple different patients showing US scans of the thyroid gland with a range of appearances of thyroid nodules. A) A benign spongiform appearing nodule. B) Cystic change in a hyperechoic nodule, also with benign appearances. C) Interrupted peripheral egg-shell calcification in a hypoechoic nodule, with suspicious appearances. D) Malignant appearing nodule with a lobulated contour and micro-calcification. E) Marked internal vascularity.

30 minutes. The ideal imaging characteristics such as low cost, and ready availability of ^{99m}Tc-pertechnetate in nuclear medicine departments make it the predominant radiopharmaceutical used to assess the thyroid pathology.

Adequate patient preparation is essential prior to the imaging study. The anti-thyroid medications should be stopped for 3—7 days prior, levothyroxine for 4 weeks, iodine-containing medicines and preparations for 4 weeks, and amiodarone for 3—6 months [52]. No CT imaging with IV contrast should be performed in the prior 1—2 months.

A normal thyroid on planar imaging should look symmetrical, with a butterfly appearance, homogeneous tracer uptake and a smooth contour. It should not extent below the sternum (this will be verified with an external radioactive sternal marker) and there will be a pyramidal lobe in approximately 10% of patients. There is normally low-grade uptake in the salivary glands and gastric mucosa if included in the field of view that can be used to visually judge if uptake in the thyroid is increased or decreased. In the case of ^{99m}Tc-pertechnetate, a semi-quantitative measurement of thyroid uptake can be calculated by measuring the counts in a region of interest drawn around the thyroid, subtracting the counts from a background region of interest and dividing this by the injected activity (activity in the syringe is measured before and after injection to approximate the injected activity). This percentage uptake is compared with the local normal uptake range. Direct assessment of thyroid uptake with [123]Iodine is more accurate and involves a small oral dose of administered activity, followed by serial measurement of counts at selected time-points, usually at 4-6 hours and 24 hours.

The functional status of thyroid nodules is visually classified as "hot," "warm," or "cold," depending on their observed uptake compared to the background gland uptake, with "hot" being above background gland activity, "warm" at a similar uptake level and "cold" having reduced or absent uptake (Fig. 20.21) [53,54]. The nodule with observed uptake should be correlated with its US appearance to stratify the risk of malignancy. Hot nodules were traditionally thought to rarely harbor malignancy. However, a recent systematic review and meta-analysis of seven observational studies observed that although, in comparison to nontoxic nodules, the odds of malignancy of hot nodules are low, it is still not zero and is higher than expected [55]. Thyroid scintigraphy can identify autonomously functioning thyroid nodules which appear hot, on a background of suppressed uptake in the rest of the gland [53,54]. In the patient with multinodular goiter, the nodules may

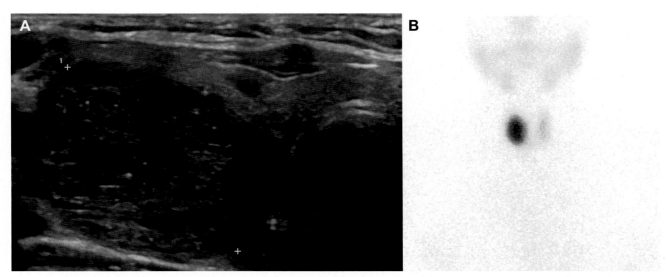

FIGURE 20.21 Thyroid images in a patient with hyperthyroidism. A) Large dominant nodule measuring 2.5 cm in the right lobe of a multinodular gland. B) ^{99m} Technetium-pertechnetate thyroid scan showing an autonomously functioning hot nodule in the right lobe with suppressed uptake in the thyroid and salivary glands.

be hyperfunctioning or hypofunctioning, leading to hyperthyroidism or hypothyroidism, or the patient may be euthyroid. Thyroid uptake scans have a nodular heterogeneous uptake, with corresponding thyroid US showing benign appearing nodules in an enlarged gland (Fig. 20.22). If hyperthyroidism is present with TSH suppression, and there are multiple focal regions of increased uptake and reduced overall gland uptake, a diagnosis of toxic multinodular goiter can be made.

In a patient with hyperthyroidism, diffuse, homogeneous thyroid overactivity with reduced uptake in the salivary glands and reduced background activity is consistent with Grave's disease. Thyroid uptake function will show values above the normal range. The thyroid US reveals an enlarged gland which may appear hyperechoic, or with a heterogeneous echo-texture without nodularity in simple cases, although there are often concomitant thyroid nodules. The gland is typically hypervascular on color Doppler imaging (Fig. 20.23) [56].

Subacute thyroiditis, originally described by Swiss surgeon Fritz de Quervain, causes destruction of follicular cells resulting in a rapid release of stored T4 and T3 leading to thyrotoxicosis. This is normally followed by transient hypo-thyroidism, although this can rarely be permanent. Gland destruction produces characteristic imaging appearances on

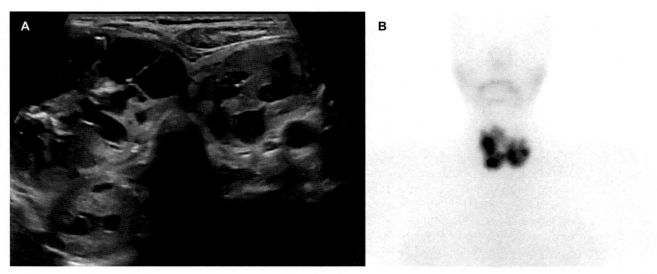

FIGURE 20.22 Toxic multinodular goiter. A) US thyroid showing a markedly enlarged gland with numerous benign appearing nodules. B) ^{99m} Technetium-pertechnetate thyroid scan showing several hot nodules mixed with cold nodules, with suppressed background uptake.

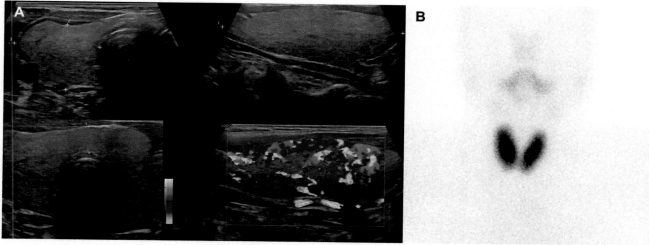

FIGURE 20.23 Grave's Disease. A) US thyroid showing an enlarged right lobe of the thyroid with a volume of 27mL and an enlarged isthmus measuring 8 mm (upper limit of normal 5 mm). There is hyperechoic gland echotexture and hypervascularity on color Doppler US. B) ^{99m} Technetium-pertechnetate thyroid scan with uptake showing markedly increased thyroid uptake (uptake function above normal range) with low background and salivary uptake, in keeping with Grave's disease.

thyroid uptake studies, where there is reduced or absent gland uptake (Fig. 20.24) [53]. This pattern is also seen in destructive thyroiditis, which may be post-partum or drug related, for example in type 2 amiodarone-induced thyroiditis or related to therapy with immune checkpoint inhibitors [57–60].

Imaging for acromegaly and AGHD

Hypertension is a frequent complication of acromegaly, present in approximately 35% of patients, and is thought to be secondary to chronic exposure to growth hormone (GH) and insulin like growth factor 1 (IGF-1) excess. This rare disease is usually caused by a GH secreting anterior pituitary adenoma (95%) with the remaining cases caused by ectopic GH-releasing hormone (GHRH) secreting neuroendocrine tumors of the lung, thyroid, pancreas, or adrenal gland [61]. Ectopic GH secreting neuroendocrine tumors (NET) are extremely rare in comparison. After initial biochemical investigations such as serum IGF-1, oral glucose tolerance test, and random GH measurement, imaging plays a crucial role in identifying the source of GH excess such as a pituitary adenoma or searching for the site of ectopic secretion.

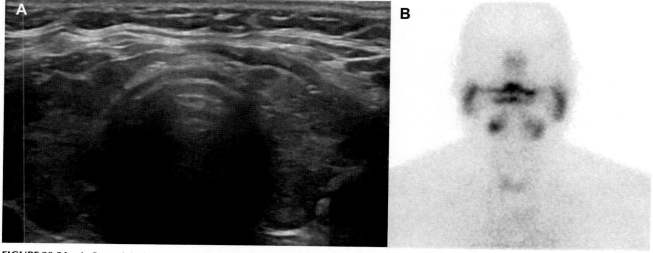

FIGURE 20.24 de Quervain's thyroiditis. A) Thyroid US scan showing an enlarged gland with heterogeneous echogenicity and nodular echotexture. B) ^{99m} Technetium-pertechnetate thyroid scan with uptake showing markedly reduced thyroid uptake (below normal range), in keeping with thyroiditis.

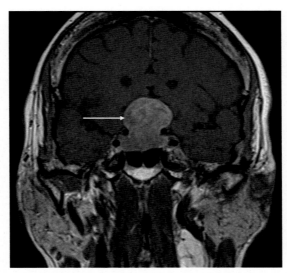

FIGURE 20.25   Coronal T1-weighted dynamic contrast-enhanced MRI of the pituitary showing a macroadenoma with suprasellar extension (*arrow*).

Adult-onset growth hormone deficiency (AGHD) is also often caused by a pituitary adenoma, with other causes such as craniopharyngioma, other brain tumors, traumatic brain injury, cranial irradiation, hypophysitis, subarachnoid hemorrhage, pituitary apoplexy, or idiopathic GH deficiency being less common [62]. The risk of hypertension is proportional to the degree of AGHD. Similarly, the degree of AGHD is proportionally related to the levels of total and LDL cholesterol, truncal fat, and waist-hip ratio, and cardiovascular mortality. These effects can be significantly improved with GH replacement.

MRI of the pituitary

To evaluate the pituitary, MRI is the preferred modality over CT due to its excellent soft tissue resolution and superior sensitivity for locating brain lesions. A pituitary macroadenoma (>1 cm) appears as an enlarged gland with increased gadolinium uptake, often with surrounding mass effect causing an enlarged sella turcica (Fig. 20.25). The less frequent observation of pituitary microadenoma (<1 cm), is hypoenhancing relative to the normal pituitary (Fig. 20.26). Pituitary MRI is also useful in following up patients after surgery or assessing lesion stability in patients on somatostatin analogues. The more common densely granulated adenomas, found in 30%−50% of acromegaly cases, usually in patients over 50 years of age, are associated with low T2 signal on MR imaging [63]. These densely granulated adenomas generally respond

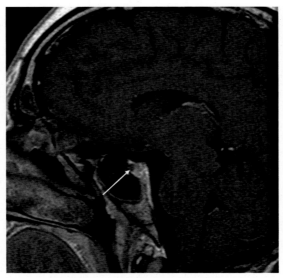

FIGURE 20.26   Sagittal T1-weighted dynamic contrast-enhanced MRI of the pituitary showing a 5 mm rounded hypoenhancing microadenoma (*arrow*).

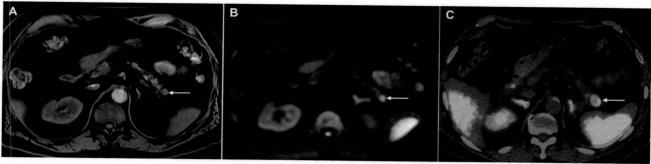

FIGURE 20.27   GNRH producing pancreatic NET. A) An axial water-only DIXON image showing a small hyperintense mass of the pancreatic tail. B) An axial high B-value diffusion-weighted image shows intense restricted diffusion in the mass. C) Axial fused image from the patient's ^{68}Ga-DOTATATE PET/CT showing intense tracer uptake, confirming a GHRH pancreatic tail NET. Note the normal background uptake in the spleen, liver, adrenal glands, and kidneys.

well to somatostatin analogues [64], in 65%−90% cases [65]. Conversely, sparsely granulated adenomas are found in 15% −35% of acromegaly cases, present in younger patients, and have high T2 signal on MRI imaging [63]. These sparsely granulated adenomas are often resistant to treatment with somatostatin analogues. Hence, lower T2 signal intensity has been shown to predict an increased response to somatostatin therapy. Molecular studies have shown that the densely granulated adenomas exclusively express SSTR2, whereas the sparsely granulated adenomas exclusively express SSTR5 [66].

If the gland appears hyperplastic, with no discrete adenoma identified, pituitary hyperplasia due to a GHRH secreting NET should be considered. First-line investigation to locate the GHRH NET is similar to the localizing study for ectopic ACTH production, usually CT of the thorax, abdomen, and pelvis, with dual phase arterial and portal venous phase CT of the abdomen. Neuroendocrine tumors and their metastases are hyper-enhancing in the arterial phase, allowing greater sensitivity in locating NETs, with an average sensitivity of 73% for the primary tumor, and 80% for liver metastases [67].

If no tumor is found on CT, functional imaging with ^{68}Ga-DOTATATE PET/CT is the most appropriate second line investigation, and more recent studies suggest an improved staging at presentation and for detection of recurrent disease (Fig. 20.27).

Summary and conclusions

Imaging is an essential component in the investigation and management of endocrine hypertension. Its role extends from detecting and characterizing hyperfunctioning endocrine lesions, assisting surgical planning, and staging malignancy where relevant. The imaging modalities and their order of use will be guided by the clinical and biochemical findings. The most frequently used modality remains CT of the chest, abdomen, and pelvis, while MRI is the imaging of choice for pituitary and spinal imaging. Scintigraphy and more specialist PET/CT imaging are reserved for complex or challenging cases. Close collaboration between the endocrinologists, endocrine surgeons, and radiologists is essential to ensure best patient outcomes.

Learning points

- CT is the work horse of adrenal imaging, with MRI reserved for young patients and pregnant women, screening in genetic disorders, and patients with contrast allergy. A homogenous nodule with intracellular lipid can be confidently diagnosed as a lipid-rich benign adenoma. Lipid poor (benign) adenomas demonstrate absolute and relative contrast washout of >60% and >40%, respectively.
- Imaging cannot differentiate between functional or nonfunctional adrenal masses.
- In patients with hyperparathyroidism, first line investigations with US neck, 4D CT, and Sestamibi SPECT/CT will localize the parathyroid adenoma in most cases.
- Thyroid ultrasound and planar scintigraphy are extremely useful in characterizing nodules and thyroiditis, and correlation with thyroid function tests is essential.
- In acromegaly patients, an MRI head is the most sensitive modality to assess for pituitary micro- or macroadenoma.
- A contrast-enhanced CT of the neck, chest, abdomen, and pelvis should be performed if an ectopic source of ACTH or GHRH is suspected, with a ^{68}Ga-DOTATATE PET/CT as the second line, if no source is found on CT.

References

[1] Velasco A, Vongpatanasin W. The evaluation and treatment of endocrine forms of hypertension. Curr Cardiol Rep 2014 Sep;16(9):528. https://doi.org/10.1007/s11886-014-0528-x. PMID: 25119722.

[2] de Silva T, Cosentino G, Ganji S, Riera-Gonzalez A, Hsia DS. Endocrine causes of hypertension. Curr Hypertens Rep 2020 Oct 20;22(11):97. https://doi.org/10.1007/s11906-020-01108-3. PMID: 33079272.

[3] de Freminville JB, Amar L. How to explore an endocrine cause of hypertension. J Clin Med 2022 Jan 14;11(2):420. https://doi.org/10.3390/jcm11020420. PMID: 35054115.

[4] Boland GW, Lee MJ, Gazelle GS, Halpern EF, McNicholas MM, Mueller PR. Characterization of adrenal masses using unenhanced CT: an analysis of the CT literature. AJR Am J Roentgenol 1998 Jul;171(1):201−4. https://doi.org/10.2214/ajr.171.1.9648789. PMID: 9648789.

[5] Boland GW, Blake MA, Hahn PF, Mayo-Smith WW. Incidental adrenal lesions: principles, techniques, and algorithms for imaging characterization. Radiology 2008 Dec;249(3):756−75. https://doi.org/10.1148/radiol.2493070976. PMID: 19011181.

[6] Boland GW. Adrenal imaging: why, when, what, and how? Part 2. What technique? AJR Am J Roentgenol 2011 Jan;196(1):W1−5. https://doi.org/10.2214/AJR.10.4205. PMID: 21178019.

[7] Blake MA, Cronin CG, Boland GW. Adrenal imaging. AJR Am J Roentgenol 2010 Jun;194(6):1450−60. https://doi.org/10.2214/AJR.10.4547. Erratum in: AJR Am J Roentgenol. 2012 May;198(5):1232. PMID: 20489083.

[8] Rodacki K, Ramalho M, Dale BM, Battisti S, de Campos RO, Giardino A, Semelka RC. Combined chemical shift imaging with early dynamic serial gadolinium-enhanced MRI in the characterization of adrenal lesions. AJR Am J Roentgenol 2014 Jul;203(1):99−106. https://doi.org/10.2214/AJR.13.11731. PMID: 24951201.

[9] Boland GW, Dwamena BA, Jagtiani Sangwaiya M, Goehler AG, Blake MA, Hahn PF, Scott JA, Kalra MK. Characterization of adrenal masses by using FDG PET: a systematic review and meta-analysis of diagnostic test performance. Radiology 2011 Apr;259(1):117−26. https://doi.org/10.1148/radiol.11100569. PMID: 21330566.

[10] Daunt N. Adrenal vein sampling: how to make it quick, easy, and successful. Radiographics 2005 Oct;25(Suppl 1):S143−58. https://doi.org/10.1148/rg.25si055514. PMID: 16227488.

[11] Young WF, Stanson AW. What are the keys to successful adrenal venous sampling (AVS) in patients with primary aldosteronism? Clin Endocrinol (Oxf) 2009 Jan;70(1):14−7. https://doi.org/10.1111/j.1365-2265.2008.03450.x. PMID: 19128364.

[12] Jakobsson H, Farmaki K, Sakinis A, Ehn O, Johannsson G, Ragnarsson O. Adrenal venous sampling: the learning curve of a single interventionalist with 282 consecutive procedures. Diagn Interv Radiol 2018 ;24(2):89−93. https://doi.org/10.5152/dir.2018.17397. PMID: 29467114.

[13] Rossi GP, Rossitto G, Amar L, Azizi M, Riester A, Reincke M, et al. Clinical outcomes of 1625 patients with primary aldosteronism subtyped with adrenal vein sampling. Hypertension 2019 Oct;74(4):800−8. https://doi.org/10.1161/HYPERTENSIONAHA.119.13463. PMID: 31476901.

[14] Vonend O, Ockenfels N, Gao X, Allolio B, Lang K, Mai K, et al. German Conn's registry. Adrenal venous sampling: evaluation of the German Conn's registry. Hypertension 2011 May;57(5):990−5. https://doi.org/10.1161/HYPERTENSIONAHA.110.168484. PMID: 21383311.

[15] Sahdev A, Kavanagh RG, Reznek RH. Adrenal imaging. In: Grainger & Allison's diagnostic radiology: a textbook of diagnostic imaging. Vol. 37. 7th edn. pp. 938−966.

[16] Sze WC, Soh LM, Lau JH, Reznek R, Sahdev A, Matson M, et al. Diagnosing unilateral primary aldosteronism - comparison of a clinical prediction score, computed tomography and adrenal venous sampling. Clin Endocrinol (Oxf). 2014 Jul;81(1):25−30. https://doi.org/10.1111/cen.12374. PMID: 24274335.

[17] Hannon MJ, Sze WC, Carpenter R, Parvanta L, Matson M, Sahdev A, Druce MR, Berney DM, Waterhouse M, Akker SA, Drake WM. Clinical outcomes following unilateral adrenalectomy in patients with primary aldosteronism. QJM 2017 May 1;110(5):277−81. https://doi.org/10.1093/qjmed/hcw194. PMID: 28180906.

[18] Fleseriu M, Auchus R, Bancos I, Ben-Shlomo A, Bertherat J, Biermasz NR, et al. Consensus on diagnosis and management of Cushing's disease: a guideline update. Lancet Diabetes Endocrinol 2021 Dec;9(12):847−75. https://doi.org/10.1016/S2213-8587(21)00235-7. PMID: 34687601.

[19] Young J, Haissaguerre M, Viera-Pinto O, Chabre O, Baudin E, Tabarin A. Management of endocrine disease: Cushing's syndrome due to ectopic ACTH secretion: an expert operational opinion. Eur J Endocrinol 2020 Apr;182(4):R29−58. https://doi.org/10.1530/EJE-19-0877. PMID: 31999619.

[20] Kiseljak-Vassiliades K, Bancos I, Hamrahian A, Habra M, Vaidya A, Levine AC, Else T. American Association of Clinical Endocrinology Disease state clinical review on the evaluation and management of adrenocortical carcinoma in an adult: a practical approach. Endocr Pract 2020 Nov;26(11):1366−83. https://doi.org/10.4158/DSCR-2020-0567. PMID: 33875173.

[21] Libé R, Bertherat J. Molecular genetics of adrenocortical tumours, from familial to sporadic diseases. Eur J Endocrinol 2005 Oct;153(4):477−87. https://doi.org/10.1530/eje.1.02004. PMID: 16189167.

[22] Jouinot A, Bertherat J. Diseases predisposing to adrenocortical malignancy (Li-Fraumeni syndrome, Beckwith-Wiedemann syndrome, and Carney complex). Exp Suppl 2019;111:149−69. https://doi.org/10.1007/978-3-030-25905-1_9. PMID: 31588532.

[23] Else T, Kim AC, Sabolch A, Raymond VM, Kandathil A, Caoili EM, Jolly S, Miller BS, Giordano TJ, Hammer GD. Adrenocortical carcinoma. Endocr Rev 2014 Apr;35(2):282−326. https://doi.org/10.1210/er.2013-1029. PMID: 24423978.

[24] Kamilaris CDC, Stratakis CA, Hannah-Shmouni F. Molecular genetic and genomic alterations in Cushing's syndrome and primary aldosteronism. Front Endocrinol (Lausanne) 2021 Mar 12;12:632543. https://doi.org/10.3389/fendo.2021.632543. PMID: 33776926.

[25] Isidori AM, Kaltsas GA, Pozza C, Frajese V, Newell-Price J, Reznek RH, Jenkins PJ, Monson JP, Grossman AB, Besser GM. The ectopic adrenocorticotropin syndrome: clinical features, diagnosis, management, and long-term follow-up. J Clin Endocrinol Metab 2006 Feb;91(2):371−7. https://doi.org/10.1210/jc.2005-1542. PMID: 16303835.

[26] Ejaz S, Vassilopoulou-Sellin R, Busaidy NL, Hu MI, Waguespack SG, Jimenez C, Ying AK, Cabanillas M, Abbara M, Habra MA. Cushing syndrome secondary to ectopic adrenocorticotropic hormone secretion: the University of Texas MD Anderson Cancer Center Experience. Cancer 2011 Oct 1;117(19):4381−9. https://doi.org/10.1002/cncr.26029. PMID: 21412758.

[27] Isidori AM, Sbardella E, Zatelli MC, Boschetti M, Vitale G, Colao A, Pivonello R, Study Group ABC. Conventional and nuclear medicine imaging in ectopic Cushing's syndrome: a systematic review. J Clin Endocrinol Metab 2015 Sep;100(9):3231−44. https://doi.org/10.1210/JC.2015-1589. PMID: 26158607.

[28] Geijer H, Breimer LH. Somatostatin receptor PET/CT in neuroendocrine tumours: update on systematic review and meta-analysis. Eur J Nucl Med Mol Imaging 2013 Oct;40(11):1770−80. https://doi.org/10.1007/s00259-013-2482-z. PMID: 23873003.

[29] Aygun N, Uludag M. Pheochromocytoma and paraganglioma: from epidemiology to clinical findings. Sisli Etfal Hastan Tip Bul 2020 Jun 3;54(2):159−68. https://doi.org/10.14744/SEMB.2020.18794. PMID: 32617052.

[30] Lenders JWM, Kerstens MN, Amar L, Prejbisz A, Robledo M, Taieb D, Pacak K, Crona J, Zelinka T, Mannelli M, Deutschbein T, Timmers HJLM, Castinetti F, Dralle H, Widimský J, Gimenez-Roqueplo AP, Eisenhofer G. Genetics, diagnosis, management, and future directions of research of phaeochromocytoma and paraganglioma: a position statement and consensus of the Working Group on Endocrine Hypertension of the European Society of Hypertension. J Hypertens 2020 Aug;38(8):1443−56. https://doi.org/10.1097/HJH.0000000000002438. PMID: 32412940.

[31] Nölting S, Bechmann N, Taieb D, Beuschlein F, Fassnacht M, Kroiss M, Eisenhofer G, Grossman A, Pacak K. Personalized management of pheochromocytoma and paraganglioma. Endocr Rev 2021 Jun;19:bnab019. https://doi.org/10.1210/endrev/bnab019. Erratum in: Endocr Rev. 2021 Dec 14; Erratum in: Endocr Rev. 2021 Dec 14;: PMID: 34147030.

[32] Ross EJ, Griffith DN. The clinical presentation of phaeochromocytoma. Q J Med 1989 Jun;71(266):485−96. PMID: 2513593.

[33] Lee KY, Oh YW, Noh HJ, Lee YJ, Yong HS, Kang EY, Kim KA, Lee NJ. Extraadrenal paragangliomas of the body: imaging features. AJR Am J Roentgenol 2006 Aug;187(2):492−504. https://doi.org/10.2214/AJR.05.0370. PMID: 16861555.

[34] Destito D, Bucolo S, Florio A, Quattrocchi C. Management of head and neck paragangliomas: a series of 9 cases and review of the literature. Ear Nose Throat J 2012 Aug;91(8):366−75. PMID: 22930086.

[35] Woo S, Suh CH, Kim SY, Cho JY, Kim SH. Pheochromocytoma as a frequent false-positive in adrenal washout CT: a systematic review and meta-analysis. Eur Radiol 2018 Mar;28(3):1027−36. https://doi.org/10.1007/s00330-017-5076-5. PMID: 29026974.

[36] Buitenwerf E, Korteweg T, Visser A, Haag CMSC, Feelders RA, Timmers HJLM, Canu L, Haak HR, Bisschop PHLT, Eekhoff EMW, Corssmit EPM, Krak NC, Rasenberg E, van den Bergh J, Stoker J, Greuter MJW, Dullaart RPF, Links TP, Kerstens MN. Unenhanced CT imaging is highly sensitive to exclude pheochromocytoma: a multicenter study. Eur J Endocrinol 2018 May;178(5):431−7. https://doi.org/10.1530/EJE-18-0006. PMID: 29467230.

[37] Pepe J, Cipriani C, Sonato C, Raimo O, Biamonte F, Minisola S. Cardiovascular manifestations of primary hyperparathyroidism: a narrative review. Eur J Endocrinol 2017 Dec;177(6):R297−308. https://doi.org/10.1530/EJE-17-0485. PMID: 28864535.

[38] Walker MD, Bilezikian JP. Endotext [Internet]. In: Feingold KR, Anawalt B, Boyce A, et al., editors. Primary Hyperparathyroidism. [Updated 2021 Apr 19]. South Dartmouth (MA): MDText.com, Inc.; 2000. Available from: https://www.ncbi.nlm.nih.gov/books/NBK278923/.

[39] Ruda JM, Hollenbeak CS, Stack Jr BC. A systematic review of the diagnosis and treatment of primary hyperparathyroidism from 1995 to 2003. Otolaryngol Head Neck Surg 2005 Mar;132(3):359−72. https://doi.org/10.1016/j.otohns.2004.10.005. PMID: 15746845.

[40] Thanseer N, Bhadada SK, Sood A, Mittal BR, Behera A, Gorla AKR, Kalathoorakathu RR, Singh P, Dahiya D, Saikia UN, Rao SD. Comparative effectiveness of ultrasonography, 99mTc-Sestamibi, and 18F-Fluorocholine PET/CT in detecting parathyroid adenomas in patients with primary hyperparathyroidism. Clin Nucl Med 2017 Dec;42(12):e491−7. https://doi.org/10.1097/RLU.0000000000001845. PMID: 28902729.

[41] Hinson AM, Lee DR, Hobbs BA, Fitzgerald RT, Bodenner DL, Stack Jr BC. Preoperative 4D CT localization of nonlocalizing parathyroid adenomas by ultrasound and SPECT-CT. Otolaryngol Head Neck Surg 2015 Nov;153(5):775−8. https://doi.org/10.1177/0194599815599372. PMID: 26248963.

[42] Mahajan A, Starker LF, Ghita M, Udelsman R, Brink JA, Carling T. Parathyroid four-dimensional computed tomography: evaluation of radiation dose exposure during preoperative localization of parathyroid tumors in primary hyperparathyroidism. World J Surg 2012 Jun;36(6):1335−9. https://doi.org/10.1007/s00268-011-1365-3. PMID: 22146947.

[43] Eslamy HK, Ziessman HA. Parathyroid scintigraphy in patients with primary hyperparathyroidism: 99mTc sestamibi SPECT and SPECT/CT. Radiographics 2008 ;28(5):1461−76. https://doi.org/10.1148/rg.285075055. PMID: 18794320.

[44] Treglia G, Sadeghi R, Schalin-Jäntti C, Caldarella C, Ceriani L, Giovanella L, Eisele DW. Detection rate of (99m) Tc-MIBI single photon emission computed tomography (SPECT)/CT in preoperative planning for patients with primary hyperparathyroidism: A meta-analysis. Head Neck 2016 Apr;38(Suppl. 1):E2159−72. https://doi.org/10.1002/hed.24027. PMID: 25757222.

[45] Krakauer M, Wieslander B, Myschetzky PS, Lundstrøm A, Bacher T, Sørensen CH, Trolle W, Nygaard B, Bennedbæk FN. A prospective comparative study of parathyroid dual-phase scintigraphy, dual-isotope subtraction scintigraphy, 4D-CT, and ultrasonography in primary hyperparathyroidism. Clin Nucl Med 2016 Feb;41(2):93−100. https://doi.org/10.1097/RLU.0000000000000988. PMID: 26447369.

[46] Huang Z, Lou C. 99mTcO4-/99mTc-MIBI dual-tracer scintigraphy for preoperative localization of parathyroid adenomas. J Int Med Res 2019 Feb;47(2):836−45. https://doi.org/10.1177/0300060518813742. PMID: 30556441.

[47] Aboagye EO, Bhujwalla ZM. Malignant transformation alters membrane choline phospholipid metabolism of human mammary epithelial cells. Cancer Res 1999 Jan 1;59(1):80−4. PMID: 9892190.

[48] Quak E, Lheureux S, Reznik Y, Bardet S, Aide N. F18-choline, a novel PET tracer for parathyroid adenoma? J Clin Endocrinol Metab 2013 Aug;98(8):3111−2. https://doi.org/10.1210/jc.2013-2084. PMID: 23788686.

[49] Michaud L, Burgess A, Huchet V, Lefèvre M, Tassart M, Ohnona J, Kerrou K, Balogova S, Talbot JN, Périé S. Is 18F-fluorocholine-positron emission tomography/computerized tomography a new imaging tool for detecting hyperfunctioning parathyroid glands in primary or secondary hyperparathyroidism? J Clin Endocrinol Metab 2014 Dec;99(12):4531−6. https://doi.org/10.1210/jc.2014-2821. PMID: 25215560.

[50] Treglia G, Piccardo A, Imperiale A, Strobel K, Kaufmann PA, Prior JO, Giovanella L. Diagnostic performance of choline PET for detection of hyperfunctioning parathyroid glands in hyperparathyroidism: a systematic review and meta-analysis. Eur J Nucl Med Mol Imaging 2019 Mar;46(3):751−65. https://doi.org/10.1007/s00259-018-4123-z. PMID: 30094461.

[51] Lee SW, Shim SR, Jeong SY, Kim SJ. Direct comparison of preoperative imaging modalities for localization of primary hyperparathyroidism: a systematic review and network meta-analysis. JAMA Otolaryngol Head Neck Surg 2021 Aug 1;147(8):692−706. https://doi.org/10.1001/jamaoto.2021.0915. PMID: 34081083.

[52] Giovanella L, Avram AM, Iakovou I, Kwak J, Lawson SA, Lulaj E, et al. EANM practice guideline/SNMMI procedure standard for RAIU and thyroid scintigraphy. Eur J Nucl Med Mol Imaging 2019 Nov;46(12):2514−25. https://doi.org/10.1007/s00259-019-04472-8. PMID: 31392371.

[53] Haugen BR, Alexander EK, Bible KC, Doherty GM, Mandel SJ, Nikiforov YE, et al. 2015 American Thyroid Association management guidelines for adult patients with thyroid nodules and differentiated thyroid cancer: the American Thyroid Association guidelines task force on thyroid nodules and differentiated thyroid cancer. Thyroid 2016 Jan;26(1):1−133. https://doi.org/10.1089/thy.2015.0020. PMID: 26462967.

[54] Intenzo C, Jabbour S, Miller JL, Ahmed I, Furlong K, Kushen M, Kim SM, Capuzzi DM. Subclinical hyperthyroidism: current concepts and scintigraphic imaging. Clin Nucl Med 2011 Sep;36(9):e107−13. https://doi.org/10.1097/RLU.0b013e3182175477. PMID: 21825836.

[55] Lau LW, Ghaznavi S, Frolkis AD, Stephenson A, Robertson HL, Rabi DM, Paschke R. Malignancy risk of hyperfunctioning thyroid nodules compared with non-toxic nodules: systematic review and a meta-analysis. Thyroid Res 2021 Feb 25;14(1):3. https://doi.org/10.1186/s13044-021-00094-1. PMID: 33632297.

[56] Castagnone D, Rivolta R, Rescalli S, Baldini MI, Tozzi R, Cantalamessa L. Color Doppler sonography in Graves' disease: value in assessing activity of disease and predicting outcome. AJR Am J Roentgenol 1996 Jan;166(1):203−7. https://doi.org/10.2214/ajr.166.1.8571877. PMID: 8571877.

[57] Epp R, Malcolm J, Jolin-Dahel K, Clermont M, Keely E. Postpartum thyroiditis. BMJ 2021 Mar 3;372:n495. https://doi.org/10.1136/bmj.n495. PMID: 33658175.

[58] Bartalena L, Bogazzi F, Chiovato L, Hubalewska-Dydejczyk A, Links TP, Vanderpump M. 2018 European Thyroid Association (ETA) guidelines for the management of amiodarone-associated thyroid dysfunction. Eur Thyroid J 2018 Mar;7(2):55−66. https://doi.org/10.1159/000486957. PMID: 29594056.

[59] George AS, Fernandez CJ, Eapen D, Pappachan JM. Organ-specific adverse events of immune checkpoint inhibitor therapy, with special reference to endocrinopathies. touchREV Endocrinol 2021 Apr;17(1):21−32. https://doi.org/10.17925/EE.2021.17.1.21. PMID: 35118443.

[60] Muller I, Moran C, Lecumberri B, Decallonne B, Robertson N, Jones J, et al. 2019 European Thyroid Association guidelines on the management of thyroid dysfunction following immune reconstitution therapy. Eur Thyroid J 2019 Jul;8(4):173−85. https://doi.org/10.1159/000500881. PMID: 31602359.

[61] Chanson P, Salenave S, Kamenicky P. Acromegaly. Handb Clin Neurol. 2014;124:197−219. https://doi.org/10.1016/B978-0-444-59602-4.00014-9. PMID: 25248589.

[62] Profka E, Rodari G, Giacchetti F, Giavoli C. GH deficiency and replacement therapy in hypopituitarism: insight into the relationships with other hypothalamic-pituitary axes. Front Endocrinol (Lausanne) 2021 Oct 19;12:678778. https://doi.org/10.3389/fendo.2021.678778. PMID: 34737721.

[63] Dehghani M, Davoodi Z, Bidari F, Moghaddam AM, Khalili D, Bahrami-Motlagh H, Jamali E, Alamdari S, Hosseinpanah F, Hedayati M, Valizadeh M. Association of different pathologic subtypes of growth hormone producing pituitary adenoma and remission in acromegaly patients: a retrospective cohort study. BMC Endocr Disord 2021 Sep 16;21(1):186. https://doi.org/10.1186/s12902-021-00850-2. PMID: 34530798.

[64] Brzana J, Yedinak CG, Gultekin SH, Delashaw JB, Fleseriu M. Growth hormone granulation pattern and somatostatin receptor subtype 2A correlate with postoperative somatostatin receptor ligand response in acromegaly: a large single center experience. Pituitary 2013 Dec;16(4):490−8. https://doi.org/10.1007/s11102-012-0445-1. PMID: 23184260.

[65] Akirov A, Asa SL, Amer L, Shimon I, Ezzat S. The clinicopathological spectrum of acromegaly. J Clin Med 2019 Nov 13;8(11):1962. https://doi.org/10.3390/jcm8111962. PMID: 31766255.

[66] Mayr B, Buslei R, Theodoropoulou M, Stalla GK, Buchfelder M, Schöfl C. Molecular and functional properties of densely and sparsely granulated GH-producing pituitary adenomas. Eur J Endocrinol 2013 Sep 12;169(4):391−400. https://doi.org/10.1530/EJE-13-0134. PMID: 23847328.

[67] Sundin A, Vullierme MP, Kaltsas G, Plöckinger U. Mallorca consensus conference participants; European Neuroendocrine Tumor Society. ENETS consensus guidelines for the standards of care in neuroendocrine tumors: radiological examinations. Neuroendocrinology 2009;90(2):167−83. https://doi.org/10.1159/000184855. PMID: 19077417.

Chapter 21

Systematic approach to the diagnosis and management of endocrine hypertension

Michael Stowasser[1], Pieter Jansen[2] and Martin Wolley[1]

[1]Endocrine Hypertension Research Centre, University of Queensland, Brisbane, QLD, Australia; [2]Department of Diabetes and Endocrinology, Princess Alexandra Hospital, Woolloongabba, QLD, Australia

Visit the *Endocrine Hypertension: From Basic Science to Clinical Practice, First Edition* companion web site at: https://www.elsevier.com/books-and-journals/book-companion/9780323961202.

Graphical Abstract

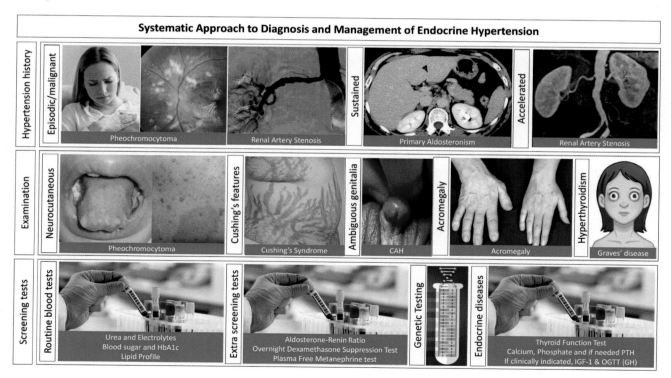

Endocrine Hypertension. https://doi.org/10.1016/B978-0-323-96120-2.00009-1

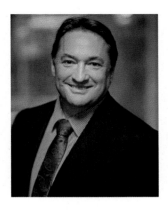

Michael Stowasser

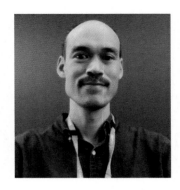

Pieter Jansen

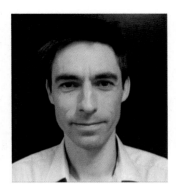

Martin Wolley

Introduction

To the patient with hypertension, the detection of an underlying, specifically treatable endocrine cause can have a profound beneficial impact. Correction of the causative entity may lead to cure or at least improvement (often marked) in hypertension control, resulting in reduced pill burden, morbidity and even mortality and improved quality of life. Furthermore, adverse consequences of hormone excess which are not necessarily dependent on blood pressure elevation may also be averted. In addition, simply solving the mystery as to why a patient has had hypertension can be a considerable comfort and relief to them. For all these reasons, the majority of hypertensive patients who are offered the opportunity to undergo screening tests for secondary endocrine causes will readily consider it. Of course, this needs to be balanced against factors such as prevalence, costs of screening, and likelihood of beneficial outcomes. For this reason, the case for widespread screening among hypertensive patients is greater for some endocrine conditions than others. For example, a growing number of investigators have advocated screening for primary aldosteronism in the great majority, and possibly all newly diagnosed hypertensives as it is common, screening requires an inexpensive blood test (the plasma aldosterone/renin ratio; ARR) and specific management has well-documented highly beneficial sequelae. Thyroid disorders and hyperparathyroidism are also common and are routinely screened in most medical settings. Greater selectivity is advocated for renovascular hypertension, in which the prevalence is somewhat less, and screening involves more costly imaging approaches, including renal artery duplex ultrasonography (which, in addition, requires substantial expertise to obtain accurate results) and CT renal angiography (which carries with it a finite risk of contrast-induced kidney injury). Although pheochromocytoma is much rarer, missing the diagnosis could have dire consequences and biochemical screening by plasma-free metanephrines or 24-hour urinary catecholamines and/or metanephrines is relatively inexpensive and straightforward, and so a case could be made for screening for this condition at least once in every hypertensive's lifetime. Against this, however, is the fact that this approach leads to the identification of not insignificant numbers of patients with mildly elevated metanephrine concentrations but who rarely turn out to have pheochromocytoma. Nonselective screening of hypertensive patients for other endocrine conditions such as Cushing's syndrome and acromegaly is likely to be of low yield due to the low prevalence of these conditions.

This chapter will attempt to provide an approach toward the diagnosis and management of various forms of endocrine hypertension with a focus on practical clinical aspects.

Primary aldosteronism (PA)

Clinical diagnosis

Symptoms and signs of PA

Almost all patients with PA are hypertensive. Rare exceptions include occasional normotensive (yet genetically positive) members of some families with inheritable forms [1,2], and others in whom PA has been heralded by hypokalemia or adrenal incidentaloma rather than hypertension [3]. Hypokalemia is present in approximately 20%−25% of patients [4,5] and may be accompanied by muscle weakness, cramping, tetany, paresthesias, palpitation, polyuria, and nocturia, the latter of which often occurs even when plasma potassium is normal. Other common symptoms in patients with PA include lethargy, impaired mental concentration, and mood disturbances [6−8].

Although uncommon, malignant hypertension can occur in PA, and the accompanying intrarenal ischemia may lead to renin levels in the unsuppressed range, which could result in the diagnosis of PA being missed [9].

During pregnancy, hypertension and biochemical manifestations of PA may be masked [10,11] due to the high circulating levels of placental progesterone (a mineralocorticoid receptor [MR] antagonist). Conversely, in other women, PA due to aldosterone producing adenoma (APA) may develop during pregnancy possibly due to (i) the presence of somatic activating mutations in *CTNNB1* (encodes β-catenin in the Wnt cell-differentiation pathway and may explain tumor development) and (ii) aberrant receptor activation of *LHCGR* (encoding lutotropin-chorionogonadotropic hormone receptor) and *GNRHR* (encoding gonadotropin releasing hormone receptor) within these APAs by high levels of human chorionic gonadotropin hormone, leading to stimulation of aldosterone production [12].

The importance of accurate assays in the diagnostic workup of PA

Highly reproducible assays are essential for all stages of the diagnostic workup of PA, including screening, confirmatory suppression testing, and adrenal venous sampling (AVS).

Concerns have been raised regarding the accuracy and reproducibility of immunoassays for serum or plasma aldosterone (which circulates at low, picomolar concentrations) and especially about the degree of specificity of the antibodies used and the need for meticulous laboratory technique. Because of this lack of specificity, newer highly accurate and reproducible methods of measuring aldosterone using high-performance liquid chromatography and tandem mass spectrometry (LC-MS/MS) generate aldosterone levels within paired samples that are substantially lower than those measured by immunoassays [13,14], necessitating adjustment of diagnostic thresholds such as the ARR and confirmatory suppression testing [15,16]. The risk of overestimation of serum or plasma aldosterone with immunoassay techniques becomes greater when concentrations are at the lower end of the reference range, presumably because other steroids which cross-react with the aldosterone antibody would be expected to make up a greater proportion of the total amount of steroid that is bound. This is particularly relevant for confirmatory suppression testing, during which "true" aldosterone concentrations in patients without PA fall to very low values, but when measured by an immunoassay with poor specificity performance characteristics, may demonstrate apparent failure to suppress (i.e., a false-positive test). The use of semiautomated technology allows high sample throughput, rapid generation of assay results, and relatively low running costs, making them suitable for the clinical setting. The initial cost outlay associated with purchasing the equipment continues to represent a barrier to wide application of LC-MS/MS but given the savings that are likely to occur through more accurate diagnosis of PA (i.e., with lower rates of false positive ARR and confirmatory suppression testing results leading to fewer unnecessary confirmatory tests and AVS procedures respectively), this situation may gradually change with time.

Accurate measurement of renin is critical for detection of PA as it has a profound influence on the ARR with small changes in absolute renin concentrations resulting in potentially large variations in the ratio [17]. Renin is most commonly measured as plasma renin activity (PRA) or of direct (or active) renin concentration (DRC). While PRA measures the amount of angiotensin I generated by the action of renin on its substrate, angiotensinogen, in a defined volume of plasma per unit of time and hence is a measure of renin enzyme activity, DRC measures the plasma concentration of the active (cleaved) form of renin. The main advantage of DRC is that it can be undertaken by automated immunometric assay [18], which is much faster and less labor intensive than PRA (which uses immunoassay or occasionally LC-MS/MS to measure angiotensin I). However, as with aldosterone assays, DRC assays tend to lack reliability and reproducibility at the lower end of the reference range, which is especially pertinent for PA in which renin levels are suppressed [19]. In the case of PRA, on the other hand, for samples with levels less than 1 ng/ml/min, reproducibility of the assay can be maintained by extending the incubation time from the recommended 90 min to 18 h [20]. Use of DRC (but not PRA) is associated with higher ARR values with the potential for false-positives during the luteal phase of the menstrual cycle or in women receiving estrogen-containing oral contraceptive or hormone replacement preparations, possibly because the concentration of angiotensinogen (substrate) increases in response to higher estrogen, and DRC falls to maintain angiotensin II concentrations in the normal range, whereas PRA remains relatively unaffected [21,22]. Automated immunometric renin assays (DRC) have, however, been reported to have better interlaboratory agreement than PRA [23].

A promising alternative to measuring renin is the mass spectrometric measurement of angiotensin II (during a period of equilibrium of formation vs. metabolism) [24] which is arguably more relevant in clinically assessing patients for the presence of angiotensin II-independent aldosterone overproduction given it is the major direct physiological hormonal modulator of adrenal cortical aldosterone synthesis (unlike renin).

Screening for PA

Screening should be considered in most patients with hypertension, and especially those with moderate to severe forms, spontaneous or diuretic induced hypokalemia, adrenal incidentaloma, sleep apnea, or a family history of early onset hypertension or cerebrovascular accident at a young age (<40 years), and all hypertensive first degree relatives of patients with PA [25]. It is no longer deemed appropriate to restrict screening to hypertensive patients with hypokalemia as this would result in up to 80% of patients with PA being missed [4]. Some investigators suggest screening of all hypertensives [26], ideally at the time of first diagnosis. Screening before commencement of antihypertensive medications avoids potentially confounding effects of these agents on renin and aldosterone levels and permits earlier institution of specific treatment with better outcomes [27].

At present, the most popular method of screening for PA involves measurement of the ARR. Demonstration of frankly elevated plasma aldosterone levels lacks sensitivity [5,28]. "Normal" aldosterone levels are commonly seen in patients with PA and should be viewed as "inappropriately normal" in the face of renin suppression which, in individuals without PA, should be accompanied by low aldosterone levels. Elevated aldosterone levels in isolation (i.e., without knowledge of the renin level) also lack specificity as they may be secondary to activation of the renin-angiotensin system (secondary hyperaldosteronism) due, for example, to treatment with diuretics or renovascular hypertension. Suppressed renin levels lack specificity, in that they are also observed in patients receiving beta-adrenergic or nonsteroidal antiinflammatory agents, ingesting a high dietary salt intake, of advanced age, or with chronic kidney disease or other varieties of low renin hypertension such as Liddle syndrome, hypertensive forms of congenital adrenal hyperplasia, familial hypertension and hyperkalemia (Gordon syndrome), the syndrome of apparent mineralocorticoid excess, ectopic adrenocorticotropin (ACTH) syndrome, deoxycortisone-secreting tumor or glucocorticoid resistance states. The ARR is much more sensitive for detection of PA than plasma potassium or aldosterone measured in isolation, and more specific than isolated renin, in that aldosterone is also suppressed is most other salt-dependent low-renin forms of hypertension and hence the ARR is not elevated.

False-positive and false-negative ARRs can result from a variety of physiological and pharmacological factors (Table 21.1), an appreciation of which aids substantially in the optimal use and interpretation of the ARR. The most common of these are antihypertensive medications, with beta-adrenoceptor blockers, clonidine, and alpha-methyldopa having the potential to cause false-positives, and diuretics (including potassium-sparing), angiotensin converting enzyme (ACE) inhibitors, angiotensin receptor blockers (ARBs) and dihydropyridine-type calcium channel blockers (CCBs) prone to cause false-negatives [29,30].

Where possible, antihypertensives known to affect the ARR should be withdrawn (for at least 4 weeks for diuretics and at least 2 weeks for other agents) prior to screening. Antihypertensive medications which appear to have minimal, if any,

TABLE 21.1 Causes for false positive and false negative plasma aldosterone/renin ratios when screening for primary aldosteronism.

Category	False positives	False negatives
Antihypertensive medications	Beta-adrenoceptor blockers Clonidine α-Methyldopa	Diuretics (including potassium-sparing) ACE inhibitors Angiotensin receptor blockers Dihydropyridine CCBs
Other medications	NSAIDs Estrogen-containing OCPs[a] Estrogen-containing HRT[a]	SSRI inhibitors
Clinical conditions	Chronic kidney disease Familial hyperkalemic hypertension	Malignant hypertension Renovascular hypertension Vomiting and diarrhea Hypokalemia
Physiological factors	High dietary sodium intake Luteal phase of menstrual cycle[a] Advanced age	Low dietary sodium intake

ACE, denotes angiotensin converting enzyme; *CCBs,* calcium channel blockers; *HRT,* hormonal replacement therapy; *NSAIDs,* nonsteroidal antiinflammatory drugs; *OCPs,* oral contraceptive preparations.
[a]*Only if renin is measured as direct renin concentration and not as plasma renin activity.*

effects on the ARR and can be used to control hypertension (where necessary) during screening and subsequent steps in the diagnostic workup of PA include [30]:

- verapamil slow release: suggested starting dose (SSD) ½ × 240 mg tablet twice daily
- hydralazine (best used in combination with verapamil SR to avoid reflex tachycardia): SSD ½ × 25 mg tablet twice daily
- prazosin: SSD ½ × 1 mg tablet twice daily
- moxonidine: SSD 200 µg one table at night.

ARR testing while patients are still on interfering medications can still be informative. For example, a normal ARR in a patient on a beta-blocker (without other interfering medications) would make PA highly unlikely, whereas a raised ARR with suppressed renin in a patient receiving an ACE inhibitor, ARB or diuretic (but not a beta-blocker) would be highly suggestive of PA.

The ARR has greater sensitivity if measured in the morning in an upright (e.g., seated) posture [31]. Cut-off values vary from laboratory to laboratory and depend, at least in part, on the assays used and the units in which aldosterone and renin are expressed. Because the ARR is mathematically highly renin-dependent, then at extremely low levels of renin (e.g., 1.5 mU/L for DRC or 0.1 ng/mL/h for PRA) the ratio may be elevated even if plasma aldosterone is very low (e.g., 110 pmol/L or 4.0 ng/dL) and clearly not compatible with PA. Under those circumstances, it is prudent to take the absolute aldosterone level into consideration (rather than simply the ratio alone) when deciding if to proceed to confirmatory suppression testing. The cut-off aldosterone level in this situation is a matter of debate. The figure used by the Endocrine Hypertension Center in Brisbane is the cut-off used for normal suppression at the conclusion of the seated saline suppression test (162 pmol/L, when measured by LC-MS/MS).

Controlling for factors that can affect the ARR or at least taking them into account enhances its usefulness in helping select patients for further diagnostic workup. The ARR also shows good within-patient reproducibility under such circumstances [32] but not when potentially interfering factors are poorly controlled [33]. Either way, the ratio should still be regarded as a screening test only and should be measured more than once before deciding whether or not to go on to confirmatory testing for PA.

Confirmatory testing for PA

The main purpose of confirmatory testing is to identify patients who, by testing positive, are definitively confirmed as having PA and are therefore candidates for undergoing AVS to determine the subtype; and conversely, to spare patients who test negative (and in whom the diagnosis of PA has therefore been excluded) from having to undergo this invasive and relatively expensive and difficult procedure.

In most cases (apart from the captopril challenge test), confirmatory testing involves measuring aldosterone during dynamic procedures designed to bring about complete suppression of circulating renin, and therefore of angiotensin II, aldosterone's normal chronic regulator. Failure to suppress aldosterone confirms autonomous aldosterone production that is relatively autonomous of angiotensin II, which is PA by definition.

The most common confirmatory tests currently in use are oral sodium loading, saline infusion, and captopril challenge testing. Fludrocortisone suppression testing (FST), although regarded by some investigators to be the most reliable, is relatively labor-intensive and requires a five-day admission to hospital and hence, is rarely performed nowadays. During FST, plasma aldosterone is measured during 4 days oral administration of fludrocortisone (0.1 mg 6 hourly) and oral salt loading (by high sodium diet and administration of slow-release sodium chloride tablets, 1800 mg three times daily with meals) [34]. Plasma potassium is maintained in the normal range by adequate slow release KCl supplementation (given 6 hourly). The FST is considered diagnostic of PA if upright (seated) 10:00 h plasma aldosterone fails to suppress to less than 6 ng/dL (165 pmol/L) when measured by immunoassay (4.8 ng/100 mL or 133 pmol/L by LC-MS/MS) at the conclusion of the test, provided that renin has been sufficiently suppressed (a prerequisite of all forms of suppression testing that involve salt loading).

For the oral salt loading test, patients are instructed to consume sufficient dietary salt to achieve a urine sodium excretion of over 200 mmol/day and are given adequate KCl supplementation to maintain normokalemia. A 24 h urinary aldosterone concentration of over 12 µg/day (33 nmol/day) on the third day is regarded as diagnostic [35].

The saline infusion test (or saline suppression test, SST) involves intravenous administration of 0.9% saline (usually 2 L over 4 h) with measurement of plasma aldosterone at the end of the infusion. Originally, this was performed while patients were maintained in the recumbent position (unlike FST). Concentrations regarded as diagnostic for PA have varied from >5 to >10 ng/dL (>140 to >280 pmol/L) [36,37]. A major advantage of this approach over FST is that it can be performed as an outpatient procedure. However, recumbent SST lacks sensitivity, especially in patients in whom plasma aldosterone demonstrates responsiveness to the assumption of upright posture as their recumbent aldosterone levels are lower than those in posture-unresponsive patients [38]. Performing SST in the seated position has been reported to result in markedly improved sensitivity for detecting PA while retaining high specificity [39]. The diagnostic cut-off for normal suppression of plasma aldosterone is < 5.8 ng/dL (<162 pmol/L) if measured by mass spectrometry [39]. A gray zone of between <6.2 ng/dL (<171 pmol/L) and 7.8 ng/dL (217 pmol/L) has been reported for plasma aldosterone measured by immunoassay [16]. However, a more recent study comparing aldosterone concentrations measured by mass spectrometry and immunoassay in the same individuals undergoing seated SST has revealed a concerning rate of overdiagnosis of PA by immunoassay using these cut-off values, most likely due to the lack of specificity of the assay for aldosterone, which becomes particularly problematic at the lower end of the reference range [40]. This has intensified calls for replacing immunoassay with mass spectrometry in laboratories offering clinical endocrine hypertension diagnostic services.

Captopril challenge testing involves measuring plasma aldosterone and renin basally and 1 or 2 h after administering 25−50 mg oral captopril, an ACE inhibitor, with the patient remaining seated throughout [41]. In subjects without PA, plasma aldosterone is suppressed (>30%) and PRA stimulated by captopril and, as a result, the ARR falls. In one commonly used protocol, the cut-off for normal suppression of plasma aldosterone is < 8.5 ng/dL (240 pmol/L) and for the ARR is < 30 (with aldosterone expressed as ng/dL and PRA as ng/mL/h) 2 h after receiving 50 mg of captopril. Because it does not involve salt loading, the captopril challenge testing avoids the potential for inducing both hypokalemia and fluid overload in patients at risk because of compromised cardiac or renal function. However, its discriminatory power has been questioned [42,43] and symptomatic hypotension can occur as a result of the blood pressure-lowering effect of captopril in upright patients.

Confirmatory testing involving salt loading may be contraindicated in patients with severe hypertension, compromised cardiac status (e.g., reduced left ventricular systolic function, marked left ventricular hypertrophy or high risk of atrial fibrillation) or renal dysfunction because of the enhanced risk of inducing potentially dangerously elevated blood pressure levels, fluid overload, or episodes of atrial fibrillation. In these circumstances, it may be reasonable to proceed directly to subtype differentiation (including AVS) or to consider a trial of medical treatment with an agent that blocks aldosterone action as an attempt to establish better hypertension control and improve cardiac function (either as a temporary measure to reduce the risk of confirmatory testing to a more acceptable level, or as long-term management of PA).

Subtype differentiation

While the morphology associated with PA is diverse, the aim of subtype differentiation from a clinical standpoint is not to attempt to distinguish the many pathological variants from each other, but to assist selection of the optimal management approach. This is achieved by:

1. genetic testing when familial PA is suspected;
2. imaging to exclude large adrenal lesions which may warrant consideration of removal because of their malignant potential and to localize adrenal veins in preparation for AVS;
3. determining whether autonomous aldosterone production is confined to one adrenal, and therefore potentially curable by unilateral adrenalectomy, or bilateral, in which case management usually involves treatment with medications which antagonize aldosterone action.

Of the various familial forms of PA, the strongest case for genetic testing can be made for FH-I (familial hyperaldosteronism type 1; glucocorticoid-remediable aldosteronism). This is because (i) it appears to be by far the most common in terms of familial forms for which a genetic basis has been found (a hybrid *CYP11B1/CYP11B2* mutation); (ii) affected individuals are at risk of severe hypertension and early death from hemorrhagic stroke unless detected and specifically treated; (iii) patients with FH-I demonstrate excellent clinical responses to glucocorticoid medications administered in small doses that do not cause Cushingoid side effects, making them the treatment of choice for this (but no other) subtype of PA; and (iv) detection heralds the need for genetic testing of other family members to identify additional individuals similarly at risk but who will also benefit greatly from timely specific glucocorticoid treatment. Genetic testing of peripheral blood DNA for FH-I involves the use of either Southern blotting or a faster PCR-based method [44,45]. The Endocrine Society recommends testing patients with onset of confirmed PA earlier than at 20 years of age and those who have a family history of PA or of strokes at young age (<40 years) [25]. Germline mutations in *CLCN2* (causing FH-II), *KCNJ5* (FH-III), and *CACNA1H* (FH-IV) have so far been reported much less frequently than hybrid gene mutations and (unlike FH-I) no specific form of treatments are yet available for these conditions. Individuals found to have FH-III due to T158A, I151S, or G151R mutations in *KCNJ5* tend to have more florid PA, often requiring bilateral adrenalectomy to control hypertension [46]. Almost all reported individuals with FH-II, FH-III, and FH-IV have had early age of onset of hypertension, so it would seem reasonable to restrict genetic testing for *CLCN2, KCNJ5,* and *CANA1H* mutations to very young patients with PA.

Adrenal imaging with CT or MRI permits detection of larger (e.g., >3 cm) mass lesions which have greater potential for malignant behavior and may warrant consideration for removal on that basis alone, or at least deserve careful follow-up. When performed with contrast, CT also allows localization of adrenal veins which can assist in successful cannulation at the time of subsequent AVS [47].

Distinguishing unilateral from bilateral PA is an important aspect of the diagnostic workup of PA as the clinical responses to unilateral adrenalectomy in patients with unilateral forms of PA are generally quite gratifying, with cure of hypertension achieved in 40%−70%, marked reductions in pill burden, and better cardiovascular outcomes and improvements in quality of life compared to patients with PA treated medically with drugs that antagonize aldosterone action [7,48−51]. AVS remains the most reliable means of differentiating these two PA subtypes but is also the most invasive and expensive test and requires considerable expertise. Clinical prediction algorithms have relied on the general observation that unilateral forms (including APA) are generally associated with more florid biochemical manifestations of PA, but the considerable degree of overlap that exists has meant that algorithms incorporating such parameters as plasma sodium and potassium, total carbon dioxide, aldosterone, renin, and the ARR have shown variable (and not very reproducible) performance characteristics [52]. Adrenal imaging by CT or MRI frequently misses APAs and can be frankly misleading by detecting nonfunctioning adrenal lesions [5,53]. Scintigraphy using labeled forms of cholesterol may detect large APAs [54] but lacks sufficient resolution to detect smaller tumors. Nuclear imaging using PET-CT with ^{11}C-metomidate has been reported to be a viable alternative or adjunct to AVS (e.g., in difficult cases) [55,56]. However, the short half-life and lack of specificity of the isotope for CYP11B2 (being a ligand also for CYP11B1) limits the current widespread application and reliability of this technique though alternatives are being investigated and are awaited with great interest [57]. Patients with APA more often show lack of responsiveness of plasma aldosterone to upright posture during posture stimulation studies and more often demonstrate elevated plasma or urinary levels of "hybrid steroids" (18-hydroxycortisol and 18-oxocortisol) compared with those with bilateral PA [58,59], but again separation is far from complete. To some extent, the phenotype regarding these two parameters among patients with APA appears to be genetically determined: APAs with somatic *KCNJ5* mutations are usually associated with posture-unresponsiveness and elevated hybrid steroid levels and vice versa for somatic *CACNA1D* (and other) mutations [60]. Although inferior to AVS, the above indicators can provide useful ancillary information, especially when AVS is unavailable, has been declined for some reason or results have been inconclusive (e.g., because of failure to cannulate one or both adrenal veins). For example, the presence of florid, hypokalemic, posture-unresponsive PA in a young patient with an obvious unilateral mass lesion on CT and elevated hybrid steroid levels (if available) would make APA highly likely.

To whom should AVS be offered and how should it be performed?

The Endocrine Society guideline [25] recommends AVS for all patients with confirmed PA who desire adrenalectomy and for whom surgery is not contraindicated. The risk of adrenal hemorrhage associated with AVS is low (less than 2% of all procedures) in experienced hands [61]. Performing AVS in the morning following overnight recumbency means an overnight stay but avoids the confounding effects of changes in posture on aldosterone concentrations and capitalizes on the higher endogenous ACTH levels (compared with later in the day), thereby ensuring that samples are collected during maximal ACTH-induced stimulation of aldosterone production. Arguably, however, these issues (and the need for overnight admission) may also be addressed by the use of exogenous ACTH stimulation, which aims to (i) maximize adrenal/peripheral venous cortisol gradients, (ii) reduce fluctuations in steroid secretion during AVS and (iii) stimulate aldosterone production by APAs and thus avoid sampling during a period of secretion "quiescence" [62]. Successful cannulation of the adrenal veins (especially the right) is challenging in inexperienced hands but tends to improve with increasing throughput. Measures which can assist in attaining high success rates include performing contrast CT scanning prior to AVS to aid in localizing the adrenal veins [47], limiting the procedure to a relatively small number of specialty radiology units within each region and radiologists within each unit to ensure high throughput for each proceduralist, collecting at least two samples from each side, and performing rapid point-of care cortisol testing to confirm correct catheter placement for collection [63]. Cortisol ratios or "gradients" between adrenal and peripheral venous samples of at least two or three (or at least five if exogenous ACTH stimulation is used) are most commonly used to indicate adequacy of AVS. Calculating the aldosterone/cortisol ratio for each adrenal and peripheral venous sample corrects for differences in dilution with nonadrenal venous blood. Criteria for lateralization vary widely from one institution to another [64] with some comparing adrenal venous aldosterone/cortisol ratios on each side with the simultaneous peripheral venous ratio (with lateralization defined as a the ratio being at least 2.5 times the peripheral on the affected side and no higher than peripheral on the other side), while others rely on the comparison of aldosterone/cortisol ratios on one side versus the other (the so-called "lateralization index") with lateralization defined as the ratio on the higher side being at least 2—4 times, depending on the center, in comparison to that on the lower side.

When the patient is suspected of having an adrenal tumor that is concomitantly secreting cortisol, the use of cortisol to "normalize" aldosterone levels may bring about misleading results. This is because the higher cortisol levels on the APA side will lead to a lowering of the ipsilateral aldosterone/cortisol ratio, while feedback suppression of ACTH due to excessive cortisol secretion results in suppression of contralateral cortisol production and consequently a rise in the aldosterone/cortisol ratio on the contralateral side, ultimately potentially culminating in loss of lateralization. In these cases, a hormone other than cortisol (e.g., metanephrine) may be used for "normalization" of aldosterone levels, although criteria for lateralization are less well defined in those circumstances [14,65]. Performing an overnight 1 mg dexamethasone suppression test (ODST) helps to identify subjects who may be candidates for measurement of metanephrine in AVS samples and should therefore be considered as part of the routine diagnostic workup of PA.

Management

Although AVS results play a major role in guiding treatment in a patient with PA, management decisions should nevertheless be tailored to the particular characteristics and wishes of the individual patient. For occasional patients who lateralize on AVS, surgical treatment may not be appropriate. Likewise, in rare patients who do not lateralize but in whom medical management has proven unsuccessful for some reason, surgery may be a reasonable consideration. All management options and their possible outcomes should be fully explained and explored with the patient and, if appropriate, their family, before a treatment is chosen.

Surgical management

In centers which use relatively strict definitions of lateralization, approximately 30% of patients with PA who undergo AVS demonstrate clear lateralization [4,5,28,34]. These patients are candidates for unilateral adrenalectomy (nowadays usually performed laparoscopically, either by an anterior or retroperitoneal approach), which results in cure of hypertension in 50%—60% and significant improvement in the remainder [28,66—69]. Centers which employ more lenient definitions report higher rates of lateralization but lower cure rates. In the Primary Aldosteronism Surgical Outcome (PASO) study, development of a consensus on criteria defining clinical and biochemical cure or improvement of PA following surgery [70] permitted a standardized framework for robust comparisons of outcomes according to a variety of potential variables (which in that study varied from <20 to >60%), including the level of experience of the center, the approach used to diagnose PA and/or to differentiate unilateral from bilateral forms, the method used to reverse the cause of excessive aldosterone production (e.g., total vs. partial adrenalectomy, surgery vs. ablation) and so forth.

Other than in a few highly specialized centers that perform "selective" sampling of adrenal vein branches [71], AVS only indicates which adrenal is excessively producing aldosterone in patients with unilateral PA, and not which part of the gland. It therefore cannot confirm with certainty whether a nodule visualized on CT scanning is actually an APA, rather than a nonsecreting nodule, which happens to be situated in the same gland as a smaller, nonvisualized autonomously secreting lesion. For this reason, the entire adrenal is almost always removed even when a discrete mass lesion is seen on CT.

In rare patients with bilateral forms of PA, inability to control hypertension at maximally tolerated doses of spironolactone (and/or amiloride) may lead to consideration of the option of unilateral adrenalectomy. In those instances, the decision as to which gland to remove should be guided by AVS (with the aim being to remove the gland that has the higher aldosterone/cortisol ratio) or CT (to identify the larger gland if the ratios are similar on both sides). Not surprisingly, the likelihood of benefit is less than with clearly lateralizing PA [72]. Surgery may also be contemplated in patients with bilateral PA in whom one adrenal contains a large mass (e.g., greater than 3—4 cm) which may warrant removal based on malignant potential. Rarely, patients with marked, bilateral adrenal hyperplasia and severe, bilateral PA (including those with severe forms of FH-III), require bilateral adrenalectomy to control hypertension and biochemical manifestations of PA [73—75].

Preoperative treatment for several weeks with an aldosterone antagonist (spironolactone or eplerenone), or epithelial sodium channel blocker (amiloride) is usually associated with a "smoother" peri-operative course in terms of blood pressure and plasma potassium control. Longer periods of such treatment may be advisable in patients with lateralizing PA whose hypertension has been particularly severe and caused substantial hypertensive heart disease in an effort to reduce operative risk by improving cardiovascular function through optimization of hypertension control, repletion of body potassium stores and blockade of direct adverse cardiovascular effects of aldosterone excess.

Immediately following unilateral adrenalectomy for APA, plasma potassium levels should be monitored closely (e.g., at least twice daily for the first 1—2 days and at least daily thereafter until discharge from hospital). Aldosterone production by the remaining adrenal gland may be markedly suppressed because of chronic suppression of renin/Angiotensin II (although this is less likely if the patient has received treatment with an agent that blocks aldosterone action in the weeks leading up to surgery). Because of this, potassium replacement should be withheld during the operation and in the first 24 h postoperatively unless concentrations drop to <3.0 mmol/L, in which case potassium replacement should be given only with extreme caution (at half the usual rate). Again, on the assumption of low aldosterone levels and thus a tendency to urinary salt wasting, postoperative fluids should be given as normal saline 1 L 12 hourly or 8 hourly. Potassium sparing diuretics (spironolactone, eplerenone and amiloride) are withheld just prior to surgery. Some or all other antihypertensives can generally be withheld, and reintroduced over the next few days if required to maintain normotension. In patients still receiving antihypertensives at discharge, gradual withdrawal of medications often continues to occur over the ensuing three to 12 months. In our Center, all operated patients have been cured of hypertension or have required substantially reduced medications following unilateral adrenalectomy.

Simultaneous autonomous overproduction of cortisol and aldosterone by an APA is being increasingly recognized [76—79]. If a patient with unilateral PA is suspected of having concomitant autonomous adrenal overproduction of cortisol, not only may the AVS protocol need to be modified (by incorporating measurement of metanephrine or some other hormone other than cortisol as discussed above), but the requirement for steroid cover perioperatively and for a variable period following surgery should be anticipated. For these reasons, there is an argument for performing overnight dexamethasone suppression testing with basal (predexamethasone) ACTH measurement on all patients undergoing diagnostic workup for PA. Failure of serum cortisol to suppress to <1.8 µg/100 mL (<50 nmol/L), accompanied by a low basal ACTH suggests concomitant autonomous adrenal overproduction of cortisol.

When present preoperatively, hypokalemia almost always resolves within days to weeks following unilateral adrenalectomy for unilateral PA. Normalization of the ARR is another reassuring sign that PA has been biochemically "cured." Blood pressure may take longer (sometimes a year or more) to return to normal but may remain elevated (but always in our experience to a lesser degree than preoperatively), even if PA has been biochemically cured, if the patient has reasons other than PA which are contributing to ongoing hypertension. Serum creatinine usually rises after surgery, and this reflects correction of the volume expanded state and glomerular hyperfiltration (caused by excessive sodium retention) that existed prior to adrenalectomy rather than a deterioration in renal function per se [80]. Patients within our center are encouraged to undergo suppression testing (previously by FST and more recently by seated SST) several months postoperatively in order to detect any autonomous aldosterone production by the remaining adrenal. By this means of assessment, preoperative lateralization on AVS by our criteria has been associated with biochemical cure of PA in over 90% and significant improvement in all remaining patients postoperatively [70]. Other reported benefits of surgery have included improvements in left ventricular mass index on echocardiography [81] and urinary albumin excretion [82], marked improvements in quality of life [7,8,51], reductions in cardiovascular morbidity and reduced mortality [48].

Medical management

In patients with PA who do not lateralize aldosterone production to one side, or who lateralize but prefer medical to surgical treatment or are unfit for surgery, treatment with specific drugs which block aldosterone action is indicated. These medications usually correct hypokalemia effectively, and potassium supplements should therefore usually be ceased when they are commenced. Overtreatment with these agents can cause volume contraction with prerenal failure, raising creatinine levels, and potentially life-threatening hyperkalaemia [34,67], which is more likely in patients who are taking other potassium-retaining agents such as ACE inhibitors, ARBs, or nonsteroidal antiinflammatory drugs (NSAIDs). They should be used with great caution in patients with existing renal impairment.

Because the onset of action of these agents on blood pressure is slow, several weeks should be allowed to elapse before assessing their full effect on blood pressure at each dose. Small doses (for example, spironolactone 12.5 mg once or twice daily, amiloride 2.5 mg once or twice daily and eplerenone 25 mg once or twice daily) should be initiated [67,83]. At these doses, these drugs are usually well tolerated. If necessary, other antihypertensive agents with more rapid onset of action could be employed during this period, and then later reduced or withdrawn.

Spironolactone, which has a steroidal structure, competitively inhibits aldosterone at the MR. Spironolactone is an inhibitor at the testosterone receptor and an agonist at the progesterone receptor (PR), and its use can therefore be associated with sex-steroid-related adverse effects, including gynecomastia and loss of libido, menstrual irregularities, and aggravation of breast fibrocystic change [84], the incidence of which are dose-related. At 12.5–50 mg daily, the incidence of gynecomastia is approximately 10%–15% [5,85] while at doses of 150 mg daily or more it exceeds 50% [86]. Combining spironolactone at lower dose with either amiloride or eplerenone can reduce the likelihood of gynaecomastia and other side effects.

Eplerenone is a newer MR antagonist that appears to be more selective for the receptor than spironolactone, and is, therefore, less likely to produce sex-steroid-related adverse effects [87]. It may also be less likely to interfere with sexual development in children. Hence, it may be particularly suited for adult patients who have demonstrated intolerance to spironolactone because of sex-steroid-related adverse effects, or in children with PA (including those with FH-I). Eplerenone is already available and being used in clinical practice. However, indications for its use in different countries vary, and in some countries, it is not approved for government-subsidized use in PA. Other, nonsteroidal MR antagonists in varying stages of development and likelihood of entering the clinical arena for the management of PA include esaxerenone and finerenone [88].

Amiloride (and the less commonly used triamterene) acts directly on the epithelial sodium channel where aldosterone exerts its effects. Because of its less potent aldosterone antagonist action and its much lower propensity to induce adverse effects, amiloride may be particularly suited to patients with milder forms of PA and to patients who are particularly concerned about the possibility of developing the sex steroid-related side effects of spironolactone.

In many patients with PA being treated medically with agents that antagonize aldosterone action, achievement of hypertension control requires the addition of other antihypertensive medications. Because of the propensity to induce or worsen hypokalemia, potassium-wasting diuretics should be generally avoided, other than in occasional patients with reduced glomerular function on aldosterone antagonists as they can help to prevent hyperkalemia in that situation. Otherwise, there is little evidence to favor one class of agents over another in this situation. Both ACE inhibitors [89,90] and calcium channel antagonists [91–93] have been shown to lower blood pressure in patients with PA.

Glucocorticoids are highly effective for the long-term treatment of FH-I. In our experience, most patients are able to maintain control of hypertension on doses of dexamethasone as low as 0.125–0.25 mg per day [94]. Hybrid gene expression is not completely suppressed at these doses, as evidenced by suppressed PRA, elevated ARR and elevated urinary 18-oxocortisol levels and tight correlation of circadian aldosterone with cortisol (rather than PRA) levels [94]. Our Center's approach is to use the lowest dose of glucocorticoid treatment required to maintain normal clinic, home and ambulatory blood pressures and normal left ventricular mass index and diastolic function on periodic echocardiographic assessments. Patients also undergo dual energy X-ray absorptiometry (DEXA) scans every 2–3 years to monitor for the development of glucocorticoid-induced osteoporosis. Spironolactone, eplerenone and amiloride are alternative options in the treatment of hypertension in FH-I. Amiloride or eplerenone may be preferable for affected children, since they avoid the potential problems of growth-retardation associated with glucocorticoids and androgen blockade with spironolactone.

Incorporation of dietary salt restriction into the management of patients with PA may help not only to lower blood pressure, but also to limit and even reverse target organ damage and morbidity through non-blood pressure-dependent means. Left ventricular mass [95] and degree of proteinuria [96] in patients with PA appear to be dependent on 24 h sodium excretion rate (as a marker of dietary salt intake).

It could be argued that treatment should strive for "complete" reversal of excessive aldosterone action rather than just normalization of potassium and blood pressure levels given that aldosterone excess is now known to have adverse cardiovascular effects that are not dependent on hypertension and hypokalemia alone. Normalization of renin levels may serve to be a better indicator in this sense, since it suggests that the dose of the MR antagonist is adequate to correct the sodium/volume expansion and is therefore providing better long-term protection against aldosterone-induced cardiovascular and renal injury (the development of which appears to be dependent on sodium balance). Indeed, recent studies have suggested better long-term clinical outcomes in medically treated patients with PA in whom renin levels have been maintained in the "unsuppressed" range [48]. However, the usefulness of monitoring of renin levels is likely to depend on whether the patient is being coadministered other medications (such as ACE inhibitors, ARBs, or beta-blockers) which also affect renin levels. In some patients, tolerability will limit the degree to which the dose of spironolactone can be increased in order to achieve normalization of renin, since even at doses of 12.5–25 mg daily, side effects (such as gynecomastia in males and menstrual irregularity in females) are not uncommon. These are not seen during treatment with amiloride or eplerenone, which therefore represent options for alternative, or additive (spironolactone "dose-sparing"), treatment in such circumstances. The serious risk of developing hyperkalemia and uremia with any agent blocking aldosterone is dose-dependent, so that initial doses should be low and only gradually increased.

Measurement of renin can also be helpful in guiding changes in management when hypertension has not yet become optimally controlled on mineralocorticoid antagonist treatment (provided, again, that the patient is not receiving other medications that are affecting renin levels). For example, if renin levels have already become "unsuppressed," it may be better to commence or increase the dose of other antihypertensive medications rather than increasing aldosterone blockade.

Aldosterone synthase inhibitors are in development and hold some promise as alternative treatment approaches for PA, but more information is required to confirm their efficacy and safety in treating PA. Remaining challenges include lack of specificity for aldosterone synthase (with evidence, for example, of reduced cortisol synthesizing capacity) and inferior treatment effect when compared to MR antagonism [97].

(For further reading about PA: refer Chapter 7).

Other mineralocorticoid forms of hypertension

Common to the conditions described in this section is hypertension caused by excessive sodium resorption via the epithelial sodium channel (ENaC) in the distal tubule, due to either:

- excessive production of mineralocorticoids other than aldosterone, leading to excessive MR activation (as in congenital adrenal hyperplasia due to 11β-hydroxylase and 17α-hydroxylase deficiency, Chrousos syndrome, and deoxycorticosterone secreting tumours)
- excessive activation of the MR in the absence of mineralocorticoid excess (as in syndrome of apparent mineralocorticoid excess or Geller syndrome) or
- excessive activity of ENaC in the absence of MR overactivation (as in Liddle syndrome).

Those with ectopic ACTH syndrome would have excessive production of both deoxycorticosterone and cortisol causing MR activation (both 1st and 2nd mechanisms). In all these conditions, as in PA, circulating levels of renin (measured as PRA or DRC) are suppressed as a result of sodium retention and there is urinary potassium and hydrogen ion wasting which can lead to hypokalemia and alkalosis. However, unlike in PA, circulating levels of aldosterone are suppressed and the ARR is not elevated.

11β-hydroxylase deficiency

Clinical diagnosis

After 21-hydroxylase deficiency, 11β-hydroxylase deficiency is the second most frequent cause of congenital adrenal hyperplasia (5%—8%) but it is a rare cause of mineralocorticoid hypertension. 11β-hydroxylase deficiency is transmitted in an autosomal recessive fashion, being caused by loss-of-function mutations affecting both alleles of *CYP11B1* which lead to partial to complete loss of 11β-hydroxylase enzyme activity [98,99]. The resulting failure of the normal conversion of 11-deoxycorticosterone (DOC) to corticosterone and of 11-deoxycortisol to cortisol [100] leads to stimulation of ACTH release, which results in adrenocortical hyperplasia and an increase in DOC production causing mineralocorticoid hypertension and increased adrenal androgen production leading to hyperandrogenism [98,101]. Severity varies markedly among affected individuals, with virilization ranging from mild to marked and hypertension from absent to severe [98,101,102].

In females, the diagnosis may be suspected because of masculinization of the external genitalia at an early age [101,103], but normal internal reproductive organs. Acne, hirsutism, rapid somatic growth during childhood with precocious puberty and short adult stature due to early closure of the epiphyses is common in both sexes. Hypertension, present in about two-thirds of patients, is associated with suppression of plasma renin and sometimes hypokalemia. Plasma cortisol and corticosterone are low while basal or ACTH-stimulated levels of DOC and 11-deoxycortisol are elevated. Unlike in PA, aldosterone levels are also low, possibly because renin is suppressed and chronic ACTH excess leads to suppression (rather than stimulation) of aldosterone production [101,103]. Unlike 11β-hydroxylase deficiency, 21-hydroxylase deficiency (which also causes virilization) is associated with signs of mineralocorticoid deficiency, with salt wasting and potassium retention [98,101—103].

Management

Hypertension normally responds well to adequate glucocorticoid therapy (for example, oral hydrocortisone 10—20 mg/m²/day divided into 2—3 doses, or dexamethasone 20—30 μg/kg/day to a maximum of 2 mg/day [100]), which suppresses ACTH and therefore lowers production of DOC. However, finding a dose that is sufficient to control androgen excess yet low enough to avoid Cushingoid side effects and growth suppression can be challenging and close clinical monitoring is required.

17α-hydroxylase deficiency

Clinical diagnosis

17α-hydroxylase deficiency is a rare cause of congenital adrenal hyperplasia (1% of patients) and mineralocorticoid hypertension [104,105] caused by loss-of-function mutations of both alleles of *CYP17*. Cortisol biosynthesis is impaired, leading to increased ACTH secretion which results in excessive production of the mineralocorticoids, DOC and corticosterone and mineralocorticoid hypertension. A characteristic clinical feature of this condition is the absence of secondary sex characteristics which results from the lack of 17α-hydroxylase and 17,20-desmolase activity and consequently, deficient formation of sex steroids. The phenotype is transmitted in an autosomal recessive fashion.

The condition is frequently recognized at the time of puberty because the association of hypertension and hypokalemia with primary amenorrhea in females, and pseudohermaphroditism with hypospadias and small testes in males. Plasma levels of 17-hydroxyprogesterone, 11-deoxycortisol and cortisol are reduced, while gonadotropins (luteinizing hormone and follicle-stimulating hormone) are increased. As in 11β-hydroxylase deficiency, plasma aldosterone levels are usually low [104,105] but sometimes normal to mildly elevated [106].

Management

Treatment consists of giving a glucocorticoid dosage sufficient to suppress ACTH secretion and hence DOC and corticosterone secretion, which usually results in control of hypertension. Supplemental sex hormone replacement therapy is usually also necessary in the young adult [104].

For detailed reading on congenital adrenal hyperplasia, please refer Chapter 9.

Primary glucocorticoid resistance (PGR) or Chrousos syndrome

Clinical diagnosis

The underlying defect in PGR is partial resistance of the human glucocorticoid receptor (hGR), resulting in chronic elevation of ACTH, adrenal hyperplasia and excessive production of ACTH-dependent steroids [107–109]. The clinical spectrum is broad, ranging from asymptomatic to severe mineralocorticoid hypertension with hypokalemia and/or severe hyperandrogenism (due to excessive production of androgens). The mineralocorticoid hypertension probably results from the combined effects of (i) excessive production of ACTH-dependent DOC and corticosterone; and (ii) markedly elevated levels of cortisol which, although relatively inactive at the hGR (and therefore failing to induce signs of Cushing's syndrome), appear to be normally active at the MR, where they exceed the capacity of the 11β-hydroxysteroid dehydrogenase type II enzyme (11β-HSD2) to render them ineffective by conversion to cortisone (see below). PGR can be sporadic or familial, with familial inheritance following either an autosomal dominant or an autosomal recessive pattern of transmission [107].

PGR is characterized clinically by increased ACTH and cortisol levels and resistance of cortisol suppression by dexamethasone, in the absence of clinical stigmata of Cushing's syndrome [108,109]. The circadian pattern of cortisol secretion is normal. The condition has been reported mainly in individuals who have presented with clinical manifestations of mineralocorticoid and/or androgen excess, and in family members who, although not necessarily symptomatic, have subsequently been found to have biochemical evidence of PGR. Plasma levels of DOC, corticosterone, and androgens such as androstenedione, dehydroepiandrosterone (DHEA), and DHEA-sulfate are variably elevated while renin (as PRA or DRC) and aldosterone levels are low [108,109].

The condition is caused by mutations within the gene encoding the glucocorticoid receptor (*NR3C1*) which impair receptor function, thereby impairing glucocorticoid signal transduction, resulting in reduced tissue sensitivity to glucocorticoids [107,108,110,111].

Management

As in 11β- and 17α-hydroxylase deficiency, treatment involves ACTH suppression by administration of glucocorticoids, but doses required to do this are higher (for example, dexamethasone 1–3 mg/day) because of resistance at the level of the receptor. Treatment is not required for asymptomatic, normotensive individuals with PGR [107].

Syndrome of apparent mineralocorticoid excess (SAME)

Clinical diagnosis

The underlying biochemical defect in SAME is reduced or absent activity of 11β-HSD2 which normally acts to "protect" the MR from activation by cortisol by converting it to cortisone, an inactive metabolite [112]. Activation of the MR by cortisol in SAME induces manifestations of mineralocorticoid excess. Congenital SAME is caused by loss-of-function mutations in *HSD11B2*, which encodes 11β-HSD2 [113–115]. While classic congenital SAME is rare and characterized by childhood onset of severe mineralocorticoid hypertension (with hypokalemic alkalosis), milder forms with less severe or later onset hypertension, and without hypokalemia, have been described [116,117]. SAME may also be acquired through the ingestion of licorice, major constituents of which (glycyrrhizic acid and its hydrolytic product glycyrrhetinic acid) are potent inhibitors of 11β-HSD2 [118]. Medical administration of carbenoxolone, the hemisuccinate derivative of glycyrrhetinic acid which was in the past used to treat peptic ulcer disease, was also associated with this syndrome [118].

SAME should be suspected in patients presenting with mineralocorticoid hypertension in association with low levels of both aldosterone and renin, and confirmed by an increased ratio of urinary metabolites of cortisol (tetrahydrocortisol and 5α-tetrahydrocortisol) to tetrahydrocortisone (THF + allo-THF/THE), or of urinary free cortisol to urinary free cortisone [119,120], reflecting reduced 11β-HSD2 activity.

Once thought to be exclusively transmitted in an autosomal recessive manner, later reports of late-onset hypertension, variably suppressed aldosterone and renin, and high urinary free cortisol to cortisone ratios in heterozygote parents of more floridly affected homozygous patients have been consistent with codominant inheritance [116,117].

Management

Dexamethasone, which does not have significant affinity for the MR, is usually effective in correcting mineralocorticoid hypertension and hypokalemic alkalosis by suppressing ACTH and cortisol, but additional antihypertensives such as spironolactone and/or amiloride may be required [112,120].

DOC-secreting tumors

Clinical diagnosis

Primary deoxycorticosteronism may be caused by adrenal adenoma or carcinoma [121–123]. Patients present with hypertension, hypokalemia and renin suppression, but unlike in PA, plasma aldosterone levels are low and plasma DOC levels are often very high. Adrenal carcinomas producing DOC may present because of the symptoms associated with a rapidly enlarging adrenal mass or metastases.

Management

Spironolactone is given before surgery. For DOC-producing adenoma, unilateral adrenalectomy has produced long-term cure [121,122]. As with other forms of adrenocortical carcinoma, the prognosis of DOC-producing carcinoma is poor, but long-term benefit from adrenalectomy has been reported [123].

Ectopic ACTH syndrome

Clinical diagnosis

In Ectopic ACTH syndrome, due, for example, to production of ACTH by bronchial carcinoids or small cell cancers of the lung, excessive sodium reabsorption and volume expansion (due to very high levels of cortisol which overload 11βHSD2 and therefore gain access to the MR as in SAME and high levels of DOC acting on the MR) leads to hypokalemia and suppression of renin (and, as a consequence, suppression of aldosterone) [124,125]. Hypertension develops if the patient lives long enough and is not too ill from the effects of the neoplasm. As in SAME, these patients have elevated ratios of cortisol to cortisone metabolites (THF + allo-THF/THE) [124,125].

Management

Where possible, the optimal treatment is rapid and complete excision of the ACTH-secreting tumor. A period of preoperative cortisol-lowering drugs may be required. If surgery is not a viable option, approaches include combinations of pharmacological agents directed against cortisol excess, bilateral adrenalectomy and antitumoral interventions (see section below on Cushing syndrome for more detail) [124].

Activating mutations of the MR or Geller syndrome

Clinical diagnosis and management

In 2000, Geller and coworkers [126] described a kindred with severe hypertension associated with suppressed renin and aldosterone levels, transmitted in an autosomal dominant fashion. Affected family members were heterozygous for a gain-of-function mutation in the gene encoding the MR, resulting in sodium retention, urinary potassium wasting and suppression of renin and aldosterone. Most affected individuals were normokalemic. All pregnancies that occurred among female carriers were complicated by marked exacerbation of hypertension, accompanied by development of hypokalemia despite undetectable aldosterone levels. Spironolactone and progesterone, normally antagonists of wild-type MR, were found to be potent agonists of the mutated gene product, explaining exacerbation of the clinical phenotype during pregnancy and excluding spironolactone (and favoring amiloride) as treatment for this clinical entity.

Liddle syndrome

Clinical diagnosis

This syndrome results from constitutive activation of ENaC caused by mutations within the genes encoding its β or γ subunits which prevent its ubiquitination and degradation [127−129]. The clinical outcomes are sodium retention and urinary potassium and hydrogen ion wasting, causing hypokalemic alkalosis with early onset severe hypertension and suppressed renin and aldosterone (due to low renin plus hypokalemia). Less florid varieties, with less severe hypertension and normal plasma potassium levels, have been described [130]. The clinical manifestations respond to treatment with ENaC antagonists but not spironolactone. Both familial and sporadic cases have been described, the former following an autosomal dominant pattern of transmission [127,129]. The condition should be suspected in patients (especially children) who present with hypertension and hypokalemic alkalosis and are found to have low renin and aldosterone levels. It can be distinguished from hypertensive forms of congenital adrenal hyperplasia, PGR, and SAME by normal levels of 17α-hydroxyprogesterone, 11-deoxycortisol and cortisol, normal ratios of free cortisol to cortisone (or metabolites) in urine, and failure to respond to dexamethasone suppression of ACTH.

Management

The hypertension and hypokalemia in Liddle's syndrome respond to amiloride or triamterene, but dietary sodium restriction is usually also necessary to maintain normotension. As with other forms of mineralocorticoid hypertension, some individuals, especially those who are older and have been hypertensive for longer periods of time, require additional antihypertensive medication to achieve control.

Familial hyperkalemic hypertension (Gordon syndrome)

Clinical diagnosis

Unlike all the above entities, Familial hyperkalemic hypertension (FHHt, Gordon Syndrome) has an autosomal dominant inheritance with salt-sensitive hypertension due to defective renal tubular function leading to sodium retention and reduced (rather than increased) potassium and hydrogen ion excretion (hyperkalemic acidosis) [131]. It is unique in that chronic hyperkalemia exists in the absence of a reduced glomerular filtration rate (GFR). Despite renin suppression, plasma aldosterone levels can be low, normal or even raised due to stimulation by elevated plasma potassium. Because of this, the ARR can be elevated and FHHt is therefore one of the causes of a "false positive" ARR when screening for PA [30]. FHHt is caused by mutations in regulators of the thiazide-sensitive Na^+-Cl^- Co-transporter, NCC, including 'With No lysine (K)' kinases (*WNK1* and *WNK4*), KeLcH-Like3 (*KLHL3*) and CULlin3 (*CUL3*) [132−134], which lead to upregulation of NCC expression. As in Liddle syndrome, significant inter- and intrapedigree phenotypic variation is observed clinically [131,135].

Management

FHHt is effectively treated by thiazide diuretics and/or dietary salt restriction [131,135].

(For further reading on various familial causes of endocrine hypertension please refer Chapters 6, 8, 9, and 10)

Pheochromocytoma and paraganglioma

Prevalence, pathophysiology and clinical presentation

Pheochromocytomas and paragangliomas (PPGL) are catecholamine releasing tumors arising from adrenal or extra-adrenal chromaffin cells. Pheochromocytoma (around 80%—85% of PPGL cases) refers to a tumor originating from the adrenal medulla, whereas paragangliomas (15%—20% of PPGL cases) are derived from paravertebral sympathetic ganglia in the thorax, abdomen or pelvis, or parasympathetic ganglia in the neck and skull base. The latter group is generally hormonally inactive [136]. PPGL is a rare diagnosis. A recent epidemiological study found a prevalence of 65 per 100,000 people [137], although autopsy studies suggest that a significant number may remain undetected during life [138]. Recent publications reported an incidence rate of 6.6 cases per million per year [139], and similar figures when expressed as age-standardized incidence rate (SIR) which allows a comparison with historical data. This evaluation detected a rise in SIR from 1.4 per million person-years in 1977 to 6.6 in 2015 [137]. This temporal change is most likely explained by an increase in early disease detection and the clinical presentation has shifted over time from the classical vignette of paroxysmal hypertension, to smaller and often asymptomatic lesions incidentally found on radiological imaging [137,140]. The pick-up rate depends on the background risk of the population that is screened. Of patients with an adrenal incidentaloma, as many as 7% is estimated to have a pheochromocytoma [141]. On the other hand, in the general hypertensive population, PPGL remains a rare cause and accounts for less than 1% of all cases [142]. Despite this, it is a diagnosis important not to miss because of the high risk of negative outcomes if the diagnosis is delayed or missed [143].

Cardiovascular events are the most significant cause for morbidity and mortality. In a retrospective analysis of 145 patients with pheochromocytoma, the incidence of cardiovascular complications was found to be as high as 19.3%. Among these, commonly reported were arrhythmias, heart failure, ischemic heart disease, and stroke [144]. The rise in blood pressure (BP) in PPGL is related to the cardiovascular actions of catecholamines, such as their vasoconstrictive effect to increase peripheral vascular resistance. The BP rise can be sustained, frequently seen in noradrenaline-dominant tumors, or paroxysmal. Orthostatic hypotension may occur with purely adrenaline-producing tumors. Dopamine-dominant tumors generally do not cause hypertension [145]. Paroxysms can occur spontaneously but may also be provoked by numerous well-known triggers such as physical activity, surgery, emotional factors and direct tumor manipulation. Furthermore, multiple drugs are known for their ability to cause a surge in catecholamine release, most notably dopamine D2 receptor antagonists (such as metoclopramide), tricyclic antidepressants, monoamine oxidase inhibitors and corticosteroids. In addition to elevation of BP, PPGL patients also display other features of BP dysregulation including greater BP variability, loss of nocturnal dipping and a high incidence of orthostatic hypotension [145].

The adverse cardiovascular risk extends beyond the hemodynamic effects of catecholamines. Catecholamine excess is characterized by dysglycemia as a result of insulin resistance, reduced insulin secretion and reduced peripheral glucose uptake [146]. In further support of this concept, a direct correlation between noradrenaline and normetanephrine with HbA1c has been described [147]. Although these observations are thought to be predominantly related to the direct metabolic effects of catecholamines, recent findings of excess glucocorticoid levels in pheochromocytoma patients suggest that glucocorticoid-mediated pathways may also play a role [148].

Another important contributor to its negative outcomes is the potential of some PPGLs to become malignant. The overall risk of metastatic disease is estimated to be around 10%—17% [143], but is significantly higher in particular genetic syndromes. The association with several clinical syndromes has been well described and over one third of PPGL cases have a germline mutation in one of the known susceptibility genes such as succinate dehydrogenase B (*SDHB*), *SDHD*, Von Hippel-Lindau (*VHL*), *RET* and Neurofibromatosis-1 (*NF-1*). Another 30%—40% of sporadic cases may furthermore have somatic mutations in a relevant gene. The actual malignancy risk depends on the specific gene and gene mutation that is involved. Of these, *SDHB* mutations carry the highest risk of malignant disease [149]. Many of the genetic syndromes are also associated with an increased risk of other tumors. An example of this is medullary thyroid cancer in multiple endocrine neoplasia type 2 (MEN2) [143]. For these reasons it is important to consider genetic testing in all PPGL cases [136]. With the advancement of next-generation sequencing technologies, the recommended pathway for genetic testing has shifted in recent years from a targeted approach based on clinical features and immunohistochemistry [136], to application of a broad panel of relevant genes [150].

Diagnosis

The initial step in diagnosis is to identify patients that require screening for PPGL. The 2014 Endocrine Society guidelines on PPGL recommend biochemical screening in patients with signs or symptoms of PPGL, especially if occurring paroxysmally, adrenal incidentaloma, a known or suspected predisposition to a genetic syndrome known to be associated with PPGL, and a previous history of PPGL [136]. The classic symptoms of PPGL are headaches, excessive sweating and palpitations, often occurring in a paroxysmal manner. However, not infrequently other, often nonspecific, manifestations can occur in PPGL such as anxiety, pallor, chest pain, and abdominal symptoms [149,151]. Geroula et al. [151] found that palpitations, hyperhidrosis, pallor, tremor and nausea, in combination with low body mass index (BMI) and elevated heart rate are key features to discriminate PPGL from non-PPGL. When combined into a clinical feature score, there was a positive correlation with urinary and plasma catecholamine levels and probability of disease, and this can be a useful tool for further risk stratification [151]. Imaging characteristics may further help in risk stratification. Contrast washout on a CT scan is considered an unreliable marker to differentiate a pheochromocytoma from an adrenal adenoma [149]. However, an attenuation value of 10 Hounsfield Units or less on an unenhanced CT scan may be sufficient to rule out a pheochromocytoma without the need for further biochemical testing [152].

Key to the biochemical diagnosis is assessment of plasma or urinary catecholamines levels. The use of the metabolites like normetanephrine, metanephrine and 3-methxotyramine (3-MT) derived from their parent hormones noradrenaline, adrenaline, and dopamine, respectively, through the action of catecholamine O-methyltransferase is recommended due to their superior diagnostic accuracy [136,149]. When plasma or urinary metanephrines are more than twofold elevated the diagnosis is likely [149,153]. On the other hand, mild-to-moderate elevations can pose a diagnostic dilemma due to a high risk of false-positive results. Common causes for false-positive results need to be considered, such as body position at the time of blood sampling. It is recommended to draw blood after at least 30 min in the supine position to prevent a posture-related rise in catecholamine levels. Any other causes for increased sympathetic activity, such as an intercurrent acute condition, heart failure or obstructive sleep apnoea, need to be carefully considered [149]. Furthermore, numerous pharmacological agents including tricyclic antidepressants, monoamine oxidase inhibitors, phenoxybenzamine, and sympathomimetics are known to cause false-positive results and should be discontinued if possible [136,149,154]. In patients with mild-to-moderate elevations of (nor)metanephrine levels, a clonidine suppression test (CST) can be helpful to exclude false positive results. The CST is based on the premise that in patients without PPGL, the administration of clonidine - a centrally acting alpha-2-adrenergic receptor agonist that reduces sympathetic catecholamine release—would result in a decrease in catecholamine levels, whereas this suppression would not be seen in patients with autonomous catecholamine release [155]. An elevated plasma normetanephrine level 3 h after an oral dose of clonidine and a less than 40% reduction from baseline is highly suggestive of PPGL [136,154]. The urinary CST can be a valuable alternative to the more widely adopted plasma CST [156].

Once the biochemical diagnosis has been established, the final step is to localize the tumor. CT or magnetic resonance imaging (MRI) scanning are commonly used modalities for anatomical localization [149]. Functional imaging such as ^{123}I-metaiodobenzylguanidine (MIBG) scintigraphy, ^{68}Ga-Dotatate Positron Emission Tomography (PET)/CT and ^{18}F-fluorodihydroxy-phenylalanine (^{18}F-FDOPA) PET scanning is of additional value, especially if the patient is at risk of multifocal or metastatic disease. This is particularly relevant when there is a (suspected) hereditary cause. The choice of modality is dependent on the context and availability. In sporadic pheochromocytoma either ^{18}F-FDOPA PET or ^{123}I-MIBG scintigraphy is recommended as first line, whereas in hereditary pheochromocytoma due to *NF-1, RET, VHL,* and *MAX* mutations ^{18}F-FDOPA PET is the modality of choice. In extraadrenal sympathetic PPGL, multifocal disease, suspected metastatic disease, *SDH* mutations, or in head-and-neck paragangliomas ^{68}Ga-Dotatate PET is the preferred imaging modality [149].

Management

Surgical management

The treatment of choice is surgical resection of the tumor. A laparoscopic approach is suitable for most patients, but an open approach is recommended for large or invasive tumors and for most paragangliomas [136]. In selected patients with bilateral pheochromocytomas who have already undergone a unilateral adrenalectomy, partial adrenalectomy or cortical sparing surgery may be considered to prevent adrenal insufficiency and the resultant need for long-term steroid replacement. This is particularly relevant for patients with hereditary PPGL such as MEN2, VHL and NF-1 who are likely to develop bilateral disease. The benefits of adrenal-sparing surgery need to be carefully balanced with the increased risk of disease recurrence and future need for reoperation and this requires an individualized and multidisciplinary approach to decision-making [136,157].

Perioperative management

Adequate blockade of catecholamines with alpha-adrenergic receptor blockers for a period of at least 7—14 days preoperatively is critical to prevent hypertensive crises, hemodynamic instability, and cardiovascular complications during surgery [136,145]. Phenoxybenzamine, a long-acting, noncompetitive, and nonselective alpha-1 and alpha-2 antagonist, is most widely used. However, short-acting, competitive, and selective alpha-1 antagonists such as doxazosin or prazosin can be used as an alternative. Studies comparing the efficacy of these agents have yielded conflicting results, but the interpretability has been limited by their retrospective and observational design [145]. In a recent randomized controlled trial, Buitenwerf et al. [158] found no difference in intraoperative duration of BP levels outside target range in PPGL patients treated preoperatively with either phenoxybenzamine or doxazosin but a score for intraoperative hemodynamic instability was significantly lower in the phenoxybenzamine group. Whether this has clinical significance is unclear. Although the authors observed no differences in perioperative cardiovascular outcomes, larger numbers are needed to answer this question with more certainty. Another point of contention has been whether preoperative alpha-blockade is indeed necessary or whether this could be safely omitted. Although a recent meta-analysis of the available literature to try and answer this question found no evidence for a benefit of alpha-blockade, the number of suitable studies was low and all were retrospective in design [159]. Therefore, the recommendation that all patients with a hormonally active PPGL should receive preoperative alpha blockade remains unchanged [136].

Beta-adrenergic receptor blockers can be used as second-line treatment but should only be initiated after adequate alpha-adrenergic blockade as inhibition of beta-2 adrenergic receptor mediated vasodilatation in the setting of ongoing alpha-adrenergic receptor mediated vasoconstriction may result in a life-threatening surge in BP [145]. CCBs may be a useful addition when BP remains inadequately controlled, when side effects limit further titration of alpha-adrenergic receptor blockers, or when a patient suffers from catecholamine-induced coronary vasospasms [160]. The tyrosine hydroxylase inhibitor alpha-methyl-paratyrosine, or metyrosine, which blocks the rate-limiting step in catecholamine synthesis, can be a further useful agent. It is not widely used due to limited availability and high costs, but can be considered in selected cases with high catecholamine levels due to large tumor size or metastatic disease and in preparation for high-risk procedures [161].

In the postoperative phase, patients may develop hypotension due to the sudden drop in catecholamine levels after successful tumor removal. This may be exacerbated by the ongoing presence of alpha-adrenergic blockade, and a catecholamine-related contraction of circulating volume [145]. A high sodium diet and an infusion of 1—2 L of normal saline in the 24 h prior to surgery are recommended to reduce the postoperative drop in BP [136].

Follow-up

After resection of a functional PPGL, it is recommended to assess levels of (nor)metanephrine and 3-methoxytyramine 2—6 weeks after surgery to confirm complete removal. Long-term follow-up should include annual clinical review and biochemistry for a period up to 10 years. In patients with risk factors for recurrence or metastatic disease, such as a young age, a known hereditary factor or the presence of a paraganglioma, lifelong surveillance is indicated. In nonfunctional PPGLs, thoraco-abdomino-pelvic imaging every 1 to 2 years for up to 10 years is advised. Chromogranin-A may be an additional useful marker to monitor in patients who have normal metanephrine and 3-MT levels [149,162]. Surveillance of patients with hereditary PPGLs furthermore needs consideration of the risk of recurrence and of extra-adrenal malignancies that may occur as part of the specific syndrome and relevant clinical, biochemical and radiological surveillance recommendations need to be applied [163].

For more detailed reading about PPGLs please refer to Chapters 2, 11, and 12.

Cushing's syndrome

Prevalence, pathophysiology and clinical presentation

Cushing's syndrome refers to a condition of excess glucocorticoids and is associated with a large number of adverse effects, increased morbidity and mortality [164]. Since pharmacological doses of corticosteroids are widely used for the treatment of a broad range of conditions, exogenous steroid use is in fact the most common cause of Cushing's syndrome

[165]. Endogenous Cushing's syndrome on the other hand is rare with an estimated incidence between 0.2 and 5 per million population per year and a prevalence between 39 and 79 per million [164].

Due to its role as a key metabolic hormone with a broad systemic action profile, cortisol excess can present with a wide variety of symptoms, signs and complications affecting almost every organ system. Well-known manifestations are weight gain and central obesity, characteristic skin changes, hirsutism and menstrual irregularities, neuropsychiatric symptoms, musculoskeletal complications (most notably osteoporosis and proximal myopathy), and multiple adverse metabolic risk factors including hypertension, glucose intolerance, and dyslipidemia [165,166]. Because many of these features are common in the general population, and the onset and progression of symptoms is often insidious, the diagnosis is frequently delayed [167]. Violaceous striae, proximal myopathy, facial plethora, easy or spontaneous bruising and un-explained osteoporosis are characteristics with a higher discriminatory value and their presence, or the presence of unusual complications for age, or multiple and progressive features should trigger further evaluation [165,168].

Untreated Cushing's syndrome is associated with a high mortality rate, and infections, cardiovascular complications, and malignancies are common causes of death [169]. Early treatment significantly improves prognosis, but does not completely mitigate excess mortality [170,171]. This is partly explained by recurrent or residual disease in some patients [170], but seems to persist even in patients with apparent successful treatment [171]. The long-term increased mortality risk is particularly related to Cushing's disease, and treated adrenal Cushing's syndrome generally has a good prognosis [170,171]. In contrast, ectopic Cushing's syndrome has a poor outcome in the majority of patients (see above within section on "other mineralocorticoid forms of hypertension") [171].

Hypertension is a very common complication of Cushing's syndrome with an estimated prevalence of 70%—85% [165,172]. On the other hand, hypercortisolism remains an uncommon secondary cause of hypertension in the general population. The prevalence of Cushing's syndrome in hypertensive patients evaluated in a general outpatient clinic was around 1% with a similar number found to have subclinical Cushing's syndrome [142]. The prevalence is likely to be higher in selected patients such as those with resistant hypertension, an unusually young age of onset, or patients with associated complications, reiterating the aforementioned principles of appropriate patient selection for screening [173]. There appears to be a tendency toward higher BP in adrenal Cushing's compared to pituitary causes [172].

Several mechanisms contribute to the pathophysiology of hypertension in states of hypercortisolism, and both direct and indirect pathways appear to be involved [172].

A key element of cortisol-induced hypertension is renal sodium and water reabsorption, and patients with Cushing's syndrome have been found to display increased expression of different sodium transporters along the nephron in urinary exosome studies [174]. Glucocorticoids influence renal sodium reabsorption through interaction with both glucocorticoid receptors (GR) and MR expressed in different parts along the nephron [175]. Their ability to activate MRs in the aldosterone-sensitive parts of the tubular system is determined by activity of the enzymes 11-beta-hydroxysteroid dehydrogenase (11β-HSD) type 1 and type 2 [175,176]. Saturation of 11β-HSD type 2 will increase the availability of cortisol to activate MRs in mineralocorticoid target tissues such as the kidney [176]. Furthermore, a reduction in plasma potassium levels can also play a contributory role to drive sodium reabsorption through activation of sodium-chloride-cotransporters (NCC) [174,177]. As a result of enhanced sodium reabsorption, renin levels are low in some, but can be inappropriately normal in others [174,178] implying that alterations at other levels of the renin-angiotensin-aldosterone system (RAAS) are involved. For instance, hypercortisolism is known to induce hepatic angiotensinogen synthesis [178,179]. In patients with nonsuppressed renin, other mechanisms may predominate, such as increased vascular responsiveness to vasopressors [174]. Older studies have indeed shown an exaggerated BP response to vasopressors such as noradrenaline [178,180], and angiotensin II (Ang II) [178,181]. The latter observation may be mediated through a glucocorticoid-induced enhancement of vascular Ang II type 1 receptor expression [182]. Elevated levels of the vasoconstrictor endothelin-1 were also postulated to be a contributing factor [183], although this relation was not confirmed in other studies [179]. Furthermore, a blunted response to different vasodilatory mediators such as atrial natriuretic peptide (ANP), nitric oxide and prosta-glandins has also been suggested [172]. More indirectly, metabolic changes including insulin resistance and hyper-insulinemia, obstructive sleep apnoea (a prevalent condition in Cushing's syndrome), and vascular dysfunction and remodeling further contribute to the development and perpetuation of hypertension in Cushing's syndrome [172].

Diagnosis

The diagnostic evaluation for Cushing's syndrome has been described in detail in the Endocrine Society guidelines [168], Chapters 13 and 14. The initial step in patients in whom a clinical suspicion exists, is to perform one of the following available screening tests: either a minimum of two measurements of 24-hour urinary free cortisol excretion, two late-night salivary cortisol measurements, or a low-dose DST. If adrenal Cushing's syndrome is suspected, the use of either a low-dose DST or late-night salivary cortisol is preferred for the initial screening. Patients with an abnormal initial test require at least one additional positive test to confirm the diagnosis. Other tests such as the dexamethasone-corticotropin releasing hormone (CRH) test may further help in the process of confirmation [168]. The next step in diagnosis is to determine whether the condition is adrenocorticotropic hormone (ACTH)-dependent or -independent. Patients with ACTH-independent Cushing's syndrome (generally caused by a cortisol-producing adrenal adenoma) account for ~20% of cases, whereas ~80% of patients with Cushing's syndrome have ACTH-dependent disease. The vast majority of these have an ACTH-producing pituitary lesion (i.e., Cushing's disease), with a small group having an ectopic ACTH-producing tumor [164]. An ACTH level below 10 pg/mL is suggestive of an adrenal origin and should be followed up by imaging of the adrenal glands. An ACTH level over 20 pg/mL indicates ACTH-dependent hypercortisolism. The high-dose DST and CRH stimulation test are dynamic tests that can assist to differentiate pituitary from ectopic ACTH production. Concordant dynamic test results in combination with a pituitary adenoma >6 mm on imaging confirms Cushing's disease. In other cases, bilateral inferior petrosal sinus sampling may be required, as the gold standard test to discriminate pituitary from ectopic Cushing's syndrome [164].

Management

Resolution or improvement of hypercortisolism is the main treatment goal in Cushing's syndrome and this is expected to also have a positive impact on BP. However, the degree of BP response is dependent on many factors including the underlying cause, treatment modality, treatment success and patient factors. If possible, surgical resection of the causative process is the preferred treatment with the highest chance of attaining cure or long-term remission. Especially in Cushing's disease, however, additional treatment may be required, either as presurgical treatment, or after surgery in case of persistent or recurrent disease, and the possibilities include radiotherapy and pharmacotherapy. Pharmacotherapeutics can target the pituitary (e.g., pasireotide or cabergoline), adrenal steroidogenesis (e.g., metyrapone, ketoconazole or mitotane), or the GR (mifepristone) [164].

Surgical management

Surgically treated patients with Cushing's syndrome (both pituitary and adrenal) show an improvement in hypertension after treatment, but its prevalence continues to be higher than in aged-matched controls [184,185]. In a retrospective analysis, it was found that 92% of surgically treated patients achieved resolution or improvement of hypertension within 12 months, and 80% did so within the first 10 days of surgery. Forty-four percent of patients had complete remission of hypertension, whereas 56% of patients had residual hypertension [185]. Furthermore, only a minority of patients with Cushing's disease restored a normal BP dipping pattern even after curative surgery [186]. Jha et al. [185] found that younger age and lower BMI were predictors for a favourable BP response. In patients with adrenal Cushing's syndrome, lower preoperative BP and shorter duration of hypertension predicted a favorable BP response 1 year after adrenalectomy [187]. In subclinical Cushing's syndrome, the cortisol level after a 1-mg DST may be another predictor of improvement in comorbid conditions including hypertension after adrenalectomy. Interestingly, a greater reduction of postoperative medication requirement was observed in patients with a post-DST cortisol between 1.8 and 3.0 mcg/dL (50 and 83 nmol/L) compared to patients with a lesser degree of cortisol suppression. It was proposed that these patients represent a milder group with a lower degree of comorbidities and possible associated irreversible target organ damage that may limit the long-term surgical outcome [188]. Although Jha et al. [189] did not find an association between duration of hypercortisolism and BP response, it is known that prolonged hypercortisolism contributes to excess long-term mortality risk after surgery. Persistence of metabolic risk factors, and long-term vascular dysfunction and remodeling are likely important factors to explain persistence of hypertension after management of hypercortisolism. Also, the alterations in the RAAS associated with hypercortisolism were found to persist long after normalization of cortisol levels [179].

Pharmacological management

Pasireotide is a somatostatin analogue (SSA) with a high affinity for somatostatin receptor subtype 5, the predominant subtype expressed in corticotroph adenomas, and has emerged as a novel treatment option for medical management of Cushing's disease [164]. Both short-acting [190], and long-acting pasireotide [191] were shown to reduce BP, even without complete normalization of cortisol. A direct effect of pasireotide on BP is further supported by experimental studies which showed that in the presence of dexamethasone, pasireotide (and octreotide) reduced the Ang II-mediated vasoconstriction in iliac arteries derived from spontaneously hypertensive rats [179]. The dopamine agonist cabergoline has also been found to be beneficial in the management of Cushing's disease. In 20 patients who had uncontrolled

Cushing's disease after pituitary surgery, 75% showed biochemical responsiveness to cabergoline after 3 months, and 50% on longer term follow-up. This was associated with an improvement in hypertension, and although the reduction in BP was more marked in treatment responders, BP still improved in patients who showed treatment escape [192].

Steroidogenesis inhibitors constitute a category of agents aimed to reduce adrenal steroid hormone synthesis. Ketoconazole is an imidazole derivative that blocks multiple adrenal steroidogenic enzymes including 11-beta-hydroxylase, 17-hydroxylase, and 18-hydroxylase. Metyrapone is an inhibitor of 11-beta-hydroxylase [193]. These agents have been shown to reduce cortisol levels in a subset of patients with Cushing's syndrome with an associated BP reduction in some [194]. The lowering of cortisol by metyrapone may result in a compensatory rise in ACTH and consequently an increase in adrenal androgens and mineralocorticoid precursors, which could in fact exacerbate hypertension and hypokalemia [193]. Other well-known steroidogenesis inhibitors are mitotane and etomidate. Mitotane is an adrenolytic agent which, due to its unfavorable side effect profile, is mainly limited to the treatment of adrenocortical carcinoma. Etomidate is another imidazole derivative with a rapid onset of action. Due to its parenteral route of administration, it is predominantly used in severe, life-threatening cortisol excess [193].

Lastly, cortisol can also be blocked at the level of its main receptor GR. Mifepristone is a GR antagonist that has been shown to improve global clinical performance in patients with Cushing's syndrome [195]. In a 24-week, open-label trial, an improvement in diastolic BP (DBP) or reduction in antihypertensives was observed in over half of the hypertensive patients with Cushing's syndrome after treatment with mifepristone, although no overall improvement in mean BP was seen. A subgroup of patients even developed a rise in BP which was associated with hypokalemia and peripheral edema [196]. It is known that GR antagonists may lead to a compensatory rise in ACTH and cortisol further contributing to MR activation via the mechanisms described previously. Mifepristone is also a potent antagonist of the progesterone receptor (PR), and endometrial thickening and irregular vaginal bleeding has been observed in women treated with this agent [196]. Relacorilant is a new selective GR modulator, which in a recent Phase II trial has shown potential in ameliorating BP in Cushing's syndrome without causing associated antiprogesterone adverse effects. The compensatory rise in ACTH and cortisol was also substantially less than with mifepristone, which may therefore reduce the risk of developing of MR-mediated hypertension and hypokalemia [197]. Further studies are awaited to determine its potential role in the treatment of hypertension in this setting.

In patients who fail to demonstrate a full response on monotherapy, combination treatment can be successful to achieve further improvement. When a step-wise approach was adopted in 17 patients with Cushing's disease using pasireotide as initial treatment, the subsequent addition of cabergoline and ketoconazole in patients with inadequate control resulted in biochemical control in the majority. This was associated with a 12, and 8 mmHg reduction in systolic BP (SBP) and DBP, respectively [198].

Multimodal treatment

The management of hypertension in Cushing's syndrome requires a multimodal approach. To address the cause of hypercortisolism is key, but most treatment modalities take time to arrange (e.g., surgery), may not result in immediate or complete restoration of eucortisolism (e.g., radiotherapy and pharmacotherapy), or may fail over time. Also, hypertension may not fully resolve after treatment for the reasons explained above. Aggressive BP management to reduce cardiovascular risk is important in all stages of the disease, from diagnosis to long-term follow-up.

Isidori et al. [172] describe a treatment algorithm for hypertension management in Cushing's syndrome to target the different pathophysiological mechanisms that are in play. In light of the significant alterations in the RAAS at multiple levels, ACE inhibitors or ARBs are considered first-line treatment. An MR antagonist such as spironolactone can be considered as second line agent, especially if hypokalemia is present, or alternatively a CCB. If this fails to control BP, alpha-adrenergic receptor antagonists or nitric oxide donors can target the increased vasoconstrictive response. Thiazide diuretics, and beta-adrenergic receptor blockers are generally used with caution due to its potential negative effects on glucose tolerance, and especially in case of thiazides, their potential to exacerbate hypokalemia but can be used in selected cases [172].

Acromegaly

Prevalence, pathophysiology, and clinical presentation

Acromegaly is a condition characterized by growth hormone (GH) excess. In the vast majority of cases this is related to a GH-producing pituitary adenoma, with GH releasing hormone (GHRH) producing tumors and ectopic GH producing tumors being extremely uncommon alternative causes [199]. Acromegaly itself is a rare disease with a reported prevalence between 2.8 and 13.7 per 100,000 people. A significant delay in diagnosis with a median time-to-diagnosis of 4.5—5 years is common due to the often-insidious onset and progression of symptoms and signs, and the high prevalence of many of its associated complications in the general population [200]. Excessive GH stimulates insulin-like growth factor 1 (IGF-1) synthesis predominantly in the liver which in turn acts on multiple target organs. Classical features such as acral enlargement, change in facial appearance, headaches and visual impairment due to a large pituitary lesion are the most frequently reported presenting symptoms, but these can be absent or subtle. When a patient presents with multiple acromegaly associated conditions, such as obstructive sleep apnoea, arthralgias, nerve entrapment syndromes, hyperhidrosis, and hypertension, this should trigger further investigations [199,200].

Acromegaly is associated with significant morbidity, mortality, and reduced quality of life due to its impact on multiple organ systems. Therefore, a rigorous assessment and management of associated comorbidities is warranted with a focus on cardiovascular, endocrine, metabolic and musculoskeletal disorders, as well as appropriate screening for malignancies [199,201]. Patients with acromegaly have an unfavorable cardiovascular risk profile due to the presence of traditional risk factors such as hypertension, type 2 diabetes mellitus and dyslipidemia [202], and a higher incidence of atrial fibrillation and congestive heart failure [203].

The relation between hypertension and acromegaly is well-known but the reported prevalence of hypertension varies widely ranging from 18% to 60% which is likely explained by differences in the populations from which the data were derived [204]. In a retrospective comparison between acromegalic patients and carefully matched healthy controls, a nearly twofold higher prevalence of hypertension was found in the patient group (46% vs. 25%) and acromegaly preferentially raised DBP [205]. Although the pathways have not been fully unraveled, multiple mechanisms are thought to be involved [204]. Acromegaly causes expansion of extracellular volume through direct actions of GH and IGF-1 on renal sodium handling [206] and indirectly through an inhibitory effect on ANP release. In addition, altered sympathetic activity, especially the loss of a normal circadian rhythm, may blunt the physiological nocturnal dip in BP. Also, acromegaly causes functional and structural cardiac and vascular changes resulting in increased vascular tone and resistance [204]. Insulin resistance and hyperinsulinemia, common features of acromegaly, may further augment these pathophysiological and structural alterations [207]. The presence of other risk factors, such as OSA, and concomitant hypopituitarism requiring exogenous steroid replacement further add to hypertension risk.

Diagnosis

When acromegaly is suspected, measurement of IGF-1 is the first step in diagnosis, and an elevated IGF-1 level in combination with typical symptoms is highly suggestive. A failure to suppress GH levels to <1 mcg/L (<1 ng/mL or <3 mIU/L) during an oral glucose tolerance test confirms the diagnosis. Pituitary imaging, preferably with a MRI scan, will usually visualize a pituitary lesion [199].

Management

Management of acromegaly requires a multimodal approach. The main goals of treatment are to achieve biochemical control of GH excess, to control tumor mass, preserve or replace pituitary function, and to manage the associated long-term complications. Transsphenoidal surgery to remove the pituitary lesion is the preferred treatment as this is the best option to achieve cure if the whole lesion can be resected. Other available treatment modalities are somatostatin analogues (SSAs), dopamine agonists, the GH receptor antagonist (pegvisomant), and (stereotactic) radiotherapy, the latter if there is residual or recurrent disease after surgery, or if surgery cannot be performed. It is of great importance to adopt a multidisciplinary approach to decide on the most appropriate management for each individual patient [199].

Although older studies had not yielded consistent evidence to show that disease control directly translates in improvements in BP [207], this has become more apparent in recent publications. In retrospective studies, disease control was found to lower BP in acromegalic patients with hypertension at baseline [208—210], but also in normotensive patients biochemical control of acromegaly was shown to prevent the incidence of hypertension [210]. A prospective study of 45 new patients with acromegaly managed with SSAs as first-line treatment showed a significant reduction in the prevalence of hypertension after 5 years of follow-up [211], further supporting the notion that disease control is directly associated with an improvement in BP. On the other hand, Gonzalez et al. [212] found no change in the prevalence of hypertension in a cohort of 522 patients with acromegaly managed with a standardized multimodal approach after a median follow-up of 7.4 years. Part of the treatment effect on BP may have been masked by the influence of aging over the follow-up period, but notably no differences were seen between those who achieved biochemical control and those who still had active disease at the completion of follow-up. Possible factors to explain these discrepant results are the influence of age, disease severity and time-to-diagnosis mediated through classical hypertension risk factors, and the accumulation of structural and irreversible target organ damage which may impact on the likelihood of complete BP remission.

When assessing the cardiovascular benefits of treatment, it is important to consider hypertension in the broader context of overall cardiovascular risk profile. In a long-term follow-up of a large cohort of acromegaly patients treated with pegvisomant, it was observed that although average BP improved on treatment, the presence of hypertension remained a significant predictor of excess mortality and associated with a higher prevalence of other risk factors such as diabetes mellitus, hyperlipidemia, and cardiovascular disease [213]. There are also indications that different treatment modalities have differential effects on cardiovascular risk factors independent of IGF-1 normalization [208]. These studies emphasize the need for continuing assessment and aggressive management of cardiovascular risk factors in long-term follow-up of treated acromegaly patients.

Limited data exist to suggest specific antihypertensive agents in this context, and the choice of agents is guided by the common comorbidities associated with acromegaly, such as diabetes mellitus and cardiomyopathy. It is therefore not surprising that ACE inhibitors and ARBs were reported to be most widely used by clinicians to treat hypertension in patients with acromegaly [214].

For further reading on acromegaly and hypertension, please refer to Chapter 15.

Thyroid disorders

Thyroid disorders are prevalent and frequently underrecognized in the general population [215]. The effects of thyroid hormones on the cardiovascular system and the role of thyroid dysfunction as a risk factor for cardiovascular disease are widely recognized [216]. Both hypo- and hyperthyroidism can lead to elevations in BP [217]. The following section will discuss the prevalence, clinical relevance, diagnostic, and management approaches of hypo- and hyperthyroidism in relation to hypertension.

Hypothyroidism

Prevalence, pathophysiology, and clinical presentation

Hypothyroidism (either subclinical or overt) is a common condition. A meta-analysis of studies on the incidence and prevalence of thyroid dysfunction in different European populations found a combined prevalence of previously diagnosed and undiagnosed hypothyroidism of 3%. In this study, up to 85% of people with thyroid dysfunction had subclinical disease [215]. There is a strong female preponderance in prevalence and incidence [215,218]. In the vast majority of patients, hypothyroidism is primary in nature. On a global scale, iodine deficiency remains the most significant causative factor. In iodine replete populations, chronic lymphocytic thyroiditis (Hashimoto's thyroiditis) is the most common cause. Other well-known reasons for primary hypothyroidism are iatrogenic causes, such as after radioactive iodine (RAI) treatment, thyroidectomy, or external beam radiation to the neck region. Further, a broad range of pharmacotherapeutic agents can cause primary hypothyroidism. Central hypothyroidism, related to pituitary or hypothalamic pathology, and peripheral hypothyroidism, which includes consumptive hypothyroidism due to increased tissue expression of the inactivating deiodinase 3 enzyme, and thyroid hormone resistance, are rare but should be considered in the relevant clinical setting [218,219].

Hypothyroidism is widely recognized as a risk factor for (predominantly diastolic) hypertension [216]. However, whether hypothyroidism is a significant cause of hypertension, especially in subclinical disease, remains a subject of debate [220]. Most evidence is derived from observational studies, with some showing positive associations [221], whereas others failed to substantiate this association [222]. A recent large cross-sectional study which included 49,433 euthyroid patients and 7719 patients with subclinical hypothyroidism confirmed a higher prevalence of hypertension in patients with subclinical hypothyroidism, and this relation was stronger for females under the age of 65 years [223]. Prospective and experimental studies further support the causative nature of this association. A systematic review and meta-analysis of nine studies showed a positive association between subclinical hypothyroidism and incident hypertension in women (OR 1.32). This association was significant only in women <65 years [224]. Fommei and Iervasi (2002) studied 12 normotensive patients with a previous thyroidectomy and performed a 24-hour ambulatory BP measurement (ABPM) 6 weeks after thyroxine withdrawal, and 2 months after reinstatement of hormone replacement. They observed that the average daytime BP was significantly higher in the thyroxine withdrawal phase compared to the replacement phase (5.1 mmHg for SBP, and 8.2 mmHg for DBP) [225].

Important factors to explain the BP rise are an increase in systemic vascular resistance (SVR) and increased arterial stiffness [216,217]. Contributors to the rise in SVR are the reduction in the physiological tri-iodothyronine (T3) mediated vasodilatory effect on vascular smooth muscle cells [226], endothelial dysfunction [227], and reduced vascular beta-adrenergic reactivity [217,228]. Hypothyroid patients were also found to have increased vascular stiffness [229]. Altered vascular reactivity and endothelial dysfunction may further play a role, as well as structural vascular changes related to long-term hypertension and dyslipidemia. As such, the increased cardiovascular risk observed in hypothyroidism is likely related to a combination of risk factors which includes not only hypertension, but also an atherogenic lipid profile [216,230]. Case detection is important, as thyroid hormone replacement was found to improve BP [221,231], carotid intima-media thickness [232], and indices for central arterial stiffness [229]. However, there is a need for randomized controlled trials to better understand the benefits of thyroid replacement on cardiovascular risk factors and outcomes [233].

Diagnosis

The diagnostic workup and management of hypothyroidism has been well-described in clinical practice guidelines [218]. In most cases, measurement of thyroid stimulating hormone (TSH) provides a reliable initial screening test for thyroid dysfunction unless central hypothyroidism is suspected, and an elevated TSH level is indicative of hypothyroidism. Subsequent assessment of tetraiodothyonine (thyroxine or T4) and tri-iodothyronine (T3) can determine whether the hypothyroidism is subclinical or overt [218].

Management

Thyroid hormone replacement with levothyroxine is the recommended treatment for hypothyroidism [234], and BP is expected to improve on adequate replacement. When antihypertensives are required, dihydropyridine CCBs and ACE inhibitors have been suggested to be beneficial in this setting [217], but the available evidence is limited. Furthermore, hypothyroidism causes a low renin, salt-sensitive form of hypertension which may respond to salt restriction and diuretics [217].

Hyperthyroidism

Prevalence, pathophysiology, and clinical presentation

Hyperthyroidism is caused by an excess of thyroid hormones. The prevalence is highly variable and depends on the population and the geographical area where it is studied with numbers ranging from 0.1% to 2.9% [235]. In a meta-analysis of epidemiological studies from Europe, a 0.75% prevalence of previously diagnosed and undiagnosed hyperthyroidism was found [215]. Similar to hypothyroidism, hyperthyroidism is more common in women than in men [215,235]. The most common causes of hyperthyroidism are Graves' disease and nodular thyroid disease with one or multiple autonomous nodules. Other well-known causes are thyroiditis (such as subacute thyroiditis and postpartum thyroiditis), and iodine-induced hyperthyroidism (Jod-Basedow effect). Primary hyperthyroidism constitutes the majority of cases and other causes such as central hyperthyroidism (TSH-oma) and ectopic thyroid hormone secretion (such as struma ovarii) are very rare [235,236].

The clinical picture of hyperthyroidism is characterized by adrenergic symptoms such as tremors, anxiety and tachycardia. Hyperthyroidism, especially if prolonged, is furthermore associated with multiple other adverse effects including weight loss, and osteoporosis [236]. Hyperthyroidism is particularly associated with an elevated risk of cardiovascular complications and severe hyperthyroidism increases the risk of heart failure, atrial fibrillation, and stroke [237]. The profound effects of hyperthyroidism on the cardiovascular system are well-known. It causes a hyperdynamic circulation with an increase in heart rate, cardiac preload, and contractility, and a decrease in SVR all contributing to an increase in cardiac output. Whether this leads to an increase in systolic BP depends on the balance between cardiac output and SVR [237]. However, other hormonal factors may alter this balance toward an increase in BP. For instance, endothelin-1 levels may rise in hyperthyroidism. Furthermore, the reduction in SVR causes activation of the renin—angiotensin—aldosterone system (RAAS) resulting in salt and water retention and increased vascular reactivity in turn leading to a further increase in cardiac preload [217,238]. Although studies on this are relatively scarce, some investigators have found that management of hyperthyroidism can lead to improvement of hypertension [239]. In subclinical disease, the evidence of an association with hypertension is more scarce and not as clear. One cross-sectional study found a higher prevalence of hypertension in subclinical hyperthyroidism (OR 2.8) [240], whereas other studies, including one prospective study, failed to confirm this association [241—243].

Diagnosis

The biochemical diagnosis of primary hyperthyroidism is confirmed when a suppressed TSH level is found with a normal or elevated T3 and/or T4 level indicating subclinical or overt hyperthyroidism. Additional investigations, including the measurement of TSH receptor antibodies, and a thyroid uptake scan may further help to establish the etiology [236].

Management

The mainstay of management is to correct the hyperthyroid state. Treatment modalities that are available include pharmacotherapy with antithyroid drugs (ATDs or thionamides), RAI treatment and surgery, each to be used in the appropriate clinical setting [236]. Antihypertensives may be indicated in situations where no specific treatment is available, such as in subacute thyroiditis, or where more rapid BP management is required. Beta-adrenergic receptor blockers are generally recommended to reduce the adrenergic effects of hyperthyroidism. The nonselective beta-adrenergic blocker propranolol has traditionally been the preferred agent of choice, due to its additional ability to block the conversion of T4 to T3. In patients with contraindications to nonselective betablockers, such as bronchospastic asthma, more selective beta1-adrenergic blockers such as atenolol or metoprolol can be used with caution [236]. Although beta-adrenergic blocker treatment is largely given for symptom control, and to reduce tachycardia and its associated cardiovascular complications, this will also assist to improve BP. In a study of 30 patients with hyperthyroidism and hypertension, a three-month treatment with propylthiouracil in combination with either metoprolol or carvedilol, a nonselective beta-adrenergic blocker and alpha1-adrenergic receptor blocker, both resulted in a significant improvement in BP and heart rate with no differences between groups [244]. When beta-blockers are contraindicated or not tolerated, nondihydropyridine CCBs such as verapamil or diltiazem can be considered [236]. Furthermore, ACE inhibitors have been suggested as a useful agent in this context [217].

Primary hyperparathyroidism

Prevalence, pathophysiology, and clinical presentation

Primary hyperparathyroidism (PHPT) is a condition defined by (semi-)autonomous secretion of parathyroid hormone (PTH) by one or multiple parathyroid glands. This generally results in elevated serum calcium levels, although cases of normocalcemic PHPT have been described. Patients can present with polyuria, polydipsia, constipation, nausea, vomiting and altered mental state, especially if calcium levels are significantly elevated. In the long run, PHPT is associated with a multitude of adverse sequelae. Well-known are the renal complications related to hypercalciuria, such as kidney stones, nephrocalcinosis, and renal impairment, and the skeletal complications, most notably osteoporosis [245].

An estimated prevalence of up to 0.9% in the general population has been reported, with a significant proportion of that remains undetected [246]. This number could be exceedingly higher when patients with normocalcemic PHPT are taken into account [247]. In the majority of patients, the disease is caused by a single parathyroid adenoma, but multiglandular disease can also occur, usually due to parathyroid hyperplasia. Female sex and advanced age are important risk factors [245]. Most cases are sporadic, but can occur as part of a familial syndrome, in particular one of the multiple endocrine neoplasia (MEN) syndromes. A familial cause should be considered in younger patients, males and multiglandular disease [248].

In addition to the complications described above, studies have shown an association between PHPT and a high prevalence of cardiovascular risk factors, such as obesity, hypertension, hyperlipidemia and type 2 diabetes mellitus, compared to the general population [249]. However, the significance of cardiovascular risk in PHPT has remained a subject of debate due to the heterogenous and observational nature of most studies, and cardiovascular risk mitigation is not currently considered an indication for surgical management of PHPT [250]. With respect to hypertension, many studies have reported an association with PHPT [249,251−254]. Although the exact mechanisms are unknown, it is suggested that alterations in the RAAS, as well as a blunted vasodilatory and enhanced vasoconstrictive response in peripheral resistance vessels to pressor hormones such as norepinephrine play a role [250,255]. It also remains unclear whether the BP rise is related to hypercalcemia, or is caused by a direct effect of PTH per se [255]. A meta-analysis of six prospective cohort studies has shown a positive correlation between PTH levels and hypertension risk [256].

Importantly, there appears to be an intimate and bidirectional relation between PTH and the RAAS [257]. Excessive aldosterone levels can cause secondary hyperparathyroidism due to induction of renal calcium and magnesium loss. Indeed, patients with primary aldosteronism are known to have higher PTH levels compared to patients with essential hypertension and PTH levels decrease after treatment of hyperaldosteronism [258]. Conversely, PTH has been shown to stimulate aldosterone synthesis via direct and indirect pathways [257]. Clinically, PHPT is associated with elevated aldosterone levels and this is ameliorated by parathyroidectomy [259]. It is thought that this interplay between PTH and aldosterone exacerbates the target-organ damage caused by the excess of either hormone alone [257].

Diagnosis

When establishing the diagnosis, an elevated serum calcium with an elevated or inappropriately normal PTH level is key. Other important biochemical measurements are serum phosphate, alkaline phosphatase activity, renal function, and vitamin D levels. Additional investigations into the presence of, or the risk for, complications should also be considered, such as a bone mineral density (DEXA) scan, a vertebral fracture assessment (VFA), a 24-hr urinary assessment for hypercalciuria, and abdominal imaging to look for renal calculi or nephrocalcinosis.

If surgery is contemplated, localization studies may aid to guide the surgical approach. Ultrasonography, a technetium-99m-labeled sestamibi scan (^{99m}Tc-sestamibi), and a four-dimensional computed tomography scan are frequently used imaging modalities for this purpose [245].

Management

Surgical management provides an opportunity for cure but is not warranted in all cases, and the indications for surgery are described in detail elsewhere [260]. Whether parathyroidectomy is effective in reducing BP has remained unresolved, and available data on this has been inconsistent and heterogeneous [255]. In a randomized controlled clinical trial, no beneficial effect on 24-hr ABPM was seen in patients with mild-to-moderate PHPT, 3 months after parathyroidectomy versus a 3-month observation period. In fact, in the treatment group, a small increase in ambulatory DBP was seen [261]. Over a longer follow up of 3.5 years after parathyroidectomy, little change in hypertension prevalence was observed in 46 PHPT patients [262]. Furthermore, Rydberg et al. [263] reported on a 5 mmHg increase in average SBP on 24-hr ABPM, 6 months after parathyroidectomy in PHPT patients with pre-existent hypertension, whereas in normotensive patients no change in average 24-hr ABPM was found. It is likely that these disparate results may be explained by a variable degree of reversibility due to the presence of other cardiovascular risk factors, duration of hypertension, and irreversible target organ damage. In the absence of clinical prognosticators to predict the postoperative BP response after parathyroidectomy, hypertension per se should not be an indication for surgery, and further studies to identify patients who would benefit from the cardiovascular perspective are needed.

Are adjustments in pharmacotherapeutics warranted in patients with concomitant PHPT and hypertension? First of all, thiazide diuretics are known to cause hypercalcemia due to its ability to increase renal tubular calcium reabsorption (thereby reducing the urinary calcium excretion). Whether this exacerbates hypercalcemia in PHPT is unknown, but in a retrospective observational study, Griebeler et al. [264] found that a high proportion of patients with thiazide-induced hypercalcemia had underlying PHPT, and thiazide use could unmask mild cases of PHPT. It was also suggested that thiazides may actually have beneficial effects on fracture risk due to reduction of hypercalciuria [264]. In the prospective Nurses' Health Study, use of loop diuretics, but none of the other antihypertensives including thiazide diuretics, was associated with a higher risk of incident PHPT [265]. Furthermore, in the study by Griebeler, a small subgroup of PHPT patients safely continued their thiazide diuretic up till definitive surgical management [264]. In the absence of any large-scale prospective data on the use of thiazide diuretics in the setting of PHPT, it is advisable to use these agents with caution.

In light of the aforementioned interaction between PTH and aldosterone, MR blockade may provide a targeted approach to reduce BP in PHPT. In a randomized clinical trial, an eight-week treatment with the MR antagonist eplerenone resulted in a significant improvement on 24-hr ABPM in patients with PHPT independent of changes in PTH [266] and MR blockade may provide an exciting new strategy to reduce the cardiovascular risk associated with PHPT that deserves further investigation.

Please refer to Chapter 16 for detailed reading on hypertension in thyroid and parathyroid disease.

Renal artery stenosis and other rare forms of renin driven hypertension

Renal artery stenosis is a common condition which, in some patients, can cause secondary hypertension. In patients with established atherosclerosis the prevalence of renal artery stenosis is high, at up to 14%—42% depending on the study [267], being more common in those with aortic or peripheral vascular disease and in patients with established chronic kidney disease. Renal artery stenosis due to fibromuscular dysplasia is typically found in younger patients, particularly females, though it can occur in other patient groups. It is important to recognize, however, that regardless of the underlying pathology, the detection of renal artery stenosis in a hypertensive patient is not sufficient in itself to establish it as the cause of the hypertension. While the coexistence of renal artery stenosis and hypertension is relatively common, cases of hypertension that are caused by renal artery stenosis (i.e. renovascular hypertension) and are therefore likely to be improved by vascular intervention are much less frequent. Other much rarer causes of renin driven hypertension include Page kidney and reninoma.

Clinical presentation

As implied above, the age and gender of the patient and presence or absence of vascular disease elsewhere or risk factors for cardiovascular disease can thus be a starting point when considering whether a patient may have renovascular hypertension. An unexplained acute kidney injury after the institution of an ACE inhibitor or ARB is commonly regarded as a potential indicator of significant renal artery disease. This typically occurs within days to weeks and is manifest by a greater than 30% rise in creatinine (often a much greater rise is seen). With significant renal arterial disease, GFR is at least partially dependent on angiotensin II mediated vasoconstriction of the efferent arteriole, and thus inhibition can cause a precipitous rise in creatinine. Severe hypertension with recurrent episodes of flash pulmonary edema is also regarded as a clinical clue suggesting bilateral renal arterial disease. In unilateral renal artery stenosis, the contralateral kidney can compensate with increased sodium excretion in the face of volume expansion (the pressure natriuresis phenomenon); however, in bilateral disease, this escape mechanism is not possible because of impaired perfusion to both kidneys.

Fibromuscular dysplasia can affect almost any arterial bed but the renal arteries are most commonly involved (75%—80% of cases) [268]. Hypertension is the most common presenting sign but flank or abdominal pain (from ischemic events or dissection) can also be a presenting symptom of renal FMD, and headaches, tinnitus, transient ischemic attacks, and strokes can be an indicator of cerebrovascular FMD. Because FMD commonly affects multiple arterial beds in individual patients (up to 2/3 of patients in one recent registry study) [269], modern guidelines suggest initial cross-sectional imaging from head to pelvis when FMD is found [270].

Renal artery bruits may be found in renal artery stenosis, and careful examination for bruits of the carotid and subclavian arteries and more widely over the abdomen for other arterial bruits is useful especially in FMD. Evidence for peripheral vascular disease in the lower limbs is also helpful in determining the overall atherosclerotic burden.

Diagnostic approach

Renal duplex ultrasound is a useful noninvasive screening method for renal arterial disease. It is, however, highly operator-dependent and although sensitivity for significant renal artery stenosis is high (up to 98%) in high-volume referral centers [271], it may not be the modality of choice in centers with less technical experience. CT angiography is less-operator dependent, has much greater spatial resolution and requires less technical expertise and in many settings is a better screening test but requires contrast administration with the risk of acute kidney injury or rarely allergic reaction. Magnetic resonance angiography (MRA) is an alternative imaging modality and can be considered where CT is contraindicated, for example because of contrast allergy. MRA however has lower sensitivity compared to CT because of lower spatial resolution and this can be important particularly in FMD which commonly affects the mid and distal renal arteries. Digital subtraction angiography is the reference standard test for diagnosis of renal artery stenosis and can be considered for diagnosis when there is a strong clinical suspicion of renal artery stenosis and particularly FMD where noninvasive imaging techniques have lower sensitivity [272]. Angiography can also be followed by angioplasty in the same procedure. Other adjunctive imaging techniques including ACE inhibitor-augmented renography using nuclear medical techniques can give additional information (including differential renal function, which may assist in assessing management options, for example, unilateral nephrectomy in the case of nonfunctioning renin-producing kidney) and have reasonable sensitivity in the right setting, but have become less popular with greater availability of highly accurate CT scanners.

The most difficult aspect of renal artery stenosis is determining if a stenosis identified on imaging is hemodynamically or functionally significant, and if intervention will result in improvement in blood pressure control or renal outcomes. Illustrating this point, randomized trials to date have failed to demonstrate a benefit to angioplasty in atherosclerotic renal artery stenosis compared to standard medical therapy [273,274]. This reflects the difficulty in determining, from imaging studies alone, which patients have a hemodynamically significant lesion. In our Center's experience, renal vein renin measurement has an important role in determining the significance of renovascular disease in terms of its contribution toward a patient's hypertension and in planning intervention. Renin secretion from a stenotic kidney that is >1.5 times higher than the contralateral kidney, especially after the administration of an ACE inhibitor, is predictive of an improvement in blood pressure after intervention, though reports vary [275,276]. It is likely that the sensitivity and specificity of the test is improved with very strict control of factors influencing the renin-angiotensin system, including avoiding RAAS blockade and diuretics, a strict low salt diet prior to the test (to stimulate renin production), control of posture on the day of the test (subjects maintain recumbency overnight until the test is complete), and collection of pre- and post-ACE inhibitor stimulated samples [276]. Performing this test in such circumstances is therefore difficult and requires an experienced unit with a strict protocol.

Management

Patients with renovascular hypertension due to FMD generally do well with angioplasty. Younger patients with a short duration of hypertension and focal FMD lesions have a particularly high chance of cure of hypertension after intervention of up to 50% in some studies [270,277—279]. Most FMD lesions respond well to angioplasty alone, with stent insertion appropriate for lesions which don't respond to angioplasty or where a dissection has complicated angioplasty. Renal artery aneurysms or very complicated disease may be better treated with a surgical approach with bypass or resection. All patients should be treated with aspirin or an alternative antiplatelet agent. Patients with renal FMD should have ongoing follow-up with measurement of renal function and a renal artery duplex initially yearly seeking evidence of progression of stenosis or recurrence after intervention.

In contrast to FMD, multiple randomized trials of angioplasty in atherosclerotic renal artery stenosis have not demonstrated consistent benefit compared to optimal medical therapy [273,274]. Limitations of the intervention trials relate mainly to the selection criteria, with exclusion of patients which most guidelines suggest would be most likely to benefit from intervention, such as patients with acute pulmonary oedema, short duration of hypertension or drug resistant hypertension. Good quality observational data suggests that intervention in patients with specific indications such as acute pulmonary edema is more likely to result in benefit [280]. Intervention for atherosclerotic disease should thus generally be reserved for those with a high likelihood of benefit, which might include patients with a short duration of hypertension, patients with drug resistant hypertension, patients with recurrent acute pulmonary edema and patients with very suggestive functional studies (such as ACE inhibitor augmented renograms or renal vein renin studies). Unlike FMD, atherosclerotic lesions generally require stent insertion due to elastic recoil, and stenting reduces rates of subsequent restenosis [281]. In addition, patients with a small kidney poorly functioning kidney (<15% split function) with lateralizing renal vein renin studies might benefit from nephrectomy of a "pressor kidney." All patients with atherosclerotic renal artery disease should have optimal cardiovascular risk factor reduction.

Page kidney

Page kidney is named after Irvine Page who demonstrated that wrapping an animal kidney in cellophane produced hypertension that responded to nephrectomy [282]. The phenomenon occurs because of external kidney compression, which activates the renin-angiotensin system likely via an ischemic mechanism. The typical patient is a young male athlete presenting after sports trauma, however contemporary case series show that kidney biopsy and transplant allograft biopsy are common causes [283]. Interestingly there can be a lag of many years between the trauma and the presentation with hypertension, though most subjects present acutely. Renin is typically high and renal vein renin studies invariably lateralize if they are performed. Patients usually respond well to decompression but nephrectomy may be required in some cases.

Reninoma

A reninoma is a benign tumor arising from juxtaglomerular cells. Cases have been sporadically reported in the literature with approximately only 100 reported to date. The typical presentation is of an adolescent or young adult with severe hypertension. There is a clear female predominance and patient presents with evidence of secondary hyperaldosteronism with normal or high renin, normal or high aldosterone, hypokalemia and a metabolic alkalosis. Ultrasound imaging may miss reninomas, but modern contrast CT will reveal most of them, which appear as well circumscribed low-density lesions. Renal vein renin studies typically lateralize strongly to the kidney in which a reninoma is present, and partial or total nephrectomy is very effective for treatment. Several case reports suggest that the direct renin inhibitor Aliskiren is also partially effective in treating reninoma though treatment breakthrough may occur [284,285]. Renal cell carcinoma and Wilm's tumor can also secrete renin [286] and histopathological examination of the tumor is important to confirm the diagnosis.

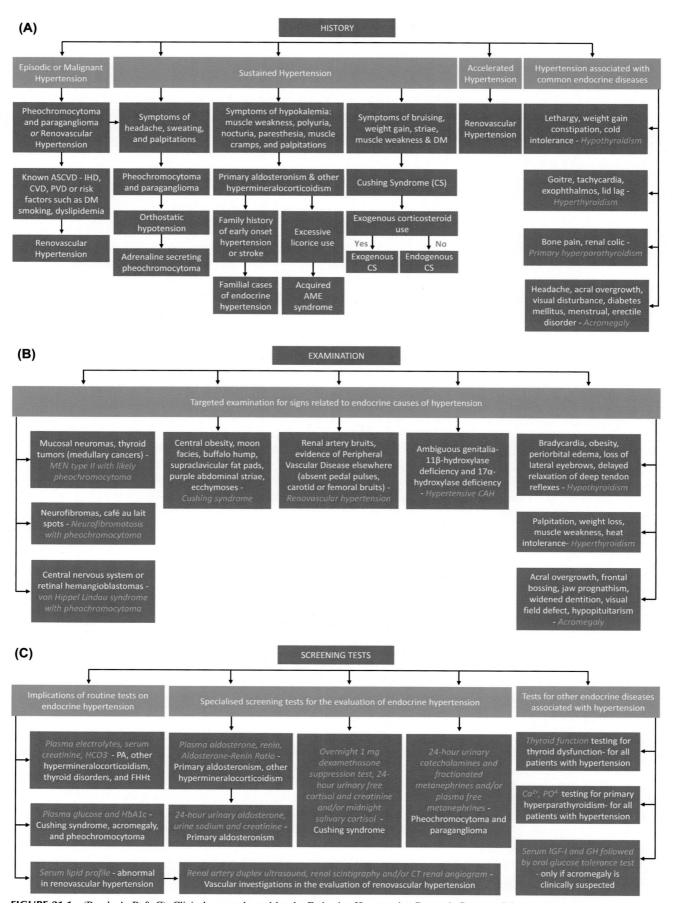

FIGURE 21.1 (Panels A, B & C). Clinical approach used by the Endocrine Hypertension Research Center at Princess Alexandra and Greenslopes Hospital for the initial diagnostic workup of patients referred with suspected endocrine hypertension, grouped according to features sought on history (A), physical examination (B), and requested screening investigations (C). *ASCVD*, denotes atherosclerotic cardiovascular disease; *CAH*, congenital adrenal hyperplasia; *CVD*, cerebrovascular disease; *DM*, diabetes mellitus; *FHHt*, familial hyperkalemia and hypertension; *IHD*, ischemic heart disease; *MEN*, multiple endocrine neoplasia; *PA*, primary aldosteronism; *PVD*, peripheral vascular disease.

Conclusion

Searching for secondary endocrine causes of hypertension can be a highly rewarding experience for both patients and physicians but requires a high index of suspicion and a systematic approach. Fig. 21.1 (Panels A, B and C) summarizes the approach used within our Center at Princess Alexandra and Greenslopes Hospital for the initial diagnostic assessment of a patient referred with suspected endocrine hypertension.

Learning points

- Consider an underlying endocrine cause of hypertension in all hypertensive patients but especially those with early onset, resistant, accelerated or malignant hypertension, or with hypokalemia, symptoms or signs of known causative endocrine conditions, incidentally discovered adrenal lesions or a family history of hypertension or stroke.
- Consider screening for PA by ARR testing in all newly diagnosed hypertensives, and in the great majority of other patients with hypertension
- Although rare, pheochromocytoma is a potentially dangerous condition and the diagnosis should not be missed, arguing for a low threshold for screening among patients with hypertension even when typical symptoms are lacking
- The demonstration of renal artery stenosis in a hypertensive patient does not necessarily establish it as the cause of hypertension: functional testing such as renal venous renin assessment can assist in selecting patients who are likely to benefit from intervention.

References

[1] Rich GM, Ulick S, Cook S, Wang JZ, Lifton RP, Dluhy RG. Glucocorticoid-remediable aldosteronism in a large kindred: clinical spectrum and diagnosis using a characteristic biochemical phenotype. Ann Intern Med 1992;116:813—20.

[2] Stowasser M, Huggard PR, Rossetti TR, Bachmann AW, Gordon RD. Biochemical evidence of aldosterone overproduction and abnormal regulation in normotensive individuals with familial hyperaldosteronism type I. J Clin Endocrinol Metab 1999;84:4031—6.

[3] Jia M, Yu H, Liu Z, et al. Normotensive presentation in primary aldosteronism: a report of two cases. J Renin Angiotensin Aldosterone Syst 2021;22(1). https://doi.org/10.1177/14703203211003780. 14703203211003780.

[4] Mulatero P, Stowasser M, Loh KC, et al. Increased diagnosis of primary aldosteronism, including surgically correctable forms, in centers from five continents. J Clin Endocrinol Metab 2004;89:1045—50.

[5] Stowasser M, Gordon RD, Gunasekera TG, et al. High rate of detection of primary aldosteronism, including surgically treatable forms, after 'non-selective' screening of hypertensive patients. J Hypertens 2003;21:2149—57.

[6] Sonino N, Tomba E, Genesia ML, et al. Psychological assessment of primary aldosteronism: a controlled study. J Clin Endocrinol Metab 2011;96:E878—83.

[7] Sukor N, Kogovsek C, Gordon RD, Robson D, Stowasser M. Improved quality of life, blood pressure, and biochemical status following laparoscopic adrenalectomy for unilateral primary aldosteronism. J Clin Endocrinol Metab 2010;95:1360—4.

[8] Tan YK, Kwan YH, Teo DCL, et al. Improvement in quality of life and psychological symptoms after treatment for primary aldosteronism: Asian Cohort Study. Endocr Connect 2021;10:834—44.

[9] Maruhashi T, Amioka M, Kishimoto S, et al. Elevated plasma renin activity caused by accelerated-malignant hypertension in a patient with aldosterone-producing adenoma complicated with renal insufficiency. Intern Med 2019;58:3107—11.

[10] Gordon RD, Tunny TJ. Aldosterone-producing-adenoma (A-P-A): effect of pregnancy. Clin Exp Hypertens A 1982;4:1685—93.

[11] Ronconi V, Turchi F, Zennaro MC, Boscaro M, Giacchetti G. Progesterone increase counteracts aldosterone action in a pregnant woman with primary aldosteronism. Clin Endocrinol (Oxf) 2011;74:278—9.

[12] Teo AE, Garg S, Shaikh LH, et al. Pregnancy, primary aldosteronism, and adrenal CTNNB1 mutations. N Engl J Med 2015;373:1429—36.

[13] Taylor PJ, Cooper DP, Gordon RD, Stowasser M. Measurement of aldosterone in human plasma by semiautomated HPLC-tandem mass spectrometry. Clin Chem 2009;55:1155—62.

[14] Peitzsch M, Dekkers T, Haase M, et al. An LC-MS/MS method for steroid profiling during adrenal venous sampling for investigation of primary aldosteronism. J Steroid Biochem Mol Biol 2015;145:75—84.

[15] Guo Z, Poglitsch M, McWhinney BC, et al. Aldosterone LC-MS/MS assay-specific threshold values in screening and confirmatory testing for primary aldosteronism. J Clin Endocrinol Metab 2018;103:3965—73.

[16] Thuzar M, Young K, Ahmed AH, et al. Diagnosis of primary aldosteronism by seated saline suppression test-variability between immunoassay and HPLC-MS/MS. J Clin Endocrinol Metab 2020;105:e477—83.

[17] Montori VM, Schwartz GL, Chapman AB, Boerwinkle E, Turner ST. Validity of the aldosterone-renin ratio used to screen for primary aldosteronism. Mayo Clin Proc 2001;76:877—82.

[18] Ferrari P, Shaw SG, Nicod J, Saner E, Nussberger J. Active renin versus plasma renin activity to define aldosterone-to-renin ratio for primary aldosteronism. J Hypertens 2004;22:377—81.

[19] Juutilainen A, Savolainen K, Romppanen J, et al. Combination of LC-MS/MS aldosterone and automated direct renin in screening for primary aldosteronism. Clin Chim Acta 2014;433:209—15.

[20] Sealey JE, Laragh JH. Radioimmunoassay of plasma renin activity. Semin Nucl Med 1975;5:189—202.

[21] Campbell DJ, Nussberger J, Stowasser M, et al. Activity assays and immunoassays for plasma renin and prorenin: information provided and precautions necessary for accurate measurement. Clin Chem 2009;55:867—77.

[22] Oelkers WK. Effects of estrogens and progestogens on the renin-aldosterone system and blood pressure. Steroids 1996;61:166—71.

[23] Morganti A. European study group for the validation of DiaSorin LDRA. A comparative study on inter and intralaboratory reproducibility of renin measurement with a conventional enzymatic method and a new chemiluminescent assay of immunoreactive renin. J Hypertens 2010;28:1307—12.

[24] Guo Z, Poglitsch M, McWhinney BC, et al. Measurement of equilibrium angiotensin II in the diagnosis of primary aldosteronism. Clin Chem 2020;66:483—92.

[25] Funder JW, Carey RM, Mantero F, et al. The management of primary aldosteronism: case detection, diagnosis, and treatment: an endocrine society clinical practice guideline. J Clin Endocrinol Metab 2016;101:1889—916.

[26] Gordon RD, Stowasser M. Primary aldosteronism: the case for screening. Nat Clin Pract Nephrol 2007;3:582—3.

[27] Zarnegar R, Young Jr WF, Lee J, et al. The aldosteronoma resolution score: predicting complete resolution of hypertension after adrenalectomy for aldosteronoma. Ann Surg 2008;247:511—8.

[28] Stowasser M, Gordon RD. Primary aldosteronism-careful investigation is essential and rewarding. Mol Cell Endocrinol 2004;217:33—9.

[29] Mulatero P, Rabbia F, Milan A, et al. Drug effects on aldosterone/plasma renin activity ratio in primary aldosteronism. Hypertension 2002;40:897—902.

[30] Stowasser M, Ahmed AH, Pimenta E, Taylor PJ, Gordon RD. Factors affecting the aldosterone/renin ratio. Horm Metab Res 2012;44:170—6.

[31] Yin G, Zhang S, Yan L, et al. One-hour upright posture is an ideal position for serum aldosterone concentration and plasma renin activity measuring on primary aldosteronism screening. Exp Clin Endocrinol Diabetes Off J German Soc Endocrinol [and] German Diabetes Assoc 2012;120:388—94.

[32] Rossi GP, Seccia TM, Palumbo G, et al. Within-patient reproducibility of the aldosterone: renin ratio in primary aldosteronism. Hypertension 2010;55:83—9.

[33] Yozamp N, Hundemer GL, Moussa M, et al. Intraindividual variability of aldosterone concentrations in primary aldosteronism: implications for case detection. Hypertension 2021;77:891—9.

[34] Gordon RD. Primary aldosteronism. J Endocrinol Invest 1995;18:495—511.

[35] Young WFJ. Primary aldosteronism: update on diagnosis and treatment. Endocrinolologist 1997;7:213—21.

[36] Kem DC, Weinberger MH, Mayes DC, Nugent CA. Saline suppression of plasma aldosterone in hypertension. Arch Intern Med 1971;128:380—6.

[37] Holland OB, Brown H, Kuhnert L, Fairchild C, Risk M, Gomez-Sanchez CE. Further evaluation of saline infusion for the diagnosis of primary aldosteronism. Hypertension 1984;6:717—23.

[38] Ahmed AH, Cowley D, Wolley M, et al. Seated saline suppression testing for the diagnosis of primary aldosteronism: a preliminary study. J Clin Endocrinol Metab 2014;99:2745—53.

[39] Stowasser M, Ahmed AH, Cowley D, et al. Comparison of seated with recumbent saline suppression testing for the diagnosis of primary aldosteronism. J Clin Endocrinol Metab 2018;103:4113—24.

[40] Eisenhofer G, Kurlbaum M, Peitzsch M, et al. The saline infusion test for primary aldosteronism: implications of immunoassay inaccuracy. J Clin Endocrinol Metab 2022;107:e2027—36.

[41] Iwaoka T, Umeda T, Naomi S, et al. The usefulness of the captopril test as a simultaneous screening for primary aldosteronism and renovascular hypertension. Am J Hypertens 1993;6:899—906.

[42] Westerdahl C, Bergenfelz A, Isaksson A, Valdemarsson S. Captopril suppression: limitations for confirmation of primary aldosteronism. J Renin Angiotensin Aldosterone Syst 2011;12:326—32.

[43] Mulatero P, Bertello C, Garrone C, et al. Captopril test can give misleading results in patients with suspect primary aldosteronism. Hypertension 2007;50:e26—7.

[44] Lifton RP, Dluhy RG, Powers M, et al. A chimaeric 11 beta-hydroxylase/aldosterone synthase gene causes glucocorticoid-remediable aldosteronism and human hypertension. Nature 1992;355:262—5.

[45] Jonsson JR, Klemm SA, Tunny TJ, Stowasser M, Gordon RD. A new genetic test for familial hyperaldosteronism type I aids in the detection of curable hypertension. Biochem Biophys Res Commun 1995;207:565—71.

[46] Scholl UI, Nelson-Williams C, Yue P, et al. Hypertension with or without adrenal hyperplasia due to different inherited mutations in the potassium channel KCNJ5. Proc Natl Acad Sci U S A 2012;109:2533—8.

[47] Daunt N. Adrenal vein sampling: how to make it quick, easy, and successful. Radiographics 2005;25(Suppl. 1):S143—58.

[48] Hundemer GL, Curhan GC, Yozamp N, Wang M, Vaidya A. Cardiometabolic outcomes and mortality in medically treated primary aldosteronism: a retrospective cohort study. Lancet Diabetes Endocrinol 2018;6:51—9.

[49] Rossi GP, Maiolino G, Flego A, et al. Adrenalectomy lowers incident atrial fibrillation in primary aldosteronism patients at long term. Hypertension 2018;71:585—91.

[50] Ahmed AH, Gordon RD, Sukor N, Pimenta E, Stowasser M. Quality of life in patients with bilateral primary aldosteronism before and during treatment with spironolactone and/or amiloride, including a comparison with our previously published results in those with unilateral disease treated surgically. J Clin Endocrinol Metab 2011;96:2904—11.

[51] Buffolo F, Cavaglia G, Burrello J, et al. Quality of life in primary aldosteronism: a prospective observational study. Eur J Clin Invest 2021;51:e13419.

[52] Kupers EM, Amar L, Raynaud A, Plouin PF, Steichen O. A clinical prediction score to diagnose unilateral primary aldosteronism. J Clin Endocrinol Metab 2012;97:3530–7.

[53] Young WF, Stanson AW, Thompson GB, Grant CS, Farley DR, van Heerden JA. Role for adrenal venous sampling in primary aldosteronism. Surgery 2004;136:1227–35.

[54] Wu MH, Liu FH, Lin KJ, Sun JH, Chen ST. Diagnostic value of adrenal iodine-131 6-beta-iodomethyl-19-norcholesterol scintigraphy for primary aldosteronism: a retrospective study at a medical center in North Taiwan. Nucl Med Commun 2019;40:568–75.

[55] O'Shea PM, O'Donoghue D, Bashari W, et al. (11) C-Metomidate PET/CT is a useful adjunct for lateralization of primary aldosteronism in routine clinical practice. Clin Endocrinol (Oxf) 2019;90:670–9.

[56] Powlson AS, Gurnell M, Brown MJ. Nuclear imaging in the diagnosis of primary aldosteronism. Curr Opin Endocrinol Diabetes Obes 2015;22:150–6.

[57] Sander K, Gendron T, Cybulska KA, et al. Development of [(18)F]AldoView as the first highly selective aldosterone synthase PET tracer for imaging of primary hyperaldosteronism. J Med Chem 2021;64:9321–9.

[58] Gordon RD, Gomez-Sanchez CE, Hamlet SM, Tunny TJ, Klemm SA. Angiotensin-responsive aldosterone-producing adenoma masquerades as idiopathic hyperaldosteronism (IHA: adrenal hyperplasia) or low-renin essential hypertension. J Hypertens Suppl 1987;5:S103–6.

[59] Satoh F, Morimoto R, Ono Y, et al. Measurement of peripheral plasma 18-oxocortisol can discriminate unilateral adenoma from bilateral diseases in patients with primary aldosteronism. Hypertension 2015;65:1096–102.

[60] Guo Z, Nanba K, Udager A, et al. Biochemical, histopathological, and genetic characterization of posture-responsive and unresponsive APAs. J Clin Endocrinol Metab 2020;105:e3224–35.

[61] Monticone S, Satoh F, Dietz AS, et al. Clinical management and outcomes of adrenal hemorrhage following adrenal vein sampling in primary aldosteronism. Hypertension 2016;67:146–52.

[62] Young WF, Stanson AW. What are the keys to successful adrenal venous sampling (AVS) in patients with primary aldosteronism? Clin Endocrinol (Oxf) 2009;70:14–7.

[63] Yoneda T, Karashima S, Kometani M, et al. Impact of new quick gold nanoparticle-based cortisol assay during adrenal vein sampling for primary aldosteronism. J Clin Endocrinol Metab 2016;101:2554–61.

[64] Rossi GP, Auchus RJ, Brown M, et al. An expert consensus statement on use of adrenal vein sampling for the subtyping of primary aldosteronism. Hypertension 2014;63:151–60.

[65] Goupil R, Wolley M, Ungerer J, et al. Use of plasma metanephrine to aid adrenal venous sampling in combined aldosterone and cortisol over-secretion. Endocrinol Diab Metab Case Rep 2015;2015:150075.

[66] Celen O, O'Brien MJ, Melby JC, Beazley RM. Factors influencing outcome of surgery for primary aldosteronism. Arch Surg 1996;131:646–50.

[67] Gordon RD, Stowasser M, Klemm SA, Tunny TJ. Primary aldosteronism and other forms of mineralocorticoid hypertension. In: Swales J, editor. Textbook of hypertension. London: Blackwell Scientific Publications; 1994. p. 865–92.

[68] Rutherford JC, Taylor WL, Stowasser M, Gordon RD. Success of surgery for primary aldosteronism judged by residual autonomous aldosterone production. World J Surg 1998;22:1243–5.

[69] Stowasser M, Klemm SA, Tunny TJ, Storie WJ, Rutherford JC, Gordon RD. Response to unilateral adrenalectomy for aldosterone-producing adenoma: effect of potassium levels and angiotensin responsiveness. Clin Exp Pharmacol Physiol 1994;21:319–22.

[70] Williams TA, Lenders JWM, Mulatero P, et al. Outcomes after adrenalectomy for unilateral primary aldosteronism: an international consensus on outcome measures and analysis of remission rates in an international cohort. Lancet Diabetes Endocrinol 2017;5:689–99.

[71] Satoh F, Morimoto R, Seiji K, et al. Is there a role for segmental adrenal venous sampling and adrenal sparing surgery in patients with primary aldosteronism? Eur J Endocrinol 2015;173:465–77.

[72] Sukor N, Gordon RD, Ku YK, Jones M, Stowasser M. Role of unilateral adrenalectomy in bilateral primary aldosteronism: a 22-year single center experience. J Clin Endocrinol Metab 2009;94:2437–45.

[73] Choi M, Scholl UI, Yue P, et al. K+ channel mutations in adrenal aldosterone-producing adenomas and hereditary hypertension. Science 2011;331:768–72.

[74] Stowasser M. Primary aldosteronism and potassium channel mutations. Curr Opin Endocrinol Diabetes Obes 2013;20:170–9.

[75] Charmandari E, Sertedaki A, Kino T, et al. A novel point mutation in the KCNJ5 gene causing primary hyperaldosteronism and early-onset autosomal dominant hypertension. J Clin Endocrinol Metab 2012;97:E1532–9.

[76] Fallo F, Bertello C, Tizzani D, et al. Concurrent primary aldosteronism and subclinical cortisol hypersecretion: a prospective study. J Hypertens 2011;29:1773–7.

[77] Fujimoto K, Honjo S, Tatsuoka H, et al. Primary aldosteronism associated with subclinical Cushing syndrome. J Endocrinol Invest 2013;36:564–7.

[78] Hiraishi K, Yoshimoto T, Tsuchiya K, et al. Clinicopathological features of primary aldosteronism associated with subclinical Cushing's syndrome. Endocr J 2011;58:543–51.

[79] Spath M, Korovkin S, Antke C, Anlauf M, Willenberg HS. Aldosterone- and cortisol-co-secreting adrenal tumors: the lost subtype of primary aldosteronism. Eur J Endocrinol 2011;164:447–55.

[80] Sechi LA, Di FA, Bazzocchi M, Uzzau A, Catena C. Intrarenal hemodynamics in primary aldosteronism before and after treatment. J Clin Endocrinol Metab 2009;94:1191–7.

[81] Rossi GP, Sacchetto A, Visentin P, et al. Changes in left ventricular anatomy and function in hypertension and primary aldosteronism. Hypertension 1996;27:1039–45.

[82] Monticone S, Sconfienza E, D'Ascenzo F, et al. Renal damage in primary aldosteronism: a systematic review and meta-analysis. J Hypertens 2020;38:3–12.

[83] Stowasser M, Gordon RD, Rutherford JC, Nikwan NZ, Daunt N, Slater GJ. Diagnosis and management of primary aldosteronism. J Renin Angiotensin Aldosterone Syst 2001;2:156–69.

[84] Lim PO, Young WF, MacDonald TM. A review of the medical treatment of primary aldosteronism. J Hypertens 2001;19:353–61.

[85] Pitt B, Zannad F, Remme WJ, et al. The effect of spironolactone on morbidity and mortality in patients with severe heart failure. Randomized Aldactone Evaluation Study Investigators. N Engl J Med 1999;341:709–17.

[86] Jeunemaitre X, Chatellier G, Kreft-Jais C, et al. Efficacy and tolerance of spironolactone in essential hypertension. Am J Cardiol 1987;60:820–5.

[87] Delyani JA. Mineralocorticoid receptor antagonists: the evolution of utility and pharmacology. Kidney Int 2000;57:1408–11.

[88] Agarwal R, Kolkhof P, Bakris G, et al. Steroidal and non-steroidal mineralocorticoid receptor antagonists in cardiorenal medicine. Eur Heart J 2021;42:152–61.

[89] Griffing GT, Berelowitz B, Hudson M, et al. Plasma immunoreactive gamma melanotropin in patients with idiopathic hyperaldosteronism, aldosterone-producing adenomas, and essential hypertension. J Clin Invest 1985;76:163–9.

[90] Mantero F, Fallo F, Opocher G, Armanini D, Boscaro M, Scaroni C. Effect of angiotensin II and converting enzyme inhibitor (captopril) on blood pressure, plasma renin activity and aldosterone in primary aldosteronism. Clin Sci (Lond) 1981;61(Suppl. 7):289s–93s.

[91] Hsueh WA. New insights into the medical management of primary aldosteronism. Hypertension 1986;8:76–82.

[92] Nadler JL, Hsueh W, Horton R. Therapeutic effect of calcium channel blockade in primary aldosteronism. J Clin Endocrinol Metab 1985;60:896–9.

[93] Carpene G, Rocco S, Opocher G, Mantero F. Acute and chronic effect of nifedipine in primary aldosteronism. Clin Exp Hypertens A 1989;11:1263–72.

[94] Stowasser M, Bachmann AW, Huggard PR, Rossetti TR, Gordon RD. Treatment of familial hyperaldosteronism type I: only partial suppression of adrenocorticotropin required to correct hypertension. J Clin Endocrinol Metab 2000;85:3313–8.

[95] Pimenta E, Gordon RD, Ahmed AH, et al. Cardiac dimensions are largely determined by dietary salt in patients with primary aldosteronism: results of a case-control study. J Clin Endocrinol Metab 2011;96:2813–20.

[96] Pimenta E, Gordon RD, Ahmed AH, et al. Unilateral adrenalectomy improves urinary protein excretion but does not abolish its relationship to sodium excretion in patients with aldosterone-producing adenoma. J Hum Hypertens 2011;25:592–9.

[97] Amar L, Azizi M, Menard J, Peyrard S, Plouin PF. Sequential comparison of aldosterone synthase inhibition and mineralocorticoid blockade in patients with primary aldosteronism. J Hypertens 2013;31:624–9.

[98] New MI. Inborn errors of adrenal steroidogenesis. Mol Cell Endocrinol 2003;211:75–83.

[99] Geley S, Kapelari K, Johrer K, et al. CYP11B1 mutations causing congenital adrenal hyperplasia due to 11 beta-hydroxylase deficiency. J Clin Endocrinol Metab 1996;81:2896–901.

[100] White PC, Curnow KM, Pascoe L. Disorders of steroid 11 beta-hydroxylase isozymes. Endocr Rev 1994;15:421–38.

[101] White PC, Speiser PW. Steroid 11 beta-hydroxylase deficiency and related disorders. Endocrinol Metab Clin North Am 1994;23:325–39.

[102] Zachmann M, Tassinari D, Prader A. Clinical and biochemical variability of congenital adrenal hyperplasia due to 11 beta-hydroxylase deficiency. A study of 25 patients. J Clin Endocrinol Metab 1983;56:222–9.

[103] New MI. Polycystic ovarian disease and congenital and late-onset adrenal hyperplasia. Endocrinol Metab Clin North Am 1988;17:637–48.

[104] Kater CE, Biglieri EG. Disorders of steroid 17 alpha-hydroxylase deficiency. Endocrinol Metab Clin North Am 1994;23:341–57.

[105] Biglieri EG, Herron MA, Brust N. 17-hydroxylation deficiency in man. J Clin Invest 1966;45:1946–54.

[106] Lee HI, Kwon A, Suh JH, et al. Two cases of 17alpha-hydroxylase/17,20-lyase deficiency caused by the CYP17A1 mutation. Ann Pediatr Endocrinol Metab 2021;26:66–70.

[107] Nicolaides NC, Charmandari E. Primary generalized glucocorticoid resistance and hypersensitivity syndromes: a 2021 update. Int J Mol Sci 2021;22:10839.

[108] Charmandari E, Kino T, Chrousos GP. Familial/sporadic glucocorticoid resistance: clinical phenotype and molecular mechanisms. Ann N Y Acad Sci 2004;1024:168–81.

[109] Chrousos GP, Vingerhoeds A, Brandon D, et al. Primary cortisol resistance in man. A glucocorticoid receptor-mediated disease. J Clin Invest 1982;69:1261–9.

[110] Malchoff DM, Brufsky A, Reardon G, et al. A mutation of the glucocorticoid receptor in primary cortisol resistance. J Clin Invest 1993;91:1918–25.

[111] Ruiz M, Lind U, Gafvels M, et al. Characterization of two novel mutations in the glucocorticoid receptor gene in patients with primary cortisol resistance. Clin Endocrinol (Oxf) 2001;55:363–71.

[112] Stewart PM, Corrie JE, Shackleton CH, Edwards CR. Syndrome of apparent mineralocorticoid excess. A defect in the cortisol-cortisone shuttle. J Clin Invest 1988;82:340–9.

[113] Wilson RC, Krozowski ZS, Li K, et al. A mutation in the HSD11B2 gene in a family with apparent mineralocorticoid excess. J Clin Endocrinol Metab 1995;80:2263–6.

[114] Stewart PM, Krozowski ZS, Gupta A, et al. Hypertension in the syndrome of apparent mineralocorticoid excess due to mutation of the 11 beta-hydroxysteroid dehydrogenase type 2 gene. Lancet 1996;347:88–91.

[115] Mune T, Rogerson FM, Nikkila H, Agarwal AK, White PC. Human hypertension caused by mutations in the kidney isozyme of 11 beta-hydroxysteroid dehydrogenase. Nat Genet 1995;10:394—9.

[116] Lavery GG, Ronconi V, Draper N, et al. Late-onset apparent mineralocorticoid excess caused by novel compound heterozygous mutations in the HSD11B2 gene. Hypertension 2003;42:123—9.

[117] Li A, Li KX, Marui S, et al. Apparent mineralocorticoid excess in a Brazilian kindred: hypertension in the heterozygote state. J Hypertens 1997;15:1397—402.

[118] Walker BR, Edwards CR. Licorice-induced hypertension and syndromes of apparent mineralocorticoid excess. Endocrinol Metab Clin North Am 1994;23:359—77.

[119] Palermo M, Shackleton CH, Mantero F, Stewart PM. Urinary free cortisone and the assessment of 11 beta-hydroxysteroid dehydrogenase activity in man. Clin Endocrinol (Oxf) 1996;45:605—11.

[120] New MI, Wilson RC. Steroid disorders in children: congenital adrenal hyperplasia and apparent mineralocorticoid excess. Proc Natl Acad Sci U S A 1999;96:12790—7.

[121] Ishikawa SE, Saito T, Kaneko K, Okada K, Fukuda S, Kuzuya T. Hypermineralocorticism without elevation of plasma aldosterone: deoxycorticosterone-producing adrenal adenoma and hyperplasia. Clin Endocrinol (Oxf) 1988;29:367—75.

[122] Wada N, Kubo M, Kijima H, et al. A case of deoxycorticosterone-producing adrenal adenoma. Endocr J 1995;42:637—42.

[123] Yamamoto A, Naroda T, Kagawa S, et al. Deoxycorticosterone-secreting adrenocortical carcinoma. Endocr Pathol 1993;4:165—8.

[124] Young J, Haissaguerre M, Viera-Pinto O, Chabre O, Baudin E, Tabarin A. Management of endocrine disease: Cushing's syndrome due to ectopic ACTH secretion: an expert operational opinion. Eur J Endocrinol 2020;182:R29—58.

[125] Stewart PM, Walker BR, Holder G, O'Halloran D, Shackleton CH. 11 beta-hydroxysteroid dehydrogenase activity in Cushing's syndrome: explaining the mineralocorticoid excess state of the ectopic adrenocorticotropin syndrome. J Clin Endocrinol Metab 1995;80:3617—20.

[126] Geller DS, Farhi A, Pinkerton N, et al. Activating mineralocorticoid receptor mutation in hypertension exacerbated by pregnancy. Science 2000;289:119—23.

[127] Warnock DG. Liddle syndrome: genetics and mechanisms of Na+ channel defects. Am J Med Sci 2001;322:302—7.

[128] Liddle GW, Bledsoe T, Coppage WS. A familial renal disorder simulating primary aldosteronism but with negligible aldosterone secretion. Trans Assoc Am Physicians 1963;26:199—213.

[129] Tetti M, Monticone S, Burrello J, et al. Liddle syndrome: review of the literature and description of a new case. Int J Mol Sci 2018;19:812.

[130] Findling JW, Raff H, Hansson JH, Lifton RP. Liddle's syndrome: prospective genetic screening and suppressed aldosterone secretion in an extended kindred. J Clin Endocrinol Metab 1997;82:1071—4.

[131] Gordon RD. Syndrome of hypertension and hyperkalemia with normal glomerular filtration rate. Hypertension 1986;8:93—102.

[132] Glover M, Zuber AM, O'Shaughnessy KM. Hypertension, dietary salt intake, and the role of the thiazide-sensitive sodium chloride transporter NCCT. Cardiovasc Ther 2011;29:68—76.

[133] Lifton RP, Gharavi AG, Geller DS. Molecular mechanisms of human hypertension. Cell 2001;104:545—56.

[134] Mabillard H, Sayer JA. The molecular genetics of Gordon syndrome. Genes (Basel) 2019;10:986.

[135] Stowasser M, Pimenta E, Gordon RD. Familial or genetic primary aldosteronism and Gordon syndrome. Endocrinol Metab Clin North Am 2011;40:343—68.

[136] Lenders JW, Duh QY, Eisenhofer G, et al. Pheochromocytoma and paraganglioma: an endocrine society clinical practice guideline. J Clin Endocrinol Metab 2014;99:1915—42.

[137] Ebbehoj A, Stochholm K, Jacobsen SF, et al. Incidence and clinical presentation of pheochromocytoma and sympathetic paraganglioma: a population-based study. J Clin Endocrinol Metab 2021;106:e2251—61.

[138] McNeil AR, Blok BH, Koelmeyer TD, Burke MP, Hilton JM. Phaeochromocytomas discovered during coronial autopsies in Sydney, Melbourne and Auckland. Aust N Z J Med 2000;30:648—52.

[139] Leung AA, Pasieka JL, Hyrcza MD, et al. Epidemiology of pheochromocytoma and paraganglioma: population-based cohort study. Eur J Endocrinol 2021;184:19—28.

[140] Kopetschke R, Slisko M, Kilisli A, et al. Frequent incidental discovery of phaeochromocytoma: data from a German cohort of 201 phaeochromocytoma. Eur J Endocrinol 2009;161:355—61.

[141] Fassnacht M, Arlt W, Bancos I, et al. Management of adrenal incidentalomas: European society of endocrinology clinical practice guideline in collaboration with the European network for the study of adrenal tumors. Eur J Endocrinol 2016;175:G1—34.

[142] Omura M, Saito J, Yamaguchi K, Kakuta Y, Nishikawa T. Prospective study on the prevalence of secondary hypertension among hypertensive patients visiting a general outpatient clinic in Japan. Hypertens Res 2004;27:193—202.

[143] Prejbisz A, Lenders JW, Eisenhofer G, Januszewicz A. Mortality associated with phaeochromocytoma. Horm Metab Res 2013;45:154—8.

[144] Zelinka T, Petrak O, Turkova H, et al. High incidence of cardiovascular complications in pheochromocytoma. Horm Metab Res 2012;44:379—84.

[145] Prejbisz A, Lenders JW, Eisenhofer G, Januszewicz A. Cardiovascular manifestations of phaeochromocytoma. J Hypertens 2011;29:2049—60.

[146] Mesmar B, Poola-Kella S, Malek R. The physiology behind diabetes mellitus in patients with pheochromocytoma: a review of the literature. Endocr Pract 2017;23:999—1005.

[147] Krumeich LN, Cucchiara AJ, Nathanson KL, et al. Correlation between plasma catecholamines, weight, and diabetes in pheochromocytoma and paraganglioma. J Clin Endocrinol Metab 2021;106:e4028—38.

[148] Constantinescu G, Langton K, Conrad C, et al. Glucocorticoid excess in patients with pheochromocytoma compared with paraganglioma and other forms of hypertension. J Clin Endocrinol Metab 2020;105:e3374—83.

[149] Lenders JWM, Kerstens MN, Amar L, et al. Genetics, diagnosis, management and future directions of research of phaeochromocytoma and paraganglioma: a position statement and consensus of the Working Group on Endocrine Hypertension of the European Society of Hypertension. J Hypertens 2020;38:1443−56.

[150] Group NGSiPS, Toledo RA, Burnichon N, et al. Consensus Statement on next-generation-sequencing-based diagnostic testing of hereditary phaeochromocytomas and paragangliomas. Nat Rev Endocrinol 2017;13:233−47.

[151] Geroula A, Deutschbein T, Langton K, et al. Pheochromocytoma and paraganglioma: clinical feature-based disease probability in relation to catecholamine biochemistry and reason for disease suspicion. Eur J Endocrinol 2019;181:409−20.

[152] Buitenwerf E, Berends AMA, van Asselt ADI, et al. Diagnostic accuracy of computed tomography to exclude pheochromocytoma: a systematic review, meta-analysis, and cost analysis. Mayo Clin Proc 2019;94:2040−52.

[153] Hirsch D, Grossman A, Nadler V, Alboim S, Tsvetov G. Pheochromocytoma: positive predictive values of mildly elevated urinary fractionated metanephrines in a large cohort of community-dwelling patients. J Clin Hypertens (Greenwich) 2019;21:1527−33.

[154] Eisenhofer G, Goldstein DS, Walther MM, et al. Biochemical diagnosis of pheochromocytoma: how to distinguish true- from false-positive test results. J Clin Endocrinol Metab 2003;88:2656−66.

[155] Bravo EL, Tarazi RC, Fouad FM, Vidt DG, Gifford Jr RW. Clonidine-suppression test: a useful aid in the diagnosis of pheochromocytoma. N Engl J Med 1981;305:623−6.

[156] Goupil R, Fountoulakis S, Gordon RD, Stowasser M. Urinary clonidine suppression testing for the diagnosis of pheochromocytoma. J Hypertens 2015;33:2286−93.

[157] Castinetti F, Taieb D, Henry JF, et al. Management of endocrine disease: outcome of adrenal sparing surgery in heritable pheochromocytoma. Eur J Endocrinol 2016;174:R9−18.

[158] Buitenwerf E, Osinga TE, Timmers H, et al. Efficacy of alpha-blockers on hemodynamic control during pheochromocytoma resection: a randomized controlled trial. J Clin Endocrinol Metab 2020;105:2381−91.

[159] Schimmack S, Kaiser J, Probst P, Kalkum E, Diener MK, Strobel O. Meta-analysis of alpha-blockade versus no blockade before adrenalectomy for phaeochromocytoma. Br J Surg 2020;107:e102−8.

[160] Pacak K. Preoperative management of the pheochromocytoma patient. J Clin Endocrinol Metab 2007;92:4069−79.

[161] Gruber LM, Jasim S, Ducharme-Smith A, Weingarten T, Young WF, Bancos I. The role for metyrosine in the treatment of patients with pheochromocytoma and paraganglioma. J Clin Endocrinol Metab 2021;106:e2393−401.

[162] Plouin PF, Amar L, Dekkers OM, et al. European Society of Endocrinology Clinical Practice Guideline for long-term follow-up of patients operated on for a phaeochromocytoma or a paraganglioma. Eur J Endocrinol 2016;174:G1−10.

[163] Rednam SP, Erez A, Druker H, et al. Von Hippel-Lindau and hereditary pheochromocytoma/paraganglioma syndromes: clinical features, genetics, and surveillance recommendations in childhood. Clin Cancer Res 2017;23:e68−75.

[164] Lacroix A, Feelders RA, Stratakis CA, Nieman LK. Cushing's syndrome. Lancet 2015;386:913−27.

[165] Sharma ST, Nieman LK, Feelders RA. Cushing's syndrome: epidemiology and developments in disease management. Clin Epidemiol 2015;7:281−93.

[166] Nieman LK. Cushing's syndrome: update on signs, symptoms and biochemical screening. Eur J Endocrinol 2015;173:M33−8.

[167] Rubinstein G, Osswald A, Hoster E, et al. Time to diagnosis in Cushing's syndrome: a meta-analysis based on 5367 patients. J Clin Endocrinol Metab 2020;105.

[168] Nieman LK, Biller BM, Findling JW, et al. The diagnosis of Cushing's syndrome: an endocrine society clinical practice guideline. J Clin Endocrinol Metab 2008;93:1526−40.

[169] Plotz CM, Knowlton AI, Ragan C. The natural history of Cushing's syndrome. Am J Med 1952;13:597−614.

[170] Graversen D, Vestergaard P, Stochholm K, Gravholt CH, Jorgensen JO. Mortality in Cushing's syndrome: a systematic review and meta-analysis. Eur J Intern Med 2012;23:278−82.

[171] Ntali G, Asimakopoulou A, Siamatras T, et al. Mortality in Cushing's syndrome: systematic analysis of a large series with prolonged follow-up. Eur J Endocrinol 2013;169:715−23.

[172] Isidori AM, Graziadio C, Paragliola RM, et al. The hypertension of Cushing's syndrome: controversies in the pathophysiology and focus on cardiovascular complications. J Hypertens 2015;33:44−60.

[173] Shimon I. Screening for Cushing's syndrome: is it worthwhile? Pituitary 2015;18:201−5.

[174] Salih M, Bovee DM, van der Lubbe N, et al. Increased urinary extracellular vesicle sodium transporters in Cushing syndrome with hypertension. J Clin Endocrinol Metab 2018;103:2583−91.

[175] Hunter RW, Ivy JR, Bailey MA. Glucocorticoids and renal Na+ transport: implications for hypertension and salt sensitivity. J Physiol 2014;592:1731−44.

[176] Stewart PM. Tissue-specific Cushing's syndrome, 11beta-hydroxysteroid dehydrogenases and the redefinition of corticosteroid hormone action. Eur J Endocrinol 2003;149:163−8.

[177] Wolley MJ, Wu A, Xu S, Gordon RD, Fenton RA, Stowasser M. In primary aldosteronism, mineralocorticoids influence exosomal sodium-chloride cotransporter abundance. J Am Soc Nephrol 2017;28:56−63.

[178] Saruta T, Suzuki H, Handa M, Igarashi Y, Kondo K, Senba S. Multiple factors contribute to the pathogenesis of hypertension in Cushing's syndrome. J Clin Endocrinol Metab 1986;62:275−9.

[179] van der Pas R, van Esch JH, de Bruin C, et al. Cushing's disease and hypertension: in vivo and in vitro study of the role of the renin-angiotensin-aldosterone system and effects of medical therapy. Eur J Endocrinol 2014;170:181−91.

[180] Heaney AP, Hunter SJ, Sheridan B, Brew Atkinson A. Increased pressor response to noradrenaline in pituitary dependent Cushing's syndrome. Clin Endocrinol (Oxf) 1999;51:293—9.

[181] Yasuda G, Shionoiri H, Umemura S, Takasaki I, Ishii M. Exaggerated blood pressure response to angiotensin II in patients with Cushing's syndrome due to adrenocortical adenoma. Eur J Endocrinol 1994;131:582—8.

[182] Sato A, Suzuki H, Murakami M, Nakazato Y, Iwaita Y, Saruta T. Glucocorticoid increases angiotensin II type 1 receptor and its gene expression. Hypertension 1994;23:25—30.

[183] Kirilov G, Tomova A, Dakovska L, Kumanov P, Shinkov A, Alexandrov AS. Elevated plasma endothelin as an additional cardiovascular risk factor in patients with Cushing's syndrome. Eur J Endocrinol 2003;149:549—53.

[184] Giordano R, Picu A, Marinazzo E, et al. Metabolic and cardiovascular outcomes in patients with Cushing's syndrome of different aetiologies during active disease and 1 year after remission. Clin Endocrinol (Oxf) 2011;75:354—60.

[185] Jha S, Sinaii N, McGlotten RN, Nieman LK. Remission of hypertension after surgical cure of Cushing's syndrome. Clin Endocrinol (Oxf) 2020;92:124—30.

[186] Pecori Giraldi F, Toja PM, De Martin M, et al. Circadian blood pressure profile in patients with active Cushing's disease and after long-term cure. Horm Metab Res 2007;39:908—14.

[187] Suzuki T, Shibata H, Ando T, et al. Risk factors associated with persistent postoperative hypertension in Cushing's syndrome. Endocr Res 2000;26:791—5.

[188] Sato H, Imamura Y, Sakamoto S, et al. Adrenalectomy in Japanese patients with subclinical Cushing syndrome: 1-mg dexamethasone suppression test to predict the surgical benefit. Int J Urol 2021;28:273—9.

[189] Lambert JK, Goldberg L, Fayngold S, Kostadinov J, Post KD, Geer EB. Predictors of mortality and long-term outcomes in treated Cushing's disease: a study of 346 patients. J Clin Endocrinol Metab 2013;98:1022—30.

[190] Pivonello R, Petersenn S, Newell-Price J, et al. Pasireotide treatment significantly improves clinical signs and symptoms in patients with Cushing's disease: results from a Phase III study. Clin Endocrinol (Oxf) 2014;81:408—17.

[191] Lacroix A, Bronstein MD, Schopohl J, et al. Long-acting pasireotide improves clinical signs and quality of life in Cushing's disease: results from a phase III study. J Endocrinol Invest 2020;43:1613—22.

[192] Pivonello R, De Martino MC, Cappabianca P, et al. The medical treatment of Cushing's disease: effectiveness of chronic treatment with the dopamine agonist cabergoline in patients unsuccessfully treated by surgery. J Clin Endocrinol Metab 2009;94:223—30.

[193] Feelders RA, Hofland LJ, de Herder WW. Medical treatment of Cushing's syndrome: adrenal-blocking drugs and ketaconazole. Neuroendocrinology 2010;92(Suppl. 1):111—5.

[194] Valassi E, Crespo I, Gich I, Rodriguez J, Webb SM. A reappraisal of the medical therapy with steroidogenesis inhibitors in Cushing's syndrome. Clin Endocrinol (Oxf) 2012;77:735—42.

[195] Katznelson L, Loriaux DL, Feldman D, Braunstein GD, Schteingart DE, Gross C. Global clinical response in Cushing's syndrome patients treated with mifepristone. Clin Endocrinol (Oxf) 2014;80:562—9.

[196] Fleseriu M, Biller BM, Findling JW, et al. Mifepristone, a glucocorticoid receptor antagonist, produces clinical and metabolic benefits in patients with Cushing's syndrome. J Clin Endocrinol Metab 2012;97:2039—49.

[197] Pivonello R, Bancos I, Feelders RA, et al. Relacorilant, a selective glucocorticoid receptor modulator, induces clinical improvements in patients with Cushing syndrome: results from a prospective, open-label phase 2 study. Front Endocrinol (Lausanne) 2021;12:662865.

[198] Feelders RA, de Bruin C, Pereira AM, et al. Pasireotide alone or with cabergoline and ketoconazole in Cushing's disease. N Engl J Med 2010;362:1846—8.

[199] Katznelson L, Laws Jr ER, Melmed S, et al. Acromegaly: an endocrine society clinical practice guideline. J Clin Endocrinol Metab 2014;99:3933—51.

[200] Lavrentaki A, Paluzzi A, Wass JA, Karavitaki N. Epidemiology of acromegaly: review of population studies. Pituitary 2017;20:4—9.

[201] Giustina A, Barkan A, Beckers A, et al. A consensus on the diagnosis and treatment of acromegaly comorbidities: an update. J Clin Endocrinol Metab 2020;105.

[202] Berg C, Petersenn S, Lahner H, et al. Cardiovascular risk factors in patients with uncontrolled and long-term acromegaly: comparison with matched data from the general population and the effect of disease control. J Clin Endocrinol Metab 2010;95:3648—56.

[203] Hong S, Kim KS, Han K, Park CY. Acromegaly and cardiovascular outcomes: a cohort study. Eur Heart J 2022;43:1491—9.

[204] Bondanelli M, Ambrosio MR, degli Uberti EC. Pathogenesis and prevalence of hypertension in acromegaly. Pituitary 2001;4:239—49.

[205] Vitale G, Pivonello R, Auriemma RS, et al. Hypertension in acromegaly and in the normal population: prevalence and determinants. Clin Endocrinol (Oxf) 2005;63:470—6.

[206] Kamenicky P, Viengchareun S, Blanchard A, et al. Epithelial sodium channel is a key mediator of growth hormone-induced sodium retention in acromegaly. Endocrinology 2008;149:3294—305.

[207] Colao A, Ferone D, Marzullo P, Lombardi G. Systemic complications of acromegaly: epidemiology, pathogenesis, and management. Endocr Rev 2004;25:102—52.

[208] Briet C, Ilie MD, Kuhn E, et al. Changes in metabolic parameters and cardiovascular risk factors after therapeutic control of acromegaly vary with the treatment modality. Data from the Bicetre cohort, and review of the literature. Endocrine 2019;63:348—60.

[209] Colao A, Terzolo M, Bondanelli M, et al. GH and IGF-I excess control contributes to blood pressure control: results of an observational, retrospective, multicentre study in 105 hypertensive acromegalic patients on hypertensive treatment. Clin Endocrinol (Oxf) 2008;69:613—20.

[210] Sardella C, Urbani C, Lombardi M, et al. The beneficial effect of acromegaly control on blood pressure values in normotensive patients. Clin Endocrinol (Oxf) 2014;81:573—81.

[211] Colao A, Auriemma RS, Galdiero M, Lombardi G, Pivonello R. Effects of initial therapy for five years with somatostatin analogs for acromegaly on growth hormone and insulin-like growth factor-I levels, tumor shrinkage, and cardiovascular disease: a prospective study. J Clin Endocrinol Metab 2009;94:3746—56.

[212] Gonzalez B, Vargas G, de Los Monteros ALE, Mendoza V, Mercado M. Persistence of diabetes and hypertension after multimodal treatment of acromegaly. J Clin Endocrinol Metab 2018;103:2369—75.

[213] Vila G, Luger A, van der Lely AJ, et al. Hypertension in acromegaly in relationship to biochemical control and mortality: global ACROSTUDY outcomes. Front Endocrinol (Lausanne) 2020;11:577173.

[214] Giustina A, Mancini T, Boscani PF, et al. Assessment of the awareness and management of cardiovascular complications of acromegaly in Italy. The COM.E.T.A. (COMorbidities Evaluation and Treatment in Acromegaly) Study. J Endocrinol Invest 2008;31:731—8.

[215] Garmendia Madariaga A, Santos Palacios S, Guillen-Grima F, Galofre JC. The incidence and prevalence of thyroid dysfunction in Europe: a meta-analysis. J Clin Endocrinol Metab 2014;99:923—31.

[216] Jabbar A, Pingitore A, Pearce SH, Zaman A, Iervasi G, Razvi S. Thyroid hormones and cardiovascular disease. Nat Rev Cardiol 2017;14:39—55.

[217] Mazza A, Beltramello G, Armigliato M, et al. Arterial hypertension and thyroid disorders: what is important to know in clinical practice? Ann Endocrinol (Paris) 2011;72:296—303.

[218] Garber JR, Cobin RH, Gharib H, et al. Clinical practice guidelines for hypothyroidism in adults: cosponsored by the American Association of Clinical Endocrinologists and the American Thyroid Association. Thyroid 2012;22:1200—35.

[219] Chaker L, Bianco AC, Jonklaas J, Peeters RP. Hypothyroidism. Lancet 2017;390:1550—62.

[220] Hofstetter L, Messerli FH. Hypothyroidism and hypertension: fact or myth? Lancet 2018;391:29—30.

[221] Saito I, Ito K, Saruta T. Hypothyroidism as a cause of hypertension. Hypertension 1983;5:112—5.

[222] Bergus GR, Mold JW, Barton ED, Randall CS. The lack of association between hypertension and hypothyroidism in a primary care setting. J Hum Hypertens 1999;13:231—5.

[223] Wang X, Wang H, Yan L, et al. The positive association between subclinical hypothyroidism and newly-diagnosed hypertension is more explicit in female individuals younger than 65. Endocrinol Metab (Seoul) 2021;36:778—89.

[224] Kim J, Prasitlumkum N, Randhawa S, Banerjee D. Association between subclinical hypothyroidism and incident hypertension in women: a systematic review and meta-analysis. J Clin Med 2021;10:3318.

[225] Fommei E, Iervasi G. The role of thyroid hormone in blood pressure homeostasis: evidence from short-term hypothyroidism in humans. J Clin Endocrinol Metab 2002;87:1996—2000.

[226] Ojamaa K, Klemperer JD, Klein I. Acute effects of thyroid hormone on vascular smooth muscle. Thyroid 1996;6:505—12.

[227] Gong N, Gao C, Chen X, Fang Y, Tian L. Endothelial function in patients with subclinical hypothyroidism: a meta-analysis. Horm Metab Res 2019;51:691—702.

[228] Silva JE, Bianco SD. Thyroid-adrenergic interactions: physiological and clinical implications. Thyroid 2008;18:157—65.

[229] Obuobie K, Smith J, Evans LM, John R, Davies JS, Lazarus JH. Increased central arterial stiffness in hypothyroidism. J Clin Endocrinol Metab 2002;87:4662—6.

[230] Luboshitzky R, Aviv A, Herer P, Lavie L. Risk factors for cardiovascular disease in women with subclinical hypothyroidism. Thyroid 2002;12:421—5.

[231] He W, Li S, Zhang JA, Zhang J, Mu K, Li XM. Effect of levothyroxine on blood pressure in patients with subclinical hypothyroidism: a systematic review and meta-analysis. Front Endocrinol (Lausanne) 2018;9:454.

[232] Zhao T, Chen B, Zhou Y, et al. Effect of levothyroxine on the progression of carotid intima-media thickness in subclinical hypothyroidism patients: a meta-analysis. BMJ Open 2017;7:e016053.

[233] Chaker L, Bianco AC, Jonklaas J, Peeters RP. Hypothyroidism and hypertension: fact or myth? - Authors' reply. Lancet 2018;391:30.

[234] Jonklaas J, Bianco AC, Bauer AJ, et al. Guidelines for the treatment of hypothyroidism: prepared by the American thyroid association task force on thyroid hormone replacement. Thyroid 2014;24:1670—751.

[235] Taylor PN, Albrecht D, Scholz A, et al. Global epidemiology of hyperthyroidism and hypothyroidism. Nat Rev Endocrinol 2018;14:301—16.

[236] Ross DS, Burch HB, Cooper DS, et al. 2016 American thyroid association guidelines for diagnosis and management of hyperthyroidism and other causes of thyrotoxicosis. Thyroid 2016;26:1343—421.

[237] Razvi S, Jabbar A, Pingitore A, et al. Thyroid hormones and cardiovascular function and diseases. J Am Coll Cardiol 2018;71:1781—96.

[238] Rivas AM, Pena C, Kopel J, Dennis JA, Nugent K. Hypertension and hyperthyroidism: association and pathogenesis. Am J Med Sci 2021;361:3—7.

[239] Prisant LM, Gujral JS, Mulloy AL. Hyperthyroidism: a secondary cause of isolated systolic hypertension. J Clin Hypertens (Greenwich) 2006;8:596—9.

[240] Walsh JP, Bremner AP, Bulsara MK, et al. Subclinical thyroid dysfunction and blood pressure: a community-based study. Clin Endocrinol (Oxf) 2006;65:486—91.

[241] Duan Y, Peng W, Wang X, et al. Community-based study of the association of subclinical thyroid dysfunction with blood pressure. Endocrine 2009;35:136—42.

[242] Cai Y, Ren Y, Shi J. Blood pressure levels in patients with subclinical thyroid dysfunction: a meta-analysis of cross-sectional data. Hypertens Res 2011;34:1098—105.

[243] Volzke H, Ittermann T, Schmidt CO, et al. Subclinical hyperthyroidism and blood pressure in a population-based prospective cohort study. Eur J Endocrinol 2009;161:615–21.

[244] Ozbilen S, Eren MA, Turan MN, Sabuncu T. The impact of carvedilol and metoprolol on serum lipid concentrations and symptoms in patients with hyperthyroidism. Endocr Res 2012;37:117–23.

[245] Bilezikian JP. Primary hyperparathyroidism. J Clin Endocrinol Metab 2018;103:3993–4004.

[246] Press DM, Siperstein AE, Berber E, et al. The prevalence of undiagnosed and unrecognized primary hyperparathyroidism: a population-based analysis from the electronic medical record. Surgery 2013;154:1232–7. discussion 1237-8.

[247] Kontogeorgos G, Trimpou P, Laine CM, Olerod G, Lindahl A, Landin-Wilhelmsen K. Normocalcaemic, vitamin D-sufficient hyperparathyroidism - high prevalence and low morbidity in the general population: a long-term follow-up study, the WHO MONICA project, Gothenburg, Sweden. Clin Endocrinol (Oxf) 2015;83:277–84.

[248] Medina JE, Randolph GW, Angelos P, et al. Primary hyperparathyroidism: disease of diverse genetic, symptomatic, and biochemical phenotypes. Head Neck 2021;43:3996–4009.

[249] Han D, Trooskin S, Wang X. Prevalence of cardiovascular risk factors in male and female patients with primary hyperparathyroidism. J Endocrinol Invest 2012;35:548–52.

[250] Pepe J, Cipriani C, Sonato C, Raimo O, Biamonte F, Minisola S. Cardiovascular manifestations of primary hyperparathyroidism: a narrative review. Eur J Endocrinol 2017;177:R297–308.

[251] Lind L, Ljunghall S. Pre-operative evaluation of risk factors for complications in patients with primary hyperparathyroidism. Eur J Clin Invest 1995;25:955–8.

[252] Tordjman KM, Yaron M, Izkhakov E, et al. Cardiovascular risk factors and arterial rigidity are similar in asymptomatic normocalcemic and hypercalcemic primary hyperparathyroidism. Eur J Endocrinol 2010;162:925–33.

[253] Letizia C, Ferrari P, Cotesta D, et al. Ambulatory monitoring of blood pressure (AMBP) in patients with primary hyperparathyroidism. J Hum Hypertens 2005;19:901–6.

[254] Kalla A, Krishnamoorthy P, Gopalakrishnan A, Garg J, Patel NC, Figueredo VM. Primary hyperparathyroidism predicts hypertension: results from the National Inpatient Sample. Int J Cardiol 2017;227:335–7.

[255] Fisher SB, Perrier ND. Primary hyperparathyroidism and hypertension. Gland Surg 2020;9:142–9.

[256] Zhang Y, Zhang DZ. Circulating parathyroid hormone and risk of hypertension: a meta-analysis. Clin Chim Acta 2018;482:40–5.

[257] Tomaschitz A, Ritz E, Pieske B, et al. Aldosterone and parathyroid hormone interactions as mediators of metabolic and cardiovascular disease. Metabolism 2014;63:20–31.

[258] Pilz S, Kienreich K, Drechsler C, et al. Hyperparathyroidism in patients with primary aldosteronism: cross-sectional and interventional data from the GECOH study. J Clin Endocrinol Metab 2012;97:E75–9.

[259] Kovacs L, Goth MI, Szabolcs I, Dohan O, Ferencz A, Szilagyi G. The effect of surgical treatment on secondary hyperaldosteronism and relative hyperinsulinemia in primary hyperparathyroidism. Eur J Endocrinol 1998;138:543–7.

[260] Bilezikian JP, Brandi ML, Eastell R, et al. Guidelines for the management of asymptomatic primary hyperparathyroidism: summary statement from the Fourth International Workshop. J Clin Endocrinol Metab 2014;99:3561–9.

[261] Ejlsmark-Svensson H, Rolighed L, Rejnmark L. Effect of parathyroidectomy on cardiovascular risk factors in primary hyperparathyroidism: a randomized clinical trial. J Clin Endocrinol Metab 2019;104:3223–32.

[262] Feldstein CA, Akopian M, Pietrobelli D, Olivieri A, Garrido D. Long-term effects of parathyroidectomy on hypertension prevalence and circadian blood pressure profile in primary hyperparathyroidism. Clin Exp Hypertens 2010;32:154–8.

[263] Rydberg E, Birgander M, Bondeson AG, Bondeson L, Willenheimer R. Effect of successful parathyroidectomy on 24-hour ambulatory blood pressure in patients with primary hyperparathyroidism. Int J Cardiol 2010;142:15–21.

[264] Griebeler ML, Kearns AE, Ryu E, et al. Thiazide-associated hypercalcemia: incidence and association with primary hyperparathyroidism over two decades. J Clin Endocrinol Metab 2016;101:1166–73.

[265] Vaidya A, Curhan GC, Paik JM, Kronenberg H, Taylor EN. Hypertension, antihypertensive medications, and risk of incident primary hyper-parathyroidism. J Clin Endocrinol Metab 2015;100:2396–404.

[266] Tomaschitz A, Verheyen N, Meinitzer A, et al. Effect of eplerenone on parathyroid hormone levels in patients with primary hyperparathyroidism: results from the EPATH randomized, placebo-controlled trial. J Hypertens 2016;34:1347–56.

[267] Zoccali C, Mallamaci F, Finocchiaro P. Atherosclerotic renal artery stenosis: epidemiology, cardiovascular outcomes, and clinical prediction rules. J Am Soc Nephrol 2002;13(Suppl. 3):S179–83.

[268] Olin JW, Froehlich J, Gu X, et al. The United States Registry for Fibromuscular Dysplasia: results in the first 447 patients. Circulation 2012;125:3182–90.

[269] Kim ESH, Olin JW, Froehlich JB, et al. Clinical manifestations of fibromuscular dysplasia vary by patient sex: a report of the United States registry for fibromuscular dysplasia. J Am Coll Cardiol 2013;62:2026–8.

[270] Gornik HL, Persu A, Adlam D, et al. First International Consensus on the diagnosis and management of fibromuscular dysplasia. Vasc Med 2019;24:164–89.

[271] Olin JW, Piedmonte MR, Young JR, DeAnna S, Grubb M, Childs MB. The utility of duplex ultrasound scanning of the renal arteries for diagnosing significant renal artery stenosis. Ann Intern Med 1995;122:833–8.

[272] Vasbinder GB, Nelemans PJ, Kessels AG, et al. Accuracy of computed tomographic angiography and magnetic resonance angiography for diagnosing renal artery stenosis. Ann Intern Med 2004;141:674–82. discussion 682.

[273] Cooper CJ, Murphy TP, Cutlip DE, et al. Stenting and medical therapy for atherosclerotic renal-artery stenosis. N Engl J Med 2014;370:13−22.

[274] Investigators A, Wheatley K, Ives N, et al. Revascularization versus medical therapy for renal-artery stenosis. N Engl J Med 2009;361:1953−62.

[275] Roubidoux MA, Dunnick NR, Klotman PE, et al. Renal vein renins: inability to predict response to revascularization in patients with hypertension. Radiology 1991;178:819−22.

[276] Goupil R, Cowley D, Wolley M, Ahmed AH, Gordon RD, Stowasser M. The utility of renal venous renin studies in selection of patients with renal artery stenosis for angioplasty: a retrospective study. J Hypertens 2015;33:1931−8. discussion 1938.

[277] Savard S, Steichen O, Azarine A, Azizi M, Jeunemaitre X, Plouin PF. Association between 2 angiographic subtypes of renal artery fibromuscular dysplasia and clinical characteristics. Circulation 2012;126:3062−9.

[278] Chen Y, Dong H, Jiang X, et al. Percutaneous transluminal angioplasty with selective stenting for the treatment of renal artery stenosis caused by fibromuscular dysplasia: 18 years' experience from the China Center for Cardiovascular Disease. Catheter Cardiovasc Interv 2020;95(Suppl. 1):641−7.

[279] Trinquart L, Mounier-Vehier C, Sapoval M, Gagnon N, Plouin PF. Efficacy of revascularization for renal artery stenosis caused by fibromuscular dysplasia: a systematic review and meta-analysis. Hypertension 2010;56:525−32.

[280] Ritchie J, Green D, Chrysochou C, Chalmers N, Foley RN, Kalra PA. High-risk clinical presentations in atherosclerotic renovascular disease: prognosis and response to renal artery revascularization. Am J Kidney Dis 2014;63:186−97.

[281] Nordmann AJ, Woo K, Parkes R, Logan AG. Balloon angioplasty or medical therapy for hypertensive patients with atherosclerotic renal artery stenosis? A meta-analysis of randomized controlled trials. Am J Med 2003;114:44−50.

[282] PAGE IH. The production of persistent arterial hypertension by cellophane perinephritis. J Am Med Assoc 1939;113:2046−8.

[283] Dopson SJ, Jayakumar S, Velez JC. Page kidney as a rare cause of hypertension: case report and review of the literature. Am J Kidney Dis 2009;54:334−9.

[284] Chao CT, Wu VC. Aliskiren for reninoma. Nephrology (Carlton) 2012;17:308−9.

[285] Rosei CA, Giacomelli L, Salvetti M, et al. Advantages of renin inhibition in a patient with reninoma. Int J Cardiol 2015;187:240−2.

[286] Kuroda N, Gotoda H, Ohe C, et al. Review of juxtaglomerular cell tumor with focus on pathobiological aspect. Diagn Pathol 2011;6:80.

Index

'*Note:* Page numbers followed by "f" indicate figures and "t" indicate tables.'

A

Acetominophen, 280–281
Acetylcholine (Ach), 55, 151
Acromegaly, 7, 219–223, 294, 350–352
  acromegaly related cardiomyopathy, 224
  characteristics of acromegaly related
    hypertension, 223–224
  and comorbidities, 224–226
    arrhythmias, 225
    atherosclerosis and mortality,
      225–226
    cardiomyopathy, 224
    diabetes mellitus, 225
    hyperlipidemia, 225
    valvulopathy, 225
  diagnosis, 351
  epidemiology, 219–220
    prevalence of hypertension in patients
      with acromegaly, 220t
  in hypertensive patients, screening for,
    226–227
  imaging for, 325–326
  management, 351–352
  pathophysiology of hypertension in,
    220–223
    impaired glucose metabolism, 223
    increased peripheral vascular resistance,
      222
    plasma volume expansion, 220–222
    sleep apnea syndrome, 223
  in pregnancy, 301–302
  prevalence, pathophysiology and clinical
    presentation, 350–351
  therapeutical options in, 227
ACROSTUDY, 226
Activation function-1 (AF-1), 40,
  42
Activation function-2 (AF-2), 40, 42
Activin, 55
Acute heart failure, 298
Adrenal adenomas, 310–311
Adrenal androgen synthesis, 39–40
  glucocorticoids, receptors, and effects of
    cardiovascular system, 40
Adrenal carcinomas, 141, 314
Adrenal computed tomography (Adrenal
  CT), 310–311
Adrenal cortical carcinoma/deoxycorticos-
  terone-secreting adrenal tumor, 303
Adrenal cortical hormones
  emerging research questions, 46–47

pathophysiological alterations in
  adrenocortical hormones and effects,
  45–46
physiological aspects, 36–44
  adrenal androgen synthesis and regulation
    in zona reticularis, 39–40
  androgens, receptors, and effects of
    cardiovascular system, 43–44
  glucocorticoid receptor, 40
  GR and blood pressure regulation, 41–42
  mineralocorticoid receptor, 42
  MR and blood pressure, 42–43
  MR and blood pressure regulation, 42
  regulation of steroidogenesis, 36–37
  zona glomerulosa
  aldosterone synthesis/steroid synthesis in,
    37–38
  cortisol synthesis and secretion/steroid
    hormone synthesis in, 38–39
Adrenal CS, 202–203
Adrenal CT scan, 282
Adrenal Cushing's syndrome, 7, 281
  areas of uncertainty/emerging concepts, 211
  autonomousutonomous cortisol secretion in
    adrenal incidentaloma, 210–211
  causes and epidemiology of, 202–203
  clinical features, 204–205
    clinical characteristics of Cushing's
      syndrome, 204t
  genetic syndromes associated with, 203
  genetics of ACTH-independent Cushing
    syndrome, 203–204
  investigations for, 206–207
    principles, strengths, and limitations with
      tests for screening of CS, 207t
  long-term outcome of, 208–210
  pathophysiology of hypertension in,
    205–206
  treatment of, 207–208
    postoperative treatment of, 208
    preoperative treatment of, 208
Adrenal disease, 2
Adrenal glands, 78–79
Adrenal hormones, and blood pressure, HPA
  axis, 57
Adrenal hyperplasia, 312–313
Adrenal incidentaloma, 154, 210
  autonomous cortisol secretion in, 210–211
Adrenal insufficiency (AI), 58
Adrenal lesions, 210, 310–311
Adrenal magnetic resonance imaging
  (Adrenal MRI), 311–312

Adrenal medulla, 21
  chromaffin cells of, 22
Adrenal medulla, 316
Adrenal metabolites, 187–188
Adrenal steroid
  hormones, 39
  synthesis pathways, 36
Adrenal steroidogenesis, 36
  inhibitors, 195
Adrenal venous sampling (AVS), 5, 95,
  312–315, 333, 337–338
  imaging for glucocorticoid excess states,
    313–315
  imaging for mineralocorticoid excess states,
    312–313
Adrenalectomy, 207
  laparoscopic, 96
  unilateral, 96
β-adrenergic blockers, 280–281
α-adrenergic blockers, 280–281
β2-adrenergic receptors, 151–152
Adrenoceptors
  modulate cell, 25
  subtypes, and associated second messenger
    systems, 23–24
β1-adrenoceptors, 24, 151–152
α1-adrenoceptors, 23, 25, 151–152
α2-adrenoceptor, 25, 151–152
  present on vascular smooth muscle and
    heart, 25
  stimulation of, 25
β2-adrenoceptor, 24–25
β3-adrenoceptor, 24, 26
Adrenocortical adenoma (ACA), 312
Adrenocortical hormones, 3
  and effects on cardiovascular homeostasis,
    45–46
Adrenocorticotrophic hormone (ACTH), 6,
  36, 91, 115, 135, 202, 269, 281, 313,
  334, 348–349
  ACTH-dependent Cushing syndrome, 6
  and ACTH-independent Cushing's
    syndrome, 185
  adrenal steroidogenesis inhibitors, 195
  antihypertensive therapy in, 190–194
  clinical presentation, screening, and
    diagnosis of, 184–185
  complications of, 189–190
  epidemiology of hypertension in,
    187
  follow up of Cushing syndrome and
    hypertension, 196

Adrenocorticotrophic hormone (ACTH)
(*Continued*)
glucocorticoid receptor blockers, 196
localization testing, 185
mechanisms of hypertension in, 187t
pathophysiology of hypertension in, 187
pituitary targeted agents, 195–196
role of medical therapy for CS in
treatment of hypertension, 195–196
treatment of Cushing's syndrome and
associated hypertension, 190
ACTH-independent Cushing's syndrome,
185, 202–203
ACTH-producing pituitary adenomas, 203
ACTH-secreting pituitary adenoma, 184
genetics of ACTH-independent Cushing
syndrome, 203–204
PET/CT to localize ectopic source of ACTH
secretion, 315–318
suppression, 285
β-adrenoreceptors, 3, 20
blockers, 155
α-adrenoreceptors, 3, 20
blockers, 155
Adult growth hormone deficiency (AGHD),
7, 229, 310, 326
impact of AGHD management on blood
pressure, 237–239
AGHD-related comorbidities, 236
atherosclerosis and mortality, 236
and comorbidities, 234–236
cardiac structure and performance, 234
impaired glucose metabolism, 236
lipids, 234–236
metabolic syndrome, 234
obesity, 234
diagnosis, 237
imaging for, 325–326
pathophysiology of hypertension in,
231–232
phenotype of AGHD and characteristics of
blood pressure profile, 232–236
screening for, 236–237
AGHD diagnosis, 237
suspect AGHD in hypertension, 236
Aging process, 265
Aldosterone, 3, 41–42, 64–66, 91–93, 116,
312, 339
aldosterone-secreting adenoma cells,
256
monogenic hypertension with aldosterone
levels, 84–85
synthase inhibitors, 341
synthesis in zona glomerulosa, 37–38
Aldosterone renin ratio (ARR), 9, 92–93,
106, 129, 284, 294, 332
confirmatory test after positive ARR, 93–95
as screening test, 92–93
patients with primary aldosteronism, 94t
Aldosterone-producing adenoma (APA), 5,
45, 79, 106, 333
Aldosterone-producing cell clusters
(APCCs), 96
Aliskiren, 69, 357

Aliskiren Trial in Type 2 Diabetes Using
Cardiorenal Endpoints (ALTITUDE),
69
Alkaline phosphatase (ALP), 258
Alpha-adrenoceptor blockers, 157
Ambulatory blood pressure monitoring
(ABPM), 220, 288–289, 352
American Academy of Pediatrics (AAP), 278,
288
Amiloride, 304, 340
amiloride-sensitive ENaC, 221
Γ-amino butyric acid, 55
Aminoglutethimide, 195
Amlodipine, 67, 297
Anatomical imaging
of PCC, 154
studies of PGL, 172–173
Androgen excess polycystic ovary syndrome
(AE-PCOS), 46
Androgen receptor-knockout (ARKO), 44
Androgen receptors (ARs), 40
Androgenic hormones, 142
Androgens
deficiency/excess states, 46
androgen excess and blood pressure, 46
and blood pressure, 46
receptors, and effects of cardiovascular
system, 43–44
Androstenedione, 115–116, 135
Ang II type 1 receptors (AT1 receptors), 256
Angiography, 141, 356
Angiotensin converting enzyme (ACE), 65,
92, 188, 256, 268, 334
ACEI, 67
ARBs *vs.*, 69
inhibitors, 67, 119
Angiotensin I (Ang I), 65, 256
Angiotensin II (Ang II), 55–56, 64–65, 91,
348
Angiotensin II type 1 receptors (AT1Rs), 37,
41
Angiotensin receptor blockers (ARBs),
68–69, 193, 334
ACEI *vs.*, 69
Angiotensinogen, 188, 256
Animal models, 54
Anion exchanger (AE1), 81
Antiangiogenic therapy, 176–177
Antidiuretic hormone (ADH), 252
Antihypertensive and Lipid-Lowering
treatment to Prevent Heart Attack
Trial (ALLHAT), 67
Antihypertensive therapy in Cushing's
syndrome, 190–194
Antithyroid drugs (ATDs), 300, 354
Aortic valve regurgitation, 225
Aplasia cutis, 300
Apnea Hypopnea Index (AHI), 265
Apnea-induced sympathetic overdrive, 268
Apparent mineralocorticoid excess (AME),
46, 78, 81, 128, 135–137, 285
clinical features, 136
epidemiology, 135
genetics, 136

investigation, 136–137
management, 137
pathophysiology, 135–136
Arginine vasopressin (AVP), 55, 142
Armadillo repeat-containing protein 5
(ARMC5), 204
Arrhythmias, 225, 298
Arterial blood pressure regulation, 54
Arterial hypertension, 64–65
Arterial stiffness, 231
Aspamandine, 66
Asymmetric dimethylarginine (ADMA), 222
Asymptomatic *RET*-mutation carriers, 159
Atelectasis, 270
Atenolol, 193
Atherosclerosis and mortality, 225–226, 236
Atherosclerotic cardiovascular disease
(ASCVD), 190–193
ATP1A1 gene, 79
ATP2B3 gene, 79
Atrial natriuretic peptide (ANP), 3, 188, 348
Atrioventricular node (AV Node), 25–26
ATRX chromatin remodeler gene (*ATRX*), 159
Attention deficit hyperactivity disorder
(ADHD), 178
Autoimmune disease, 253
Autonomic failure, catecholamines and,
31–32
Autonomic nervous system, HPA axis and,
56
Autonomous cortisol secretion (ACS),
57–58
Autonomous cortisol secretion in adrenal
incidentaloma, 210–211
Autosomal dominant HTNB, 84
Autosomal recessive disorders, 114
Averbuch scheme, 176–177

B

B-cell leukemia, 141
Baroreflex, 31
Beckwith-Wiedemann syndrome (BWS), 314
Berlin Questionnaire, 266
Beta adrenergic blockers, 298
Beta-adrenergic receptor blockers, 347
11-beta-hydroxysteroid dehydrogenase (11-β-
HSD), 348
Bilateral adrenal hyperplasia (BAH), 312
Bilateral adrenalectomy, 109, 196, 207
Bilateral macronodular adrenal hyperplasia
(BMAH), 190, 203
Biochemical manifestations of PA, 333
Biochemical testing of PCC, 153–154
Biological clock system, 56
Birth defects, 300
"Block and replace" therapy, 300
Blood pressure (BP), 3, 55, 78, 90, 96,
119–121, 170, 218, 251, 278, 339,
345
impact of AGHD management on, 237–239
androgen deficiency and, 46
androgen excess and, 46
catecholamines on, 25–26
effect of disease activity on, 227

impact of acromegaly therapies treatment on BP, 228t
emerging research questions, 46–47
HPA axis, adrenal hormones, and, 57
pathophysiological alterations in adreno cortical hormones and effects, 45–46
phenotype of AGHD and characteristics of, 232–236
physiological aspects, 36–44
  adrenal androgen synthesis and regulation in zona reticularis, 39–40
  androgens, receptors, and effects of cardiovascular system, 43–44
  glucocorticoid receptor, 40
  GR and, 41–42
  mineralocorticoid receptor, 42
  MR and, 42
  MR and, 42–43
  regulation of steroidogenesis, 36–37
physiology of, 54–55
  CRH and AVP and POMC, 55
  POMC, 54–55
regulation, 3–9, 54
zona glomerulosa
  aldosterone synthesis/steroid synthesis in, 37–38
  cortisol synthesis and secretion/steroid hormone synthesis in, 38–39
Blood vessels, 24–25
  GH and IGF-1 in, 218
Body mass index (BMI), 223, 265, 278, 345
Bromocriptine, 195–196, 287

C

CACNA1D gene, 79, 110
CACNA1H gene, 79, 99, 109, 140
Calcium, 25
  channel blockers, 155, 157, 295, 297
Calcium channel blockers (CCBs), 334
Calcium-sensing receptors (CaSRs), 255
Calmodulin kinases (CAMKs), 37–38
cAMPresponsive element binding protein (CREB), 37
Cancer Genome Atlas, 168
Captopril, 93–95
  test, 295
Captopril challenge testing, 336
Captopril Prevention Project trial (CAPPP trial), 67
Cardiac fibrosis, 70
Cardiac MRI, 229
Cardiac surgeons, 175–176
Cardiac ultrasound, 227
Cardiogenic shock, 298
Cardiology/European Society of Hypertension (ESC/ESH), 67
Cardiomyocytes, 24
Cardiomyopathy, 224
Cardiovascular comorbidities, 223–226
Cardiovascular complications, 226
Cardiovascular disease (CVD), 2, 40, 204–205, 223
  impact of parathyroidectomy in hypertension and, 258

impact of treatment of hypothyroidism on hypertension and, 253
Cardiovascular events, 45, 225, 345
Cardiovascular homeostasis
  pathophysiological alterations in adreno cortical hormones and effects on, 45–46
    AME, 46
    androgen deficiency/excess states, 46
    glucocorticoid excess states, 45
    mineralocorticoid excess states, 45–46
Cardiovascular protection in hypertension, 67
Cardiovascular system, 24
  androgens, receptors, and effects of, 43–44
  glucocorticoids, receptors, and effects of adrenal androgen synthesis, 40
    GR and blood pressure regulation, 41–42
  physiology of, 250
Carney complex, 142–143, 203, 314
  clinical features, 143
  epidemiology, 142
  genetics, 143
  investigations, 143
  management, 143
  pathophysiology, 143
Carotid body tumors (CBTs), 166
Carotid Doppler examination, 237
Carpal tunnel syndrome, 287
Catechol-O-methyl transferase (COMT), 22–23, 28
Catecholamine-induced cardiomyopathies (CICMPs), 24
Catecholamines, 3–9, 20, 151, 310, 347
  and autonomic physiology, 20–26
    adrenoceptors, subtypes, and associated second messenger systems, 23–24
    on blood pressure, neuroendocrine effects of, 25–26
    on metabolic regulation, 26
    metabolism of, 22–23
    synthesis, storage, and regulation of, 20–22
  biologic effects, 26–32
    and alterations in renal physiology, 31
    and autonomic failure, 31–32
    cardiotoxic effects of, 29–31
    catecholamines effecton vascular hemodynamics, 26–28
    deleterious cardiac effects of excess catecholamines, 28
    deleterious vascular effects of, 31
    dilated cardiomyopathy, 29–31
    hypertrophic cardiomyopathy, 29
    and organs, 31
    PPGLs and excess catecholamine states, 28
  epinephrine, 151
  excess states, 28
    deleterious cardiac effects of, 28
    imaging for, 316–317
  norepinephrine, 151
  producing tumors, 280–281
    diagnosis, 280–281

pheochromocytomas and paragangliomas in children, 280
Cementoplasty techniques, 177
Central hypothyroidism, 352
Central nervous system (CNS), 31, 281
Cerebrovascular accidents (CVAs), 107
Cerebrovascular complications, 226
Chemical shift imaging (CSI), 311–312
Chemotherapy, 158
  PGL, 176–177
Childhood hypertension, 278
Childhood-onset of GHD (CO-GHD), 229
Children
  biochemical phenotype of mineralocorticoid excess in, 283–286
  Cushing's syndrome in, 280
  endocrine hypertension in, 8, 279
    biochemical phenotype of mineralocorticoid excess in children, 283–286
    catecholamine producing tumors, 280–281
    clinical presentation of, 280–288
    congenital adrenal hyperplasia and hypertension in children, 286
    Cushing's syndrome in children, 280
    diagnostic approach to endocrine hypertension in children, 288–289
    endocrine hypertension in children, 279
    etiology of secondary hypertension in children and adolescents, 279t
    excessive growth hormone production, 286–287
    management of, 290
    primary *vs.* secondary hypertension in children, 278–279
    thyroid and parathyroid disorders and hypertension in children, 287–288
  primary *vs.* secondary hypertension in, 278–279
Chloride voltage-gated channel 2 (ClC-2), 79, 108, 139
Chlortalidone, 67
Choanal atresia, 300
Cholecystokinin, 55
Cholesterol esters, 36
Choline, 320–321
Chromaffin cells, 167
Chromogranin A (CgA), 154
Chromogranin-A, 347
Chromosome 12 (12q24), 140
Chromosome 16 (16q22), 136
Chromosome 3 (3q27), 139
Chromosome 7 (7p22), 140
Chronic catecholamine, 152
Chronic inflammation driven by hypoxia, 267
Chronic kidney disease, 2
Chrousos syndrome, 78, 128–129, 142, 144, 342
  clinical diagnosis, 342
  clinical features, 142
  epidemiology, 142
  genetics, 142

Chrousos syndrome (*Continued*)
  investigations, 142
  management, 142
  management, 342
  pathophysiology, 142
*CLCN*2 gene, 79
Clinical prediction score (CPS), 312–313
Clonidine suppression test (CST), 346
Cluster of differentiation 282 (CD282), 68
Cold shock domain-containing E1 (*CSDE*1),
    151
Composite Pheochromocytoma/
    paraganglioma Prognostic Score
    (COPPS), 153
Computed tomography (CT), 95, 172,
    206–207, 281, 295, 310
Congenital adrenal hyperplasia (CAH), 5, 78,
    114, 128, 134–135, 283–284, 286
  17α-hydroxylase deficiency, 119–120
  11β-hydroxylase deficiency, 118–119
  in children, 286
  clinical features, 135
  epidemiology, 134
  genetics, 114–116, 134
    congenital adrenal hyperplasia and
      relation to hypertension, 115t
  investigation, 135
  management, 135
  overtreatment of, 120–121
  pathophysiology, 134
  of hypertension in, 116–118
  suspect of, 121
Congenital disorders, 46
Conn's disease/syndrome, 90–91
Conn's syndrome. *See* Primary aldosteronism
    (PA)
Conservative surgery, 141
Continuous positive airway pressure (CPAP),
    189, 269–270
Contrast-enhanced computed tomography
    (Contrast-enhanced CT), 154,
    316–317
Coronary artery disease, 225
Cortical-sparing adrenal surgery, 157
Corticosterone, 142, 187–188, 341
Corticotrophin-releasing hormone (CRH), 39,
    55, 142, 184, 348–349
Cortisol, 57, 142, 188, 339, 342–343, 350
  biosynthesis, 342
  cortisol-induced hypertension, 348
  cortisol-lowering medical therapy, 208
  cortisol-lowering medical treatment,
    207
  cortisol-producing adrenal adenoma,
    202–203
  synthesis in zona fasciculata, 38–39
Cortisol binding globulin (CBG),
    184
Cosyntropin test, 58–60
Craniopharyngioma, 326
*CTNNB*1 gene, 79–80
Cullin-RING ligase (CRL), 83
Culprit gene, 109
Curative surgery, PGL, 175–176

Cushing syndrome (CS), 2, 45, 55–56, 99,
    108, 119, 139, 143, 184, 294, 310,
    332, 347–350
  ACTH-dependent Cushing syndrome, 6
  Adrenal Cushing's syndrome, 7
  in children, 280
    diagnostic evaluations, 280–281
  diagnosis, 348–349
  management, 349–350
    multimodal treatment, 350
    pharmacological management, 349–350
    surgical management, 349
  in pregnancy, 295–297
  prevalence, pathophysiology and clinical
    presentation, 347–348
Cushing's disease (CD), 6, 57, 187, 202,
    281
Cyclic adenosine monophosphate (cAMP),
    24, 36, 84, 91, 255–256
Cyclic adenosine monophosphate/protein
    kinase A pathway (cAMP/PKA
    pathway), 36
Cyclic guanosine monophosphate (cGMP),
    26
Cyclophosphamide, vincristine, and
    dacarbazine (CVD), 158
*CYP*11*B*1 gene, 80, 106–107, 115,
    118–119, 138
*CYP*11*B*2 gene, 80, 106–107, 115, 138
*CYP*21*A*2 gene, 91, 115
Cytochrome *b*5, 38
  and POR, 40
Cytochrome P450 oxidoreductase deficiency
    (POR deficiency), 114

D

Decarboxylase, 28
Defective cortisol, 285
Definitive diagnostic tests, 295
Dehydroepiandrosterone (DHEA), 38,
    115–116, 135, 285, 303, 342
Dehydroepiandrosterone sulfate (DHEAS),
    185, 285
Deoxycorticosterone (DOC), 114, 142,
    187–188, 195, 286, 303
  deoxycorticosterone-secreting adrenal
    tumour, 303
11-deoxycortisol (DOC), 135, 342
  DOC-secreting tumors, 343
    clinical diagnosis, 343
    management, 343
11-deoxycortisone, 135
Desensitization of adrenergic receptors, 168
Dexamethasone, 99, 139, 185, 285, 343
Dexamethasone suppression test (DST), 184,
    206, 282, 337–338
Diabetes, 297
Diabetes mellitus, 208, 225
Diabetics Exposed to Telmisartan and
    Enalapril (DETAIL), 69
Diacylglycerol, 25
Diagnosis
  clinical diagnosis
    11β-hydroxylase deficiency, 341

17α-hydroxylase deficiency, 342
  DOC-secreting tumors, 343
  ectopic ACTH syndrome, 343
  familial hyperkalemic hypertension, 344
  liddle syndrome, 344
  PA, 332–338
  PGR or chrousos syndrome, 342
  SAME, 343
Diagnostic imaging of PCC, 154–155
  anatomical imaging, 154
  functional imaging, 155
Diastolic BP (DBP), 223–224, 350
Dihydrolipoamide S-succinyl transferase
    (*DLST*), 150–151, 168
Dihydrolipoamide S-succinyltransferase
    (*DLST*)
3,4 dihydroxyphenylacetic acid (DOPAC), 22
3,4 dihydroxyphenylglycol (DHPG), 22
Dilated cardiomyopathy, 29–31
Direct renin concentration (DRC), 9, 333
Direct renin inhibitors, 69
Disease process, 187
DNA hypermethylation, 168
DNA methyltransferase (*DNMT3A*), 168
DNA-binding domain (DBD), 40
Dopamine, 3, 28, 280
  dopamine-dominant tumors, 345
  receptors, 3, 20, 24
Dopamine β-hydroxylase (DBH), 21, 28
Dopaminergic phenotype, 151
Doxazocin, 298
Doxazosin, 193
Drugs, 155, 297
Dual RAAS inhibition, 69
Dual tracer SPECT/CT imaging, 320
Dual-energy X-ray absorptiometry (DEXA),
    258
Dynorphin, 55
Dyslipidaemia, 225

E

Echocardiography, 237
Ectopic ACTH secretion (EAS), 281
Ectopic ACTH syndrome, 343–344
  clinical diagnosis, 343
  management, 343–344
Ectopic ACTH-producing tumors, 202
Ectopic CS, 202
Egl-9 prolyl hydroxylase one and 2
    (*EGLN*1/2), 150–151, 168, 280
Electrocardiography, 237
Electroencephalogram (EEG), 266
Encephalin, 55
Endocrine, 90
Endocrine disorders in pregnancy, 294
Endocrine homeostasis, 3–4
Endocrine hypertension, 2–9, 90, 106, 128
  ACTH-dependent Cushing syndrome, 6
  Adrenal Cushing's syndrome, 7
  adrenocortical hormones and BP regulation,
    3
  CAH and hypertension, 5
  catecholamines and blood pressure
    regulation, 3–9

in children, 8
in children, 279
diagnosis and management of
   acromegaly, 350–352
clinical presentation, 356
Cushing's syndrome, 347–350
diagnostic approach, 356–357
familial hyperkalemic hypertension,
   344–345
management, 357
mineralocorticoid forms of, 341–347
PA, 332–341
page kidney, 357
PHPT, 354–355
PPGL, 345–346
renal artery stenosis and rare forms of
   renin driven hypertension, 355–357
reninoma, 357
thyroid disorders, 352–354
FH, 5
genetic testing
   for familial hyperaldosteronism, 11–13
   for familial PPGL, 10–11
in growth hormone excess and deficiency, 7
HPA axis and blood pressure regulation,
   3–4
imaging for patients with, 8–9
inherited disorders of, 129–131, 130t, 132t
monogenic hypertension, 4
obesity, insulin resistance, and obstructive
   sleep apnea, 7–8
PA, 4–5
paragangliomas and hypertension, 6
pheochromocytomas and hypertension, 6
in pregnant woman, 8
primary hypertension *vs.* secondary
   hypertension, 2–3
RAAS and blood pressure regulation, 4
recent trends/emerging concepts, 9
systematic approach for diagnosis and
   management of, 9
in thyroid disease and hyperparathyroidism,
   7
Endocrine Society (ES), 92
Endocrinopathies, 8
Endogenous CS, 184, 202
etiologies of, 203
Endoplasmic reticulum-associated
   degradation (ERAD), 39
Endothelial dysfunction, 222, 231
Endothelial nitric oxide synthase (eNOS), 26,
   218
Endothelial sodium channels (EnNaCs),
   66–67
Endothelin-1 (ET-1), 46, 188
Epidemiology of hypertension in Cushing's
   syndrome, 185
Epinephrine, 3, 22, 24, 55
Episodic hypertension, 298
Epithelial sodium channel (ENaC), 66,
   80–81, 131, 187–188, 219, 283,
   285, 303, 341
Eplerenone, 97, 108, 193, 295, 340
Epworth Sleepiness Scale, 266

Erythropoietin (EPO), 188
Esmolol, 298
Essential hypertension, 4
Estrogen receptors (E2), 40
Estrogens, 55
Ethacrynic acid, 193
Etomidate, 195, 297
European Registry on CS (ERCUSYN), 208
European Society of Endocrinology clinical
   practice guideline, 154
Eutrophic remodeling, 222
Event-free survival (EFS), 158
External beam radiation therapy (EBRT),
   158
Extracellular signal-regulated kinase 1/2
   (ERK 1/2), 42
Extracellular-signal-regulated (ERK), 151

F

^{18}F-labeled fluorodihydroxyphenylalanine
   (18F-FDOPA)-PET/CT, 155
False-negative ARRs, 334
False-positive ARRs, 334
Familial Adenomatous Polyposis (FAP), 314
Familial hyperaldosteronism (FH), 5, 45–46,
   78–79, 98, 106, 128, 304
   FH-2, 108, 139
      clinical features and investigations, 108,
       139
      diagnostic evaluation, 108
      epidemiology, 139
      genetics, 139
      management, 108, 139
      pathophysiology, 108, 139
   FH-3, 109, 139–140
      clinical features, 109, 140
      diagnostic evaluation, 109
      epidemiology, 139
      genetics, 140
      investigations, 140
      management, 109, 140
      pathophysiology, 109, 140
   FH-4, 109–110, 140
      clinical features, 110
      diagnostic evaluation, 110
      management, 110
      pathophysiology, 109
   FH1, 45, 106–108, 138–139
      clinical features, 107, 138
      diagnostic evaluation, 107–108
      epidemiology, 138
      genetics, 138
      investigations, 139
      management, 108, 139
      pathophysiology, 106–107, 138
   genetic testing for, 11–13
   pathophysiology of, 106
   subtypes of, 106–110
      emerging research questions/future
       research, 110
      FH type 1, 106–108
      FH type 2, 108
      FH type 3, 109
      FH type 4, 109–110

PASNA syndrome, 110
Familial hyperkalemic hypertension (FHHt),
   78, 83, 344–345
   clinical diagnosis, 344
   management, 344–345
Familial hyperparathyroidism
   genetic testing for, 10–11
   syndrome, 258
Familial hypocalciuric hypercalcemia (FHH),
   10–11
Familial isolated pituitary adenoma (FIPA),
   12–13, 286–287
Familial isolated primary hyperparathyr-
   oidism (FIPH), 300
Familial PGL syndromes, 280
Familial pheochromocytoma, 141–142
Familial PPGL, genetic testing for, 10–11
Familial primary generalized glucocorticoid
   resistance, 128
^{18}F-FDOPA PET/CT, 155
Felodipine, 193
Fetal loss risk, 297
^{18}FFluorodopamine (18F-FDA), 155
Fibroblast Growth Factor Receptor 1
   (*FGFR*1), 151
Fibromuscular dysplasia, 356
Finerenone, 97–98
Flash pulmonary edema, 356
Flow mediated dilatation (FMD), 225
Fludrocortisone suppression testing (FST),
   335
Fludrocortisone test, 295
^{18}Fluorine-Fluorodeoxyglucose positron
   emission tomography/CT (18F-FDG
   PET/CT), 155
^{18}F-fluorodihydroxy-phenylalanine (^{18}F-
   FDOPA), 346
4D computed tomography (4D CT), 319
Fractures, 204–205
Framingham Heart Study, 264
Fumarate hydratase (*FH*), 150–151, 280
Fumarate hydrogenase (*FH*), 168
Functional imaging
   modalities, 155
   of PCC, 155
   using radioisotopes, 322–323
   studies of PGL, 172–173
Functional PGLs, 166–167
Furosemide, 193

G

G-protein-coupled potassium channel 4, 109
G-protein-coupled receptor kinases (GRKs),
   24
G-protein-coupled receptors (GPCRs), 20, 23
^{68}Ga-DOTA-SSA PET/CT, 155
^{68}Ga-DOTA-SSA, 155, 173
^{68}Ga-DOTATATE PET/CT, 155
^{68}Ga/^{90}Y/^{177}Lu-DOTA-SSA analogs, 158
Galanin, 55
^{68}Gallium DOTATATE, 315
Gastrointestinal stromal tumor (GIST), 10
Geller syndrome, 78, 81–83, 137, 144, 286,
   304

Geller syndrome (*Continued*)
activating mutations of, 344
clinical diagnosis and management, 344
clinical features, 137
epidemiology, 137
genetics, 137
investigation, 137
management, 137
pathophysiology, 137
Genetic syndromes associated with adrenal
Cushing syndrome, 203
Genetics
of ACTH-independent Cushing syndrome,
203—204
of paragangliomas, 168
paraganglioma-associated clusters, genes,
and syndromes and clinical
characteristics, 169t
testing, 106, 134, 281
for familial hyperparathyroidism, 10—11
for familial PPGL, 10—11
for FH, 106
genetic testing for familial
hyperaldosteronism especially GRA,
11—13
"Genomic" process, 36
Genotype-phenotype correlations, 151
German Pegvisomant Observational Study,
223—224
Germline mutations, 106, 168, 280
Gestational hypertension, 298, 300
Glomerular filtration rate (GFR), 219, 343
Glucocorticoid receptor (GR), 40—42,
187—188
blockers, 196
and effects on cardiovascular system, 41—42
Glucocorticoid response elements (GREs),
40
Glucocorticoid-Remediable Aldosteronism
(GRA), 45, 80, 98, 106—107, 128,
138, 283—284
Glucocorticoids, 42, 45, 47, 91—92, 98, 119,
139, 188—190, 281, 310, 340, 348
deficiency, 119—120
excess states, 45
imaging for, 313—315
glucocorticoid resistance syndrome, 78
glucocorticoid-mediated hypertension, 193
receptors, and effects of cardiovascular
system
adrenal androgen synthesis, 40
GR and blood pressure regulation, 41—42
suppressible aldosteronism, 138—139
clinical features, 138
epidemiology, 138
genetics, 138
investigations, 139
management, 139
pathophysiology, 138
therapy, 139
treatment, 117
Glucose metabolism, 223, 236
Glutamic-oxaloacetic transaminase (*GOT2*),
150—151

*GNA*11 gene, 79
GNAQ gene, 79
Gordon syndrome, 78, 83, 129, 137—138,
344—345
clinical features, 138
epidemiology, 137
genetics, 138
investigation, 138
management, 138
pathophysiology, 137
GR knock out (GRKO), 41
Grading of Adrenal Pheochromocytoma and
Paraganglioma (GAPP), 153
Graves' disease, 254, 287
Growth hormone (GH), 218, 325, 350—351
disorders, 279
hypertension in growth hormone excess and
deficiency, 7
physiological effects, 218—219
therapy, 237—239
Growth hormone deficiency (GHD), 7,
189—190, 218
hypertension and, 229—232
Growth hormone-releasing hormone
(GHRH), 231, 325, 350—351

H
24-h urine tetrahydrocortisol (THF), 285
1H-nuclear magnetic resonance (1H-NMR
spectrometry), 172
Harvey rat sarcoma viral oncogene homolog
(*HRAS*), 151, 280
Hashimoto's thyroiditis, 287, 352
Heart, 25
Hepatoblastoma, 141
High resolution flourodeoxy glucose positron
emission tomography (FDG PET),
282, 312
High-dose dexamethasone suppression test,
282
Highly sensitive C-reactive protein (hs-CRP),
267
Histamine, 55
Histone subunit gene (*H3F3A*), 168
Homeostasis model of insulin resistance
(HOMA-IR), 268
Homeostatic Model Assessment for Insulin
Resistance (HOMA), 232
Hormonal disorders, and hypertension, HPA
axis, 57—60
Hormone replacement therapy (HRT), 265
Hormone-sensitive lipase (HSL), 36
Hounsfield Units (HU), 154, 206—207
*HSD*11*B*2 gene, 285
Human adrenal cortex, 36
Human arterial endothelial cells, 195
Human chorionic gonadotropin (hCG), 300
Human Chorionic Somatomammotropin. *See*
Human Placental Lactogen (hPL)
Human glucocorticoid receptor (hGR), 342
Human Placental Growth Hormone Variant
(HGH-V), 301
Human Placental Lactogen (hPL), 301
Human vascular smooth muscle cells, 66

Hybrid gene expression, 340
Hybrid steroids, 106—108, 139, 337
Hydrocortisone, 99, 118, 120, 135, 284
Hydronephrosis, 300
18-hydroxycortisol, 98, 106—107, 139
20-hydroxyeicosatetraenoic acid, 47
11β-hydroxylase deficiency (11β-OHD), 78,
115, 118—119, 135, 286, 341
clinical diagnosis, 341
clinical presentations, 118
diagnostic approach for, 118—119
management, 341
management algorithm, 119
therapeutic targets, 119
17α-hydroxylase deficiency (17α-OHD), 78,
81, 114, 117, 119—121, 134—135,
342
clinical diagnosis, 342
clinical presentations, 119—120
diagnostic approach, 120
management, 342
management algorithm, 120
therapeutic targets, 120
21-α-hydroxylase deficiency, 135
17α-hydroxylase/17,20-lyase (17OH), 5
deficiency, 286
11β-hydroxylase (11βOH), 5, 117, 135
deficiencies, 134
enzyme, 115
17α-hydroxylase, 5, 38, 117
21-hydroxylase (21OH), 5
deficiency, 114—115, 341
17-hydroxypregnenolone, 117
17-hydroxyprogesterone, 342
11β-hydroxysteroid dehydrogenase type 2
(11βHSD2), 57, 129, 135—136,
187—188, 205, 285, 342
3β-hydroxysteroid dehydrogenase type 2
(3βHSD2), 5, 39—40
deficiency, 114
17β-hydroxysteroid dehydrogenase-5
(HSD5), 40
3β-hydroxysteroid dehydrogenase (3β-HSD),
37
Hypercalcemia, 257, 287
Hypercortisolism, 349
Hyperkalemia, 70—71, 96, 116
Hyperkalemic metabolic acidosis, 78
Hyperlipidemia, 225
Hyperparathyroidism
hypertension in, 7
parathyroid disease, 255—258
thyroid disease, 250—255
Hyperparathyroidism jaw tumour syndrome
(HPT-JT syndrome), 300
Hyperparathyroidism-jaw tumor syndrome
(HPTJTS), 10—11, 258
Hyperpolarization-activated cyclic
nucleotide-gated (HCN), 25—26
Hypertension (HTN), 2, 6, 28, 31, 41, 45,
78, 81—83, 90, 108, 115—116, 120,
128, 142, 184, 208, 225, 229—232,
278, 332, 341, 348, 356
acromegaly and, 219—223

acromegaly and hypertension, 219–223
CAH and, 5
in children, 286
  obesity, insulin resistance, and OSA
    associated with hypertension in
    children, 287–288
  thyroid and parathyroid disorders and,
    287–288
in Cushing's syndrome, 350
  epidemiology of, 185
  pathophysiology of, 187
epidemiology, 219–220
  prevalence of hypertension in patients
    with acromegaly, 220t
epidemiology of paragangliomas and,
  166–167
  clinical and pathologic features of head
    and neck HNPGLs, 167t
GH and IGF-1 physiological effects,
  218–219
  GH and IGF-1 in blood vessels, 218
  role of GH and IGF-1 in kidney, 219
  role of GH and IGF-1 in myocardium,
    218
growth hormone deficiency and, 229–232
growth hormone deficiency and
  hypertension, 229–232
  epidemiology, 229, 230t
  pathophysiology of hypertension in
    AGHD, 231–232
in growth hormone excess and deficiency, 7
HPA axis, various hormonal disorders, and,
  57–60
management, 229
of PA, 333
paragangliomas and, 6
parathyroid disease, 255–258
impact of parathyroidectomy in hypertension
  and cardiovascular disease, 258
pathophysiology in acromegaly, 220–223
  impaired glucose metabolism, 223
  increased peripheral vascular resistance,
    222
  plasma volume expansion, 220–222
  sleep apnea syndrome, 223
pathophysiology of hypertension and HPA
  axis, 55–60
pathophysiology of hypertension in adrenal
  Cushing syndrome, 205–206
pathophysiology of hypertension in AGHD,
  231–232
  endothelial dysfunction, 231
  increased sympathetic activity, 231–232
  insulin resistance, 232
  vitamin D deficiency, 232
pathophysiology of hypertension in primary
  hyperparathyroidism, 255–256
pathophysiology of hypertension in thyroid
  dysfunction, 251–252
pathophysiology of paraganglioma and,
  167–168
phenotype, 223–226
phenotype and cardiovascular comorbidities,
  223–226

acromegaly and comorbidities, 224–226
characteristics of acromegaly related
  hypertension, 223–224
phenotype of AGHD and characteristics of
  blood pressure profile, 232–236
  AGHD and comorbidities, 234–236
  main AGHD-related comorbidities,
    236
pheochromocytomas and, 6
RAAS blocking agents and cardiovascular
  protection in, 67
role of medical therapy for CS in treatment
  of, 195–196
screening for acromegaly in hypertensive
  patients, 226–227
  suspect acromegaly in hypertensive
    patients, 226–227
screening for AGHD, 236–237
  subclinical or overt hypothyroidism and
    associated, 253
  suspect AGHD in, 236
suspect of CAH in patients with, 121
thyroid disease, 250–255
in thyroid disease and hyperparathyroidism,
  7
treatment, 227–229, 237–239
  effect of disease activity on blood
    pressure, 227
  hypertension management, 229
  impact of AGHD management on blood
    pressure, 237–239, 238t
  therapeutical options in acromegaly, 227
treatment of Cushing's syndrome and
  associated, 190
  medications for treatment of HTN or CS,
    191t–193t
impact of treatment of hypothyroidism on
  hypertension and cardiovascular
  disease, 253
  clinical features, 253–254
  epidemiology, 253–255
  investigation and management, 254–255
  treatment of hyperthyroidism on
    hypertension and cardiovascular
    disease, 1 impact of, 255
Hypertension with brachydactyly (HTNB),
  84
Hyperthyroidism, 251, 353–354
  diagnosis, 355
  imaging for, 322
  management, 355
  in pregnancy, 300–301
  prevalence, pathophysiology and clinical
    presentation, 353
  diagnosis, 354
  management, 354
Hypertriglyceridemia, 234–236
Hypertrophic cardiomyopathy, 29
Hypertrophic remodeling, 222
Hypokalemia, 93, 96, 117–120, 297, 332
Hypokalemic alkalosis, 136
  monogenic hypertension with, 79–83
Hypokalemic metabolic alkalosis, 78, 108
Hypopituitarism, 303

Hypopituitary Control and Complications
  Study (HypoCCS), 234
Hypothalamic–pituitary–adrenal axis (HPA
  axis), 3–4, 39, 54, 142, 208, 269,
  282, 294
  pathophysiology of hypertension and HPA
    axis, 55–60
    adrenal hormones, and blood pressure, 57
    and autonomic nervous system, 56
    and metabolic syndrome, 57
    various hormonal disorders, and
      hypertension, 57–60
  physiology of, 54–55
    CRH and AVP and POMC, 55
    POMC, 54–55
Hypothalamic–pituitary–gonadal axes (HPG
  axes), 8
Hypothalamo–pituitary–thyroid axis,
  physiology of, 250
Hypothalamus, 3
Hypothyroid patients, 353
Hypothyroidism, 252, 352–353
  imaging for, 322
  in pregnancy, 300–301
  prevalence, pathophysiology and clinical
    presentation, 352–353
  diagnosis, 353
  management, 353
  impact of treatment of hypothyroidism on
    hypertension, 253
Hypoxia, chronic inflammation and oxidative
  stress driven by, 267
Hypoxia-induced factor 2α (HIF2A),
  150–151, 168, 280
Hypoxia-inducible factors (HIFs), 150–151

I

^{131}I-MIBG targeting norepinephrine
  transporter system, 158
iKCNJ5 gene, 79
Imaging
  for acromegaly and AGHD, 325–326
  for catecholamine excess states, 316–317
  for glucocorticoid excess states, 313–315
  for hyperthyroidism and hypothyroidism,
    322
  for mineralocorticoid excess states,
    312–313
  for patients with endocrine hypertension
    4D CT, 319
    adrenal CT, 310–311
    adrenal MRI, 311–312
    AVS, 312–315
    MRI of pituitary, 326–327
    neck ultrasound, 318
    PET/CT to localize ectopic source of
      ACTH secretion, 315–318
    PET/CT with 18-fluorine labeled choline
      analogues, 320–322
    planar scintigraphy, 322–326
    SPECT/CT imaging with 99mTc-
      sestamibi, 319–320
    thyroid ultrasound, 322
  for primary hyperparathyroidism, 317–318

Imetaiodobenzylguanidine (MIBG), 346
Incidentaloma, 92
Indapamide, 193
[111]Indium octeotide scan, 315
Inferior petrosal sinus sampling (IPSS), 185, 282
Inferior vena cava (IVC), 95
Initial screening, 282
Inositol triphosphate (IP3), 25
Insulin resistance, 7–8, 189, 232
   associated with hypertension in children, 287–288
   insulin resistance-mediated metabolic dysfunction, 264
   OSA and, 268–269
Insulin-like growth factor 1 (IGF-1), 189–190, 218, 269, 287, 301, 325, 350–351
Insulin-like growth factor-1 receptor (IGF-1R), 66–67
Intercellular Adhesion Molecule-1, 66
Interleukin-1 (IL-1), 55
Interleukin-1β (IL-1β), 42
Interleukin-6 (IL-6), 66
Interleukins, 267
Interventional radiological techniques, 177
Intima-media thickness (IMT), 225
[123]Iodine-labeled metaiodobenzylguanidine (^{123}I-MIBG), 9, 141
   scintigraphy, 155
Iron regulatory protein 1 (IRP1), 150–151, 168
Isocitrate dehydrogenase 1 (IDH1), 150–151, 168
Isolated and paired ventricular ectopic beats, 225
Isolated GHD, 232
Isolated Micronodular Adrenocortical Disease (iMAD), 314–315
Isosorbide mononitrate, 193

J

Jugulotympanic PGLs (JTPGLs), 166
Juxtaglomerular cell tumors (JGCT), 140–141

K

Kallikrein, 188
KCNJ5 gene, 79–80, 109
Ketoconazole, 195, 350
Kidney, role of GH and IGF-1 in, 219
Kidney-specific isoform (KS-WNK1), 83–84
KIMS, 229
Kinase signaling-related molecular groups, 168
Krebs cycle, 168
   Krebs cycle-related PPGL, 150–151

L

L-aromatic amino acid, 28
L-type voltage-gated calcium channels (L-type VGCCs), 25–26

Labetalol, 155
Lanreotide, 287
Laparoscopic adrenalectomy, 96, 281
Laparoscopic surgery, 96
Late night salivary cortisol (LNSC), 184, 206, 282
Lateralization index, 337–338
Leptin, 268
Levoketoconazole, 195
Levothyroxine, 353
Li Fraumeni syndrome (LFS), 314
Liddle syndrome, 78, 80–81, 128–129, 131–134, 285, 303, 344
   clinical diagnosis, 344
   clinical features, 131
   epidemiology, 131
   genetics, 131
   investigations, 131
   management, 131–134, 344
   pathophysiology, 131
Ligand-binding domain (LBD), 40
Liothyronine, 253
Lipids, 234–236
   lipid-poor adenomas, 311–312
   lipid-rich adenomas, 311–312
Liquid chromatography coupled with tandem mass spectrometry (LS-MS/MS), 93, 118–119, 154, 333
Load-dependent remodelling method, 29
Local ablative therapy, 177
Locoregional approaches, 158
Losartan Intervention For Endpoint reduction in hypertension trial (LIFE trial), 68
Low bone mineral density, 257
Low renin
   hypertension, 119–120
   monogenic hypertension with, 79–83
   and raised aldosterone, 79–80
   and reduced aldosterone, 80–83
   and variable aldosterone, 83–84
Low-density lipoproteins (LDLs), 225, 253
^{177}Lu-DOTATATE, 177
Lynch syndrome, 314

M

Macronodular BHA, 314–315
Magnetic resonance (MR), 95
Magnetic resonance angiography (MRA), 356
Magnetic resonance imaging (MRI), 141, 154, 172, 206–207, 281, 295, 310, 346
Malate dehydrogenase 2 (MDH2), 150–151, 168, 280
Malignant lesions, 310–311
Malignant metastases, 310–311
Malignant potential for PGLs, 166, 168
Malignant ventricular tachyarrhythmia, 225
Mammalian target of rapamycin (mTOR), 151
Management
   Cushing's syndrome, 349–350
   PA, 338–341
   PPGL, 346–347

Mas-1. See Mediated by specific receptor (MasR)
Massive macronodular adrenocortical disease (MMAD), 202–203, 314–315
Mastermind-like transcriptional coactivator 3 (MAML3), 151
Maternal complications associated with hypercalcemia, 299
Matrix metalloproteinase-9 (MMP-9), 46–47
McCune-Albright syndrome, 203, 286–287
Mediated by specific receptor (MasR), 66
Medical therapy, 227
   for CS, 190
      in treatment of hypertension, role of, 195–196
   of PA, 96–98
Medical treatment of hypercortisolemia, 190
Melanocortin type-2 receptor (MC2R), 36
Melanocyte stimulating hormones (MSHs), 54
Membrane polarity, 38
MER Proto-Oncogene Tyrosine Kinase (MERTK), 151, 168
MET receptor tyrosine kinase (MET), 151
Metabolic acidosis, 83
   hyperkalemic metabolic acidosis, 78
Metabolic alkalosis
   hypokalemic metabolic alkalosis, 78
Metabolic regulation, catecholamines on, 26
Metabolic syndrome (MetS), 57, 234
   components and cut-off values proposed by NCEP, criteria used in studies, 235t
Metabolic syndrome, 264
   HPA axis and, 57
Metaiodobenzylguanidine scintigraphy (MIBG scintigraphy), 315
Metanephrine, 346
Metastatic paragangliomas, PGL, 176
Metastatic PCC, 152
Methimazole, 300
3-methoxytyramine (3MT), 151, 154, 346
Methyldopa, 297
Metoclopramide, 178
Metyrapone, 195, 350
Mifepristone, 196, 297, 350
Mineralocorticoid receptor (MR), 40, 42, 57, 66, 108, 129, 281, 285
   and blood pressure, 42–43
   regulation, 42
Mineralocorticoid receptor antagonists (MRAs), 70–71, 92, 137, 285, 295
Mineralocorticoids, 47, 91–92, 310
   biochemical phenotype of mineralocorticoid excess in children, 283–286
   AME, 285
   Geller syndrome, 286
   GRA, 284
   Liddle syndrome, 285
   primary aldosteronism, 284
   primary generalized glucocorticoid resistance, 285
   pseudohypoaldosteronism type II, 285–286
   stepwise approach in evaluation of pediatric hypertension, 283t

excess states, 45–46
  imaging for, 312–313
forms of hypertension, 341–347
  11β-hydroxylase deficiency, 341
  17α-hydroxylase deficiency, 342
  activating mutations of MR or Geller
    syndrome, 344
  DOC-secreting tumors, 343
  ectopic ACTH syndrome, 343–344
  Liddle syndrome, 344
  PGR or chrousos syndrome, 342
  SAME, 343
mineralocorticoid-sparing synthetic
    glucocorticoids, 285
Minimally invasive parathyroidectomy, 258
Minimally invasive surgery, 157, 175–176
Mitochondrial glutamicoxaloacetic
    transaminase (GOT2), 168
Mitogenactivated protein kinase/ERK kinase
    (MEK/ERK kinase), 36, 151
Mitotane, 195, 297, 350
Molecular clusters, 150
Monoamine oxidase (MAO), 22
Monoamine oxidase inhibitors, 280–281
Monocyte Chemoattractant Protein-1, 66
Monogenic hypertension, 4, 78, 106
  associated with elevated PAC and PRA,
    140–141
    renin-secreting JGCT, 140–141
  associated with high PAC and low PRA,
    138–140
    FH-1, 138–139
    FH-2, 139
    FH-3, 139–140
    FH-4, 140
  associated with normal PAC and low PRA,
    137–138
    pseudohypoaldosteronism type II,
      137–138
  associated with normal PAC and PRA,
    141–143
    Carney complex, 142–143
    familial pheochromocytoma and
      paragangliomas, 141–142
    primary generalized glucocorticoid
      resistance, 142
  associated with suppressed PAC and PRA,
    131–137
    AME, 135–137
    CAH, 134–135
    Geller syndrome, 137
    laboratory evaluation of, 133t
    Liddle syndrome, 131–134
    management of, 134t
  classification of, 79f
  genetics of, 79–85
  with hypokalemic alkalosis, low renin
    and raised aldosterone, 79–80
    and reduced aldosterone, 80–83
    and variable aldosterone, 83–84
  with normokalemia and normal renin and
    aldosterone levels, 84–85
  syndromes, 78
⁹⁹mTc-MIBI, 319–320

Multinodular goiter (MNG), 253–254
Multiple endocrine neoplasia (MEN), 258,
    280, 354
  MEN1, 10–11, 203, 256–257, 314
  MEN2, 141, 155, 345
    MEN2-related PCCs, 155
    MEN2a/MEN2b, 298, 316
Multiplex ligation dependent probe analysis
    (MLPA), 10
Mutation-driven oncogenic process, 159
Myc-associated factor X (MAX), 151, 280
Myocardium, role of GH and IGF-1 in, 218
α-myosin heavy chain (α-MHC), 250
β-myosin heavy chain (β-MHC), 250

N

N-terminal domain (NTD), 42
N-terminal transactivation domain (NTD), 40
Na⁺-Cl⁻Co-transporter (NCC), 83, 137
National Cholesterol Education Program's
    Adult Treatment Panel III (NCEP),
    234
National Comprehensive Cancer Network,
    177
National Institute of Health (NIH), 155
Natriuretic peptides (NPs), 65–66
Neck ultrasound, 318
Neprilysin, 65–66
Nervous system, 92
Neuroectodermal syndromes, 316
Neuroendocrine tumors (NET), 325, 327
Neurofibromatosis type 1 (NF1), 280, 314,
    316, 345
Neurofibromin 1 genes (NF1 genes), 150
Neurogenic orthostatic hypotension, 32
Neurogenic tumors, 172
Neuropeptide Y (NPY), 55
Next Generation Sequencing (NGS), 5, 157
Nifedipine, 297
Nitric oxide (NO), 3, 41, 65–66, 188, 218
    pathway, 222
Nitric oxide synthase (NOS), 41
Nocturnal hypoxia, 268
Nocturnal negative intrathoracic pressure,
    cardiac effects of, 268
Nondippers, 221–222
"Nongenomic" cell signaling process, 36
Nonload-dependent remodelling method, 29
Nonneoplastic Cushing's syndrome (NCS),
    55–56
Nonneoplastic hypercortisolism, 185
Nonrapid eye movement sleep (NREM
    sleep), 266
Nonselective alpha blocker, 298
Nonsteroidal antiinflammatory drugs
    (NSAIDs), 339
Norepinephrine, 3, 21–22, 24, 26, 55, 167
Norepinephrine transporter (NET), 21–22
Normal androgen synthesis, 43
Normetanephrine, 346
Normocalcemic primary hyperparathy-
    roidism, 257
Normokalemia, monogenic hypertension
    with, 84–85

NR3C1 gene, 81
NR3C2 gene, 42
Nuclear factor-kB (NF), 66
Nuclear receptor (NR), 40
Nuclear scans, 299
NUCLEUS tractus solitarius (NTS), 21

O

O-6-methylguanine-DNA methyltransferase
    (MGMT), 158
Obesity, 7–8, 57, 234
  associated with hypertension in children,
    287–288
  obesity-related sequelae, 264
  OSA and, 265
Obstructive sleep apnea (OSA), 7–8, 264
  diagnosis of, 266
    grading of severity of obstructive sleep
      apnea, 266t
  epidemiology of, 264–265
  and insulin resistance, 268–269
  management of, 269–271
    conservative management, 270
    CPAP, 270
    oral appliances, 271
    surgical management, 271
    weight loss therapies, 271
  and obesity, 265
  OSA associated with hypertension in
    children, 287–288
  OSA-related sympathetic overdrive,
    268
  pathophysiology of, 266–268
    activation of RAAS, 268
    cardiac effects of nocturnal negative
      intrathoracic pressure, 268
    chronic inflammation and oxidative stress
      driven by hypoxia, 267
    nocturnal fluid shifts, 267–268
    nocturnal sympathetic overdrive,
      266–267
Obstructive sleep apnea syndrome (OSAS),
    92
Octreatate, 315
Octreotide, 287
Omphalocele, 300
Open surgery, 281
OSA-related secondary hypertension
    (ORSH), 8, 264
Osilodrostat, 195
Osteosynthesis techniques, 177
Overnight dexamethasone-suppression test
    (Overnight DST), 282
Overt hyperthyroidism, 253–254
Overt hypothyroidism and associated
    hypertension, 253
Overt primary hypothyroidism, 253
18-oxcortisol, 98, 106–107, 139
Oxidative stress driven by hypoxia,
    267
Oxidative stress-responsive gene 1 (OSR1),
    83
2-oxoglutarate-malate carrier (SLC25A11),
    150–151, 168

P

PA with seizures and neurological abnormalities syndrome (PASNA), 5, 110
Page kidney, 357
Palliative surgery, PGL, 176
Pancreas, 175
Pancreatic neuroendocrine tumours (pNETs), 315
Paragangliomas (PGLs), 3, 6, 24, 141—142, 150, 166, 280, 316, 345—346
  anatomical and functional imaging studies, 172—173
  areas of uncertainty/emerging research, 179
  biochemical investigations, 171—172, 171t—172t
  clinical features, 141
  clinical presentation, 168—170, 170t—171t
  epidemiology, 141
    clinical and pathologic features of head and neck HNPGLs, 167t
    of hypertension and, 166—167
  follow-up care of patients with, 177
  genetics and pathophysiology, 141
  genetics of, 168
  and hypertension, 6
  investigations, 141
  management, 142
    children, 177—178
    elderly, 178
    pregnancy, 178
    in special populations, 177—178
  pathophysiology of hypertension and, 167—168
  perioperative medical management of, 173—175
  radionuclide therapy, 177
    local ablative therapy, 177
  surgery for management of, 175—177
    curative surgery, 175—176
    metastatic paragangliomas, 176
    palliative surgery, 176
    systemic therapy, 176—177
Paralytic ileus, 176
Parasympathetic ganglia of the head and neck region (HNPGLs), 166
Parathyroid carcinoma, 256—257
Parathyroid cells, 256
Parathyroid chief cells, 255
Parathyroid disease, 255—258
  bidirectional relation between renin—angiotensin—aldosterone system and PTH, 256—258
  clinical features of primary hyperparathyroidism, 257
  epidemiology of PHPT, 256—257
  investigation and management, 258
  parathyroidectomy impact in hypertension and cardiovascular disease, 258
  pathophysiology of hypertension in primary hyperparathyroidism, 255—256
  physiology of parathyroid hormone action, 255
  suspect PHPT in hypertensive subjects, 258

Parathyroid disorders and hypertension in children, 287—288
Parathyroid hormone (PTH), 287, 354
  bidirectional relation between, 256—258
Parathyroid hormone-related peptide (PTHrP), 84, 299
Parathyroid hyperplasia, 317—318
Parathyroid scintigraphy, 299
Parathyroidectomy, 258, 287
  impact in hypertension and cardiovascular disease, 258
Paraventricular nucleus (PVN), 54
Paroxysmal atrial fibrillation, 225
Paroxysms, 345
Pasireotide, 195, 349—350
Pathophysiological mechanisms, 252
Pegvisomant, 223, 287
Peptide receptor radionuclide therapy (PRRT), 155, 159
Percutaneous ablation, 158
Peri-operative managemen, 96
Perindopril, 67
Peripheral vascular resistance, 222
Peroxisome proliferator-activated receptor gamma (PPARγ), 193—194
Pharmacologic agents, 287
Pharyngeal muscle tonicity, 271
Phenoxybenzamine, 142, 298, 347
Phenylethanolamine-N-methyltransferase (PNMT), 21, 151
Pheochromocytoma of Adrenal Gland Scaled Score rading system (PASS grading system), 153
Pheochromocytomas (PCC), 3, 150, 168, 280, 294, 310
  areas of uncertainty/emerging concepts, 159
  clinical presentation, 153
    clinical score for likelihood of PCC, 153t
  diagnostic workup, 153—157
    biochemical testing, 153—154
    diagnostic imaging, 154—155
    MEN2 and VHL PCCs, 155
    molecular diagnosis, 157
  follow-up, 159
  and hypertension, 6
  locoregional approaches, 158
    EBRT, 158
  management, 157
    presurgical and surgical management of PCC, 157
  molecular and genetic aspects of, 150—153
    clinical and biochemical characteristics of PCC, 151, 152t
    metastatic risk, 152—153
    pathophysiology, 151—152
    tumor clusters, 150—151
  systemic therapy, 158—159
    agents, 159
    chemotherapy, 158
    radionuclide therapy, 158
    TKI, 158—159
Pheochromocytomas (PCCs), 150, 310—311, 316
  PCC-related malignancy, 152

Pheochromocytomas and paragangliomas (PPGLs), 24, 150, 166, 280, 289, 316, 345—346
  in children, 280
  diagnosis, 346
  and excess catecholamine states, 28
  management, 346—347
    follow-up, 347
    perioperative management, 347
    surgical management, 346—347
  in pregnancy, 298
  prevalence, pathophysiology and clinical presentation, 345
  syndromes, 298
Phosphatidylinositol 3-kinase (PI3K) /Protein kinase B, 151
Phosphodiesterase 2A gene (*PDE2A* gene), 110
Phosphodiesterase 3B gene (*PDE3B* gene), 110
Pigmented Nodular Adrenocortical Disease (PPNAD), 143
Pioglitazone, 193—194
Pituitary
  adenoma, 202
  macroadenoma, 326—327
  MRI of, 326—327
  targeted agents, 195—196
Planar scintigraphy, 322—326
  imaging for acromegaly and AGHD, 325—326
Plasma aldosterone concentration (PAC), 9, 92, 129, 284
  monogenic hypertension
    associated with elevated PAC and PRA, 140—141
    associated with high PAC and low PRA, 138—140
    associated with normal PAC and low PRA, 137—138
    associated with normal PAC and PRA, 141—143
    associated with suppressed PAC and PRA, 131—137
Plasma catecholamine concentrations, 221—222
Plasma cortisol, 341
Plasma fractionated metanephrines, 281
Plasma membrane calcium ATPase (PMCA3), 79
Plasma potassium, 335
Plasma renin, 85
Plasma renin activity (PRA), 9, 93, 128, 284, 333
  monogenic hypertension
    associated with elevated PAC and PRA, 140—141
    associated with high PAC and low PRA, 138—140
    associated with normal PAC and low PRA, 137—138
    associated with normal PAC and PRA, 141—143
    associated with suppressed PAC and PRA, 131—137

Plasma volume expansion, 220—222
Plasma-free metanephrines, 154
Pneumocystis jiroveci pneumonia (PJP), 189
Pneumocystis jirovecii, 58
Pneumonia, 270
Poly(ADPribose polymerase) (PARP inhibitors), 176—177
Polycystic ovary syndrome (POCS), 268
Polysomnography, 266
Portal venous contrast (PV contrast), 310—311
Positron-emission tomography (PET), 282, 346
   PET-based techniques, 173
   PET/CT to localize ectopic source of ACTH secretion, 315—318
      catecholamine excess states, imaging for, 316—317
      primary hyperparathyroidism, imaging for, 317—318
   PET/CT with 18-fluorine labeled choline analogues, 320—322
      imaging for hyperthyroidism and hypothyroidism, 322
Postoperative treatment of adrenal CS, 208
Postpartum thyroiditis, 254
Potassium, 91
   stimulate aldosterone, 91
Prazosin, 298
Preauricular sinuses, 300
Prednisone, 99, 139
Predominantly epinephrine, 26
Pregnancy, 8, 294
   endocrine hypertension in
      acromegaly in pregnancy, 301—302
      adrenal cortical carcinoma/ deoxycorticosterone-secreting adrenal tumor, 303
      Cushing syndrome in pregnancy, 295—297
      familial hyperaldosteronism, 304
      Geller syndrome, 304
      hyperthyroidism and hypothyroidism in pregnancy, 300—301
      hypopituitarism, 303
      Liddle's syndrome, 303
      of PA, 333
      PPGL in pregnancy, 298
      primary hyperaldosteronism in, 294—295, 299—300
      rare causes of, 302
Pregnant woman, endocrine hypertension in, 8
Preoperative treatment of adrenal CS, 208
Presurgical management of PCC, 157
Primary aldosteronism (PA), 2, 4—5, 57, 79, 90, 106, 294, 332—341
   ARR as screening test, 92—93
   clinical diagnosis, 332—338
      accurate assays in diagnostic workup of, 333
      AVS, 337—338
      confirmatory testing for, 335—336
      screening for, 334—335, 334t
      subtype differentiation, 336—337

symptoms and signs of, 332—333
   confirmatory test after positive ARR, 93—95
   epidemiology of, 92
   familial forms of, 98—99
      FH, 98t
   laparoscopic surgery and peri-operative managemen, 96
   management, 338—341
      medical management, 339—341
      surgical management, 338—339
   medical therapy of, 96—98
   renin—angiotensin—aldosterone system, 91—92
   subtyping in, 95—96
Primary aldosteronism, 45—46, 284, 312
Primary aldosteronism, seizures, and neurological abnormalities syndrome (PASNA syndrome), 99, 106, 110
Primary Aldosteronism Surgical Outcome (PASO), 338
Primary bilateral macronodular adrenocortical hyperplasia (PBMAH), 202—204, 314—315
Primary deoxycorticosteronism, 343
Primary generalized glucocorticoid resistance, 142, 285
Primary glucocorticoid resistance (PGR), 342
   clinical diagnosis, 342
   management, 342
Primary hyperaldosteronism in pregnancy, 294—295
   antihypertensives and safety categorization on use in pregnancy, 295t
Primary hyperparathyroidism (PHPT), 250, 256—257, 287, 294, 299—300, 310, 317—318, 354—355
   clinical features of, 257
   epidemiology of, 256—257
   imaging for, 317—318
   pathophysiology of hypertension in, 255—256
   prevalence, pathophysiology and clinical presentation, 354—355
Primary hypertension, 2—3, 78
   in children, 278—279
Primary neurodegenerative autonomic disorders, 31—32
Primary Pigmented Nodular Adrenal Hyperplasia (PPNAD), 203, 314—315
Primary tumors, 170
PRKACA mutation, 204
Progesterone, 120, 294
Progesterone receptor (PR), 40, 339—340
Progression-free survival (PFS), 158
Proopiomelanocortin (POMC), 54—55
Propylthiouracil, 300
Prostacyclin, 188, 218
Prostaglandin E2, 188
Protein kinase A (PKA), 24, 143, 203
Protein kinase B (PKB), 26, 151
Protein kinase C (PKC), 26, 37—38
Proton pump inhibitors (PPIs), 172
"Pseudo-Cushing's" syndrome, 55—56, 185

Pseudohypoaldosteronism type II (PHAII), 78, 83, 137—138, 285—286
Pseudohypoxia-related molecular groups, 168
Pseudohypoxic
   group, 168
   molecular signature, 150—151
   PPGL, 150—151
Psychiatric illness, 204—205
Pulse wave velocity (PWV), 225

R
Radioactive iodine therapy (RAI therapy), 253
Radionuclide therapy, 158, 177
Radiopharmaceuticals, 322—323
Radiotherapy, 227
Raised aldosterone, monogenic hypertension with, 79—83
Rapid eye movement (REM), 288
   REM sleep, 266
Ras/Raf/MEK/ERK kinase cascade, 151
Reactive oxygen species (ROS), 46
Really interesting new gene (RING), 83
Relacorilant, 350
Renal artery bruits, 356
Renal artery stenosis, 355—357
Renal cell carcinoma (RCC), 10
Renal duplex ultrasound, 356
Renal manifestations, 257
Renal outer medullary potassium (ROMK), 80—81
Renal parenchymal disease, 2
Renal physiology, catecholamines and alterations in, 31
Renal sympathetic nerve activity (RSNA), 31
Renin, 65, 92—93, 333
   measurement of, 340—341
   monogenic hypertension with, 84—85
Renin-angiotensin—aldosterone system (RAAS), 3—4, 46, 57, 64—65, 91—92, 129, 188, 221, 252, 264, 281, 283, 294, 334, 348, 353
   ACE inhibitors, 67
   ACEI *vs.* ARBs, 69
   activation of, 268
   Ang II and Aldo, 65t
   ARBs, 68—69
   bidirectional relation between, 256—258
   direct renin inhibitors, 69
   dual RAAS inhibition, 69
   mineralocorticoid receptor antagonists, 70—71
   physiological aspects of, 65—66
   RAAS, inflammation, and remodeling, 66—67
   RAAS blocking agents and cardiovascular protection in hypertension, 67
Renin-secreting JGCT, 140—141
   clinical features, 140
   epidemiology, 140
   genetics, 140
   investigations, 141
   management, 141
   pathophysiology, 140
Reninoma, 357

Renovascular hypertension, 332, 357
Resistant hypertension, 90
RET genes, 150
Retinoic acid, 196
Retroperitoneal approach, 295
Rosiglitazone, 193—194
Rostral ventrolateral medulla (RVLM), 21

S

S-adenosyl-L-methionine, 21
SAHB gene, 142
SAHC gene, 142
SAHD gene, 142
Saline infusion test, 93—95, 335—336
Saline loading test, 295
Saline suppression test (SST), 335—336
Salivary cortisol, 282
Sarcomas, 172
Sarcoplasmic reticulum calcium adenosine
    triphosphatase (SERCA), 250
*SCNN*1A gene, 131
*SCNN*1B gene, 131
*SCNN*1G gene, 131
Scoring system, 153
Screening for PA, 334—335, 334t
SDHA gene, 142
SDHB genes, 280
Secondary hyperaldosteronism, 284
Secondary hypertension, 2—3, 226, 288
    in children, 278—279
Secondary hypothyroidism, 253
Secretion/steroid hormone synthesis in zona
    fasciculata, 38—39
Serotonin, 55
Serum IGF-1, 325
Serum potassium, 120
Serum-and glucocorticoid-inducible protein
    kinase 1 (SGK-1), 42
Sex steroid-producing adrenal tumors, 58
Sick sinus syndrome, 225
Single photon emission computed
    tomography (SPECT), 173
    SPECT/CT imaging with 99mTc-sestamibi,
        319—320
Sinoatrial node (SA Node), 25—26
Sleep apnea syndrome, 2, 189, 223
Small cell lung cancer (SCLC), 315
Small VCPinteracting protein (SVIP), 39
Smooth muscle cells, 222
Sodium chloride cotransporter (NCC),
    187—188, 285—286, 348
Sodium diet, 131
Sodium-calcium exchanger (NCX), 188, 250
Sodium-dependent phosphate transport
    protein 2A (NaPi-2a), 219
Somatostatin, 55
Somatostatin analogues (SSAs), 227, 302,
    349—351
Somatostatin receptor 2 (SSTR2), 315
Somatostatin receptor analogues (SSA), 155
Somatostatin receptors (SSTR), 158, 173
    SSTR based radionuclide therapy, 158, 173
Spironolactone, 97, 108, 131, 285, 295,
    339—340, 343

Sporadic PPGLs, 151
Standardized incidence rate (SIR), 345
Standardized mortality ratio (SMR), 168,
    209—210
Ste20-related proline—alanine-rich kinase
    (SPAK), 83
Steroid metabolome, 95
Steroid synthesis in zona glomerulosa,
    37—38
Steroidogenesis
    inhibitors, 350
    regulation of, 36—37
Steroidogenic acute regulatory protein
    (StAR), 5, 36, 114
Steroidogenic pathways, 36
Stiff endothelial cell syndrome (SECS),
    66—67
STOPBANG Questionnaire, 266
Stress system, 56
Subacute thyroiditis, 254, 324—325
Subclinical hyperaldosteronism, 92
Subclinical hypothyroidism (SCH), 253—254,
    300—301
    and associated hypertension, 253
Substance P (SP), 55
Succinate dehydrogenase (SDH), 280
    SDH mutation related syndromes, 298
Succinate dehydrogenase B (SDHB), 345
succinate dehydrogenase complex assembly
    factor-2 (SDHAF2), 150—151, 168
Succinate dehydrogenase genes (*SDHx*
    genes), 150, 152, 155, 168, 173, 177
Succinate dehydrogenase subunits, 150—151
Suggested starting dose (SSD), 335
Sulfotransferase 2A1 (SULT2A1), 40
Supine hypertension, 31—32
Suppressed renin, 284
Supraventricular tachycardia, 225
Surgery, 298, 355
Surgical adrenalectomy, 45—46
Surgical management of PCC, 157
Surgical resection, 157—158
Sympathetic nervous system, 21—22, 188,
    221—222
Sympathetic PGLs, 166—167
Sympathomimetic agents, 280—281
Syndrome of apparent mineralocorticoid
    excess (SAME), 343
    clinical diagnosis, 343
    management, 343
Systemic drugs, 159
Systemic therapy, 158—159
    chemotherapy, 176—177
    PGL, 176—177
Systemic vascular resistance (SVR), 353
Systolic BP (SBP), 350
Systolic hypertension, 287

T

Tachycardia, 254
Takotsubo cardiomyopathy, 28
Technetium, 254
99m Technetium-sestamibi, 319—320
Temozolomide (TMZ), 158, 176—177

1,4,7,10-tetraazacyclododecane-1,4,7,10-
    tetraacetic acid (DOTA), 315
5α-tetrahydrocortisol (5αTHF), 285
Tetrahydrocortisone (THE), 285
Thermal-ablation techniques, 177
Thiazide-sensitive NCCT, 285—286
Thiazides, 193
Thionamide antithyroid drugs (Thionamide
    ATDs), 254—255
Thromboembolic disease, 204—205
Thyroglobulin, 253
Thyroid disease, 250—255
    hypertension in, 7
    pathophysiology of hypertension in thyroid
        dysfunction, 251—252
    physiology of hypothalamo—pituitary—
        thyroid axis and cardiovascular system,
        250
    subclinical or overt hypothyroidism and
        associated hypertension, 253
        clinical features, 253
        epidemiology, 253
        hypothyroidism impact on hypertension
            and cardiovascular disease, 253
        investigation and management, 253
        suspect hypothyroidism and
            hyperthyroidism in hypertensive
            subjects, 255
Thyroid disorders, 2, 352—354
    and hypertension in children, 287—288
    hyperthyroidism, 353—354
    hypothyroidism, 352—353
Thyroid dysfunction, pathophysiology of
    hypertension in, 251—252
Thyroid hormones, 250, 353
    disorders, 279
    thyroid hormone-related disorders, 300
Thyroid peroxidase (TPO), 253, 287
Thyroid stimulating hormone (TSH), 353
Thyroid stimulating immunoglobulins (TSI),
    287
Thyroid ultrasonography, 254
Thyroid ultrasound, 322
Thyroid-stimulating hormone (TSH), 250
Thyroidectomy, 254—255, 300
Thyroiditis, 322
Thyrotoxicosis, 287
Thyroxine, 287
Thyroxine—binding globulin (TBG), 300
Toll-like receptors 2 (TLR2), 68
Toxic megacolon, 176
Transforming growth factor-β (TGF-β), 42
Transmembrane protein 127 (*TMEM*127),
    151
Transsphenoidal surgery (TSS), 190, 227,
    282
Triamterene, 193
Tricyclic antidepressants, 155, 280—281
Triiodothyronine (T3), 287, 353
TSH Receptor antibodies (TRAb), 287, 300
Tuberous sclerosis, 316
Tumor
    catecholamine producing, 280—281
    clusters, 150—151

radiologic evaluation to locate, 281
Tumor necrosis factor-α (TNF-α), 42, 55, 66, 267
Type 2 diabetes mellitus (T2DM), 268
Tyrosine, 20–21
Tyrosine hydroxylase, 20–21, 28
Tyrosine kinase inhibitors (TKIs), 158–159, 176–177

U

Ultrasonography (USG), 298, 310
    of neck, 299
Ultrasound (US), 317–318
Uncertain significance (VUS), 10
Unilateral adrenalectomy, 96, 207
United States Preventive Services Task Force, 278
Untreated hypothyroidism, 300–301
Urinary free cortisol (UFC), 184, 206, 282
Urine sodium excretion, reduction in, 189
Uvulopalatopharyngoplasty (UPPP), 271

V

Vagal PGLs (VPGLs), 166
Vaginoplasty, 135

Valsartan Antihypertensive Longterm Use Evaluation (VALUE), 68
Valvulopathy, 225
Vanillylmandelic acid (VMA), 171
Vascular bed, 24–25
Vascular endothelial cells (VECs), 41
Vascular endothelial growth factor (VEGF), 46, 189
Vascular endothelium, 218
Vascular hemodynamics, catecholamines effect on, 26–28, 27t
Vascular remodeling of resistance arteries, 222
Vascular smooth muscle ATP-sensitive potassium channel (KATP), 218
Vascular smooth muscle cells (VSMCs), 25, 41
Vascular surgeons, 175–176
Vasodilators, 188
Vasodilatory agents, 218
Venous thromboembolic (VTE), 189
Ventricular tachycardia, 225
Verapamil, 295
Very low-density lipoprotein (VLDL), 225
Vitamin D deficiency, 232–233
Von Hippel Lindau genes (VHL genes), 150–151, 280, 298, 345

VHL PCCs, 155
VHL tumor suppressor, 168
VHL/EPAS1, 150–151
Von Hippel-Lindau disease (VHL disease), 141, 280, 316

W

Water house–Friderichsen syndrome, 58
Weight loss therapies, 271
Werner's syndrome, 314
Wilms' tumor, 141
WNK genes, 137
Wnt-related molecular groups, 168

X

X-linked acrogigantism (X-LAG), 12–13, 286–287

Z

Zona glomerulosa, 91
    aldosterone synthesis/steroid synthesis in, 37–38
    cortisol synthesis and secretion/steroid hormone synthesis in, 38–39
    regulation in, 39–40